THE SURVEY HANDBOOK

THE SURVEY KIT

Purpose: The purposes of this 9-volume Kit are to enable readers to prepare and conduct surveys and become better users of survey results. Surveys are conducted to collect information by asking questions of people on the telephone, face-to-face, and by mail. The questions can be about attitudes, beliefs, and behavior as well as socioeconomic and health status. To do a good survey also means knowing how to ask questions, design the survey (research) project, sample respondents, collect reliable and valid information, and analyze and report the results. You also need to know how to plan and budget for your survey.

Users: The Kit is for students in undergraduate and graduate classes in the social and health sciences and for individuals in the public and private sectors who are responsible for conducting and using surveys. Its primary goal is to enable users to prepare surveys and collect data that are accurate and useful for primarily practical purposes. Sometimes, these practical purposes overlap the objectives of scientific research, and so survey researchers will also find the Kit useful.

Format of the Kit: All books in the series contain instructional objectives, exercises and answers, examples of surveys in use and illustrations of survey questions, guidelines for action, checklists of do's and don'ts, and annotated references.

Volumes in The Survey Kit:

1. **The Survey Handbook**
   Arlene Fink

2. **How to Ask Survey Questions**
   Arlene Fink

3. **How to Conduct Self-Administered and Mail Surveys**
   Linda B. Bourque and *Eve P. Fielder*

4. **How to Conduct Interviews by Telephone and in Person**
   James H. Frey and *Sabine Mertens Oishi*

5. **How to Design Surveys**
   Arlene Fink

6. **How to Sample in Surveys**
   Arlene Fink

7. **How to Measure Survey Reliability and Validity**
   Mark S. Litwin

8. **How to Analyze Survey Data**
   Arlene Fink

9. **How to Report on Surveys**
   Arlene Fink

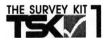

THE SURVEY KIT 1

THE SURVEY HANDBOOK

ARLENE FINK

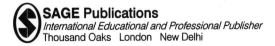

SAGE Publications
International Educational and Professional Publisher
Thousand Oaks   London   New Delhi

For information address:

 SAGE Publications, Inc.
2455 Teller Road
Thousand Oaks, California 91320
E-mail: order@sagepub.com

SAGE Publications Ltd.
6 Bonhill Street
London EC2A 4PU
United Kingdom

SAGE Publications India Pvt. Ltd.
M-32 Market
Greater Kailash I
New Delhi 110 048 India

Printed in the United States of America

Library of Congress Cataloging-in-Publication Data

Main entry under title:

The survey kit.
    p. cm.
    Includes bibliographical references.
    Contents: v. 1. The survey handbook / Arlene Fink — v. 2. How to ask survey questions / Arlene Fink — v. 3. How to conduct self-administered and mail surveys / Linda B. Bourque, Eve P. Fielder — v. 4. How to conduct interviews by telephone and in person / James H. Frey, Sabine Mertens Oishi — v. 5. How to design surveys / Arlene Fink — v. 6. How to sample in surveys / Arlene Fink — v. 7. How to measure survey reliability and validity / Mark S. Litwin — v. 8. How to analyze survey data / Arlene Fink — v. 9. How to report on surveys / Arlene Fink.
    ISBN 0-8039-7388-8 (pbk. : The survey kit : alk. paper)
    1. Social surveys. 2. Health surveys. I. Fink, Arlene.
HN29.S724   1995
300'.723—dc20   95-12712

This book is printed on acid-free paper.

95 96 97 98 99 10 9 8 7 6 5 4 3 2 1

Sage Production Editor: Diane S. Foster
Sage Copy Editor: Joyce Kuhn
Sage Typesetter: Janelle LeMaster

Contents

The Survey Handbook:
Learning Objectives

The major goal of this handbook is to introduce you to the skills and resources you need to conduct a survey. The skills include identifying specific survey objectives, designing studies and sampling respondents, developing reliable and valid self-administered questionnaires and interviews, administering the survey, and analyzing and reporting the results. The handbook also aims to teach you how to organize surveys and estimate their costs and contains examples of management plans the budgets.

The specific objectives are:

■ Identify the characteristics of high-quality surveys

■ Describe the usefulness in surveys of specific objectives, straightforward questions, sound research design, sound choice of population or sample, reliable and valid instruments, appropriate analysis, accurate reporting of results, and reasonable resources

■ Distinguish between four types of survey instruments

■ Define reliability and its characteristics

■ Define validity and its characteristics

■ Interpret data from open-ended questions using the "liked best / liked least" method

- Distinguish between the uses of figures and tables in survey results

- Describe the activities that constitute a "typical" survey

- List the questions to ask in pilot tests

- Relate survey costs to needs for personnel and time for the survey

- Understand the relationships between time, scope, and quality in survey design and implementation

- Understand the contents and characteristics of survey budget presentations

1 What Is a Survey? When Do You Use One?

A survey is a system for collecting information to describe, compare, or explain knowledge, attitudes, and behavior. Surveys involve setting objectives for information collection, designing research, preparing a reliable and valid data collection instrument, administering and scoring the instrument, analyzing data, and reporting the results.

Surveys are taken of political and consumer choices, use of health services, numbers of people in the labor force, and opinions on just about everything from aardvarks to zyzyvas. Individuals, communities, schools, businesses, and researchers use surveys to find out about people by asking questions about feelings, motivations, plans, beliefs, and personal backgrounds. The questions in survey instruments are typically

1

arranged into mailed, taped, or self-administered questionnaires (on paper or on a computer) and into in-person (face-
to-face) or telephone interviews.

Surveys are a prominent part of life in many major indus-
trialized nations, particularly the United States. The absurdity
of some survey questions are symbolized in the following
cartoon.

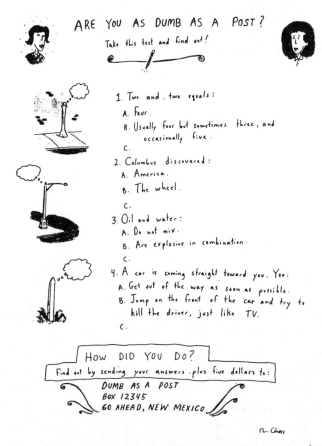

Drawing by R. Chast published in the February 10, 1986 issue of *The New
Yorker* (p. 43). © 1986 by The New Yorker Magazine, Inc. Reprinted by
permission.

U.S. elections are always accompanied by a flood of polls. Polling is a major type of survey but far from the only kind. Other types of surveys are now widely used in conjunction with a variety of projects and activities. As Example 1.1 shows, surveys are used in very diverse settings, such as deciding on the perfect painting and making public policy regarding the environment.

EXAMPLE 1.1
Art and Sea Otters: Two Surveys

Survey on Art

What would a genuine people's art look like? Can artists make paintings that truly reflect the tastes of the American public? To find out, two artists conducted a phone survey of 1,001 adults. The following are some of the questions they asked:

- Do you prefer pictures from a long time ago, like Lincoln or Jesus?
- Which do you think you like better, a painting of one person or a painting of a group of people?
- Would you rather see paintings of outdoor scenes or indoor scenes?
- If you had to name one color as your favorite, what would it be?
- Would you say you prefer paintings in which the person or people are nude, partially clothed, or fully clothed?

(Excerpts from "The Perfect Painting," by Richard B. Woodward in February 20, 1994 issue of the *New York Times Magazine*, pp. 36-37. Copyright © 1994 by the New York Times Company. Reprinted by permission.)

Survey on Sea Otters

How much is a Pacific sea otter's life worth—not as someone's pet but as a wild animal that will never be studied by scientists or frolic in front of tourists? Could the U.S. government find out how much they would voluntarily pay to keep the otter safe from unnatural hazards?

Until recently, such abstract questions have mostly been grist for academic debate. But now federal regulators are under orders from Congress and the courts to figure ways to measure losses to people not directly affected by environmental problems like oil spills or haze in national parks. The first set of guidelines, from the National Oceanic and Atmospheric Administration, is due later this month [September 1993] and is widely expected to support the use of survey-based techniques.

[Excerpts from "Economic Watch; Disputed New Role for Polls: Putting a Price Tag on Nature," by Peter Passell in September 6, 1993 issue of the *New York Times*, p. A1. Copyright © 1993 by the New York Times Company. Reprinted by permission.]

A surveyor's job can be very rewarding in its variety and in intellectual challenges. What does the typical survey expert need to know? One way to answer the question is to consider the requirements for getting a job as a surveyor.

Example 1.2 is an excerpt from a typical advertisement for an employment opportunity that might appear in the classified advertisement section of a newspaper.

EXAMPLE 1.2
A Job in a Survey Center

Project Coordinator

Assisting the department director in carrying out applied survey research, your duties will include: formulating study designs and sampling frames; . . . developing instruments; supervising data collection, entry, and manipulation; application of descriptive and inferential statistics; interpreting results and preparing reports.

The "duties" specified in the advertisement are typical skills required to conduct surveys. This book introduces all of them: study design and sampling; survey instrument development, with emphasis on asking straightforward questions and developing reliable and valid instruments (including in-person and telephone interviews and self-administered questionnaires); data collection and statistical analysis and interpretation; and report preparation. The book also discusses how to plan surveys and prepare a budget for them.

The best surveys have these features:

- Specific objectives
- Straightforward questions
- Sound research design
- Sound choice of population or sample
- Reliable and valid survey instruments
- Appropriate analysis
- Accurate reporting of survey results
- Reasonable resources

Survey Objectives:
Measuring Hoped-For Outcomes

What should the survey ask? What information should it collect? You must know the survey's objectives to answer these questions. An objective is a statement of the survey's hoped-for outcomes. Example 1.3 contains three objectives for a survey of educational needs.

EXAMPLE 1.3
Illustrative Objectives for a
Survey of Educational Needs

1. Identify the most common needs for educational services
2. Compare needs of men and women
3. Determine the characteristics of people who benefit most from services

---

A specific set of objectives like these suggests a survey that asks questions about the following:

Objective 1: Educational needs

Sample survey question: Which of the following skills would you like to have?

Objective 2: Gender

Sample survey question: Are you male or female?

Objective 3, first part: Characteristics of survey participants

Sample survey questions: What is your occupation? What was your household income last year? How much television do you watch? How many books do you read in an average month?

Objective 3, second part: Benefits

Sample survey question: To what extent has this program helped you improve your job skills? (In this example, you can infer that one benefit is improvement in job skills.)

Suppose you add these objectives:

EXAMPLE 1.4
More Objectives for a
Survey of Educational Needs

4. Compare younger and older parents in their needs for education in managing a household and caring for a child
5. Determine the relationship between parents' education and method of disciplining children for mild, moderate, and severe infractions

---

If you add objectives to the survey, you may need to add questions to the instrument. To collect information for the new objectives, for example, you need to ask about the following:

- Parents' age
- How parents manage their household
- How parents care for their children

- Level of parents' education
- Methods for disciplining children for mild, moderate, and severe infractions

When planning a survey and its instrument, define all potentially imprecise or ambiguous terms in the objectives. For the objectives above, the imprecise terms are needs; educational services; characteristics; benefit; younger and older; household management; child care; discipline methods; and mild, moderate, and severe infractions. Why are these terms ambiguous? No standard definition exists for any of them. What are needs, for example, and of the very long list that you might create, which are so important that they should be included on the survey? What is discipline? In a later section, this chapter discusses how focus groups and consensus panels can be used to determine a survey's objectives and help define and clarify their meaning.

Survey objectives can also be converted into questions or hypotheses to be researched by a change in sentence structure, as illustrated in Example 1.5 with Survey Objectives 4 and 5 listed earlier (Example 1.4).

EXAMPLE 1.5
Survey Objectives, Research Questions, and Hypotheses

Survey Objective 4

To compare younger and older parents in their needs to learn how to manage a household and care for a child

Survey Research Question: How do younger and older parents compare in their needs to learn how to manage a household and care for a child?

Research Hypothesis: No differences exist between younger and older parents in their needs to learn how to manage a household and care for a child.

Survey Objective 5

To determine the relationship between parents' education and method of disciplining children for mild, moderate, and severe infractions

Survey Research Question: What is the relationship between parents' education and method of disciplining children for mild, moderate, and severe infractions?

Research Hypothesis: No relationship exists between parents' education and method of disciplining children for mild, moderate, and severe infractions.

If you achieve Survey Objective 4 or answer its associated question or properly test its associated hypothesis, you will provide data on younger and older parents' needs to learn to manage a household and care for a child. Similarly, with Survey Objective 5, you will provide data on the relationship between education and methods of discipline. The difference between stating a survey's purpose as an objective and as a question is a relatively minor change in sentence form from statement to question. Hypothesis testing is a different matter because it requires the rigorous application of the scientific method. **State survey objectives as hypotheses only when you are sure that your research design and data quality justify your doing so.**

For more on hypothesis testing, see **How to Analyze Survey Data** (Vol. 8 in this series).

WHERE DO SURVEY OBJECTIVES ORIGINATE?

The objectives of a survey can come from a defined need. For example, suppose a school district is concerned with finding out the causes of a measurable increase in smoking among students between 12 and 16 years of age. The district calls on the Survey Research Department to design and implement a survey of students. The objective of the survey—to find out why students smoke—is defined for the surveyors and is based on the school district's needs.

The objectives of a survey can also come from reviews of the literature and other surveys. The literature refers to all published and unpublished public reports on a topic. Systematic reviews of the literature tell you what is currently known about a topic; using the available data you can figure out the gaps that need to be filled.

The objectives of a survey can also come from experts. Experts are individuals who are knowledgeable about the survey or will be affected by its outcomes or are influential in implementing its findings. Experts can be surveyed by mail or telephone or brought together in meetings. Two types of meetings that are sometimes used to help surveyors identify objectives, research questions, and research hypotheses are **focus groups** and **consensus panels.** A focus group usually contains up to 10 people. A trained leader conducts a carefully planned discussion in a permissive atmosphere to obtain participants' opinions on a defined area of interest. A consensus panel may contain up to 14 people. The panel should be led by a skilled leader in a highly structured setting. For example, consensus participants may be required to read documents and rate or rank preferences. Example 1.6 illustrates how focus groups and consensus panels can be useful in identifying survey objectives.

EXAMPLE 1.6
Identifying Survey Objectives:
Focus Groups and Consensus Panels

Focus Group

A 10-member group—5 students, 2 parents, and 3 teachers—was asked to help identify the objectives of a survey on teenage smoking. The group met for 2 hours in a classroom at the Middle School. The group was told that the overall goal of the survey was to provide the school district with information on why children start smoking. What information should the survey collect? What types of questions should be on the survey to encourage children to provide honest, and not just acceptable, answers? The focus group recommended a survey that had at least two major objectives:

- Determine the effects of cigarette advertising on smoking behavior
- Compare smoking behavior among children with and without family members who smoke

Consensus Panel

A two-round consensus panel was conducted to help identify the objectives of a survey to find out why children start smoking. The panel consisted of 10 members with expertise in survey research, smoking behavior among children, health professionals, students, and teachers.

In the first round, panelists were provided with a list of potential survey objectives and asked to rate each on two dimensions: their importance and the feasibility of obtaining honest answers to questions pertaining to the objective. The ratings were analyzed to identify objectives that were rated very important *and* definitely feasible. The following table shows a portion of the rating sheet.

	Importance					Feasibility				
Survey Objective	Scale: 5 = Very important; 3 = Somewhat important; 1 = Very unimportant (circle *one* choice for each objective)					Scale: 5 = Definitely feasible; 3 = Somewhat feasible; 1 = Definitely not feasible (circle *one* choice for each objective)				
To determine the effects of cigarette advertising on smoking behavior	5	4	3	2	1	5	4	3	2	1
To compare smoking behavior among children with and without family members who smoke	5	4	3	2	1	5	4	3	2	1

In the second round of the consensus process, panelists met for a half-day and discussed the first round's ratings. After their discussion, the panelists rated the objectives a second time. Objectives were chosen for the survey that at least 8 of the 10 panelists agreed were very important and also definitely feasible.

Straightforward Questions and Responses

Because questions are the focus of many surveys, learning how to ask them in written and spoken form is essential. A straightforward question asks what it needs in an unambiguous way and extracts accurate and consistent information. Straightforward questions are purposeful, use correct grammar and syntax, and call for one thought at a time with mutually exclusive questions.

TYPES OF QUESTIONS

Purposeful questions. Questions are purposeful when the respondent can readily identify the relationship between the intention of the question and the objectives of the survey. A respondent is the person who answers the questions on a survey instrument. Sometimes, the survey instrument writer has to spell out the connection between the question and the survey, as illustrated in Example 1.7.

EXAMPLE 1.7
Purposeful Questions:
The Relationship Between the
Question and the Survey's Objective

Survey Objective: To find out about reading habits in the community

Survey Question: In what year were you born?

Comment: The relationship between the question and the objective is far from clear.

The surveyor should place a statement just before the question that says something like "In this survey of reading habits, we want to be able to compare readers of different ages and backgrounds so that we can better meet the needs of each. The next five questions are about age, education, and living arrangements."

Concrete questions. A concrete question is precise and unambiguous. Adding a dimension of time and defining words can help concretize the question, as shown in Example 1.8.

EXAMPLE 1.8
Concrete Questions

Less Concrete: How would you describe your mood?

More Concrete: In the past 3 weeks, would you say you were generally happy or generally unhappy?

Comment: Adding a time period (3 weeks) and defining mood (generally happy and generally unhappy) adds precision to the question.

Complete sentences. Complete sentences express one entire thought. Look at Example 1.9.

EXAMPLE 1.9
Complete Sentences

Poor: Place of birth?

Comment: Place of birth means different things to different people. I might give the city in which I was born, but you might tell the name of the hospital.

Better: Name the city and state in which you were born.

Make sure that all questions are reviewed by experts and a sample of potential respondents. You should do this even if you are using a survey that someone else has used successfully. The reason is that your respondents may have different reading levels and interests than did users of a previous survey.

Open and closed questions. Questions can take two primary forms. When they require respondents to use their own words, they are called **open.** When the answers or responses are preselected for the respondent, the question is termed **closed.** Both types of questions have advantages and limitations.

An open question is useful when the intricacies of an issue are still unknown, in getting unanticipated answers, and for describing the world as the respondent sees it—rather than as the questioner does. Also, some respondents prefer to state their views in their own words and may resent the questioner's preselected choices. Sometimes, when left to their own devices, respondents provide quotable material. The disadvantage is that unless you are a trained anthropologist or qualitative researcher, responses to open questions are often difficult to compare and interpret. Consider the question in Example 1.10.

EXAMPLE 1.10
Three Possible Answers
to an Open Question

Question: How often during the past week were you bored?
Answer 1: Not often
Answer 2: About 10% of the time
Answer 3: Much less often than the month before

Open questions provide answers that must be catalogued and interpreted. Does 10% of the time (Answer 2) mean not often (Answer 1)? How does Answer 3 compare to the other two?

Some respondents prefer closed questions because they are either unwilling or unable to express themselves while being surveyed. Closed questions are more difficult to write than open ones, however, because the answers or response choices must be known in advance. But the results lend themselves more readily to statistical analysis and interpretation, and this is particularly important in large surveys because of the number of responses and respondents. Also, because the respondent's expectations are more clearly spelled out in closed questions (or the surveyor's interpretations of them), the answers have a better chance of being more reliable or consistent over time. Example 1.11 shows a closed question.

EXAMPLE 1.11
A Closed Question

How often during the past week were you bored? Circle **one.**

Always	1
Very often	2
Fairly often	3
Sometimes	4
Almost never	5
Never	6

TYPES OF RESPONSES

The choices given to respondents for their answers may take three forms. The first is called **nominal** or **categorical.** (The two terms are sometimes used interchangeably.) Categorical or nominal choices have no numerical or preferential values. For example, asking respondents if they are male or female (*or* female or male) asks them to "name" themselves as belonging to one of two categories: male or female.

The second form of response choice is called **ordinal.** When respondents are asked to rate or order choices, say, from very positive to very negative, they are given ordinal choices. The third form of response choice, **numerical,** asks for numbers such as age (e.g., number of years) or height (e.g., number of meters).

Nominal, ordinal, and numerical response choices are illustrated in Example 1.12.

EXAMPLE 1.12
Three Questions About Movies

1. *Nominal:* Which of these movies have you seen? Please circle yes *or* no for each choice. (The response choices are categorized as yes/no.)

	Yes (1)	No (2)
Gone With the Wind	1	2
Schindler's List	1	2
Casablanca	1	2
Chariots of Fire	1	2
Police Academy 1	1	2
Star Wars	1	2

2. *Ordinal:* How important has each of the following films been in helping form your image of modern life? Please use the following scale to make your rating:

> 1 = Definitely unimportant
> 2 = Probably unimportant
> 3 = Probably important
> 4 = Definitely important
> 9 = No opinion/Don't know

Movie	Please *circle* one for each film				
Gone With the Wind	1	2	3	4	9
Schindler's List	1	2	3	4	9
Casablanca	1	2	3	4	9
Chariots of Fire	1	2	3	4	9
Police Academy 1	1	2	3	4	9
Star Wars	1	2	3	4	9

3. *Numerical:* What is your date of birth?

                      19
_____ _____   _____
Month   Day   Year

Each of the questions in Example 1.12 produces different information. The first question asks respondents to tell if they have seen each of six films. The second question asks the respondents to use a continuum to indicate how important each of the six films is to them. This continuum has been divided into four points (with a "no opinion/don't know" option). The third question asks respondents to specify the month, day, and year of their birth.

Survey questions typically use one of three measurement classifications, as illustrated by the three questions in Example 1.12. The first question in Example 1.12, for instance, asks respondents to tell whether or not they fit into one of two categories: saw this movie or did not see this movie. Data or measures like these have no natural numerical values, and they are called nominal or categorical (the names are placed into categories, say, of yes or no). A hypothetical survey finding that uses nominal data results in numbers or percentages, as follows:

> More than 75% of the respondents saw at least one movie or play on the list, but no one saw all six. Of 75 respondents, 46 (61.3%) indicated they had seen *Star Wars*, the most frequently seen movie.

The second measurement pattern, represented by the second question in Example 1.12 is called ordinal. Responses are made to fit on a continuum or scale that is ordered from positive (*very important*) to negative (*very unimportant*). The information from scales like this is called ordinal because an ordered set of answers results. Ordinal data, for example, consist of the numbers and percentages of people who select each point on a scale. In some cases, you may find it expedient to compute the average response: the average rating of importance across all respondents. Sample survey results might take a form like this:

> Of 75 respondents completing this question, 43
> (57.3%) rated each movie as definitely or probably
> important. The average ratings ranged from 3.7 for
> *Star Wars* to 2.0 for *Police Academy 1*.

Surveys often ask respondents for numerical data. In Example 1.12, respondents are asked for their birth date. From the date, you can calculate each respondent's age. Age is considered a numerical and continuous measure, starting with zero and ending with the age of the oldest person in the survey. When you have numerical data, you can perform many statistical operations. Typical survey findings might appear as follows:

> The average age of the respondents was 43 years. The
> oldest person was 79, and the youngest was 23. We found
> no relation between age and ratings of importance.

For more informations on questions, see **How to Ask Survey Questions** (Vol. 2 in this series). Objectives of that volume are the following:

- Understand a survey's cultural, psychological, economic, and political context by:

  - Identifying specific purposes
  - Preparing appropriately worded, meaningful questions for participants
  - Clarifying research and other objectives
  - Determining a feasible number of questions
  - Standardizing the questioner
  - Standardizing the response choices

- Ask valid questions that:

  - Make sense to the respondent
  - Are concrete
  - Use time periods that are related to the importance of the question
  - Use conventional language
  - Use short and long questions appropriately
  - Use loaded words cautiously
  - Avoid biasing words
  - Avoid two-edgers
  - Avoid negative phrasing

- Compare the characteristics and uses of closed and open questions

- Distinguish among response formats that use nominal, ordinal, and numerical measurement

- Identify correctly prepared questions

■ Correctly ask questions by:

- Using response categories that are meaningfully grouped

- Choosing an appropriate type of response option

- Balancing all responses on a scale

- Selecting neutral categories appropriately

- Determining how many points to include on a rating scale

- Deciding on where to place the positive or negative end of the scale

- Determining the proper use of skip patterns

■ Applying special questioning techniques to survey behaviors, knowledge, attitudes, and demographics

2 Sound Survey Design

A design is a way of arranging the environment in which a survey takes place. The environment consists of the individuals or groups of people, places, activities, or objects that are to be surveyed.

Some designs are relatively simple. A fairly uncomplicated survey might consist of a 10-minute interview on Wednesday with a group of 50 children to find out if they enjoyed a given film, and if so, why. This survey provides a description or portrait of one group's opinions at a particular time—a cross section of the group's opinions—and its design is called cross-sectional.

More complicated survey designs use environmental arrangements that are experiments, relying on two or more groups of participants or observations. When the views of randomly constituted groups of 50 children each are compared three times, for example, the survey design is experimental. Definitions of the major survey designs follow.

■ Experimental

Experimental designs are characterized by arranging to compare two or more groups, at least one of which is experimental. The other is a control (or comparison) group. An experimental group is given a new or untested, innovative program, intervention, or treatment. The control is given an alternative (e.g., the traditional program or no program at all). A group is any collective unit. Sometimes, the unit is made up of individuals with a common experience, such as men who have had surgery, children who are in a reading program, or victims of violence. At other times, the unit is naturally occurring: a classroom, business, or hospital.

Concurrent controls in which participants are randomly assigned to groups. **Concurrent** means that each group is assembled at the same time. For example, when 10 of 20 schools are randomly assigned to an experimental group while, at the same time, 10 are assigned to a control, you have a randomized controlled trial or true experiment.

Concurrent controls in which participants are not randomly assigned to groups. These are called nonrandomized controlled trials, quasi-experiments, or nonequivalent controls.

Self-controls. One group is surveyed at two different times. These require premeasures and postmeasures and are called longitudinal or before-after designs.

Historical controls. These make use of data collected for participants in other surveys.

Combinations. These can consist of concurrent controls with or without pre- and postmeasures.

■ Descriptive

Descriptive designs produce information on groups and phenomena that already exist. No new groups are created. Descriptive designs are also called **observational** designs.

Cross sections. These provide descriptive data at one fixed point in time. A survey of American voters' current choices is a cross-sectional survey.

Cohorts. These forward-looking, or **prospective,** designs provide data about changes in a specific population. Suppose a survey of the aspirations of athletes participating in the 1996 Olympics is given in 1996, 2000, and 2004. This is a cohort design, and the cohort is 1996 Olympians.

Cohort designs can also be **retrospective,** or look back over time (a historical cohort) if the events being studied actually occurred before the onset of the survey. For example, suppose a group of persons was diagnosed 10 years ago with Disease X. If you survey their medical records to the present time, you are using a retrospective cohort.

Case controls. These retrospective studies go back in time to help explain a current phenomenon. At least two groups are included. When first you survey the medical records of a sample of smokers and nonsmokers of the same age, health, and socioeconomic status and then compare the findings, you have used a case-control design.

For more information on survey designs, see **How to Design Surveys** (Vol. 5 in this series). Objectives of that volume are the following:

- Describe the major features of high-quality survey systems

- Identify the questions that structure survey designs

- Distinguish between experimental and observational designs

- Explain the characteristics, benefits, and concerns of these designs:

  - Concurrent controls with random assignment

  - Concurrent controls without random assignment

  - Self-controls

  - Historical controls

  - Cross-sectional designs

  - Cohort designs

  - Case-control designs

- Identify the risks to a design's internal validity

- Identify the risks to a design's external validity

Sound Survey Sampling

A sample is a portion or subset of a larger group called a population. Surveys often use samples rather than populations. A good sample is a miniature version of the population—just like it, only smaller. The best sample is **representative,** or a model of the population. A sample is representative of the population if important characteristics (e.g., age, gender, health status) are distributed similarly in both groups. Suppose the population of interest consists of 1,000 people, 50% of whom are male, with 45% over 65 years of age. A representative sample will have fewer people, say, 500, but it must also consist of 50% males, with 45% over age 65.

No sample is perfect. Usually, it has some degree of bias or error. To ensure a sample whose characteristics and degree of representation can be described accurately, you must start with very specific and precise survey objectives. You also must have clear and definite eligibility, apply sampling methods rigorously, justify the sample size, and have an adequate response rate.

ELIGIBILITY CRITERIA

The criteria for inclusion in a survey refer to the characteristics of respondents who are eligible for participation in the survey; the exclusion criteria consist of characteristics that rule out certain people. You apply the inclusion and exclusion criteria to the target population. Once you remove from the target population all those who fail to meet the inclusion criteria and all those who succeed in meeting the exclusion criteria, you are left with a study population consisting of people who are eligible to participate. Consider the illustrations in Example 2.1.

EXAMPLE 2.1
Inclusion and Exclusion Criteria:
Who Is Eligible?

Research Question: How effective is QUITNOW in helping smokers to stop smoking?

Target Population: Smokers

Inclusion Criteria

- Between the ages of 10 and 16 years
- Smoke one or more cigarettes daily
- Have an alveolar breath carbon monoxide determination of more than eight parts per million

Exclusion Criterion: If any of the contraindications for the use of nicotine gum are applicable

Comment: The survey's results will only apply to the respondents who are eligible to participate. If a smoker is under 10 years of age or over 16, then the survey's findings may not apply to these people. Although the target population is smokers, the inclusion and exclusion criteria have defined their own world or study population of "people who smoke."

The survey in Example 2.1 sets boundaries for the respondents who are eligible. In so doing, they are limiting the generalizability of the findings. Why deliberately limit applicability?

A major reason for setting eligibility criteria is that to do otherwise is simply not practical. Including everyone under age 10 and over 16 in the survey of smokers requires additional resources for administering, analyzing, and interpreting data from large numbers of people. Also, very young and older teenage smokers may be different in their needs and motivations. Setting inclusion and exclusion criteria is an efficient way of focusing the survey on only those people from whom you are equipped to get the most accurate information or about whom you want to learn something.

Rigorous Sampling Methods

Sampling methods are usually divided into two types. The first is called probability sampling. Probability sampling provides a statistical basis for saying that a sample is representative of the study or target population.

In probability sampling, every member of the target population has a known, nonzero probability of being included in the sample. Probability sampling implies the use of random selection. Random sampling eliminates subjectivity in choosing a sample. It is a "fair" way of getting a sample.

The second type of sampling is nonprobability sampling. Nonprobability samples are chosen based on judgment regarding the characteristics of the target population and the needs of the survey. With nonprobability sampling, some members of the eligible target population have a chance of being chosen and others do not. By chance, the survey's findings may not be applicable to the target group at all.

PROBABILITY SAMPLING

Simple random sampling. In simple random sampling, every subject or unit has an equal chance of being selected. Members of the target population are selected one at a time and independently. Once they have been selected, they are not eligible for a second chance and are not returned to the pool. Because of this equality of opportunity, random samples are considered relatively unbiased. Typical ways of selecting a simple random sample are using a table of random numbers or a computer-generated list of random numbers and applying it to lists of prospective participants.

The advantage of simple random sampling is that you can get an unbiased sample without much technical difficulty. Unfortunately, random sampling may not pick up all the elements of interest in a population. Suppose you are conducting a survey of patient satisfaction. Consider also that you have evidence from a previous study that older and younger patients usually differ substantially in their satisfaction. If you choose a simple random sample for your new survey, you might not pick up a large enough proportion of younger patients to detect any differences that matter in your particular survey. To be sure that you get adequate proportions of people with certain characteristics, you need stratified random sampling.

Stratified random sampling. A stratified random sample is one in which the population is divided into subgroups or "strata," and a random sample is then selected from each subgroup. For example, suppose you want to find out about the effectiveness of a program in caring for the health of homeless families. You plan to survey a sample of 1,800 of the 3,000 family members who have participated in the program. You also intend to divide the family members into groups according to their general health status (as indicated by scores on a 32-item test) and age. Health status and age are the strata.

How do you decide on subgroups? The strata or subgroups are chosen because evidence is available that they are related to the outcome—in this case, care for health needs of homeless families. The justification for the selection of the strata can come from the literature and expert opinion.

Stratified random sampling is more complicated than simple random sampling. The strata must be identified and justified, and using many subgroups can lead to large, unwieldy, and expensive surveys.

Systematic sampling. Suppose you have a list with the names of 3,000 customers, from which a sample of 500 is to be selected for a marketing survey. Dividing 3,000 by 500 yields 6. That means that 1 of every 6 persons will be in the sample. To systematically sample from the list, a random start is needed. To obtain this, a die can be tossed. Suppose a toss comes up with the number 5. This means the 5th name on the list would be selected first, then the 11th, 17th, 23rd, and so on until 500 names are selected.

To obtain a valid sample, you must obtain a list of all eligible participants or members of the population. This is called the **sampling frame.** Systematic sampling should not be used if repetition is a natural component of the sampling frame. For example, if the frame is a list of names, systematic sampling can result in the loss of names that appear infrequently (e.g., names beginning with X). If the data are arranged by months and the interval is 12, the same months will be selected for each year. Infrequently appearing names and ordered data (January is always Month 1 and December Month 12) prevents each sampling unit (names or months) from having an equal chance of selection. If systematic sampling is used without the guarantee that all units have an equal chance of selection, the resultant sample will not be a probability sample. When the sampling frame has no inherently recurring order, or you can reorder the list or adjust the sampling intervals, systematic sampling resembles simple random sampling.

Cluster sampling. A cluster is a naturally occurring unit (e.g., a school, which has many classrooms, students, and teachers). Other clusters are universities, hospitals, metropolitan statistical areas (MSAs), cities, states, and so on. The clusters are randomly selected, and all members of the selected cluster are included in the sample. For example, suppose that California's counties are trying out a new program to improve emergency care for critically ill and injured children. If you want to use cluster sampling, you can consider each county as a cluster and select and assign counties at random to the new emergency care program or to the traditional one. The programs in the selected counties would then be the focus of the survey.

Cluster sampling is used in large surveys. It differs from stratified sampling in that with cluster sampling you start with a naturally occurring constituency. You then select from among the clusters and either survey all members of the selection or randomly select from among them. The resulting sample may not be representative of areas not covered by the cluster, nor does one cluster necessarily represent another.

NONPROBABILITY SAMPLING

Nonprobability samples do not guarantee that all eligible units have an equal chance of being included in a sample. Their main advantage is that they are relatively convenient, economical, and appropriate for many surveys. Their main disadvantage is that they are vulnerable to selection biases. Two uses of nonprobability sampling are illustrated in Example 2.2.

EXAMPLE 2.2
Sample Reasons for Using
Nonprobability Samples

Surveys of Hard-to-Identify Groups

A survey of the goals and aspirations of members of teenage gangs is conducted. Known gang members are asked to suggest at least three others to be interviewed.

Comment: Implementing a probability sampling method among this population is not practical because of potential difficulties in obtaining cooperation from and completing interviews with all eligible respondents.

Surveys in Pilot Situations

A questionnaire is mailed to 35 nurses who participated in a workshop to learn about the use of a computer in treating nursing home patients with fever. The results of the survey will be used in deciding whether to sponsor a formal trial and evaluation of the workshop with other nurses.

Comment: The purpose of the survey is to decide whether to formally try out and evaluate the workshop. Because the data are to be used as a planning activity and not to disseminate or advocate the workshop, a nonprobability sampling method is appropriate.

The following are three commonly used nonprobability sampling methods.

Convenience sampling. A convenience sample consists of a group of individuals that is ready and available. For example, a survey that relies on people in a shopping mall is using a convenience sample.

Snowball sampling. This type of sampling relies on previously identified members of a group to identify other members of the population. As newly identified members name others, the sample snowballs. This technique is used when a population listing is unavailable and cannot be compiled. For example, surveys of teenage gang members and illegal aliens might be asked to participate in snowball sampling because no membership list is available.

Quota sampling. Quota sampling divides the population being studied into subgroups such as male and female and younger and older. Then you estimate the proportion of people in each subgroup (e.g., younger and older males and younger and older females).

Sample Size

The size of the sample refers to the number of units that needs to be surveyed to get precise and reliable findings. The units can be people (e.g., men and women over and under 45 years of age), places (e.g., counties, hospitals, schools), and things (e.g., medical or school records).

When you increase the sample's size, you increase its cost. Larger samples mean increased costs for data collection (especially for interviews), data processing, and analysis. Moreover, increasing the sample size may divert attention from other sampling activities like following up on eligible people who fail to respond. The diversion may actually increase total sampling error. It is very important to remember that many factors affect the amount of error or chance variation in the sample. Besides nonresponse, these include the design of a sample. If the sample design deviates from simple random sampling, relies on cluster sampling, or does not use probability sampling, then the total error will invariably decrease the quality of the survey's findings. The size of the sample, although a leading contender in the sampling error arena, is just one of several factors to consider in coming up with a "good" sample.

The most appropriate way to produce the right sample size is to use statistical calculations. These can be relatively complex, depending on the needs of the survey. Some surveys have just one sample, and others have several. Like most survey activities, sample size considerations should be placed within a broad context.

Response Rate

All surveys hope for a high response rate. The response rate is the number who respond (numerator) divided by the number of *eligible* respondents (denominator). No single response rate is considered the standard. In some surveys, between 95% and 100% is expected; in others, 70% is adequate. Consider the following two surveys in Example 2.3.

EXAMPLE 2.3
Two Surveys and Response Rates

1. According to statistical calculations, the Domestic Violence Commission needs a sample of 100 for their mailed survey. Based on the results of previous mailings, a refusal rate of 20% to 25% is anticipated. To allow for this possibility, 125 eligible people are sent a survey.

2. A sample of employees at United Airlines participates in an interview regarding their job satisfaction. A 100% response is achieved.

The first survey described in Example 2.3 uses past information to estimate the probable response rate. The survey **oversamples** in the hope that the desired number of respondents will participate. Oversampling can add costs to the survey but is often necessary.

Practically all surveys are accompanied by a loss of information because of **nonresponse.** These nonresponses may introduce error bias into the survey's results because of differences between respondents and others in motivation and other potentially important factors. It is very frustrating and costly to send out a mail survey only to find that half the addressees have moved. As a guide to how much oversampling is necessary, anticipate the proportion of people who, although otherwise apparently eligible, may not turn up in the sample. For mail surveys, this can happen if the addresses are outdated and the mail is undeliverable. With telephone interviews, respondents may not be at home. Sometimes, people cannot be interviewed in person because they suddenly become ill.

Unsolicited surveys receive the lowest fraction of responses. A 20% response for a first mailing is not uncommon. With effort, response rates can be elevated to 70% or even 80%. These efforts include follow-up mailings and use of graphically sophisticated surveys and monetary and gift incentives like pens, books, radios, music and videotapes, and so on.

Nonresponse to an entire survey introduces error or bias. Another type of nonresponse can also introduce bias: item nonresponse, which occurs when respondents or survey administrators do not complete all items on a survey form. This type of bias occurs when respondents do not know the answers to certain questions or refuse to answer them because they believe them to be sensitive, embarrassing, or irrelevant. Interviewers may skip questions or fail to record an answer. In some cases, answers are made but are later rejected because they appear to make no sense. This can happen if the respondent misreads the question or fails to record all the information called for. For example, respondents may leave out their year of birth and just record the month and date.

To promote responses, minimize response bias, and reduce survey error, use these guidelines.

Guidelines for Promoting Responses, Minimizing Response Bias, and Reducing Error

- Use trained interviewers. Set up a quality assurance system for monitoring quality and retraining.

- Identify a larger number of eligible respondents than you need in case you do not get the sample size you need. Be careful to pay attention to the costs.

- Use surveys only when you are fairly certain that respondents are interested in the topic.

- Keep survey responses confidential or anonymous.

- Send reminders to complete mailed surveys and make repeat phone calls.

- Provide gift or cash incentives (and keep in mind the ethical implications of what some people think of as "buying" respondents).

- Be realistic about the eligibility criteria. Anticipate the proportion of respondents who may not be able to participate because of survey circumstances (e.g., incorrect addresses) or by chance (they suddenly become ill).

For more information on sampling, see **How to Sample in Surveys** (Vol. 6 in this series). Objectives of that volume are the following:

■ Distinguish between target populations and samples

   − Identify research questions and survey objectives

   − Specify inclusion and exclusion criteria

   − Choose the appropriate probability and nonprobability sampling methods:

      ☐ Simple random sampling

      ☐ Stratified random sampling

      ☐ Systematic sampling

      ☐ Cluster sampling

      ☐ Convenience sampling

      ☐ Snowball sampling

      ☐ Quota sampling

      ☐ Focus groups

■ Understand the logic in estimating standard errors

■ Understand the logic in sample size determinations

■ Understand the sources of error in sampling

■ Calculate the response rate

3 Reliable and Valid Survey Instruments

A reliable survey instrument is consistent; a valid one is accurate. For example, an instrument is reliable if each time you use it (and assuming no intervention), you get the same information. Reliability or the consistency of information can be seriously imperiled by poorly worded and imprecise questions and directions. If an instrument is unreliable, it is also invalid because you cannot have accurate findings with inconsistent data. Valid survey instruments serve the purpose they were intended to and provide correct information. For example, if a survey's aim is to find out about mental health, the results should be consistent with other measures of mental health and inconsistent with measures of mental instability. Valid instruments are always reliable, too.

41

Four Types of Survey Instruments

Survey instruments take four forms: self-administered questionnaire, interview, structured record review, and structured observation. Each is discussed in turn.

SELF-ADMINISTERED QUESTIONNAIRES

A self-administered questionnaire consists of questions that an individual completes by oneself. Self-administered questionnaires can be mailed or completed "on site," say, on a computer or by hand in a classroom, waiting room, or office. As an example, consider a student who is given a printed form with 25 questions on it about future career plans. The student is told to complete the questionnaire at home and return it to the teacher on Friday. Another type of self-administered questionnaire is the computerized or computer-assisted survey. This type of self-administered survey asks the respondent to give answers to questions directly on the computer. A typical computer-assisted survey presents the questions and the choices on a screen and the respondent uses a keyboard (or voice) to answer the question, as illustrated by this example:

[sample text on screen]

Who is the author of *Macbeth*?
WORDSWORTH
SHAKESPEARE
NOBEL
MACARTHUR

Use up and down arrows to point.
Use space to select
Use left and right arrows to go forward and backward
Hit enter to go to next question
Hit pq to go to previous question

INTERVIEWS

An interview requires at least two people: one to ask the questions (the interviewer) and one to respond (the interviewee). (Group interviews are possible.) Interviews can take place on the telephone, face-to-face, or using television. An example of an interview is when a psychologist directly asks clients to describe their family background and writes the answers on a specially prepared form.

For more about mail, telephone, and in-person surveys, see **How to Conduct Self-Administered and Mail Surveys** and **How to Conduct Surveys by Telephone and in Person** (Vols. 3 and 4, respectively, in this series). Objectives of those volumes are the following:

For Volume 3: **How to Conduct Self-Administered and Mail Surveys**

- Describe the types of self-administered questionnaires

- Identify the advantages and disadvantages of self-administered questionnaires

- Decide whether a self-administered questionnaire is appropriate for your survey question

- Determine the content of the questionnaire

- Develop questions for a "user-friendly" questionnaire

- Pretest, pilot-test, and revise questions

- Format a "user-friendly" questionnaire

■ Write advance letters and cover letters that motivate and increase response rate

■ Write specifications that describe the reasons for and sources of the questions on the questionnaire and the methodology used in administering the study

■ Describe how to develop and produce a sample, identify potential resources for a sample, organize the sample, determine sample sizes, and increase response rate

■ Inventory materials and procedures involved in mail and self-administered surveys

■ Describe follow-up procedures for nonrespondents, methods of tracking a respondent, and number and timing of follow-up attempts

■ Describe how returned questionnaires are processed, edited, and coded

■ Describe data entry

■ Describe how records are kept

■ Estimate the costs of a self-administered or mailed survey

■ Estimate personnel needs for a self-administered or mailed survey

■ Fully document the development and administration of the questionnaire and the data collected with it

For Volume 4: **How to Conduct Interviews by Telephone and in Person**

- Choose the most appropriate interview mode (telephone or in person) for specific surveys

- Write specific questions with structured interviewer instructions

- Employ appropriate question-writing techniques based on whether the interview will be done by telephone or in person

- Construct useful visual aids

- Organize a flowing interview script that considers possible question order effects

- Write an informative introductory statement

- Write a preletter

- Write a script for a precall

- Design an eligibility screen

- Write and appropriately place transition statements

- Write a job description for an interviewer

- Develop an interviewer training manual

- Design an interviewer training session

- Describe the role of a supervisor

STRUCTURED RECORD REVIEWS

A structured record review is a survey that uses a specially created form to guide the collection of data from financial, medical, school, and other records. An example of a structured record review is the use of a form to collect information from school attendance records on the number and characteristics (e.g., age, reading level) of students who are absent 4 or more weeks each semester.

STRUCTURED OBSERVATIONS

A structured observation collects data visually and is designed to guide the observer in focusing on specific actions or characteristics. For example, two visitors to school would be participating in a structured observation if both are asked to count and record the number of computers they see, look for the presence or absence of air conditioning, and measure the room's area in square feet.

Reliability

A reliable survey instrument is one that is relatively free from "measurement error." Because of this "error," individuals' obtained scores are different from their true scores, which can only be obtained from perfect measures. What causes this error? In some cases, the error results from the measure itself: It may be difficult to understand or poorly administered. For example, a self-administered questionnaire on the value of preventive health care might produce unreliable results if its reading level is too high for the teenaged mothers who are to use it. If the reading level is on target but the directions are unclear, the measure will be unreliable. Of course, the surveyor could simplify the language and clarify the directions and still find measurement error. This is because measurement error can also come directly from the examinees. For example, if teenaged mothers are asked to complete a questionnaire and they are especially anxious or fatigued, their obtained scores could differ from their true scores.

Four kinds of reliability are often discussed: stability, equivalence, homogeneity, and inter- and intrarater reliability.

STABILITY

Stability is sometimes called test-retest reliability. A measure is stable if the correlation between scores from one time to another is high. Suppose a survey of students' attitudes was administered to the same group of students at School A in April and again in October. If the survey was reliable and no special program or intervention was introduced, then, on average, we would expect attitudes to remain the same. The major conceptual difficulty in establishing test-retest reliability is in determining how much time is permissible between the first and second administration. If too much time elapses, external events might influence responses for the second administration; if too little time passes, the respondents may remember and simply repeat their answers from the first administration.

EQUIVALENCE

Equivalence, or alternate-form reliability, refers to the extent to which two items measure the same concepts at the same level of difficulty. Suppose students were asked a question about their views toward technology before participating in a new computer skills class and again 2 months after completing it. Unless the surveyor was certain that the items on the surveys were equal, more favorable views on technology after the second administration could reflect the survey's language level (for example) rather than improved views. Moreover, because this approach to reliability requires two administrations, a problem may arise concerning the appropriate interval between them.

When testing alternate-form reliability, the different forms may be administered at separate time points to the same population. Alternatively, if the sample is large enough, it can be divided in half and each alternate form administered to half the group. This technique, called the split-halves method, is generally accepted as being as good as administering the different forms to the same sample at different time points. When using the split-halves method, you must make sure to select the half-samples randomly.

HOMOGENEITY

Homogeneity refers to the extent to which all the items or questions assess the same skill, characteristic, or quality. Sometimes, this type of reliability is referred to as internal consistency. Cronbach's coefficient alpha, which is basically the average of all the correlations between each item and the total score, is often calculated to determine the extent of homogeneity. For example, suppose a surveyor created a questionnaire to find out about students' satisfaction with Textbook A. An analysis of homogeneity will tell the extent to which all items on the questionnaire focus on satisfaction.

Some variables do not have a single dimension. Student satisfaction, for example, may consist of satisfaction with school in general, their school in particular, teachers, classes, extracurricular activities, and so on. If you are unsure of the number of dimensions expressed in an instrument, a factor analysis can be performed. This statistical procedure identifies "factors" or relationships among the items or questions.

INTER- AND INTRARATER RELIABILITY

Interrater reliability refers to the extent to which two or more individuals agree. Suppose two individuals were sent to a clinic to observe waiting times, the appearance of the waiting and examination rooms, and the general atmosphere. If the observers agreed perfectly on all items, then interrater reliability would be perfect. Interrater reliability is enhanced by training data collectors, providing them with a guide for recording their observations, monitoring the quality of the data collection over time to see that people are not "burning out," and offering a chance to discuss difficult issues or problems. *Intrarater reliability* refers to a single individual's consistency of measurement, and this, too, can be enhanced by training, monitoring, and continuous education.

Validity

Validity refers to the degree to which a survey instrument assesses what it purports to measure. For example, a survey of student attitude toward technological careers would be an invalid measure if the survey only asked about their knowledge of the newest advances in space technology. Similarly, an attitude survey will not be considered valid unless you can prove that people who are identified as having a good attitude on the basis of their responses to the survey are different in some observable way from people who are identified as dissatisfied.

Four types of validity are often discussed: content, face, criterion, and construct.

CONTENT

Content validity refers to the extent to which a measure thoroughly and appropriately assesses the skills or characteristics it is intended to measure. For example, a surveyor who is interested in developing a measure of mental health has to first define the concept ("What is mental health?" "How is health distinguished from disease?") and then write items that adequately contain all aspects of the definition. Because of the complexity of the task, the literature is often consulted either for a model or for a conceptual framework from which a definition can be derived. It is not uncommon in establishing content validity to see a statement like "We used XYZ cognitive theory to select items on mental health, and we adapted the ABC role model paradigm for questions about social relations."

FACE

Face validity refers to how a measure appears on the surface: Does it seem to ask all the needed questions? Does it use the appropriate language and language level to do so? Face validity, unlike content validity, does not rely on established theory for support.

CRITERION

Criterion validity compares responses to future performance or to those obtained from other, more well-established surveys. Criterion validity is made up two subcategories: predictive and concurrent.

- *Predictive validity:* Extent to which a measure forecasts future performance. A graduate school entry examination that predicts who will do well in graduate school has predictive validity.

- *Concurrent validity:* Demonstrated when two assessments agree or a new measure is compared favorably with one that is already considered valid. For example, to establish the concurrent validity of a new survey, the surveyor can either administer the new and validated measure to the same group of respondents and compare the responses or administer the new instrument to the respondents and compare the responses to experts' judgment. A high correlation between the new survey and the criterion means concurrent validity. Establishing concurrent validity is useful when a new measure is created that claims to be better (shorter, cheaper, fairer).

CONSTRUCT

Construct validity is established experimentally to demonstrate that a survey distinguishes between people who do and do not have certain characteristics. For example, a surveyor who claims constructive validity for a measure of satisfaction will have to prove in a scientific manner that satisfied respondents behave differently from dissatisfied respondents.

Construct validity is commonly established in at least two ways:

1. The surveyor hypothesizes that the new measure correlates with one or more measures of a similar characteristic (convergent validity) and does not correlate with measures of dissimilar characteristics (discriminant validity). For example, a surveyor who is validating a new quality-of-life survey might posit that it is highly correlated with another quality-of-life instrument, a measure of functioning, and a measure of health status. At the same time, the surveyor would hypothesize that the new measure does not correlate with selected measures of social desirability (the tendency to answer questions so as to present yourself in a more positive light) and of hostility.

2. The surveyor hypothesizes that the measure can distinguish one group from the other on some important variable. For example, a measure of compassion should be able to demonstrate that people who are high scorers are compassionate but that people who are low scorers are unfeeling. This requires translating a theory of compassionate behavior into measurable terms, identifying people who are compassionate and those who are unfeeling (according to the theory), and proving that the measure consistently and correctly distinguishes between the two groups.

For more information on reliability and validity, see **How to Measure Survey Reliability and Validity** (Vol. 7 in this series). Objectives of that volume are the following:

■ Select and apply reliability criteria, including

– Stability or test-retest reliability

– Alternate-form reliability

– Internal consistency reliability

– Interobserver reliability

– Intraobserver reliability

■ Select and apply validity criteria, including

– Content validity

– Criterion validity

– Construct validity

■ Understand the fundamental principles of scaling and scoring

---

- Create and use a codebook for survey data

- Pilot-test new and established surveys

- Address cross-cultural issues in survey research

Appropriate Survey Analysis

Surveys use conventional statistical and other scholarly methods to analyze findings. Statistics is the mathematics of organizing and interpreting numerical information. The results of statistical analyses are descriptions, relationships, comparisons, and predictions, as shown in Example 3.1.

EXAMPLE 3.1
Statistical Analysis and Survey Data

A survey is given to 160 people to find out about the number and types of movies they see. The survey is analyzed statistically to accomplish the following:

- Describe the backgrounds of the respondents
- Describe the responses to each of the questions
- Determine if a connection exists between the number of movies seen and number of books read during the past year
- Compare the number of books read by men with the number read by women
- Find out if gender, education, or income predicts how frequently the respondents read books

Illustrative results of the above goals of statistical analysis are as follows:

- *Describe respondents' background.* Of the survey's 160 respondents, 77 (48.1%) were men, with 72 of all respondents (48%) earning more than $50,000 per year and having at least two years of college. Of the 150 respondents answering the question, 32 (21.3%) stated that they always or nearly always attended movies to escape daily responsibilities.

- *Describe responses.* Respondents were asked how many movies they see in an average year, and if they preferred action or romance. On average, college graduates saw 10 or more movies, with a range of 2 to 25. The typical college graduate prefers action to romance.

- *Determine relationships between number of books read and movies seen.* Respondents were asked how many books they read in the past year. The number of books they read and the number of movies they saw were then compared. Respondents who read at least five books in the past year saw five or more movies.

- *Comparisons.* The percentage of men and women who saw five or more movies each year was compared, and no differences were found. On average, women's scores on the Value of Film Survey were statistically significantly higher and more positive than men's, but older men's scores were significantly higher than older women's.

- *Predicting frequency.* Education and income were found to be the best predictors of how frequently people go to the movies. Respondents with the most education and income, for example, saw the fewest movies.

In the first set of results, the findings are tallied and reported as percentages. A **tally,** or **frequency count,** is a computation of how many people fit into a category (men or women, under and over 70 years of age, saw five or more movies last year or did not). Tallies and frequencies take the form of numbers and percentages.

In the second set of results, the findings are presented as averages ("on average," "the typical" moviegoer). When you are interested in the center, such as the average, of a distribution of findings, you are concerned with **measures of central tendency. Measures of dispersion,** or spread, like the range, are often given along with measures of central tendency.

In the third set of results, the survey reports on the relationships between number of books read and movies seen. One way of estimating the relationship between two characteristics is through **correlation.**

In the fourth set of results, comparisons are made between men and women. The term **statistical significance** is used to show that the differences between them are statistically meaningful and not due to chance.

In the fifth set of results, survey data are used to "predict" frequent moviegoing. In simpler terms, predicting means answering a question like "Of all the characteristics on which I have survey data (e.g., income, education, types of books read, types of movie seen), which one or ones are linked to frequent moviegoing? For instance, does income make a difference? Education? Income and education?"

What methods should you use to describe, summarize, compare, and predict? Before answering that question, you must answer four others: Do the survey data come from nominal, ordinal, or numerical scales or measures? How many independent and dependent variables are there? What statistical methods are potentially appropriate? Do the survey data fit the requirements of the methods? Nominal, ordinal, and numerical measures have already been discussed, so the next section deals with independent and dependent variables.

INDEPENDENT AND DEPENDENT VARIABLES

A **variable** is a measurable characteristic that varies in the population. Weight is a variable, and all persons weighing 55 kilograms have the same numerical weight. Satisfaction with a product is also a variable. In this case, however, the numerical scale has to be devised and rules created for its interpretation. For example, in Survey A, product satisfaction is measured on a scale from 1 to 100, with 100 representing perfect satisfaction. Survey B, however, measures satisfaction by counting the number of repeat customers. The rule is that at least 15% of all customers must reorder within a year to demonstrate satisfaction.

Your choice of method for analyzing survey data is always dependent on the type of data available to you (nominal, ordinal, or numerical) and on the number of variables involved. Some survey variables are termed **independent,** and some are termed **dependent.**

Independent variables are also called "explanatory" or "predictor" variables because they are used to explain or predict a response, outcome, or result—the dependent variable. The independent and dependent variables can be identified by studying the objectives and target of the survey, as illustrated in Example 3.2.

EXAMPLE 3.2
Targets and Variables

Objective: To compare elementary school students in different grades regarding (a) opinions on the school's new science program and (b) attitudes toward school

Target: Boys and girls in Grades 3 through 6 in five elementary schools

Independent Variables: Gender, grade level, school

Characteristics of Survey: To get gender, ask if male or female; ask students to write in grade level and name of school.

Type of Data: All nominal

Dependent Variables: Opinion of new science program and attitudes toward school

Characteristics of Survey: To get opinions on new science program, ask for ratings of like and dislike (e.g., from *like a lot* to *dislike a lot*); to learn about attitudes, use the Attitude Toward School Rating Scale.

Type of Data: Both ordinal

When choosing an appropriate analysis method, you begin by deciding on the purpose of the analysis and then you determine the number of independent and dependent variables and whether you have nominal, ordinal, or numerical data. When these activities are completed, you can choose an analysis method. Example 3.3 shows how this works.

EXAMPLE 3.3
Choosing an Analysis Method

Survey Objective: To compare boys and girls in terms of whether they do or do not support their school's new dress code

Number of Independent Variables: One (gender)

Type of Data: Nominal (boys, girls)

Number of Dependent Variables: One (support dress code)

Type of Data: Nominal (support or do not support)

Possible Method of Analysis: Logistic regression, a statistical method used when the behavior of interest has two outcomes—support or do not support.

In Example 3.3, the choice of analytic method is labeled "possible." The appropriateness of the choice of a statistical method depends on the extent to which you meet the method's **assumptions** about the characteristics and quality of the data. In the examples above, too little information is given to help you decide on whether the assumptions are met.

For more information on how to analyze data from surveys, see **How to Analyze Survey Data** (Vol. 8 in this series). Objectives of that volume are the following:

■ Learn the use of analytic terms, such as the following:

  – Distribution

  – Critical value

  – Skew

  – Transformation

  – Measures of central tendency

  – Dispersion

  – Variation

  – Statistical significance

  – Practical significance

- *p* value
- Alpha
- Beta
- Linear
- Curvilinear
- Scatterplot
- Null hypothesis

■ List the steps to follow in selecting an appropriate analytic method

■ Distinguish between nominal, ordinal, and numerical scales and data so as to:

- Identify independent and dependent variables

- Distinguish between the appropriate uses of the mean, median, and mode

- Distinguish between the appropriate uses of the range, standard deviation, percentile rank, and interquartile range

- Understand the logic in and uses of correlations and regression

- Learn the steps in conducting and interpreting hypothesis tests

- Compare and contrast hypothesis testing and the use of confidence intervals

- Understand the logic in and uses of the chi-square distribution and test

- Understand the logic in and uses of the *t* test
- Understand the logic in and uses of analysis of variance
- Read and interpret computer output

How to Analyze Data From Open-Ended Questions: One Qualitative Approach

A very common use of a survey is to find out if people are satisfied with a new product, service, or program. Their opinions provide important insights into why new ideas or ways of doing things do or do not get used.

One open-ended set of questions that is particularly appropriate for determining satisfaction requires collecting information about what people like best (LB) about the product or service and what they like least (LL). Here's how the LB/LL method works:

Step 1. Ask respondents to list what is good and what is bad. Always set a limit on the number of responses: "List at least one thing, but no more than three things, you like best about your participation in the focus group." If respondents cannot come up with three responses, they can leave blank spaces or write "none." If they give more than three, you can keep or discard the extras, depending on the information you need.

Instead of asking about the conference as a whole, you may want to focus on some particular aspect: "List at least one thing, but no more than three things, you like best about the instructional materials handed out before the focus group discussion."

Step 2. Once you have all the responses, the next step is to categorize and code them. To do this, you can create categories based on your review of the responses, or you can create categories based on past experience with similar services, products, or activities.

Try to keep the categories as precise as possible—that is, more categories rather than fewer—because it is easier to combine them later if necessary than it is to break them up.

Suppose these were answers that focus group participants gave to the question on what they liked least about the activity:

- Some people did all the talking.
- The leader didn't always listen.
- I couldn't say anything without being interrupted.
- Too much noise and confusion.
- Some members of the group were ignored.
- The leader didn't take control.
- I didn't get a chance to say anything.
- Meles and Petrus were the only ones who talked.
- The leader didn't seem to care.
- I couldn't hear myself think.

You might then categorize and code these answers, as shown in Example 3.4.

EXAMPLE 3.4
Response Categories

Category	Code
Leader didn't listen (ignored participants; didn't seem to care)	1
Some people monopolized discussion (did all the talking; couldn't say anything; Meles and Petrus were the only ones who talked)	2
Disorderly environment (too much noise; leader didn't take control; couldn't hear myself think)	3

Now match your codes and the responses, as shown in Example 3.5.

EXAMPLE 3.5
Group Member Responses

Response	Code
Member A Instructor didn't always listen.	1
I couldn't hear myself think.	3
I couldn't say anything without being interrupted.	2
Member B Leader didn't always listen.	1
Leader didn't take control when things got noisy.	3
The leader ignored some members.	3
Member C I didn't get a chance to say anything.	2

To make sure you assigned the codes correctly, you should establish their reliability. Bring in another rater. Do the two of you agree? In other words, are the ratings reliable? If not, negotiate the differences or redo the codes.

Step 3. When you are satisfied about the reliability, the next step is to count the number of responses for each code. Example 3.6 shows how to do this for 10 focus group participants.

EXAMPLE 3.6
Number of Responses for Each Code

Participant	Codes			
	1	2	3	Total
A	1	1	1	3
B	1	—	2	3
C		2	1	3
D		1	2	3
E		3	—	3
F		2	1	3
G		2	1	3
H		2	1	3
I		3	2	5
J		1	—	1

Look at the number of responses in each category. The 10 focus group members listed 30 things they liked least about the discussion group. Seventeen of the 30 (more than 50%) were assigned to the same category, Code 2, and the surveyor could justly argue that, based on the data, what the participants tended to like least about the focus group was that some people monopolized the discussions and others did not get a chance to say anything.

Next, count the *number* of participants whose answers were assigned to each code—for example, only Participants A and B gave answers that were coded 1 (see Example 3.7).

EXAMPLE 3.7
Participants' Response Pattern

Code	Number of Participants Listing a Response Assigned to This Code	Which Participants?
1	2	A and B
2	9	All but B
3	8	All but E and J

Look at the number of focus group participants whose responses fit each category. Because 8 or 9 of the 10 participants gave responses that fell into the same categories (Codes 2 and 3), their opinions probably represent those of the entire group. It is safe to add that the participants also disliked the disorderly atmosphere that prevailed during the focus groups. They complained that the noise made it hard to think clearly, and the leader did not take control.

When respondents agree with one another, there will be few types of answers, and these will be listed by many people. If respondents disagree, many different kinds of answers will turn up on their lists, and only a few people (fewer than 10%) will be associated with each type.

Interpreting LB/LL data gets more complex when you have many participants and responses to categorize. Suppose, for example, you asked 100 participants to indicate which aspects of a health education program they liked best.

First, you must decide on your response categories and assign each one a code. Then try this:

1. Put the codes in rank order. That is, if the largest number of participants chose responses that are assigned to Code 3, list Code 3 first.

2. Calculate the percentage of students assigned to each code. If 40 of 100 students made responses that were assigned to Code 3, then the calculation would be 40%.

3. Count the number of responses assigned to each code.

4. Calculate the percentage of responses assigned to each code. If 117 responses from a total of 400 were assigned to Code 3, then 29.25%, or *117/400*, of responses were for Code 3.

5. Calculate the cumulative percentage of response by adding the percentages together: 29.25% + 20.25% = 49.50%.

The table in Example 3.8 summarizes these steps with some hypothetical survey data.

EXAMPLE 3.8
Summary of Responses

Response Categories (codes arranged in rank order)	% 100 Participants Assigned to Each Code	No. of 400 Responses Assigned to Each Code	% Respondents Assigned to Each Code	Cumulative % Responses Assigned to Each Code
3	40	117	29.25	29.25
4	34	81	20.25	49.50
7	32	78	19.50	69.00
8	20	35	8.75	77.75
10	17	30	7.50	85.25
1	15	29	7.25	92.50
6	10	14	3.50	96.00
2	5	10	2.50	98.50
9	3	5	1.25	99.75
5	1	1	0.25	100.00

What does this table tell you?

- The highest number and percentages of participants and responses were assigned to Code 3, followed by responses assigned to Code 4.
- Nearly 50% of all responses (49.50%) were assigned Codes 3 and 4.

- Of the 10 coded response categories, more than three fourths (77.75%) were encompassed by 4 codes: 3, 4, 7, and 8.

- Five codes—3, 4, 7, 8, and 10—accounted for nearly all responses (92.50%).

Accurate Survey Reports

Fair and accurate reporting means staying within the boundaries set by the survey's design, sampling methods, data collection quality, and analysis. Accurate survey reports require knowledge of how to use lists, charts, and tables to present data.

LISTS

Lists are used to state survey objectives, methods, and findings. The following illustrations (Example 3.9) of these uses of lists come from a formal talk about a survey of job satisfaction conducted with part-time employees.

EXAMPLE 3.9
Surveys and Lists

1. To State Survey Objectives

   Survey of Part-Time Employees: Purposes

   TO FIND OUT ABOUT
   - Quality of life
   - Characteristics of office environment
   - Reasons for part-time employment

2. To Describe Survey Methods

   Seven Tasks
   - Conduct focus groups
   - Identify specific objectives
   - Set inclusion and exclusion criteria
   - Adapt the PARTEE Survey
   - Pilot-test and revise PARTEE
   - Train interviewers
   - Administer the interviews

3. To Report Survey Results or Findings

   PARTEE'S Results

   62% STATE THAT PART-TIME EMPLOYMENT HAS
   IMPROVED THE QUALITY OF THEIR LIVES.
   - No difference between men and women
   - No difference between younger and older respondents

   32% OF EMPLOYEES ARE ALMOST ALWAYS SATISFIED.
   - Men more satisfied
   - No difference between younger and older respondents

Lists are simple to follow and so are very useful in survey reports.

CHARTS

A figure is a method of presenting data as a diagram or chart. Pie, bar, and line charts are figures. Each has its uses and rules of preparation, as illustrated below. The pie chart shown in Figure 3–1 is used to describe a survey's responses in percentages.

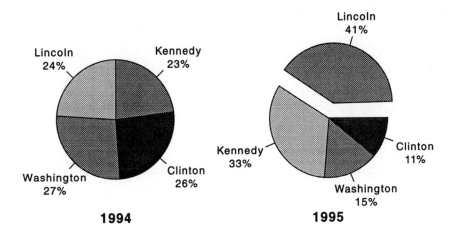

Figure 3–1. Attitude Toward School

As you see, the pie chart is given a title and an explanation of the source of data—telephone interviews. The "slices" show you that the response rates in all four schools were fairly equal proportionately in 1994, ranging from 23% to 27%. In 1995, Lincoln substantially increased its responses, so the range was much wider (from 11% to 41%), and the proportions were less similar among the schools.

Figure 3–2 shows a bar chart. Bar charts (or graphs) depend on a horizontal X-axis and a vertical Y-axis. On the X-axis, you can put nearly all types of data (e.g., names, years, time of day, and age). The X-axis usually has data on the independent variable. The Y-axis represents the unit of measurement, or dependent variable (e.g., dollars, scores, and number of people responding).

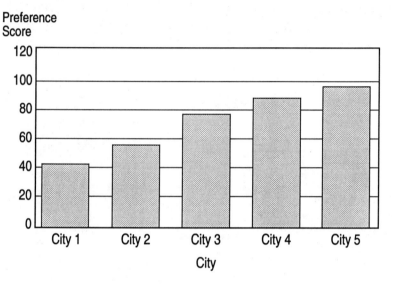

Figure 3–2.   Housing Commission Mail Survey

Bar charts are used in survey reports because they are relatively easy to read and interpret. The bar chart in Figure 3–2 shows the results of a study of housing preferences in five cities. Notice that the chart has a title ("Housing Preferences in Five Cities"), both the X-axis and the Y-axis are labeled (cities and preference score), and the source of data (Housing Commission Mail Survey) is given.

Figure 3–3 shows a line chart in which men's and women's job satisfaction is compared over a 10-year period.

Score

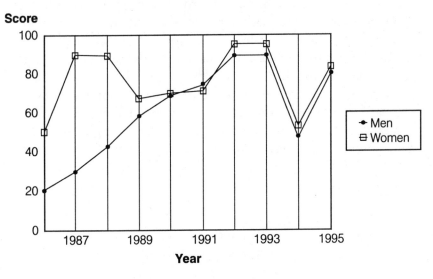

Figure 3–3. Job Satisfaction: A 10-Year Study
SOURCE: The Job Satisfaction Inventory (Higher scores are better)

Because two groups (men and women) are involved in the job satisfaction survey, a key (or legend) to the meaning of the bars is given. The chart shows that men's satisfaction has been lower than women's for 9 of the 10 years. Only in 1991 were the positions reversed and men appeared slightly more satisfied than women.

TABLES

Tables are also frequently used in survey reports. Their major use is to summarize data about respondents and their responses and to compare survey results at one or more times.

Suppose you are responsible for surveying workers in an experiment to find out if their health habits can be improved through an on-the-job health promotion program. One of Company A's two factories is randomly assigned to the experimental program. The other is assigned to the control condition, which consists of free lectures at the company's gym; attendance at the lectures is voluntary. The survey's main objectives are to describe and compare the participants in each program and to compare their health habits (e.g., willingness to exercise regularly) before entering the program, immediately after, and 2 years later. If you achieve the survey's objectives, you will produce tables that look like the empty "shells" in Example 3.10.

EXAMPLE 3.10
Shell Tables to Describe,
Compare, and Illustrate Changes

Description of participants in the experimental and control groups

The table will contain the number (*n*) and percentage of the sample (%) in the experimental group and in the control group of different ages (years), with varying exposures to education, who are male or female, and who speak primarily English, Russian, Spanish, or some other language at home.

	Experimental Group		Control Group	
	n	%	n	%
Age (years)				
Over 55				
45 - 55				
35 - 44				
34 or less				
Education (type of school last attended)				
Graduate school				
College				
High school (or equivalent)				
Gender				
Female				
Male				
Primary language spoken at home				
English				
Russian				
Spanish				
Other (specify)				

Changes over time in the experimental and control groups:
Willingness to exercise regularly

The shell table below is set up to show comparisons among scores on the 25-question Exercise Inventory for the number of people (*n*) in the experimental group and in the control group.

	Average Scores on Exercise Inventory	
Timing	Experimental Group (*n* =)	Control Group (*n* =)
Before program participation		
Immediately after		
2 years after		

When should tables be used? They are especially useful in written reports because they provide detailed information for the reader. Technically oriented people also like them in oral presentations. Unfortunately, little information is available to conclusively guide you in the choice of charts versus tables. If you need to make a visual impact, then charts are appropriate. If you want to illustrate your points with numbers, then tables are appropriate. Often, a mixture of tables and charts is presented in a single report.

For more about survey reports, see **How to Report on Surveys** (Vol. 9 in this series). Objectives of that volume are the following:

■ Prepare, interpret, and explain lists, pie charts, and bar and line charts

■ Prepare, interpret, and explain tables

■ Identify survey report contents for:

— Oral presentations

— Written presentations

— Technical and academic audiences

— General audiences

■ Prepare slides

■ Prepare transparencies

■ Explain orally the contents and meaning of a slide or transparency

■ Explain in writing the contents and meaning of a table or figure

■ Explain orally and in writing the survey's objectives, design, sample, psychometric properties, results, and conclusions

■ Review reports for readability

■ Review reports for comprehensiveness and accuracy

4 Reasonable Resources

A survey's resources are reasonable if they adequately cover the financial costs of and time needed for the survey. This includes the costs of, and time for, hiring and training staff, preparing and validating the survey form, administering the survey, and analyzing, interpreting, and reporting the findings.

How much does it cost to conduct a survey? How can I be sure that I have an adequate amount of resources (time and money) to conduct my survey? These questions are often asked by novice surveyors and experts alike. They can be answered by obtaining the answers to seven other questions:

1. What are the survey's major tasks?

2. What skills are needed to complete each task?

3. How much time do I have to complete the survey?

4. How much time does each task take?

5. Whom can I hire to perform each task?

6. What are the costs of each task?

7. What additional resources are needed?

The meaning of each of these questions and how to answer them are discussed and illustrated in the sections that follow.

What Needs to Be Done?

A survey is a system for collecting information. It often involves deciding on the objectives of the survey, developing a survey instrument, designing a study and identifying the sample, administering the survey, and analyzing and reporting the results. The following is a checklist of typical survey tasks. It may be used as a guide in determining your own survey's tasks. Each of the tasks on the checklist is then explained.

Checklist of Typical Survey Tasks

✓ **Identify the survey's objectives.**

- Conduct focus groups to identify the objectives

- Obtain official approval of the objectives

- Conduct a review of the literature to define terms and justify theory underlying questions

✓ **Design the survey.**

- Choose a survey design (e.g., descriptive or experimental)
- Decide on a sample

✓ **Prepare the survey instrument.**

- Identify existing and appropriate instruments
- Conduct a literature review
- Contact other surveyors
- Adapt some or all questions on existing instruments
- Prepare a new instrument

✓ **Pilot-test the instrument.**

- Identify the sample for the pilot test
- Obtain permission for the pilot test
- Analyze the pilot-test data
- Revise the instrument to make it final

✓ **Administer the survey.**

- Hire staff
- Train staff
- Monitor the quality of administration
- Retrain staff
- Send out mail, supervise the questionnaire, conduct interview
- Follow up

✓ **Organize the data.**

- Code responses
- Consult with programmer
- Train data enterers
- Enter the data into a computer
- Run a preliminary analysis
- Clean the data
- Prepare a codebook

✓ **Analyze the data.**

- Prepare an analysis plan
- Analyze the psychometric properties of instrument
- Analyze the results of the survey

✓ **Report the results.**

- Write the report
- Have the report reviewed
- Modify the report based on the reviews
- Prepare slides, transparencies
- Present the report orally

Getting Each Survey Task Done

IDENTIFICATION OF SURVEY OBJECTIVES

The survey's objectives are its particular purposes or hoped-for outcomes. In general, surveys can be used to describe, compare, or explain knowledge, attitudes, and behavior. For example, a survey can be designed to describe customer satisfaction in Stores A and B, compare satisfaction in A and B, and explain why satisfaction is higher in A than in B.

What are the particular objectives of a survey? For example, in a customer satisfaction survey, should the survey's aim be to compare younger and older persons in their satisfaction? Should information be collected about education or region of the country so that satisfaction can be compared among people with differing levels of education who live in various parts of the country? Methods for answering questions like these include conducting "focus" groups or reviewing the literature.

Once you have identified the survey's objectives, you should certify them "officially." For example, suppose you intend to survey customers and compare men and women of differing educational attainment. Does this meet the needs of the users of the survey? One way to find this out is to create an advisory group of users of the survey. This group may consist of 3 to 5 people who can assist you in keeping the survey on target.

Example 4.1 illustrates how objectives were set for a survey of responses to natural disasters.

EXAMPLE 4.1
Setting Survey Objectives:
What Needs to Be Done?

The Center for Natural Disease Control and Prevention plans to survey victims of floods, fires, earthquakes, and tornados. A mailed questionnaire will be supplemented with interviews. Data from the survey are to be used to determine how to most effectively respond to victims immediately after a natural disaster. What should the survey want to find out? In other words, what should its objectives be?

The survey team first conducts a review of the literature for the definition of the term "victim" and to determine if other surveys of disaster victims are available, and if so, what their objectives are. The team then convenes a six-member focus group that consists of three people who have lived through one or more natural disasters, a psychiatrist whose expertise is in treating people with posttraumatic stress syndrome, and two members of the Agency for Emergency Relief.

Based on the review of the literature and the focus group results, the survey team decides to use a mail survey. The literature reviews and focus groups also result in setting the following four survey objectives:

1. Describe psychological damage associated with the disaster

2. Describe physical damage to person, home, business, school, and so on

3. Identify needs for services during the disaster (for victims of fires and floods)

4. Identify needs for services immediately and 6 months after the disaster

The list of objectives is sent for approval to the Advisory Board, which recommends that Objective 4 be amended to read as follows:

> 4. Identify needs for services within 3 months of the disaster and 12 to 18 months after.

DESIGN OF SURVEY

The objectives of the survey guide the design. For example, if a survey objective is to identify needs for services within 3 months of a natural disaster and 12 to 18 months after, then you know that you must conduct a longitudinal survey or one that collects data over time (in this case, twice: within 3 months of the disaster and then between 12 and 18 months after the disaster). If the objective is to make comparisons, then the survey's design will include two or more groups of respondents.

The next issue that must be resolved is whether you plan to survey everyone or just a sample. If you sample, you must decide on a sampling strategy. Look at Example 4.2.

EXAMPLE 4.2
Survey Design:
What Needs to Be Done?

The Center for Natural Disaster Control and Prevention's survey team decides to conduct a mail survey of a cohort of victims in three states: California, Missouri, and Tennessee. A cohort is a group of respondents that shares an experience (e.g., loss of their home to an earthquake) that is central to the objectives of a survey.

Four cohorts will be surveyed. In California, there will be two: fire victims and earthquake victims; in Missouri, flood victims; and in Tennessee, tornado victims. To find out how many people should be in each cohort, the survey team's statistician conducts a special analysis and finds that at least 50 people are needed in each cohort. Because the study is a longitudinal survey, the statistician recommends having 75 in each cohort, assuming that as many as 25 people may drop out, move, or become inaccessible because of illness or other reasons.

PREPARATION OF SURVEY INSTRUMENT

Once the objectives are set, the survey instrument has to be created. The literature and other surveyors should be consulted to find out if other instruments are available.

If you are lucky, you may find a survey instrument that is designed to collect data that meet the needs of your survey's objectives and that also can be obtained, administered, and scored in a timely and efficient way. You still must check to see that the instrument is appropriate for your population. Is the reading level appropriate? Does the survey ask for all the information you need? Has it been tried out with a population similar to your own? Can you obtain the survey instrument in time? Will you have to pay, and can you afford the price? If you decide to adopt an instrument that is already in use, check the directions to the user and administrator to make sure that they are satisfactory for your purposes.

The most important consideration in adapting a survey instrument is whether it is the type you need. If you want to conduct telephone interviews but the instrument is in the form of a self-administered questionnaire, you must be sure you have the resources to translate it from one type of survey to the other.

If you decide to prepare some or all of your own instrument, you should outline the content, select the response formats (e.g., ratings on a scale from *very positive* to *very negative*) and prepare rules for administration and scoring.

In Example 4.3, a survey team prepares a self-administered questionnaire to find out about people's reactions to natural disasters.

EXAMPLE 4.3
Preparing a Self-Administered Questionnaire: What Needs to Be Done?

The survey team reviews the literature on natural disasters. They focus on reports published by government emergency agencies to identify survey instruments. Twenty appropriate survey instruments are identified: 15 are obtained within the 1-month period allocated for the literature review. None of the surveys is considered wholly appropriate; however, 10 contain at least one question that may be adapted or used in its entirety.

The team prepares an outline of the survey's content and decides to ask questions that have the following format:

Where were you when the earthquake struck? *Please circle ONE response.*

My own home	Yes	No
Someone else's home	Yes	No
Traveling on a city street	Yes	No
Traveling on the freeway	Yes	No
In an office building	Yes	No
In a restaurant	Yes	No
Other (specify)	Yes	No

PILOT-TESTING OF INSTRUMENT

A pilot test is an opportunity to try out an instrument well before it is made final. In a pilot test, you should monitor the ease with which respondents complete the questionnaire and also its ease of administration and scoring.

Usually, you need 10 or more people who are willing to complete the survey. Ask them if they understand the directions for completing the survey and each question and whether the wording in each question and the place to mark responses are clear. Verify the logistics of administering the survey instrument. This is particularly important with interviews. Can interviewers follow the directions that are on the survey form? How long does it take for them to record responses? Do they know what to do with completed interviews? For example, how many should be completed before they are returned to the survey team's office? How many phone calls should be made before giving up on a potential respondent? Use the following questions to guide pilot testing.

Questions to Ask When
Pilot-Testing Survey Instruments

Mail and other self-administered questionnaires:

- Are instructions for completing the survey clearly written?
- Are questions easy to understand?
- Do respondents know how to indicate responses (e.g., circle or mark the response; use a special pencil; use the space bar)?
- Are the response choices mutually exclusive?
- Are the response choices exhaustive?

- If a mail questionnaire, do respondents understand what to do with completed questionnaires (e.g., return them by mail in a self-addressed envelope; fax them)?
- If a mail questionnaire, do respondents understand when to return the completed survey?
- If a computer-assisted survey, can respondents correctly use the commands?
- If a computer-assisted survey, do respondents know how to change (or "correct") their answers?
- If an incentive is given for completing the survey, do respondents understand how to obtain it (e.g., it will automatically be sent upon receipt of completed survey; it is included with the questionnaire)?
- Is privacy respected and protected?
- Do respondents have any suggestions regarding the addition or deletion of questions, the clarification of instructions, or improvements in format?

Telephone interviews:

- Do interviewers understand how to ask questions and present options for responses?
- Do interviewers know how to get in-depth information, when appropriate, by probing respondents' brief answers?
- Do interviewers know how to record information?
- Do interviewers know how to keep the interview to the agreed-on time limit?
- Do interviewers know how to return completed interviews?
- Are interviewers able to select the sample using the agreed-on instructions?
- Can interviewers readily use the phone logs to record the number of times and when potential respondents were contacted?

- Do interviewees understand the questions?

- Do interviewees understand how to answer the questions (e.g., pick the top two; rate items according to whether they agree or disagree)?

- Do interviewees agree that privacy has been protected? Respected?

Face-to-face interviews:

- Do interviewers understand how to ask questions and present options for responses?

- Do interviewers know how to get in-depth information, when appropriate, by probing respondents' brief answers?

- Do interviewers know how to record information?

- Do interviewers know how to keep the interview to the agreed-on time limit?

- Do interviewers know how to return completed interviews?

- Do interviewees understand the questions?

- Do interviewees understand how to answer the questions (e.g., pick the top two; rate items according to whether they agree or disagree)?

- Do interviewees agree that privacy has been protected? Respected?

For pilot testing to be effective, you should use respondents who are similar to those who will be asked to participate in the survey. If the survey is targeted to parents of teenaged children, for example, then parents of teenaged children should constitute the pilot test sample.

Use the results of the pilot test to revise the survey instrument and logistics. Sometimes, a pilot test is conducted more than once; this is costly. A field test is a minitrial of the actual survey. For example, a field test of a survey of teenagers' use of health services may take place in one state. The results would then be used to guide any revisions. The final version of the instrument might then be used in a national survey.

ADMINISTRATION OF SURVEY

The survey's administration includes mailing the survey instrument, supervising its use (say, in a classroom), or conducting an interview. To properly administer a telephone survey requires the interviewer to ask questions, record answers, keep records, stay within a time limit, and respect the respondent. To administer a mail survey means packaging the questionnaire (e.g., by including a self-addressed, stamped envelope and ensuring that respondents have enough time to complete all questions), following up with people who do not respond by the due date, and, in some situations, handling rewards and incentives for completed surveys.

A poorly administered survey invariably leads to garbled responses and a poor response rate. To ensure high-quality administration, the staff should be trained and monitored. When hiring staff members, decide on the skills they must have in advance of training. For example, do you want people who can speak a certain language? Who can work between certain hours? Be sure to take the time to train the staff. Have formal training sessions, give each trainee a written manual, and provide practice in conducting interviews. Monitor the results. Observe a sample of interviews, for instance. If they are unsatisfactory, then retrain the interviewers.

ORGANIZATION OF DATA

Organizing survey data means starting with the responses to the survey instrument (the data) and entering them into the computer. To do this, you must assign codes or numbers to all anticipated responses. If the survey instrument is to be completed anonymously or confidentially, you must assign a unique identification number to each respondent. To facilitate direct computer entry, survey questions should be precoded. That is, codes should be assigned to all potential responses before any data are collected. Data enterers should be trained so that data are entered with minimum errors.

ANALYSIS OF DATA

Plan the analysis after you have the survey objectives and know if the data will be nominal, ordinal, or numerical, and if you can explain and justify the quality of the data. Suppose Surveyor 1 wants to compare boys and girls in their willingness to choose future careers in politics. Suppose also that in the analysis willingness is determined by the number of positive answers to a self-administered questionnaire and that a score of 100 is considered twice as good as a score of 50. If the survey data are high quality (e.g., all respondents answer all survey questions on a valid measure) and the data are numerical and continuous, then a *t* test might be the appropriate analytic method to use to make the comparison. Suppose, however, that Surveyor 2 takes a different approach to analyzing the extent of willingness to choose a career in politics. Surveyor 2 decides that positive willingness is a score of 50 or greater and negative willingness is a score of 49 or less. Assuming the data can be dichotomized, Surveyor 2 might use a chi-square analysis to compare the number of boys and girls with scores of 49 and below and those with scores of 50 and above.

Besides providing survey results (e.g., data on how boys and girls compare in their willingness to choose careers in politics), the analysis can be used to determine the survey instrument's psychometric properties. How do you demonstrate that a score of 100 is twice as good as a score of 50, as posited in Survey 1? To prove that a survey has a scale with equal intervals (e.g., a score of 5 is half the value of a score of 10) requires the kind of analytic proof that psychometricians can provide. Psychometricians are skilled in statistically interpreting a survey's reliability and validity.

REPORT OF RESULTS

Once the data are available, surveyors typically write and disseminate reports or present them orally. In any case, a first draft is rarely acceptable, and reviews and revisions are necessary. In oral reports, slides, overhead transparencies, and other visual aids are often prepared to facilitate the audience's understanding of the survey's message.

Who Will Do It, and What Resources Are Needed? Personnel, Time, and Money

A survey happens because one or more persons are responsible for completing the required tasks. In a very small survey, one or two persons may be in charge of planning the survey design, developing the survey instrument, administering it, analyzing the data, and reporting the results. In larger surveys, teams of individuals with differing skills are involved. Sometimes, a survey is planned and conducted by the staff with the assistance of consultants who are called in for advice or to complete very specific activities.

First, you need to plan the activities and tasks that need to be completed. Once this is accomplished, you then decide on the skills required for each task. Next, you decide on the specific personnel or job descriptions that are likely to get you as many of the skills you need as efficiently as possible. For example, suppose your survey design requires someone with experience in training interviewers and writing survey questions. You may just happen to know someone who needs a job and has both skills, but if you do not know the right person, knowing the skills needed will help you target your employment search.

The specific resources needed for each survey will vary according to its size and scope and the number of skills and personnel needed to accomplish each task. Table 4–1 illustrates the types of skills and resources for a "typical" survey. An explanation of the example follows.

Table 4–1
Typical Survey Tasks, Skills, and Resources

Survey Task	Skills Needed	Other Resources
Identify survey objectives	Conduct focus groups	Honorariums for participants Transportation for participants Room rental for meeting Refreshments Materials to guide discussion
	Convene advisors	Honorariums Telephone Mail
	Conduct literature reviews	Librarian Reproduction of materials Standardization of forms for recording contents of literature Computer time for searches Training reviewers

Survey Task	Skills Needed	Other Resources
Design survey	Know alternative research designs and their implementation Have technical expertise in selecting sampling methods, determining sample size, and selecting sample	Research design expert Computer expert Software Hardware
Prepare survey instrument	Conduct literature reviews Have ability to write questions Have knowledge of the survey's topic Have knowledge of how to assemble questions into an instrument	Same as those needed for survey design Questionnaire expert
Pilot-test survey instrument	Have ability to analyze pilot-test data Have ability to interpret data in order to revise pilot-tested instrument and make it final	Room rental to administer the survey Refreshments for pilot-test sample
Administer survey	*Interviews* Ask questions in standardized, efficient manner Record answers in a standardized, efficient manner Have ability to monitor *Mail* Understand logistics of mailed surveys (e.g., include self-addressed return envelope) Have ability to monitor	Questionnaire expert Training materials expert Expert trainers Room for training Materials for training Materials for retraining Telephones Telephone time Incentives to complete interview Postage Paper Graphics consultant Incentives for completion

$\rightarrow$

Survey Task	Skills Needed	Other Resources

Organize data	Code data
	Enter data
	Clean data
	Prepare codebook
		Programmer
		Consultant in data
		  analysis (e.g., what to
		  do with missing data)

Analyze data	Select appropriate data-
	  analytic methods
	Perform data analysis
	Select appropriate
	  psychometric analysis
	Conduct appropriate
	  psychometric analysis
		Programmer
		Statistician
		Software
		Hardware

Report results	Write report
	Prepare slides,
	  transparencies
	Present report
		Duplicating report
		Dissemination (e.g., mail)
		Travel to orally present
		  report
		Honorariums for
		  reviewers
		Editorial consultant
		Slide preparation expert

Survey Tasks, Skills, and Resources: An Explanation

1. *Identify survey objectives.*

A first task requires identifying the survey's objectives. If you use focus groups, you need special expertise in conducting them and interpreting the results. Sometimes, focus group participants are remunerated financially; almost always, they receive refreshments. Other costs that might be incurred are renting a meeting room, transporting the participants, and preparing materials such as literature reviews and survey questionnaires.

A surveyor may decide to use an advisory group to help in obtaining certification of the survey and its objectives. This may require payment of honorariums, transportation to and from a meeting, and the costs of telephone and mail conference calls.

Conducting a literature review as an aid in identifying a survey's objectives requires expertise in identifying relevant sources of information from a variety of places (e.g., the library and public and private agencies), abstracting the information, and displaying the results in a useable fashion. If more than one person is involved in abstracting information, then a standardized form should be prepared so that the same types of information are required from the abstractors; special expertise is needed to prepare abstraction forms. Additionally, the abstractors should be trained by experienced educators to use the form, and the quality of their review should be monitored. Training can take place more than once; depending on the survey, 1 hour or 2 days may be needed. For example, a 2-day training session is not unusual in large surveys of the literature regarding effective social programs and medical treatments.

2. *Design the survey.*

To design a survey requires expertise in research methodologies. For example, research knowledge is essential in deciding on the appropriate intervals in longitudinal studies, determining the inclusion and exclusion criteria for the survey, and for choosing appropriate and meaningful comparison groups.

Sampling is usually considered one of the most technical of all survey tasks because knowledge of statistics is essential in deciding on a sample size, choosing and implementing a sampling technique, and determining the adequacy and representativeness of the sample. Large survey teams include experts in research design and sampling; smaller surveys sometimes rely on expert consultation.

Whenever technical activities take place, it is wise to check on the adequacy of the hard- and software available to the survey team. If it is not appropriate, computers or programs may need to be purchased. In some cases, the existing computer facilities are adequate, but special expertise, like programming, is needed so that the special needs of the survey are met.

3. *Prepare the survey instrument.*

If the survey instrument is to be adapted from an already existing instrument, expertise is needed in conducting literature reviews to find out if any potentially useful instruments are available. Sometimes, a reasonably good survey is available: Why spend time and money to prepare an instrument if a valid one exists? It helps to have experience in the subject matter being addressed by the survey and to know who is working in the field and might either have instruments or questions or know where and how to get them.

Selecting items or rewording them to fit into a new survey requires special skills. You must be knowledgeable regarding the survey respondents' reading levels and motivations to complete the survey and have experience writing survey questions and placing them in a questionnaire.

Preparing an entirely new instrument is daunting. A job description for an instrument writer would call for excellent writing skills and knowledge of the topic of the survey.

4. *Pilot-test the instrument.*

Pilot testing means having access to a group of potential respondents that is willing to try out a survey instrument that may be difficult to understand or complete. Expertise is needed in analyzing the data from the pilot test, and experience in interpreting respondents' responses is essential. Additional knowledge is needed in how to feasibly incorporate the findings of the pilot test into a more final version of the survey instrument.

Pilot testing may be very simple, say, a 1-hour tryout by a teacher in the classroom, or very complicated, involving many people, training, room rental, and so on. Also, the survey instrument, even in pilot-test format, must be prepared in a readable, user-friendly format. Assistance with graphics may be useful.

5. *Administer the survey.*

Face-to-face and telephone interviews require skilled personnel. Interviewers must be able to elicit the information called for on the survey instrument and record the answers in the appropriate way. Interviewers must be able to talk to people in a courteous manner and listen carefully. Also, they must talk and listen efficiently. If the interview is to last no longer than 10 minutes, the interviewer must adhere to that schedule. Interviews become increasingly costly and even unreliable when they exceed their planned times.

Mailed questionnaires also require skilled personnel. Among the types of expertise required is the ability to prepare a mailing that is user friendly (e.g., includes a self-addressed envelope) and the skill to monitor returns and conduct follow-ups with those not responding.

Expertise is needed in defining the skills and abilities needed to administer the survey and in selecting people who are likely to succeed. Training is key to getting reliable and valid survey data. For example, a poorly trained telephone interviewer is likely to get fewer responses than a well-trained interviewer. Because of the importance of training, many large surveys use educational experts to assist them in designing instructional materials and programs.

In large and long-term surveys, quality must be monitored regularly. Are interviewers continuing to follow instructions? Who is forgetting to return completed interviews at the conclusion of each 2-day session? If deficiencies in the survey process are noted, then retraining may be necessary.

Telephone interviews, of course, require telephones. Survey centers have phone banks or systems for computer-assisted, random-digit dialing. Face-to-face interviews require space for privacy and quiet. Mailed surveys can consume quantities of postage and paper. All types of surveys may include monetary and other incentives to encourage respondents to answer questions.

6. *Organize the data.*

Organizing the data means programming, coding, and data entry. Programming requires relatively high-level computer skills. Coding can be very complicated, too, especially if response categories are not precoded. Training and computer skills are needed to ensure that data enterers are expert in their tasks. Finally, data cleaning can be a highly skilled task involving decisions regarding what to do about missing data, for example.

7. *Analyze the data.*

Appropriate and justifiable data analysis is dependent on statistical and computer skills. Some surveys are very small and require only the computation of frequencies (number and percentages) or averages. Most, however, require comparisons among groups or predictions and explanations of findings. Furthermore, surveys of attitudes, values, beliefs, and social and psychological functioning also require knowledge of the statistical methods for ascertaining reliability and validity. When data analysis becomes complex, statistical consultation may be advisable.

8. *Report the results.*

Writing the report requires communication skills, including the ability to write and present results in tables and figures. Oral presentations require ability to speak in public and to prepare slides or transparencies. It helps to have outside reviewers critique the report; time must be spent on the critique and any subsequent revisions. Expenses for reports can mount if many are to be printed and disseminated.

TIME, SCOPE, AND QUALITY

Ideally, surveyors prefer to make their own estimates of the amount of time needed to complete the survey. Unfortunately, most surveys have a due date that must be respected.

The amount of time available for the survey is a key factor in the survey's size, scope, and quality and costs. Time limits your hiring choices to people who can complete each task within the allotted time, places boundaries on the survey's design and implementation, may affect the survey's quality, and is a determinant of the survey's costs. Example 4.4 compares two surveys to show the links among time, scope, quality, and costs.

EXAMPLE 4.4
Connections Between Time, Scope, Quality, and Costs in Surveys

Six elementary schools have joined together as a consortium to sponsor a survey to find out why young children start smoking. Among the questions the survey is to answer are these: Do children smoke because their friends do? Do parents smoke and thus serve as a negative model of adult behavior? How influential is advertising? What types of programs, events, or activities are most likely to be effective in teaching young children about the dangers of smoking?

The Consortium Board meets every 6 months. The Board plans to use the survey's results as a basis for determining whether an antismoking program should be undertaken, and if so, what format it might take.

Case Study 1

The Board gives approval for the survey at its September meeting and requires that findings be presented within 6 months in time for its next meeting in March. The survey team's schedule looks like this:

Month 1: Identify objectives and previously used surveys. Conduct a review of the published literature to assist in identifying reasonable aims for the survey. The literature will be used also in helping to locate other surveys that might be appropriate for use in the present survey. (Six months is considered too short a time to develop and properly pilot-test an entirely new instrument.)

Months 1 and 2: Ensure that the sample is readily attainable. The survey team plans to compile a list of families of children in all six schools and make sure that the addresses are current. All children will be included in the survey.

Month 2 and 3: Prepare, pilot-test, and revise the survey.

Month 4: Mail the survey and follow up when necessary.

Month 5: Clean, enter, and analyze the data.

Month 6: Write the report and prepare an oral presentation.

Comments: The survey team must hire an experienced reviewer because the literature on children and smoking is voluminous; sophisticated skills are necessary to efficiently identify and select the highest-quality, relevant articles and instruments. Skilled literature reviewers cost more to hire than unskilled ones who are trained and supervised. The relatively short time line prevents the team from targeting the survey directly to its own specific population and, with just 1 month for cleaning, entering, and analyzing the data and preparing a written and oral report, requires experienced, skilled (and relatively costly) individuals.

Also, unless items and instruments are available that are demonstrably applicable (e.g., same issues are covered in the appropriate language level), the survey's quality will be compromised.

Case Study 2

The Board gives approval for the survey at its September meeting and requires that findings be presented within 1 year in time for its September meeting. This is what the survey team plans:

Month 1: Identify the survey's objectives. Conduct a literature review and focus groups. Use the focus groups to target the survey's objectives and to determine if the survey should be an interview or a questionnaire.

Month 2: Design the survey. Ensure that the sample list is up-to-date and that all children are included on the list.

Month 3: Prepare the survey instrument.

Month 4: Pilot-test the instrument.

Month 5: Revise the instrument and have it reviewed.

Month 6: Administer the survey and conduct follow-ups.

Month 7: Enter and clean the data, and prepare the codebook.

Month 8: Analyze the data.

Month 9: Write the report.

Month 10: Have the report reviewed.

Month 11: Revise the report.

Month 12: Prepare the final written report and oral presentation.

Comments: The longer time line permits the addition of a focus group for identifying the survey's objectives, a review of the sampling list for accuracy, reviews of the report, and preparation of a codebook.

No guarantees exist that the longer time line will
produce a better and more valid survey than the shorter
time line. The longer time line is likely to cost more
because of the longer length of employment for the team
and the additional activities.

SURVEY BUDGETS

How much does a survey cost? This is a two-edged question.
A quick answer is that the survey costs exactly the amount of
money that has been allocated for it. This can range from $100
to the millions of dollars allocated for the U.S. Census. If you
have $5,000 to conduct a survey, well, that is what you have.
The only issue is whether you can conduct a survey that you
believe will have valid findings, given that amount of money.

Another answer to the question regarding the cost of a
survey is related to an ideal or the amount of money and time
you need to do a first-rate job. As a surveyor, you are likely to
encounter both situations: a. The price is "set," and b. You set
the price. Only experience can really tell you if 10 or 15 days
is enough to finish task X, and whether person Y is worth the
price you are required to pay.

In the next few examples, we assume that when asked to
prepare a budget, you are left to your own devices (common
enough in government and foundation funding and in business
applications, just to name two situations you may encounter).
Being left on your own, however, does not mean that a survey
can be as expensive as you think you need it to be. On the
contrary, everyone loves a bargain. Whatever the cost, you
must be prepared to justify your budget, often in written form.
Is 10 days enough of Jones's time, for example? Is Jones worth

$5,000 per hour? To justify Jones's time, you will have to demonstrate that he or she is an experienced, even genius, survey developer who is definitely able to complete the task within the time allotted.

How do you calculate the costs of a survey? To answer this question, you must specify all of the survey's activities and tasks, when the activity will be completed, who will be involved in completing each task, how many days each person will spend on each task, the cost-per-hour for each staff person, other direct costs, and indirect costs. Use the following checklist to guide you in calculating costs and preparing survey budgets.

Costs of a Survey: A Checklist

✓ **Learn about direct costs. These are all the expenses you will incur *because* of the survey. These include all salaries and benefits, supplies, travel, equipment, and so on.**

✓ **Decide on the number of days (or hours) that constitute a working year. Commonly used numbers are 230 days (1,840 hours) and 260 days (2,080 hours). You use these numbers to show the proportion of time or "level of effort" given by each staff member.**

Example: A person who spends 20% time on the project (assuming 260 days per year) is spending .20 × 260, or 52 days or 416 hours.

✓ **Formulate survey tasks or activities in terms of months-to-complete each.**

Example: Prepare survey instrument during Months 5 and 6.

✓ **Estimate the number of days (or hours) you need each person to complete each task.**

Example: Jones, 10 days; Smith, 8 days. If required, convert the days into hours and compute an hourly rate (e.g., Jones: 10 days, or 80 hours).

✓ **Learn each person's daily (and hourly) rate.**

Example: Jones, $320 per day, or $40 per hour; Smith, $200 per day, or $25 per hour.

✓ **Learn the costs of benefits (e.g., vacation, pension, and health)—usually a percentage of salaries. Sometimes, benefits are called labor overhead.**

Example: Benefits are 25% of Jones's salary. For example, the cost of benefits for 10 days of Jones's time is 10 × 320 per day × .25, or $800.

✓ **Learn the costs of other expenses that are incurred specifically for *this* survey.**

Example: One 2-hour focus group with 10 participants costs $650. Each participant gets a $25 honorarium for a total of $250; refreshments cost $50; a focus group expert facilitator costs $300; the materials costs $50 for reproduction, notebooks, name tags, and so on.

✓ Learn the indirect costs, or the costs that are incurred to keep the survey team going. Every individual and institution has indirect costs, sometimes called overhead or general and administrative costs (G and A). Indirect costs are sometimes a prescribed percentage of the total cost of the survey (e.g., 10%).

> *Example:* All routine costs of doing "business," such as workers' compensation and other insurance; attorney's and license fees; lights, rent, and supplies, such as paper and computer disks.

✓ If the survey lasts more than 1 year, build in cost-of-living increases.

✓ In for-profit consultation and contracting, you may be able to include a "fee." The fee is usually a percentage of the entire cost of the project and may range from about 3% to 10%.

✓ Be prepared to justify all costs in writing.

> *Example:* The purchases include $200 for 2,000 labels (2 per student interviewed) @ .10 per label and $486 for one copy of MIRACLE software for the data management program.

The following discussion tells you how to put the checklist into practice.

Direct Costs: Salaries

1. *Determine survey tasks, months to complete, and number of days for each task.*

Suppose the School Consortium (Example 4.4) asks the survey team to plan and prepare a 12-month budget for its Stop Smoking Survey. The team—which consists of Beth Jones, Yuki Smith, and Marvin Lee—begins its budget preparation process by preparing a chart that contains a description of the tasks to be accomplished, the months during which the tasks will be performed and completed, and the number of days the staff will need to complete each task. This is illustrated in Example 4.5.

EXAMPLE 4.5
Tasks, Months, and Staff Days

Task	Month	Staff Members	Number of Days Spent by Each Staff Member on Task	Total Number of Days Needed for All Staff Members to Complete Task
Identify objectives: Conduct literature review	1	Smith	20	35
		Jones	10	
		Lee	5	
Identify objectives: Organize and conduct focus groups	1	Jones	10	15
		Lee	5	

Task	Month	Staff Members	Number of Days Spent by Each Staff Member on Task	Total Number of Days Needed for All Staff Members to Complete Task
Design the survey	2	Lee	15	20
		Smith	5	
Prepare the survey	3	Lee	20	50
		Jones	15	
		Smith	15	
Pilot-test the instrument	4	Lee	15	35
		Smith	10	
		Jones	10	
Revise the instrument	5	Lee	10	15
		Smith	5	
Administer the survey	6	Lee	10	20
		Smith	10	
Enter and clean data; prepare codebook	7	Lee	10	28
		Smith	3	
		Jones	15	
Analyze the data	8	Lee	15	30
		Jones	15	
Write the report	9	Lee	15	25
		Smith	5	
		Jones	5	

→

Task	Month	Staff Members	Number of Days Spent by Each Staff Member on Task	Total Number of Days Needed for All Staff Members to Complete Task
Have report reviewed	10	Lee	5	5
Revise the report	11	Lee	10	10
Prepare final report and oral presentation Written report	12	Lee	15	35
		Smith	10	
		Jones	10	
Oral presentation	12	Lee	5	15
		Smith	5	
		Jones	5	

This chart enables the survey team to tell how long each task will take and how much staff time will be used. For example, 35 days of staff time is needed to prepare the final report and oral presentation. Soon, the days of staff time will be converted into costs. Obviously, many days of staff time is costlier than fewer days.

Preparing a chart like this is essential. First, it helps you decide where you may need to trim the budget. For example, do Smith and Jones really need to spend 10 days each on the preparation of the final report and oral presentation? What will Lee be doing during the 5 days the report is being reviewed in Month 10? The chart is also useful because it tells you how much time each person is going to be needed for the particular project. For example, Marvin Lee will be working 155 days.

Assuming 260 days is 1 year, Marvin will be spending nearly 60%, or two thirds, of his time on this project. If Marvin also has other projects and very limited time, you may want to ask "Where can we trim Marvin's time and still get the job done?"

Direct Costs: Resources

Practically all surveys require secretarial and clerical support. These persons may also receive benefits if they are employed for a certain percentage of time. (The percentage may vary.) Secretarial and clerical support are sometimes (not always) considered direct costs. You also need to identify any special resources needed for this survey. The following is a potential list of additional resources that are needed for the Stop Smoking Survey to find out about children and smoking.

Task	Special Resources
Review literature	Reproduction of reports and surveys; reproduction of forms for abstracting content of literature
Conduct focus groups	Honorariums for participants; refreshments; notebooks for participants' materials
Design the survey	Honorariums for clerical staff for assistance in reviewing addresses
Prepare the survey instrument	Graphics specialist to help format the questionnaire
Administer the survey	Postage for one original and one follow-up mailing; printing costs for questionnaire
Enter the data	Trained data enterer
Analyze the data	Programmer, statistical consultation
Prepare the report	Paper for multiple copies of the report; graphic specialist for tables
Present the report orally	Program for setting up slides; slide-preparation expert to prepare them for use

Budgets can be prepared for specific activities, individual staff members, and the entire survey. Example 4.6 illustrates the contents that are included in survey budgets. The associated monetary figures are not included because they vary so much from place to place and over time, that information presented at this time may appear ridiculously low (or high) depending on where the survey is conducted and the value of the dollar. Also, Example 4.6 uses a general format for recording budgetary information. If you have all the needed information, you will not have trouble translating from this particular format to another.

EXAMPLE 4.6
Contents of a Budget for
Activities, Staff, and Entire Survey

This is a budget for a 1-year mailed questionnaire.

Budget Contents for an Activity: Present Report Orally

Direct Costs	Cost	Total
Survey personnel		
Marvin Lee—15 days		
Beth Jones—10 days		
Yuki Smith—10 days		
Secretarial support—15 days		
Personnel subtotal		
Benefits (percentage of the subtotal)		
Marvin Lee		
Beth Jones		
Yuki Smith		
Benefits subtotal		

Other direct costs
    Consultant: Slide preparation
    Purchases: MIRACLE software
       Other direct costs subtotal

Indirect costs
    10% of direct costs
        TOTAL BUDGET FOR TASK

Budget Contents for Staff: Marvin Lee

Direct costs
    Days spent on survey: 155
    Salary per day
Indirect costs
    Benefits
       Total for Marvin Lee

Total Budget

Direct Costs   Cost   Total

Survey personnel
    Marvin Lee—155 days
    Beth Jones—95 days
    Yuki Smith—88 days
    Secretarial support—165 days
       Personnel subtotal

Benefits (percentage of the subtotal)
    Marvin Lee
    Beth Jones
    Yuki Smith
       Benefits subtotal

Other direct costs
   Consultants:
      Lanita Chow, Slide preparation
      Graphics artist: To be named
      ABC Data Entry, Inc.
      John Becke, Programmer
      Edward Parker, Statistician
      Purchases: MIRACLE software
      Paper

Other direct costs
   Reproduction of reports, surveys, and forms
   Honorariums
   Postage for survey mailings
   Printing
      Other direct costs subtotal

Indirect costs
   10% of direct costs
      TOTAL BUDGET

BUDGET JUSTIFICATION

Budgets are often accompanied by a justification of any or all of the following: choice of personnel, amount of time they are to spend on a task or on the project, salaries, other direct costs, indirect costs, and any fees or purchases of equipment and supplies. Example 4.7 contains samples of budget justifications for staff, focus groups, and purchase of software.

EXAMPLE 4.7
Budget Justification

Staff

Marvin Lee will be the leader of the survey team and spend 155 days (or 63%) of his professional time on the project. Dr. Lee has conducted local and national surveys, the most recent of which is the Elementary School Behavior Questionnaire (ESB). For the ESB, he successfully performed many of the tasks required in the present study including the conduct of literature reviews and focus groups and survey design, sampling, instrument preparation, data analysis, and report writing. He has worked as a surveyor for this institution for 10 years. His salary is based on his experience and education and is consistent with the salary schedule described in our handbook (which is on file).

Focus Groups

Focus groups are planned to assist in determining the objectives of the survey. We are aiming for 10 participants: 3 children, 2 parents, 2 teachers, 1 health professional, and 2 school administrators. Each will get an honorarium of $XX for a total of $XXX. Each participant will have a specially designed notebook with materials for discussion. Each notebook is $XX to produce, and 10 will cost $XXX. Light refreshments include cookies and soft drinks at $X per person, for a total of $XX.

MIRACLE is a multipurpose graphics program that permits camera-ready slide preparation. Comparison shopping (estimates upon request) found the least expensive price to be $XX.

HOW TO REDUCE COSTS

One of the most difficult aspects of budget preparation is usually performed after the bottom line—the total—is calculated. The reason is that during the first try, we include everything we think we need—and probably then some. Invariably, the budget needs trimming. The following are recommended ways to reduce the costs of a survey.

Guidelines for Reducing Survey Costs

- Shorten the duration of data collection.
- Reduce the number of follow-ups.
- Limit pilot testing to fewer respondents. (If you pilot-test 10 or more in federally funded surveys, you will need to get "clearance" —permission to proceed—from the appropriate federal agency. Nine or fewer in your pilot test also saves time and money.)
- Shorten instrument preparation time by adapting items and ideas from other surveys.
- Keep the instrument brief to reduce interviewer and respondent time.
- Use nonfinancial incentives, such as certificates of appreciation, to reward respondents.
- Use less expensive staff for day-to-day activities.
- Save expensive staff for consultation and leadership.
- Comparison shop for all supplies and equipment.
- Reduce the number of activities.
- Shorten the amount of time each activity takes.
- Use transparencies rather than slides for oral presentations.

Exercises

1. List three sources of survey objectives.

2. Make this question more concrete:

   How would you describe your health?

3. Rewrite these questions so that they are more appropriate for a survey.

   a. Age?

   b. How tall are you?

4. Name the type of sampling used in the following examples:

   Example A: The school has an alphabetical list of 300 students, 60 of which will be asked to participate in a new reading program. The surveyor tosses a die and comes up with the number 3. Starting with the 3rd name on the list and continuing with the 8th, 13th, and so on, she continues sampling until she has 60 names.

Example B: Four of the schools are assigned to the experimental and three to the control group.

Example C: The teachers are asked to give the survey to 10 colleagues.

5. Name four types of survey instruments.

6. Tell whether each of the following statements is true or false.

   a. A reliable survey is one that is relatively free from measurement error.

   b. A reliable survey is nearly always valid.

   c. Test-retest reliability is sometimes called internal consistency reliability.

   d. New Survey A, a measure of self-esteem, has content validity when people who score well on it also score well on Survey B, an older and valid measure of self-esteem.

   e. Construct validity is an appropriate term for a measure of hostility that accurately discriminates between hostile and nonhostile persons.

7. Tell whether each of the following must be considered or can be ignored in choosing a method of analyzing survey data.

	Must be considered (1)	Can be ignored (2)
a. Whether data are nominal, ordinal, or numerical	1	2
b. Reliability of data collection	1	2
c. Validity of data collection	1	2
d. Assumptions of the analysis method	1	2
e. Validity of the research design	1	2
f. Whether the survey is an interview or self-administered questionnaire	1	2

8. What are eight main survey tasks?

9. List 10 questions to ask when pilot-testing mail and other self-administered questionnaires.

10. List 10 questions to ask when pilot-testing telephone interviews.

11. List 8 questions to ask when pilot-testing face-to-face interviews.

ANSWERS

1. The literature, defined needs, and experts

2. In the past month, how often have you felt ill?

3. a. What is your birth date? OR How old were you on your **last** birthday?

   _____ years old

   b. How tall are you in inches?

   _____ inches

4. Example A: Systematic sampling

   Example B: Cluster sampling

   Example C: Snowball sampling

5. a. Interviews (telephone and in person)

   b. Self-administered questionnaires (mail and individual)

   c. Structured observations

   d. Structured record reviews

6. a. true

   b. false

   c. false

   d. false

   e. true

7. a. must be considered

   b. must be considered

   c. must be considered

   d. must be considered

   e. must be considered

   f. can be ignored

8. Identify survey objectives, design the survey, prepare the survey instrument, pilot-test the instrument, administer the survey, organize the data, analyze the data, report the results.

9. *Mail and other self-administered questionnaires*

   1. Are instructions for completing the survey clearly written?

   2. Are questions easy to understand?

   3. Do respondents know how to indicate responses (e.g., circle or mark the response; use a special pencil; use the space bar)?

   4. Are the response choices mutually exclusive?

   5. Are the response choices exhaustive?

   6. If a mail questionnaire, do respondents understand what to do with completed questionnaires (e.g., return them by mail in a self-addressed envelope; fax them)?

   7. If a mail questionnaire, do respondents understand when to return the completed survey?

   8. If a computer-assisted survey, can respondents correctly use the commands?

   9. If a computer-assisted survey, do respondents know how to change (or "correct") their answers?

10. If an incentive is given for completing the survey, do respondents understand how to obtain it (e.g., it will automatically be sent on receipt of completed survey; it is included with the questionnaire)?

11. Is privacy respected and protected?

12. Do respondents have any suggestions regarding the addition or deletion of questions, the clarification of instructions, or improvements in format?

10. *Telephone interviews*

1. Do interviewers understand how to ask questions and present options for responses?

2. Do interviewers know how to get in-depth information, when appropriate, by probing respondents' brief answers?

3. Do interviewers know how to record information?

4. Do interviewers know how to keep the interview to the agreed-on time limit?

5. Do interviewers know how to return completed interviews?

6. Are interviewers able to select the sample using the agreed-on instructions?

7. Can interviewers readily use the phone logs to record the number of times and when potential respondents were contacted?

8. Do interviewees understand the questions?

9. Do interviewees understand how to answer the questions (e.g., pick the top two; rate items according to whether they agree or disagree)?

10. Do interviewees agree that privacy has been protected? Respected?

11. *In-person interviews*

1. Do interviewers understand how to ask questions and present options for responses?

2. Do interviewers know how to get in-depth information, when appropriate, by probing respondents' brief answers?

3. Do interviewers know how to record information?

4. Do interviewers know how to keep the interview to the agreed-on time limit?

5. Do interviewers know how to return completed interviews?

6. Do interviewees understand the questions?

7. Do interviewees understand how to answer the questions (e.g., pick the top two; rate items according to whether they agree or disagree)?

8. Do interviewees agree that privacy has been protected? Respected?

Suggested Readings

Afifi, A. A., & Clark, V. (1990). *Computer-aided multivariate analysis*. New York: Van Nostrand Reinhold.

Textbook on multivariate analysis with a practical approach. Discusses data entry, data screening, data reduction, and data analysis. Also explains the options available in different statistical packages.

American Psychological Association. (1985). *Standards for educational and psychological testing*. Washington, DC: Author.

Classic work on reliability and validity and the standards that testers should achieve to ensure accuracy.

Babbie, E. (1990). *Survey research methods*. Belmont, CA: Wadsworth.

Fundamental reference on how to conduct survey research. Good examples of survey questions with accompanying rules for asking questions.

Baker, T. L. (1988). *Doing social research*. New York: McGraw-Hill.
A "how to," with examples.

Bradburn, N. M., & Sudman, S. (1992). The current status of questionnaire design. In P. N. Biemer, R. M. Groves, L. E. Lyberg, N. A. Mathiowetz, & S. Sudman (Eds.), *Measurement errors in surveys*. New York: John Wiley.
Addresses many of the major issues in designing questionnaires and asking questions.

Braitman, L. (1991). Confidence intervals assess both clinical and statistical significance. *Annals of Internal Medicine, 114,* 515-517.
This brief article contains one of the clearest explanations anywhere of the use of confidence intervals and is highly recommended.

Campbell, D. T., & Stanley, J. C. (1963). *Experimental and quasi-experimental designs for research*. Chicago: Rand McNally.
The classic book on differing research designs. "Threats" to internal and external validity are described in detail. Issues pertaining to generalizability and how to get at "truth" are important reading.

Converse, J. (1987). *Survey research in the United States*. Berkeley: University of California Press.
An overview and good examples of how surveys are used in the United States. Helpful in understanding the context of survey research.

Converse, J. M., & Presser, S. (1986). *Survey questions: Handcrafting the standardized questionnaire* (Quantitative Applications in the Social Sciences: A Sage University Papers series, 07-063). Beverly Hills, CA: Sage.
All you need to know on how to put a standardized questionnaire together.

Cook, D. C., & Campbell, D. T. (1979). *Quasi-experimentation: Design and analysis issues for field settings.* Boston: Houghton Mifflin.

Discusses the issues that arise in fieldwork and quasi-experimentation. Helps bring together issues that link design, sampling, and analysis.

Dawson-Saunders, B., & Trapp, R. G. (1990). *Basic and clinical biostatistics.* Englewood Cliffs, NJ: Prentice Hall.

A basic and essential primer on the use of statistics in medicine and medical care settings. Explains study designs, how to summarize and present data, and discusses sampling and the main statistical methods used in analyzing data.

Dillman, D. A. (1978). *Mail and telephone surveys: The total design method.* New York: John Wiley.

The special issues associated with mail and telephone surveys are reviewed.

Fink, A. (1993). *Evaluation fundamentals: Guiding health programs, research, and policy.* Newbury Park, CA: Sage.

Many of the skills needed by survey researchers are shared by program evaluators. Discusses design, sampling, analysis, and reporting.

Fink, A., & Kosecoff, J. (1985). *How to conduct surveys: A step by step guide.* Beverly Hills, CA: Sage.

Gives many examples of survey questions and contains rules and guidelines for asking questions.

Fowler, F. J. (1993). *Survey research methods.* Newbury Park, CA: Sage.

Chapter 6 deals with designing and evaluating survey questions, including defining objectives.

Fowler, F. J., & Mangione, T. W. (1990). *Standardized survey interviewing: Minimizing interviewer related error.* Newbury Park, CA: Sage.

Contains good survey question examples and tells how to minimize error by standardizing the questioner and the questionnaire.

Frey, J. H. (1989). *Survey research by telephone.* Newbury Park, CA: Sage.

Gives excellent examples of questions and how to get the information you need from telephone surveys.

Hambleton, R. K., & Zaal, J. N. (Eds.). (1991). *Advances in educational and psychological testing.* Boston: Kluwer Academic.

Important source of information on the concepts of reliability and validity in education and psychology.

Henry, G. T. (1990). *Practical sampling.* Newbury Park, CA: Sage.

Excellent source of information about sampling methods and sampling errors. Although statistical knowledge helps, this book is worth reading even if the knowledge is basic.

Kalton, G. (1983). *Introduction to survey sampling.* Beverly Hills, CA: Sage.

Excellent discussion of survey sampling. It requires understanding of statistics.

Kish, L. (1965). *Survey sampling.* New York: John Wiley.

This book is a classic and often consulted in resolving issues that arise when implementing sampling designs.

Kraemer, H. C., & Thiemann, S. (1987). *How many subjects? Statistical power analysis in research.* Newbury Park, CA: Sage.

Complexity of statistical power analysis is thoroughly discussed. Requires an understanding of statistics.

Lavrakas, P. J. (1987). *Telephone survey methods: Sampling, selection, and supervision.* Newbury Park, CA: Sage.

Excellent source of information on all aspects of telephone (and other) survey methods.

McDowell, I., & Newell, C. (1987). *Measuring health: A guide to rating scales and questionnaires.* New York: Oxford University Press.

Provides numerous examples of health measurement techniques and scales available to the survey researcher interested in health. Also discusses the validity and reliability of important health measures.

Miller, D. C. (1991). *Handbook of research design and social measurement.* Newbury Park, CA: Sage.

Discusses and defines all possible components of social research. Part 6 has selected sociometric scales and indexes and is a very good source of questions pertaining to social status, group structure, organizational structure, job satisfaction, community, family and marriage, and attitudes.

Morris, L. L., Fitzgibbon, C. T., & Lindheim, E. (1987). How to measure performance and use tests. In J. L. Herman (Ed.), *Program evaluation kit* (2nd ed.). Newbury Park, CA: Sage.

Excellent discussion of reliability and validity in measuring students' performance.

Norusis, M. J. (1983). *SPSS introductory statistics guide*. Chicago: SPSS, Inc.

This manual accompanies a statistical package for the social sciences. It contains an overview and explanation of the logic behind most of the statistical methods commonly used in the social sciences. The manual also presents and explains statistical output.

Pfeiffer, W. S. (1991). *Technical writing*. New York: Macmillan.

Provides useful tips on the details of putting together formal reports. Discusses the cover and title page, table of contents, and executive summary. Also contains rules for preparing charts and giving oral presentations.

Siegel, S. (1956). *Nonparametric statistics for the behavioral sciences*. New York: McGraw-Hill.

Classic textbook on nonparametric statistics.

Schuman, H., & Presser, S. (1981). *Questions and answers in attitude surveys*. New York: Academic Press.

Raises and addresses many of the important issues in designing questions about attitudes. Contains good examples.

Sudman, S., & Bradburn, N. M. (1982). *Asking questions*. San Francisco: Jossey-Bass.

Very good source for examples of how to write questions pertaining to knowledge, attitudes, behavior, and demographics.

About the Author

ARLENE FINK, PhD, is Professor of Medicine and Public Health at the University of California, Los Angeles. She is on the Research Advisory Board of UCLA's Robert Wood Johnson Clinical Scholars Program, a health research scientist at the Veterans Administration Medical Center in Sepulveda, California, and president of Arlene Fink Associates. She has conducted evaluations throughout the United States and abroad and has trained thousands of health professionals, social scientists, and educators in program evaluation. Her published works include nearly 100 monographs and articles on evaluation methods and research. She is coauthor of *How to Conduct Surveys* and author of *Evaluation Fundamentals: Guiding Health Programs, Research, and Policy* and *Evaluation for Education and Psychology*.

HOW TO ASK
SURVEY
QUESTIONS

THE SURVEY KIT

Purpose: The purposes of this 9-volume Kit are to enable readers to prepare and conduct surveys and become better users of survey results. Surveys are conducted to collect information by asking questions of people on the telephone, face-to-face, and by mail. The questions can be about attitudes, beliefs, and behavior as well as socioeconomic and health status. To do a good survey also means knowing how to ask questions, design the survey (research) project, sample respondents, collect reliable and valid information, and analyze and report the results. You also need to know how to plan and budget for your survey.

Users: The Kit is for students in undergraduate and graduate classes in the social and health sciences and for individuals in the public and private sectors who are responsible for conducting and using surveys. Its primary goal is to enable users to prepare surveys and collect data that are accurate and useful for primarily practical purposes. Sometimes, these practical purposes overlap the objectives of scientific research, and so survey researchers will also find the Kit useful.

Format of the Kit: All books in the series contain instructional objectives, exercises and answers, examples of surveys in use and illustrations of survey questions, guidelines for action, checklists of do's and don'ts, and annotated references.

Volumes in The Survey Kit:

1. **The Survey Handbook**
   Arlene Fink

2. **How to Ask Survey Questions**
   Arlene Fink

3. **How to Conduct Self-Administered and Mail Surveys**
   Linda B. Bourque and *Eve P. Fielder*

4. **How to Conduct Interviews by Telephone and in Person**
   James H. Frey and *Sabine Mertens Oishi*

5. **How to Design Surveys**
   Arlene Fink

6. **How to Sample in Surveys**
   Arlene Fink

7. **How to Measure Survey Reliability and Validity**
   Mark S. Litwin

8. **How to Analyze Survey Data**
   Arlene Fink

9. **How to Report on Surveys**
   Arlene Fink

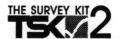

THE SURVEY KIT

TSK 2

HOW TO ASK
SURVEY
QUESTIONS

ARLENE FINK

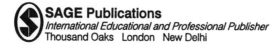

SAGE Publications
International Educational and Professional Publisher
Thousand Oaks London New Delhi

For information address:

SAGE Publications, Inc.
2455 Teller Road
Thousand Oaks, California 91320
E-mail: order@sagepub.com

SAGE Publications Ltd.
6 Bonhill Street
London EC2A 4PU
United Kingdom

SAGE Publications India Pvt. Ltd.
M-32 Market
Greater Kailash I
New Delhi 110 048 India

Printed in the United States of America

Library of Congress Cataloging-in-Publication Data

Main entry under title:

The survey kit.
    p. cm.
    Includes bibliographical references.
    Contents: v. 1. The survey handbook / Arlene Fink — v. 2. How to ask survey questions / Arlene Fink — v. 3. How to conduct self-administered and mail surveys / Linda B. Bourque, Eve P. Fielder — v. 4. How to conduct interviews by telephone and in person / James H. Frey, Sabine Mertens Oishi — v. 5. How to design surveys / Arlene Fink — v. 6. How to sample in surveys / Arlene Fink — v. 7. How to measure survey reliability and validity / Mark S. Litwin — v. 8. How to analyze survey data / Arlene Fink — v. 9. How to report on surveys / Arlene Fink.
    ISBN 0-8039-7388-8 (pbk. : The survey kit : alk. paper)
    1. Social surveys. 2. Health surveys. I. Fink, Arlene.
HN29.S724   1995
300'.723—dc20   95-12712

This book is printed on acid-free paper.

95 96 97 98 99 10 9 8 7 6 5 4 3 2 1

Sage Production Editor: Diane S. Foster
Sage Copy Editor: Joyce Kuhn
Sage Typesetter: Janelle LeMaster

Contents

How to Ask Survey Questions:
Learning Objectives

The aim of this book is to guide the reader in preparing and using reliable and valid survey questions. The following specific objectives are stated in terms of aspirations for the reader.

- Understand a survey's cultural, psychological, economic, and political context by:

  - Identifying specific purposes
  - Preparing appropriately worded, meaningful questions for participants
  - Clarifying research and other objectives
  - Determining a feasible number of questions
  - Standardizing the questioner
  - Standardizing the response choices

- Ask valid questions that:

  - Make sense to the respondent
  - Are concrete
  - Use time periods that are related to the importance of the question
  - Use conventional language
  - Use short and long questions appropriately
  - Use loaded words cautiously

- Avoid biasing words
- Avoid two-edgers
- Avoid negative phrasing
- Compare the characteristics and uses of closed and open questions
- Distinguish among response formats that use nominal, ordinal, and numerical measurement
- Identify correctly prepared questions

■ Correctly ask questions by:

- Using response categories that are meaningfully grouped
- Choosing an appropriate type of response option
- Balancing all responses on a scale
- Selecting neutral categories appropriately
- Determining how many points to include on a rating scale
- Deciding where to place the positive or negative end of the scale
- Determining the proper use of skip patterns

■ Apply special questioning techniques to survey knowledge, attitudes, and demographics

1 Asking Questions: A Matter of Context

Asurvey is a system for collecting information to describe, compare, or explain knowledge, attitudes, and practices or behavior. Surveys are taken of political and consumer choices, use of health services, numbers of people in the labor force, and opinions on just about everything from aardvarks to zyzyvas.

Individuals, communities, schools, businesses, and researchers use surveys to find out about people by asking questions about feelings, motivations, plans, beliefs, and personal backgrounds. The questions are typically arranged into mailed or self-administered questionnaires and into in-person (face-to-face) or telephone interviews. Because **questions** are

1

the focus of many surveys, learning how to ask them in written and spoken form is essential.

The way you ask survey questions prescribes the answers, as you can see from Example 1.1.

EXAMPLE 1.1
The Relationship Between
Questions, People, and Information

Three survey experts were invited to present the results of their survey "American Views on Taxation." Expert A's presentation was entitled "Most Americans Support Increased Taxes for Worthy Purposes." Expert B's speech was called "Some Americans Support Increased Taxes for Worthy Purposes." Expert C's talk was named "Few Americans Support Increased Taxes for Worthy Purposes." A review of the talks and original surveys revealed three questions:

Expert A's: Would you support increased taxes to pay for education programs for very poor children?

Expert B's: Would you support an increase in your taxes to pay for education programs for very poor children?

Expert C's: Would you support a 10% increase in your taxes to pay for education programs for very poor children?

As you can see, three surveyors with competing agendas can come up with entirely different questions, responses, and interpretations.

Surveys are used as a source of information in research and evaluation studies and in planning programs and setting policy in health, education, business, and government. This book focuses on guidelines for asking questions for all these survey uses.

The selection and wording of questions are strongly influenced by the survey's context: its purposes, who asks the questions, how they are asked, who answers them, and the characteristics of respondents and responses. Consider the two surveys in Example 1.2.

EXAMPLE 1.2
Survey Questions and Their Context

Survey 1

Lancaster, a community of about 150,000 people, is planning programs to prevent child abuse and family violence. The community intends to conduct a survey in which families are asked to identify their problems and to suggest solutions to them. The results will be used to guide the development of programs to prevent and treat alcohol use, social isolation, and unemployment. These problems and others like them are known to be prevalent in the community. Research has linked them to abuse and violence.

Parents with school-age children in 4 of the city's 10 school districts will be mailed a survey questionnaire to complete in the privacy of their homes. The survey, which focuses on educational needs, takes 20 minutes to complete and is written in the five languages most commonly spoken in the community. All responses are anonymous. Respondents are given statements and asked to rate on a scale from 1 to 4 whether they strongly agree, agree, disagree, or strongly disagree with each. The questionnaire has been endorsed by prominent members of the community and the city.

Survey 2

The Children's Clinic is a school-based clinic in a very low-income area of a large city. The clinic intends to conduct a survey in which families and teachers are asked to identify children's health problems (including medical and psychosocial issues) that the clinic might address. A sample of parents, teachers, health professionals, and children will be interviewed in person. The interview will take 30 minutes and will be conducted in English and Spanish. About half the questions will use ratings and rankings; the remainder will allow respondents to give answers in their own words. All responses will be confidential. A report of the results will be available in 12 months.

The two surveys described in Example 1.2 are different in several ways. These differences influence the choice, characteristics, and number of questions, as shown in Example 1.3.

EXAMPLE 1.3
Two Surveys

	Survey 1: A Mailed Questionnaire Concerning Child Abuse	Survey 2: Interviews About the Services of a School-Based Clinic	Effect on Questions
Purpose	Identify needs and solutions to guide program development	Identify needs to guide focus of clinic services	Survey 1: Questions are about education Survey 2: Questions are about health
Respondents	Parents of school-age children	Parents, teachers, health professionals, and children	Survey 1: Questions posed are for parents only Survey 2: Questions posed are for people of differing roles and ages
Surveyor	Self-administered, mailed questionnaire contains the questions	Interviewers ask face-to-face questions	Survey 1: Questions must be easily read and understood without outside assistance Survey 2: Questions must be worded so that they can be understood orally

	Survey 1: A Mailed Questionnaire Concerning Child Abuse	Survey 2: Interviews About the Services of a School-Based Clinic	Effect on Questions
Responses	Closed: Ratings are made on a scale from 1 to 4	Some questions use ratings and rankings; the remainder rely on the respondent's own words	Survey 1: Responses can be translated on a scale from 1 to 4 Survey 2: Half the responses will come from ratings and rankings; the remainder will be in participants' own words
Timing	Survey takes 20 minutes	Survey takes 30 minutes	Survey 1: Respondents may not return questionnaires, or they many not answer all questions Survey 2: Time must be allocated for reading and interpreting respondents' answers
Resources	Need translation into five languages Survey must be printed and mailed	Need translation into English and Spanish Interviewers must be hired and trained	Survey 1: Expertise is needed in five languages Survey 2: Expertise is needed in two languages
Privacy	All responses will be anonymous	All responses will be confidential (codes will replace names)	Survey 1: "Sensitive" questions (e.g., about drug use and sexual habits) are more likely to be answered Survey 2: Must be a little more "careful" with sensitive questions as respondents can be traced

The two surveys described in Examples 1.2 and 1.3 aim to guide the development of programs and the focus of services to prevent child abuse and family violence and to promote health. The first survey is for parents only; the second is for parents, teachers, health professionals, and children. Because the first survey is self-administered, the questions must be worked on until they are understandable by respondents without assistance from the survey team. The results of the second survey will require the surveyors to have special expertise in interpretation and classification of the responses that are given in the participants' own words. The first survey will need resources for printing and mailing; the second will need funding for hiring and training interviewers. Because the first survey is anonymous, the surveyors may be able to ask questions about topics that named respondents might be reluctant to discuss. Confidential answers remove some of the anonymity and so may reduce the respondents' frankness. The first survey needs to be translated into five languages; the second survey is to be given in English and Spanish.

A survey's purpose, surveyors, and respondents (along with other considerations) must be fully understood before you begin to write questions. The following is a checklist to use in identifying and understanding a survey's context.

Checklist for
Deciding the Survey's Context

✓ **Identify the survey's specific purposes.**

The purpose of a survey is its hoped-for outcomes. Usually, you have a general purpose in mind, say, to find out about job satisfaction, preferences for certain products, or voting plans. If you are concerned with job satisfaction, for example, the survey should focus on that topic. Questions about previous jobs, hobbies, personal background, and so on may not be relevant.

✓ Clarify the terms used to state the survey's purpose.

In Example 1.2, the first survey's questions focus on educational needs. This term is very general. Educational needs may include completing high school and obtaining vocational training as well as acquiring specific skills like how to be a parent, to cook, and to manage money.

The second survey in Example 1.2 is about the health needs of children. Definitions of health are far from uniform and vary according to culture. To select appropriate and usable definitions for a survey, you can review what is known and published about a topic. You can also define the term yourself. The problem with creating your own definition is that others may not be convinced of its validity. Sometimes, it is best to adopt a respected definition and even, if possible, an already tested set of questions.

Choices regarding the focus and definitions used in survey questions are sometimes made when you know its specific objectives.

✓ Be sure to have the specific objectives of the survey in place.

The specific objectives refer to the precise information the survey is to collect. Sometimes, the objectives take the form of research hypotheses or questions. At other times, the objectives are written as statements. Consider these sample objectives for Survey 1 (Example 1.2):

1. Identify the most common needs for educational services
2. Determine the extent to which differences exist among the needs of parents of differing ethnicities/races
3. Determine the extent to which differences exist in needs between men and women
4. Identify if parents are willing to participate in job retraining programs
5. Find out if parents are satisfied with their current educational status

A specific set of objectives like these suggests a survey that asks questions about the following:

- Educational needs (Objective 1)
- Ethnicity/race (Objective 2)
- Gender (Objective 3)
- Willingness of respondents to participate in job retraining (Objective 4)
- Satisfaction with current educational status (Objective 5)

Suppose another surveyor added these objectives:

6. Compare younger and older parents in their needs to learn how to manage a household and care for a child
7. Determine the relationship between parents' education and method of disciplining children for mild, moderate, and severe infractions

To collect information for the new objectives, Survey 1 would need to add questions on the following:

- Age of parents
- How parents manage their household
- How parents care for their children

- Level of parents' education
- Methods for disciplining children for mild, moderate, and severe infractions

Before preparing a survey, all potentially imprecise or ambiguous terms used in the survey's specific questions have to be clarified or defined. For the questions above, the imprecise terms are: needs; educational services; ethnicity/race; willingness; satisfaction; younger and older; effective household management; effective child care; discipline; and mild, moderate, and severe infractions. Why are these terms ambiguous? No standard definition exists for any of them. What are needs, for example, and of the very long list that you might create, which will be included on the survey? What is effective child care? What is discipline? How do you distinguish satisfied from dissatisfied parents?

EXERCISE

The following are four sample specific objectives for Survey 2 (Example 1.2):

1. Find out where children usually receive their health care
2. Identify barriers to using preventive health services, such as vaccinations
3. Identify if differences exist in the health care needs of younger and older children of differing ethnicities/races.
4. Compare the health status of boys and girls of differing ethnicities/races

   □ Add at least three more objectives
   □ Describe the data that the survey must collect to meet all seven objectives (the first four above and the three you have added)

❑ List all terms that will need to be defined or clarified before good questions can be written

■ SUGGESTED ANSWERS ■

Two additional objectives:

5. Compare the barriers to use of health services among older and younger parents whose children will use the clinic
6. Determine if respondents are satisfied with the quality of the health services their children currently receive

Data to be collected:

- Barriers to the use of health services
- Age
- Ethnicity/race
- Health status
- Satisfaction with quality of health services

Definitions and clarifications needed:

- Health services
- Barriers
- Younger and older
- Ethnicity/race
- Health status
- Satisfaction

✓ **Know the respondents.**

Questions should be written so that they encompass your needs for data, but they must also be formulated so that respondents can answer them easily and accurately. Check the appropriateness of the language level. Reading abilities may vary considerably even for the same survey. For example, a survey of parents in a school district may include some people who read extremely well and others who read poorly. If so, you will have to decide how to state the questions to maximize the number of respondents who can read and comprehend all questions.

Make sure that respondents have sufficient knowledge to answer the questions. Facing unanswerable questions is extremely frustrating for the respondent. In a survey to find out about the quality of education, many people may not be able to answer a question like the following:

> What role should the Department of Curriculum and Instruction play in setting educational standards for this community?

Unless told, many people might not know about the department's current authority, how it is administered, and how it has been designed to fit into the community. They may not have a clue about the department's role. In their frustration, they may guess or they may refuse to answer the question or any other question on the survey.

Survey respondents may also have difficulty answering questions that ask them about past or future actions and behaviors. For example, if you ask relatively healthy survey respondents about their health exactly 1 year ago on this date, they may have forgotten because they have no compelling reason to dwell on their health. Also, if you ask people to tell you who they will elect to the Board of Education in 6 months, they may not yet know. Asking respondents to compare their behavior to that of others sometimes results in confusion. Asking employees to compare the adequacy of child care at your company to that provided by other firms, for example, is likely to produce poor results unless you are certain that your employees are familiar with the child-care practices of other companies.

✓ **Carefully match what you need to know against the time you have to find out.**

The number of questions to include in a survey depends largely on the amount of time available for the survey. A half-hour interview is usually able to include more questions than a 10-minute interview. The number of questions in a survey also depends on what you need to know and how many questions are needed for adequate measurement.

Suppose that in Example 1.2, Survey 1, the survey of parents is allotted 20 minutes. Suppose also that it is supposed to cover 10 topics: educational needs; ethnicity/race; gender; willingness of respondents to participate in job retraining; satisfaction with current educational status; age of parents; how parents manage their household; how parents can care for their children; level of parents' education; and methods for disciplining children for mild, moderate, and severe infractions. The surveyor can ask one or more questions to cover each topic or ask 10 questions about any single topic. To decide on which questions to ask, you must balance what you need to know (the specific objectives), the number of questions needed to cover each topic covered by the objective, and the amount of time available for the survey.

A good way to get started in determining the number of questions for each topic is to make a chart like the one shown in Example 1.4.

EXAMPLE 1.4
Topics, Number of Questions, and Information Collected

Topic	Number of Questions	Information Collected
Educational level	1	Last year of school completed
Educational needs	10	Whether had training for specific jobs (e.g., sales, nurses aide, etc.)
Ethnicity/race	1	African American, White but not Latino, Latino/Latina, Chinese, Southeast Asian, Other
Gender	1	Male/Female
Satisfaction with current educational status	1	Yes, no
Willingness to participate in job retraining	1	If needed: yes, no, do not know, or not sure
Age	1	Whether under 18 years of age, between 18 and 20, between 21 and 30, and over 30
Managing a household	6	Manage financial affairs (e.g., balance checkbook, shop for food for a week, monitor household repairs)
Caring for the child	5	Doctor's visits, supervise school work, know names of friends
Discipline methods	8	Methods (e.g., talking, hitting, yelling) for mild (e.g., not answering a question), moderate (e.g., coming home more than an hour late), and severe (e.g., not coming home at all) infractions
Total	35	

Remember that Survey 1 (Example 1.2) is to last 20 minutes. To find out if the 35 questions can be answered in the 20 minutes available, the survey must be tried out in advance of use with potential respondents or people just like them. To determine if the questions adequately cover the topics, you can ask experts, search other surveys, and conduct statistical analyses to find out if parents who are known to cope well answer the questions differently from parents who are known to cope poorly.

✓ Standardize the surveyor.

The ideal standardized surveyor asks questions the same way every time. When two surveyors who are conducting the same survey are indistinguishable from one another in their delivery and findings, they are standardized.

Standardized surveyors can take human form, as in face-to-face or telephone interviews, or they can take the form of a self-administered questionnaire. A self-administered questionnaire can be mailed to respondents or completed in a specially designated area such as a clinic waiting room, a classroom, or a personnel office. Example 1.5 illustrates the use of standardized surveyors.

EXAMPLE 1.5
Standardized Surveyors

1. A survey of parents is conducted to find out if they are willing to participate in a program to prevent child abuse and neglect. A 25-item questionnaire is mailed to 200 parents. The questionnaire was tried out with 50 parents before it was considered

suitable. The original version had 35 questions, but that was considered by parents to take too much time to answer. Questions were omitted if 10 or more parents either would not or could not complete them. All questions are accompanied by four choices, and the respondent is to circle the one "best" answer.

2. Interviews were conducted to compare the views of managers and sales staff regarding a program to introduce more flexible hours for employees. The Human Resources Department trained five of its staff to conduct the interviews. The training took 6 hours, and quality checks of a sample of interviews were made to ensure that each interviewer followed very strict question-asking guidelines.

✓ **Standardize the response format.**

A standardized format asks each respondent to select from a list of preset choices. Example 1.6 distinguishes between standardized formats and other types.

EXAMPLE 1.6
Standardized and Other Response Formats

Standardized Format

Directions: To what extent do you agree with the following statements about the purpose of pretesting self-administered survey questionnaires? In a pretest, a draft of the survey is tried out with a sample of people, and their reviews are incorporated into the final version. *Circle one choice for each statement.*

Purpose of Pretesting?	Strongly Agree (1)	Agree (2)	Disagree (3)	Strongly Disagree (4)	No Opinion (5)
To find out if the questions are appropriate for the respondents	1	2	3	4	5
To determine if any questions are misleading	1	2	3	4	5
To examine whether surveyors can appropriately use the survey forms	1	2	3	4	5
To determine if the information obtained by the survey is reliable	1	2	3	4	5
To determine if the information obtained by the survey is valid	1	2	3	4	5

Not Standardized

Directions: Explain the extent of your agreement with the following statement:

"Self-administered questionnaires should be tried out in advance of their use to see if they provide consistent and accurate data. An advance trial means testing the logistics of the survey (the ease with which the interviewers can record responses) as well as the survey form itself."

Write your explanation here:

Some people may have difficulty with standardized question-and-response formats. They may object to the structure or be unfamiliar with it. When this happens, the surveyor should try to find another standardized format that is acceptable to the respondents or look for an alternative way of getting the information. One way that is currently in use is to tape the questionnaire. This seems to have the effect of making the structure more palatable.

✓ **Remember that questions are asked in a social, cultural, and economic context.**

In the two survey situations illustrated in Example 1.2, the survey instruments are to be translated from English into another language. To ensure that you are asking questions that are meaningful to people speaking that language, rely on survey experts and potential respondents to help with the wording of the questions. Remember also to budget time and money for these activities.

Another contextual factor to consider is whether the answers will be anonymous. If so, you may be posing different kinds of questions than you would otherwise. Surveyors agree generally that more "sensitive" questions can be asked about personal behaviors and beliefs in anonymous surveys (where the identity of the respondent is not known) than can be asked in confidential surveys or in those in which the respondent's name is common knowledge.

Guidelines for
Asking Survey Questions

The following are guidelines for asking survey questions. You may find that in your survey some guidelines are more important than others.

ASK PURPOSEFUL QUESTIONS

Purposeful questions are those that are logically related to the survey's objectives. In a survey about airline travel, respondents will expect questions about the food, service, on-time record, and so on. If questions are asked that do not seem to be about airline travel (they are about age or reading habits, for instance), explain the reason for them: "Some of our questions are about your background and preferences so that we can examine whether Uniting Airlines is meeting the needs of all its passengers."

ASK CONCRETE QUESTIONS

A concrete question is precise and unambiguous. Questions are precise and ambiguous when, without prompting, two or more potential respondents agree on the words used in the question. For example, suppose you want to find out about people's perceptions of their health and you ask them to describe it. A person who is generally well but has been sick this past week might answer differently from another individual who was desperately ill all year but is now feeling better. To help make a question more concrete, add a time period:

Less concrete: How would you describe your health?

More concrete: In the past 3 months, how would you describe your health?

The more detail you can provide, the more reliable the answer is likely to be. For example, in providing a time period, avoid asking about usual or typical behavior. Instead, provide a specific time period, as illustrated in Example 1.7.

EXAMPLE 1.7
Using Specific Time Periods
to Make Questions More Concrete

Poor: How often do you exercise in a typical week?

Better: How often did you exercise during the past week? (Start with today's date and count back 7 days.)

Detailed questions alway help produce reliable answers. For example, if you are surveying responses to a play, rather than just asking a general question about enjoyment of the play, decide on the components of the play that are the most important to the survey, as in these examples.

Less concrete: Did you enjoy the play?

More concrete: Did you enjoy the first act of the play?

Even more concrete: Did you find the comedy scenes in the play's first act funny?

EXERCISE

Make these three questions more concrete and describe how you improved specificity.

1. How satisfactory was your stay at the hotel?
2. What is the best way to improve health care?
3. Which restaurants do you eat in most frequently?

■ POSSIBLE ANSWERS ■

1. How satisfactory was room service during your stay at the hotel?

   The question has been made more specific by focusing on room service.

2. What is the best way to improve the quality of preventive health care?

   "Improve" has been clarified to concentrate on the quality of preventive care.

3. In the past 3 months, which New York restaurants did you eat in most frequently?

   A time period and a place have been set: in the past 3 months and New York, respectively.

USE TIME PERIODS THAT ARE RELATED
TO THE IMPORTANCE OF THE QUESTION

Periods of a year or more can be used for major life events like the purchase of a house, occurrence of serious illness, birth of a child, or death of a parent. Periods of a month or less should be used for questions that are less important. Asking people to remember relatively unimportant events over long periods of time leads to too much guessing. You do not want the period to be too short either because the event in question may not have occurred during the interval. Example 1.8 illustrates good and poor use of time periods in survey questions.

EXAMPLE 1.8
Use of Time Periods in Survey Questions

Poor: How long did it usually take for you to fall asleep during the past 6 months?

Comment: Too much time has probably elapsed for the respondent to recall accurately. Also, the amount of time to fall asleep may have varied considerably, making estimation a truly difficulty task.

Better: How long did it usually take for you to fall asleep during the past 2 weeks?

Poor: In reference to your car accident of a year ago, how many visits have you made to a physician in the past 6 weeks?

Comment: The number of visits made to the doctor in the past 6 weeks is probably different from the number made in the first weeks after the accident.

Better: In reference to your car accident of a year ago, look at the following list and tell how many visits you have made to a physician.

USE CONVENTIONAL LANGUAGE

A survey is not a conversation. To get accurate information, survey questions rely on standard grammar, punctuation, and spelling. You should use words that maximize understanding for everyone in the survey. This is often difficult to do. All questions should be reviewed and tested by people who are proficient in reading and speaking the language in which the survey is written, content experts, and potential respondents.

Guidelines for Using Conventional Language When Asking Survey Questions

The following are guidelines for using conventional language in surveys.

USE COMPLETE SENTENCES

Complete sentences, whether as statements or questions, express a clear and complete thought, as illustrated in Example 1.9.

EXAMPLE 1.9
Using Complete Sentences and Questions

Poor: Place of residence?

Comment: Place of residence means different things to different people. For example, I might answer Los Angeles, but another respondent might say California, the United States, or 15 Pine Road.

Better: What is the name of the city where you currently live?

Poor: Accidents among children are . . .

Comment: This statement is unclear. A respondent might say "terrible," "the leading cause of death among children under the age of 12 years," "underreported," "a public health problem," and so on.

Better: Indicate the extent of your agreement with the statement "Accidents among children are a public health problem in the United States."

AVOID ABBREVIATIONS

You should avoid abbreviations unless you are certain that they are commonly understood. Most people probably are familiar with USA and FBI; many would be familiar with the abbreviations for their cities, states, provinces, universities, and so on. But don't count on it. If in doubt, spell it out, as shown in Example 1.10.

EXAMPLE 1.10
Avoiding Abbreviations

Poor: In your view, does USC provide a liberal arts education worth its yearly tuition?

Comment: If this question is being asked of many Californians, USC will stand for the University of Southern California. But for others, USC can mean University of South Carolina or University of Southern Connecticut.

Better: In your view, does the University of South Charleston provide a liberal arts education worth its yearly tuition?

AVOID SLANG AND COLLOQUIAL EXPRESSIONS

Slang and colloquialisms should be avoided because they go out of fashion quickly and not everybody keeps up with the newest expressions. Some exceptions exist. You may want to use slang for a survey of a homogeneous group who share a special language, such as workers in the same job or profession, people with similar health or social problems, and teenagers.

The problem in using slang and colloquialisms is that if you plan to report the results of the survey to a general audience, you need to translate the slang. Less than expert translation may result in loss of meaning.

BE CAREFUL OF JARGON
AND TECHNICAL EXPRESSIONS

Survey questions should avoid jargon and technical terms (see Example 1.11). If you have reason to believe that your group is homogeneous and familiar with the terms, you can use them. However, you must then be concerned with how understandable a wider audience will find the results.

EXAMPLE 1.11
Avoiding Jargon and Technical Terms

Poor: Should a summative evaluation of Head Start be commissioned by the U.S. government?

Comment: The term "summative evaluation" is used among some specialists in program evaluation. It means a review of the activities and accomplishments of a completed program or of one that has been in existence for a long time.

Better: Should the U.S. government commission a history of Head Start to review its activities and accomplishments?

HAVE THE QUESTIONS REVIEWED BY EXPERTS

Experts are individuals who are knowledgeable about survey question-writing or the subject matter addressed by a survey. Experts can tell you which survey questions appear too complex to be administered easily and too long or too difficult to be answered accurately.

HAVE THE QUESTIONS REVIEWED
BY POTENTIAL RESPONDENTS

Potential respondents are people who are eligible for the survey. Eligible people are the population or sample that you want to hear from. For example, if you plan to survey teens in high school to find out about their eating habits, then the reviewers should be high school teenagers. A review by potential respondents helps guarantee that the survey's questions are meaningful and inclusive of all important ideas.

ADOPT OR ADAPT QUESTIONS THAT HAVE
BEEN USED SUCCESSFULLY IN OTHER SURVEYS

A great many survey questions are available to the public. Among these are questions asked by the U.S. Census. Questions like these have already been reviewed and used and shown to collect accurate information. Use them for your survey, when appropriate.

USE SHORTER QUESTIONS WHEN YOU
NEED TO SAVE TIME, MINIMIZE READING,
OR ARE SATISFIED WITH BRIEF ANSWERS

Shorter questions save time and require relatively little reading. They also tend to provide less detailed information. Longer questions often provide background information to respondents and help them recall or think about why they did something or hold a particular view.

Short: Have you ever traveled to another country? If yes, how important was the scenery in your decision to take a trip?

Long: Travel to other countries has become increasingly popular in this country. Have you ever traveled to another country? If yes, you might have traveled to other countries to enjoy their scenery. How important was the scenery in deciding to take a trip?

Long questions are useful in getting information on sensitive concerns (e.g., health and sexual habits) and socially controversial issues (e.g., gun control and substance abuse). When using longer questions in self-administered questionnaires, consider the time they take to ask or read and answer. Example 1.12 shows the use of a longer question.

EXAMPLE 1.12
Longer Questions

"A diagnosis of prostate cancer can have a profound effect on the quality of life of older men and their families. At least three treatments are available to men with prostate cancer: observation, surgery, and radiation. Your husband (partner) has chosen surgery. How much influence did you have in your husband's (partner's) choice of treatment?"

USE LOADED QUESTIONS, IF NECESSARY, BUT BE CAUTIOUS

Surveyors sometimes deliberately load a question to get information on embarrassing or controversial topics. The purpose of the loading is to encourage respondents to give a "true" response rather than just one that is socially acceptable. Two kinds of loading are often used, as illustrated in Example 1.13.

EXAMPLE 1.13
Loaded Questions Used in
Prompting the Respondent

1. *You are not alone.* Parents get really angry at their children sometimes. In the past week, have you been really angry at your son?

2. *You are in the best company.* Many prominent people have publicly admitted that they have sought help for problems related to alcohol abuse. In the past year, have you been to see a physician or other health professional because you thought you were drinking too much?

Use loaded questions with caution. People may see through them, get annoyed, and either not answer the question or answer it inaccurately.

AVOID BIASING WORDS AND PHRASES

Biasing words and phrases elicit emotional responses that may have little to do with the issues addressed by the survey. They are considered biasing because they trigger an emotional response or a prejudice. Some words and expressions like this are abortion, pro-life, creationism, secular humanism, and people's right to bear arms.

The bias in words tends to change with time. "Socialist" and "communist" now rarely evoke much emotional response in the United States, although they did so for 50 years. Other words and phrases simply die out, are discarded, or replaced. Drug addict, for example, has been replaced by substance abuser (or user).

Bias may arise if the surveyor does not fully understand the culture and values of the respondents and asks questions that are inadvertently offensive. To guard against this possibility, all questions must be reviewed and pilot tested before they are used.

AVOID TWO-EDGED QUESTIONS

A two-edged question contains two ideas. An example is "Do you think we should continue to use tax money to support arts and sports programs in the public schools?" This question is really twofold: "Do you think we should continue to use tax money to support art programs?" and "Do you think we should continue to use tax money to support sports programs?" Certainly, some people would support the arts programs, some the sports, others both, and still others neither. No matter what the respondent answers, however, you will not know what he or she means. To avoid asking two-edged questions, check the use of the word "and" in the question.

AVOID NEGATIVE QUESTIONS

Negative questions are difficult for many respondents to answer because they require an exercise in logical thinking. For example, suppose a question asked respondents if they agreed or disagreed with the statement "The United Nations should not have more authority to intervene in a nation's military affairs." Some respondents will fail to read the word "not." Others will first translate the negative into the positive and ask "Do I think the United Nations should have more authority to intervene in a nation's military affairs?" If you do use a negative, be sure to emphasize the negative word: "The United Nations should **NOT** have more authority to intervene in military affairs."

2 Keep Questions Closed or Open Them Up?

Questions take one of two primary forms. When they require respondents to use their own words, they are called open. When they are preselected for the respondent, they are called closed. In general, closed questions are considered more efficient and reliable than open questions for getting information from groups of people. Both types have advantages and limitations.

Open Questions

An open question allows respondents to give answers in their own way. These questions are useful in getting unanticipated answers and for describing the world as the respondent really sees it rather than how the researcher does. Some respondents also prefer to state their views in their own words. Sometimes, the responses provide quotable material. The responses to open questions, however, are often difficult to compare and interpret. Consider the question in Example 2.1.

EXAMPLE 2.1
Open Question and Three Answers

Question: How often during the past month did you find yourself having difficulty trying to calm down?

Answer 1: Not often

Answer 2: About 10% of the time

Answer 3: Much less often than the month before

Open questions provide answers that must be catalogued and interpreted. Does 10% of the time (Answer 2) mean not often (Answer 1)? How does Answer 3 compare to the other two? Open questions are used primarily in making decisions about individuals rather than groups. Experts in qualitative research are experienced in cataloguing and interpreting open questions.

Closed Questions

Closed questions are more difficult to write than open ones because the answers or response choices must be known in advance. However, some respondents prefer closed questions because they are either unwilling or unable to express themselves while being surveyed. Finally, closed questions produce standardized data that can be analyzed statistically. Statistical analysis is essential in making sense of survey data for groups of people (e.g., teams, schools, teens, the elderly, Americans). Also, because the respondent's expectations are more clearly spelled out, the answers have a better chance of being more reliable or consistent over time. Closed questions are easy to standardize. Example 2.2 shows a closed question.

EXAMPLE 2.2
Closed Question

How often during the past month did you find yourself having difficulty trying to calm down?

(Circle **one** number)

Always	1
Very often	2
Fairly often	3
Sometimes	4
Almost never	5
Never	6

How do you decide when to use open and closed questions? The following checklist can be used in choosing which type to ask.

Checklist for Deciding Between
Open and Closed Questions

	✓ If yes, use OPEN	✓ If yes, use CLOSED
Purpose	Respondents' own words are essential (to please respondent, to obtain quotes, to obtain testimony)	You want data that are rated or ranked (on a scale of very poor to very good, for example) and you have a good idea of how to order the ratings in advance
Respondents' characteristics	Respondents are capable of providing answers in their own words Respondents are willing to provide answers in their own words	You want respondents to answer using a prespecified set of response choices
Asking the question	You prefer to ask only the open question because the choices are unknown	You prefer that respondents answer in their own words
Analyzing the results	You have the skills to analyze respondents' comments even though answers may vary considerably You can handle responses that appear infrequently	You prefer to count the number of choices
Reporting the results	You will provide individual or grouped verbal responses	You will report statistical data

3 Responses: Choices and Measurement

When respondents give answers in their own words, the questions are open. When the spectrum of possible answers is provided to the respondent, the question is closed. Open questions consist of the question alone. Closed questions consist of the question and the response choices.

Response Choices

The choices given to respondents for their answers may take several forms. One form is called nominal or categorical. (The two terms are often used interchangeably.) Categorical choices

35

have no numerical or preferential values. For example, asking respondents if they are male or female calls for categorical choices: Two categories are named—male and female. The second type of response choice is called ordinal. Respondents who are asked to rate or order choices (say, from very positive to very negative) are given ordinal choices. Numerical response choices call for numbers, such as age or height.

Categorical, ordinal, and numerical response choices are illustrated in Example 3.1.

EXAMPLE 3.1
Three Common Response Choices

1. **Categorical (or nominal):** *Name* or *categorize* your astrological sign. Check *one* only.

[ ] Aquarius	[ ] Leo
[ ] Pisces	[ ] Virgo
[ ] Aries	[ ] Libra
[ ] Taurus	[ ] Scorpio
[ ] Gemini	[ ] Sagittarius
[ ] Cancer	[ ] Capricorn

2. **Ordinal:** Tell into which of the following age groups, *given in order from youngest to oldest,* you fit best. Circle *yes* or *no* for each.

Years of Age	Yes (1)	No (2)
Under 25	1	2
25 - 30	1	2
31 - 40	1	2
41 - 55	1	2
56 - 65	1	2
Over 65	1	2

3. **Numerical:** As of your most recent birthday, *what number of years tells* how old you are?

_____ years old

The first question asks for the name or category of astrological signs and implicitly provides information on the month in which each respondent was born. A survey result might be "At least 34% of respondents are Aries, who were born between March and April." The second question is different in the information it provides because it results in a hierarchy. A sample result might be "At least 50% of the sample is under 50, but only 5% is over 65 years of age." The third question uses a number to determine age. A survey result might be "The average age is 26 years."

Which format should you use? To decide, you must first know what each can do for your survey.

Consider the three questions in the next example, Example 3.2. These questions have been designed for a survey whose main purpose is to guide curriculum development in colleges. As in Example 3.1, the three types of response choices are represented: categorical, ordinal, and numerical.

Suppose the objectives of the survey in Example 3.2 are these:

- Identify books and plays that are considered important reading for graduates.
- Examine the relationship between the books and plays people read and those they rate as being important.
- Examine the relationship between respondents' age and the books and plays they rate most and least important.

EXAMPLE 3.2
Three Questions
About Important Literature

1. **Nominal or categorical:** Which of these books or plays have you read? Circle yes or no for each choice.

Have you read each of these?	Yes (1)	No (2)
Oedipus Rex	1	2
Pride and Prejudice	1	2
The Vicar of Wakefield	1	2
Bible	1	2
Moby Dick	1	2
The Glass Menagerie	1	2

2. **Ordinal:** How important to a college graduate's education is each of the following books and plays? Use the following scale to make your rating:

> 1 = Definitely unimportant
> 2 = Probably unimportant
> 3 = Probably important
> 4 = Definitely important
> 5 = No opinion/Don't know

Books/Plays	Circle ONE for each literary work				
Oedipus Rex	1	2	3	4	5
Pride and Prejudice	1	2	3	4	5
The Vicar of Wakefield	1	2	3	4	5
Bible	1	2	3	4	5
Moby Dick	1	2	3	4	5
The Glass Menagerie	1	2	3	4	5

3. **Numerical:** What is your date of birth?

_____ _____ 19 _____

Month   Day   Year

Each of the questions in Example 3.2 produces a different kind of information. The first question asks respondents to tell if they have read each of six works of literature. The second question asks the respondent to use a continuum to indicate how important each of the six works is. This continuum has been divided into four points (with a "no opinion/don't know" option). The third question asks respondents to specify the month, day, and year of their birth.

Survey questions typically require three basic tasks of respondents, use three "scales," and produce three measurement patterns or types of data. The three questions in Examples 3.1 and 3.2 represent the three tasks, scales, and data.

The first question in Example 3.2 asks respondents to tell whether or not they fit into one of two categories: read this book or did not read this book. Data or measures like these have no natural numerical values and are called **categorical** or **nominal.** A hypothetical survey finding that uses categorical data might take this form: "Over 75% of the respondents read at least one book or play on the list, but no one read all six. Of 75 respondents, 46 (61.3%) indicated they had read the *Bible,* the most frequently read book."

Categorical measures result in counts and frequencies expressed as numbers and percentages.

The second measurement pattern, represented by the second question in Example 3.2, is called **ordinal.** A response is made to fit on a continuum or scale that is ordered from positive (very important) to negative (very unimportant). The information from scales like this is called ordinal because an ordered set of answers results. Ordinal data consist of the numbers and percentages of people who select each point on the scale. In some cases, you may find it expedient to compute the average response: the average rating of importance across all respondents. Sample survey results might take a form like this: "Of 75 respondents completing this question, 43 (57.3%) rated each book or play as definitely or probably important. The average ratings ranged from 3.7 for the *Bible* to 2.0 for *The Vicar of Wakefield.*"

Surveys often ask respondents for **numerical** data. In Example 3.2, respondents are asked for their birth date. From the date, you can calculate each respondent's age. Age is considered a numerical and continuous measure, starting with zero and ending with the age of the oldest person in the survey. When you have numerical data, you can perform many statistical operations. Typical survey findings might appear as follows: "The average age of the respondents was 43 years. The oldest person was 79 years, and the youngest was 23. We found no relation between age and ratings of importance."

CATEGORICAL OR NOMINAL MEASURES: HOW TO GET THEM

The first question in Example 3.2 asks respondents to answer yes or no regarding whether they read a named book or play. "Yes" and "no" are categories into which the responses must be placed. Other commonly used response categories are "present" or "absent" and "applies" or "does not apply." If you ask 100 respondents the name of the country of their birth, and 20 answer France and 80 say the United States, you have categorical data that can be described this way:

	Yes	No
Born in France?	20	80
Born in the United States?	80	20

When you ask people the name of their country of birth, astrological sign, ethnicity, and so on, you are collecting categorical data. In this case, it is also called nominal because the name determines the category.

Questions about gender and race/ethnicity produce nominal or categorical information, as shown in Example 3.3.

EXAMPLE 3.3
Nominal or Categorical Data From Surveys

1. Indicate your gender by circling the appropriate number.

	Yes (1)	No (2)
Female	1	2
Male	1	2

2. Which best describes your race/ethnicity? Circle *one* choice only.

Race/Ethnicity	Yes (1)	No (2)
White, not Latino	1	2
Latino	1	2
African American	1	2
Native American	1	2
Asian		
(please specify_____)	1	2

Other examples of nominal or categorical measures are questions like these:

- Which of the following medical problems do you have? Hypertension; diabetes; low back pain.
- Are you currently married? Living with someone but not married? Not currently married and not living with someone? Married but living alone?
- Do you have a BA? MA? MEd? MSW? PhD? MD?

CATEGORICAL RESPONSES AND WHO'S ELIGIBLE

Nominal or categorical responses put respondents into categories such as male or female, Native American or African American. Questions asking respondents to categorize or name themselves are used to get demographic information and help decide who should be included (or excluded) from a survey. Suppose you are planning to ask people to rate the importance of six books or plays. To get accurate information, you want to survey people who know what they are doing. You might decide to exclude potential respondents who have read only four or fewer. A question asking for categorical answers would then be appropriate:

- Which of the following books have you read? Check all that apply.

> _____ *Pride and Prejudice*
> _____ *The Vicar of Wakefield*
> _____ *Bible*
> _____ *Moby Dick*
> _____ *Madame Bovary*

The responses to "check all that apply" questions are almost always categorical. The reason is that each check means "Yes, I belong in the category." Each category or choice that is left blank is assumed to mean "No, I do not belong."

CATEGORICAL RESPONSES ARE EXCLUSIVE

Categorical response choices should be mutually exclusive. Compare the following good and poor questions and response categories.

Poor: Which of the following best describes you?

	Yes (1)	No (2)
Professional	1	2
Registered nurse	1	2
Nurse practitioner	1	2
Administrator	1	2
Nurse midwife	1	2

Comment: The categories for the responses are not mutually exclusive. The choice "professional" can include all of the remaining categories. A nurse practitioner, a registered nurse, a nurse midwife, and an administrator can be considered professionals. To confuse matters even more, the nurse practitioner, administrator, and nurse midwife may all be registered nurses.

Better: Which of the following apply to you? Answer yes *or* no for each category.

	Yes (1)	No (2)
Nurse practitioner	1	2
Administrator	1	2
Registered nurse	1	2
Nurse midwife	1	2

CATEGORICAL RESPONSES ARE INCLUSIVE

Categorical response categories should be inclusive and exhaustive. Include all categories on which you hope to get information. The following are illustrations of two questions that might be asked in a survey of lawyers to identify how many of them had specific expertise in various kinds of legal problems.

Poor: Which **one** of the following best describes your primary expertise?

[ ] Landlord-tenant problems
[ ] Consumer problems
[ ] Traffic cases
[ ] Other (specify) _____

Comment: These categories are not exhaustive. The survey is likely to produce more responses in the "other" category than in the three that are listed.

> *Better:* Which **one** of the following best describes your primary expertise?

[ ] Landlord-tenant problems
[ ] Consumer problems
[ ] Traffic cases
[ ] Small claims
[ ] Misdemeanors
[ ] Felony cases
[ ] Wills
[ ] Personal injury claims
[ ] Domestic relations
[ ] Adoption
[ ] Tax
[ ] Real estate
[ ] Bankruptcy
[ ] Poverty
[ ] Other (specify) _____

CATEGORICAL RESPONSES AND MEANING

A major issue in asking questions that produce categorical responses is how to group responses so that they are meaningful. A general rule is to use groups that make sense in the survey and that also will be useful when you report the results of the survey. Suppose you were conducting a survey of elderly people and you wanted to know how many in your survey fell into certain categories or age groups. You could frame your question as in Example 3.4.

EXAMPLE 3.4
Question for Older People

Which best describes your age group? Circle **one** choice only.

Age Group	Yes (1)	No (2)
65 - 74	1	2
75 - 84	1	2
85 - 95	1	2
Over 95	1	2

The question and responses used above are fairly standard. If you look at surveys of older persons, you will find that the response groups used in the question are typical. One good way to be sure you are using meaningful categories is to adapt or adopt those used in other surveys. Already existing and in-use choices tend to make reporting easier because they are familiar.

Existing response choices may not always suffice to meet the needs of a particular survey; then, of course, you must create your own. Question 2 in Example 3.3 used standard racial/ ethnic terms to describe categories for a survey of prenatal care and low income in Northern California. At the time of the survey (1992), these groupings accounted for 98% of women who were likely to be in any survey of prenatal care in the geographic region. Terms change over time, and so the ones in the question may seem out of place or time just a few years later. Be cautious in using questions from other surveys and standard terms for job descriptions, names of countries, and income groups. These terms change.

Example 3.5 shows two questions about age that might be used in a study of music listening.

EXAMPLE 3.5
Choosing Response Choices

1. We conducted a survey to compare teens and others in their music-listening habits. We asked this question:

Which best describes your age? Circle **one.**

Years of Age	Yes (1)	No (2)
12 or younger	1	2
13 - 14	1	2
15 - 17	1	2
18 - 21	1	2
22 - 30	1	2
31 or older	1	2

2. We conducted a survey to compare the music-listening habits of people of differing ages. We asked the following question:

Which best describes your age? Circle **one.**

Years of Age	Yes (1)	No (2)
20 or younger	1	2
21 - 30	1	2
31 - 40	1	2
41 - 50	1	2
51 - 60	1	2
61 or older	1	2

The purpose of Question 1 is to produce information for comparing teens and nonteens. All people 31 or older are grouped together.

The aim of Question 2 is to obtain data for comparing people of differing ages. The groupings assume that

1. Music-listening habits vary according to age decade (e.g., 31-40 and 51-60), and

2. All people under 20 years of age have similar listening habits and all those 61 and older have similar listening habits OR

3. The differences in music-listening habits between people under 20 and between those 61 and older are not important for the survey's purposes.

Questions With Ordered Responses: How to Get Ordinal Data Using Common Rating Scales

Questions that ask respondents to order their responses are ordinal measures. Question 2 in Example 3.2 is a typical ordinal measure. In the question, respondents are asked to create an order by rating importance on a scale from 1 to 4. In so doing, they are making an implicit statement about the relative importance of one literary work ("definitely important") over another ("definitely not important.") When responses are ordered or placed in ordered groupings along one dimension, you have ordinal data. The most familiar kinds of ordinal data come from scales like the following:

- Strongly agree, agree, neither agree nor disagree, disagree, strongly disagree
- Excellent, very good, good, fair, poor
- Always, very often, fairly often, sometimes, almost never, never

■ Completely satisfied, very satisfied, somewhat satisfied, somewhat dissatisfied, very dissatisfied, completely dissatisfied

Ordinal measures are extremely common in surveys. In fact, typical surveys tend to have more ordinal measures than any other kind. When asking questions that require respondents to order their answers, you need to be concerned with the content of the choices, the number of choices, whether to include a middle point and a "do not know" response, and a range of grammatical and other issues including how the question looks on a page or sounds when spoken in person or on the telephone. Tune in on a conversation between two surveyors about ordered responses:

Surveyor A: I am conducting a survey of anxiety and depression in the workplace. I'd like to ask "In the past month, how often has feeling depressed interfered with doing your job?" What response choices can I use so that I can compare the number of people who feel depressed most often with the number of people who feel depressed least often?

Surveyor B: You need a set of response choices that are ordered on a scale ranging from "often" to "not often."

A: What scales are available?

B: You have several options. You can use a simple 3-point scale with response choices like "often," "sometimes," "never"; a 4-point scale like "nearly all the time," "some of the time," "a little of the time," "almost none of the time"; a 6-point scale like "all of the time," "most of the time," "a good bit of the time," "some of the time," "little of the time," "none of the time." You can also create longer scales if you want. I can even think of situations in which discrete numerical categories might be appropriate. These categories could be "100% of the time," "between 50% and 100% of the time," and "less than 50% of the time."

A: How do I make my decision?

B: Before I answer, I want to raise some issues to consider in asking respondents to order their responses, such as whether to include a middle point ("neither agree nor disagree," for example) and whether to include a "don't know" or "no opinion" choice.

A: Do you know of some guidelines for me to use in asking this type of question and determining response choices?

B: You're in luck. I just came across a set.

Guidelines for Asking Closed Questions and Determining Ordered Responses or Scales

USE A MEANINGFUL SCALE

A meaningful scale is one that makes sense in terms of the survey's specific objectives. In the preceding conversation, Surveyor A wants to compare people in terms of the frequency of their depression. Surveyor B has suggested a number of response choices. To choose among them, Surveyor A can do any or all of the following:

- Ask potential respondents which scale is best.
- Ask other surveyors to help select a scale.
- Try one or more scales on a preliminary basis and select the one that gives a good "spread" of answers (you do not want everyone to choose just one point on the scale) and is meaningful to the respondent.

CONSIDER FIVE TYPES OF RESPONSE OPTIONS

Endorsement: Definitely true, true, don't know, false, definitely false

Frequency: Always, very often, fairly often, sometimes, almost never, never

Intensity: None, very mild, mild, moderate, severe

Influence: Big problem, moderate problem, small problem, very small problem, no problem

Comparison: Much more than others, somewhat more than others, about the same as others, somewhat less than others, much less than others

---

EXERCISE

Surveyor A wants to study the frequency with which depression interferes with job performance. Suppose the surveyor asks you for a question that results in comparative information. Write the question.

■ ANSWER ■

Compared to your usual performance on the job, how has your depression affected your performance in the past 4 weeks?

Please circle ONE response

Much worse than usual	1
Somewhat worse than usual	2
About the same as usual	3
Somewhat better than usual	4
Much better than usual	5

BALANCE ALL RESPONSES

A scale is balanced when the two endpoints mean the opposite of one another and the intervals between the points on the scale are about equal. "Much worse" (see the preceding exercise) is the opposite of "much better," and the meaning of the interval between "much worse" and "somewhat worse" is similar in degree to that of "somewhat better" and "much better." "About the same as usual" appears to fit in the middle. Of course, language is imprecise, and the intervals may be less equal than they appear on the face of it. That's why all questions should be tried out before they are used. Examples of how to balance scales follow:

#1　*Poor:*
  　　Yes, constantly
  　　Yes, very often
  　　Yes, once
  　　No, never
  　Better:
  　　Yes, constantly
  　　Yes, very often
  　　Yes, fairly often
  　　Yes, a couple of times
  　　Yes, once
  　　No, never

#2　*Poor:*
  　　Very happy
  　　Somewhat happy
  　　Neither happy nor unhappy
  　　Not very happy
  　Better:
  　　Very happy
  　　Happy
  　　Somewhat happy
  　　Neither happy nor unhappy
  　　Somewhat unhappy
  　　Unhappy
  　　Very unhappy

USE A NEUTRAL RESPONSE
CATEGORY ONLY IF IT IS VALID

Provide a neutral category only when you are sure it is a valid response. A neutral category is either a middle point (neither happy nor unhappy) or "no opinion," "don't know." Some surveyors believe that neutral choices provide respondents with an excuse for not answering the question. If not answering is a possibility, pretest the question with and without the neutral choices and compare the results. How many responses cluster around the middle point? Do some respondents resent not having a middle point? As part of the pretesting process, ask the respondents about the scale. Did they encounter any problems in using it? Would another set of responses be more appropriate?

USE 5- TO 7-POINT RATING SCALES

Current thinking suggests that 5- to 7-point scales are adequate for the majority of surveys that use ordered responses. Self-administered questionnaires and telephone interviews should probably use 4 or 5. In-person interviews should use visual aids for scales with 5 or more points on them, such as the following sample:

MUCH WORSE THAN USUAL	1
SOMEWHAT WORSE THAN USUAL	2
ABOUT THE SAME AS USUAL	3
SOMEWHAT BETTER THAN USUAL	4
MUCH BETTER THAN USUAL	5

Conclusive evidence supporting odd or even scales is unavailable. Use odd or even depending on the survey's needs.

PUT THE NEGATIVE END
OF THE SCALE FIRST

Consider putting the negative end of the scale first for questions that are potentially embarrassing or about socially undesirable behaviors or attitudes, as illustrated in Example 3.6.

EXAMPLE 3.6
Putting the Negative End of the Scale
First When Questions May Be Embarrassing

How much do these statements apply to you? Circle **one** number for each line.

Embarrassing Statement	Very Much (4)	Much (3)	A Fair Amount (2)	A Little (1)	Not at All (0)
I find that my clothes do not fit.	4	3	2	1	0
I am uncomfortable with the changes in my body.	4	3	2	1	0
I frequently feel anxious.	4	3	2	1	0

In this question, the negative end of the scale means agreeing that the statement applies "very much." If you put the positive end first (that is, the statement applies "not at all"), people may just select that as the least embarrassing option. Deciding which end of the scale to place first is most important in face-to-face interviews and least important in anonymous self-administered and other mail surveys. If the survey deals with a problem the respondent thinks is important, the direction of the scale may not count at all. If the questions above, for example, are asked of cancer patients, you do not have to worry as much about directionality as you do if the questions are meant for teens.

KEEP QUESTIONNAIRES UNCLUTTERED
AND EASY TO COMPLETE

Present the question in an uncluttered, easy-to-complete way in self-administered questionnaires (including mail questionnaires). This can be achieved by following the rules in Example 3.7.

EXAMPLE 3.7
Rules for Presenting
an Uncluttered Question

1. Tell the respondent how and where to mark the responses.

Emphasize any special tasks or requirements in the question, as shown below:

Example

Considering your reading habits, **during the past year** how often did you read the following newspapers, journals, and magazines? Circle **one** for each choice.

Periodical	Never (1)	Rarely (2)	Sometimes (3)	Frequently (4)	Always (5)
New York Times	1	2	3	4	5
Wall Street Journal	1	2	3	4	5
Cosmopolitan	1	2	3	4	5
New England Journal of Medicine	1	2	3	4	5
Sports Illustrated	1	2	3	4	5

2. *Avoid questions with skip patterns in self-administered questionnaires.*

   A skip pattern is a question that you expect does not apply to all participants. If you must use skip patterns, set them off as clearly as possible, as shown below:

Example

14. Have you had **two years or more in your life** when you felt depressed or sad most days, even if you felt OK sometimes?

   [ ] No → **GO TO QUESTION 15**
   [ ] Yes _____
              ↓

              14A. Have you felt depressed or sad much of the time in the **past year?**

                   [ ] Yes
                   [ ] No

3. *Organize responses so that they are readable.* Consider the following:

   Poor: To what extent do you agree or disagree with the following statements?

      1. Each day of work feels as if it will never end.

      ___ Strongly agree ___ Undecided ___ Agree ___ Disagree
      ___ Strongly disagree

2. Most of the time I have to force myself to go to work.

[ ] Strongly agree   [ ] Undecided
[ ] Agree   [ ] Disagree
        [ ] Strongly disagree

Item 1 is poor because the lines before the choices sometimes appear as if they are after the choices. For example, the line that precedes "agree" is also right next to "strongly agree." Item 2 is poor because the choices are not aligned, and the logic of the scale disappears.

Better:

	Strongly Agree (1)	Agree (2)	Undecided (3)	Disagree (4)	Strongly Disagree (5)
Each day of work feels as if it will never end.	1	2	3	4	5
Most of the time I have to force myself to go to work.	1	2	3	4	5

QUESTIONS SHOULD BE WRITTEN SO THAT
INTERVIEWERS CAN DISTINGUISH BETWEEN
WORDS READ TO RESPONDENTS AND WORDS
THAT ARE INSTRUCTIONS/OPTIONS (Example 3.8).

EXAMPLE 3.8
Distinguishing Between Words for
Respondents, Instructions, and Options

Which of the following have you (or SOMEONE IN YOUR FAM-
ILY) done in the last year with a neighbor? HAND RESPONDENT
CARD A. CODE YES OR NO FOR EACH ITEM ANSWERED.

	Yes (1)	No (2)
Stopped and talked when we met	1	2
Had dinner together at their home or ours	1	2
Had dinner together at a restaurant	1	2
Watched their home when on vacation, or they watched ours	1	2

In this example, the use of capitalized bold letters tells the
interviewer to give the respondent an option: (or SOMEONE
IN YOUR FAMILY). The question for respondents is in regular
letters, and the instructions are capitalized. Notice that the
interviewer is asked to present Card A to the respondent.
Face-to-face or in-person interviewers use cards that contain
the scale and its definition when respondents are asked to
select from among five or more choices. Telephone interviewers
read the choices before asking the question and repeat them
for each question.

USE RANKINGS ONLY IF RESPONDENTS
CAN SEE OR EASILY REMEMBER ALL CHOICES.

Rankings or rank-order scales are a type of ordinal measure in which choices are placed in order from the highest to the lowest (or the other way around). The rank of students in a college senior class is important to graduate school admissions committees, for example. The following is typical of questions asking respondents to rank their preferences:

- Select the **three** most important books or plays for reading by U.S. college graduates from the following list.

   Oedipus Rex
   Pride and Prejudice
   The Vicar of Wakefield
   Bible
   Moby Dick
   The Glass Menagerie
   Other (specify) _____

   Put your choices here.
       Top Choice:
       Second Choice:
       Third Choice:

In telephone interviews, ranking should be limited to two or three alternatives at a time. In self-administered surveys and face-to-face interviews in which visual aids can be used, respondents should not be asked to rank more than five alternatives. If you insist on many alternatives, you can have respondents choose the top two or three and the bottom two or three.

Numerical Measures

Numerical measures ask respondents to produce numbers, as illustrated in Example 3.9.

EXAMPLE 3.9
Numerical Measures

1. How many of the following books and plays have you read?

    Oedipus Rex
    Pride and Prejudice
    The Vicar of Wakefield
    Bible
    Moby Dick
    The Glass Menagerie
    Number of books and plays I have read: _____

2. IF YOU HAVE READ THE *BIBLE:*
   How old were you when you first read the *Bible?*

    _____ years old

---

3. How important to a college graduate's education is each of the following books and plays? **Cross out** the one number that best describes your opinion of importance. The meaning of the numbers is as follows:

> 1 = Very important
> 8 = Neither important nor unimportant
> 15 = Very unimportant

Example

Hamlet 1 2 ✗ 4 5 6 7 8 9 10 11 12 13 14 15

This person has assigned the reading of *Hamlet* a rating of 3.

Cross out **ONE** number

Oedipus Rex	1	2	3	4	5	6	7	8	9	10	11	12	13	14	15
Pride and Prejudice	1	2	3	4	5	6	7	8	9	10	11	12	13	14	15
The Vicar of Wakefield	1	2	3	4	5	6	7	8	9	10	11	12	13	14	15
Bible	1	2	3	4	5	6	7	8	9	10	11	12	13	14	15
Moby Dick	1	2	3	4	5	6	7	8	9	10	11	12	13	14	15
The Glass Menagerie	1	2	3	4	5	6	7	8	9	10	11	12	13	14	15

The first question asks respondents to record the number of books and plays they have read. The numbers produced by questions like this are called discrete. Other examples of discrete data are number of pregnancies, accidents, employees, patients, and so on. The second question asks for age. Age can start with zero and go up to the end of the human lifespan. The numbers produced by questions like this are called continuous. Other examples of continuous data are weight, height, years of survival, and scores on a test.

Sometimes, numerical data are classified as interval or ratio. With interval data, the distance between numbers or points have a real meaning. The most commonly quoted example is the Fahrenheit temperature scale. The 10-point difference between 70° and 80° is the same as the 10-point difference between 40° and 50°. Ratio measurements have a true zero, as in the Kelvin temperature scale. Fifty kelvins is half as warm as 100 kelvins. Because the Fahrenheit scale has an arbitrary zero, 40° is not half as hot as 80°. In practice, very few interval scales exist, and statistically, interval and ratio data tend to be treated the same. The term "numerical scales" or "measures" avoids confusion.

The third question in Example 3.9 asks the respondent to choose a number along a continuum. A similar way to obtain numerical data is through the use of rating scales that are presented along a printed line. In the following, respondents are asked to place an "X" on the line to describe the extent of their pain:

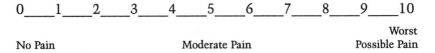

0_____1_____2_____3_____4_____5_____6_____7_____8_____9_____10

No Pain   Moderate Pain   Worst Possible Pain

Scales like this lend themselves to reports like this: "At least 47% of respondents indicated that they had moderate pain (markings of 4, 5, or 6), whereas 10% had the worst possible pain (marking of 10)."

To aid in interpretation, decide on a length for the line, say, 10 centimeters or 10 inches. Then you can measure where along the line each respondent makes a mark and compute averages and other statistics. If one person places a mark at 1 inch (the low end of the scale), another at 1.3 inches, and a third at 3.3 inches, the average among the three respondents would be $1 + 1.3 + 3.3 = 5.6/3 = 1.866$.

4

Knowledge, Attitudes, and Behavior: Additional Tips When Creating Survey Questions

Although it is conventional in some fields, such as health, to think of measuring knowledge first and then attitudes and behavior, surveys tend to focus on attitudes.

Feelings and Intensity: Getting at the Attitude

An attitude is a general way of thinking, such as being liberal or conservative or being hostile or peaceable. The term "attitude" is often used to mean the same as opinion, belief, preference, feeling, and value. The following are typical of survey questions about attitudes:

- Do you favor gun control?
- Should the federal government do more to equalize income differences between the rich and the poor?
- How satisfied are you with your job?
- Which of the following are essential goals of a democratic society?
- Which description comes closest to defining the quality of your life?
- How healthy do you feel?
- Which is the best solution to illegal immigration?
- Do you favor an increase in taxes to support educational programs for very poor children?

Attitudes are very complex entities and difficult to define and measure. What are the characteristics that consistently and accurately distinguish liberals from conservatives? Does a universal definition of quality of life exist? Aspects of these questions are philosophical, but scientific and technical methods are available for producing attitude scales that are valid for specific survey needs. These methods are used by psychometricians to examine the statistical properties of questions to find out if they consistently and accurately distinguish people with the attitude from those without.

Attitudes are often contrasted with knowledge and behavior. How you feel about gun control laws, what you know about gun control laws, and what you personally do about guns may or may not be related logically.

Most survey experts agree that if you are interested in measuring concepts like political stance, religiosity, satisfaction (with job or quality of life or health) and you are not in a position to do a scientific experiment to validate the questions, you should use already existing and proven questions. These can be found through library searches of books and journals; by contacting college and university departments of medicine, public health, sociology, political science, and psychology; and by asking colleagues and associates to lend you their questions and measures. Books are available that contain attitudinal questions, but no central, updated clearinghouse exists. The fact is that finding attitude questions and scales is hard work. It can be costly in terms of the amount of time you have to spend to identify the right agency with the right questions. In some cases, payment is required. If you plan to use questions from existing surveys, check on who owns the copyright and whether you need the authors' permission to reproduce some or all questions.

Once you have identified one or more questions that meet the needs of your survey, check carefully to make certain that each is suitable for your survey's respondents. Is the language level appropriate? Does it truly ask what you need to know? You should have any borrowed questions reviewed and pretested.

A good way to pretest questions is to ask respondents to tell you in their own words what the question means to them. Tune in on the following dialogue with two potential survey respondents:

Surveyor: We are conducting a survey to find out if you are satisfied with your health care. Question one asks you to rate the importance of accessible care. The scale you will use has five response choices: definitely important, important, probably important, probably not important, and no opinion. Please tell me in your own words what this question means.

Respondent 1: You are asking me to tell you if I think getting an appointment with a doctor when I need one is important to me.

Respondent 2: To me, accessible care means not having to travel long distances and being able to park when you get there.

Surveyor: Based on what you have said, I see that the term "accessibility" is unclear at the present. The survey needs at least three questions to measure accessible care. The first will ask about the ease of getting an appointment, and the second and third will address time to travel and parking, respectively. I also plan to clearly define the response choices. For example, a response of a "very important" to a listed consideration would be one that must be addressed or you would choose to go elsewhere for care.

It often helps to think of attitude questions as having at least two components: how respondents feel and how strongly they feel (or believe). This is illustrated in Example 4.1.

EXAMPLE 4.1
Feelings and Intensity
in Attitude Questions

Edith Wilson, Eleanor Roosevelt, and Hillary Rodham Clinton, each of them the spouse of a U.S. president, have had considerable influence on U.S. policy. In general, do you approve of the role these spouses have played? Check **one** choice.

[ ] Approve (**ask A**)
[ ] Do not approve (**ask A**)
[ ] Do not care/No opinion (**stop**)

How strongly do you feel about it? Check **one** choice.

[ ] Very strongly
[ ] Fairly strongly
[ ] Not very strongly

Recall and Time: Getting at Behavior

Behavior refers to what respondents actually do. The following are examples of survey questions about respondents' behavior:

- Which of the following magazines and newspapers do you read at least once a month?
- How often do you exercise?
- Did you vote in the last election?
- How frequently do you go to church?
- In the past 3 years, how often did you apply for federal grants?

All questions about behavior are concerned with time, duration, or frequency. The preceding questions specify time periods: at least once a month, how frequently, the last election, and within the past 3 years.

Choose time periods that meet the survey's needs and that make sense to the respondent. You can obtain reliable information about events and activities that occurred years ago if they are important. People remember births, deaths, marriage, divorce, buying their first house, and so on. They also remember what they were doing at the time of great historical events like wars and assassinations and during natural disasters like fires, floods, and earthquakes. For most other events, do not expect people to remember past one year's time. You can, however, use yearly periods primarily for summary information:

- About how much money did you spend on vacations away from home in the past year?
- In the past 12 months, how often did you go for bicycle rides of 5 or more miles?

Asking respondents to give specific information over a long period of time leads to omissions:

Poor: In the past year, which of the following items of children's clothing did you buy from Outdoors Clothing Company?

Comment: Unless respondents have bought very few items of clothes for their children or buy exclusively from Outdoors Clothing Company, they might very easily forget.

Better: In the past 3 months, which of the following items of children's clothes did you buy from Outdoors Clothing Company?

Very short periods of time can adversely affect the accuracy or validity of an answer to a question about behavior:

Poor: In the past week, how often did you buy coffee, tea, bottled water, diet soda, or regular soda?

Comment: A question like this may produce invalid results because people may not have purchased any of the items during the past week. Nevertheless, because they do purchase and use them regularly, they may overreport by indicating a purchase in the past week that really occurred the week before.

Better: In the past 3 weeks, how often did you buy coffee, tea, bottled water, diet soda, or regular soda?

Because questions about behavior have a time element, you are dependent on respondents' ability to recall. To jog the memory, use lists, as illustrated in Example 4.2.

EXAMPLE 4.2
Using a List to Help Respondents
Remember Their Actions

This question is about your leisure activities. Since last January, did you do any of these activities? Check **yes** or **no** for each.

	Yes (1)	No (2)
Go to a movie	1	2
Eat out for pleasure	1	2
Window shop	1	2
Go to the theater	1	2

$\rightarrow$

	Yes (1)	No (2)
Read for pleasure	1	2
Go for a run	1	2
Go for a hike	1	2
Ride a bicycle	1	2
Go fishing	1	2
Do gardening	1	2

The advantage of a list is its capacity for reminding respondents of events they may have forgotten. To be maximally helpful, the list should be inclusive. An inclusive list can go on for many pages, which is confusing and boring. One way to get around the long-list problem is to divide a question into its component parts, as illustrated in Example 4.3.

EXAMPLE 4.3
Dividing the Question:
How to Avoid Long Lists and
Still Get the Behaviors You Need

1. Since last January, have you participated in any of the following activities? Answer **yes** or **no** for each.

Shopping for pleasure	1	2	If **yes**, answer Question 3
Religious groups	1	2	If **yes**, answer Question 5

2. Since last January, did you play any of the following sports? Answer **yes** or **no** for each sport.

	Yes (1)	No (2)
Basketball	1	2
Baseball	1	2
Football	1	2
Bowling	1	2
Other—please name:	1	2
Other—please name:	1	2

By presenting a list to respondents, you may encourage them to use only the categories in the survey, and this may result in a loss of information. To avoid losing information, you can add an "other" category as is done in Question 2 in Example 4.3. By adding this option, you are including an open question and must be prepared to interpret and catalogue the answers.

EXERCISE

Will the questions in Examples 4.2 and 4.3 produce categorical, ordinal, or numerical data?

■ ANSWER ■

Categorical

Regulating Difficulty and Threat: Getting at Knowledge

Knowledge questions are included in surveys to achieve the following objectives:

- Determine if people have enough knowledge about a topic to warrant asking their opinion about it
- Identify gaps in knowledge that warrant education, advertising, or publicity or other kinds of information campaigns
- Help explain attitudes and behavior

Example 4.4 illustrates the three main uses of knowledge questions.

EXAMPLE 4.4
Using Knowledge Questions in Surveys

The University Medical Center is concerned that women are not routinely getting Pap smears. These screening tests are essential for early diagnosis of cervical cancer. A survey is taken of all women who come for gynecological services in a one-year period.

1. *Knowledge of a Topic.* A primary survey purpose is to find out what women know. Accordingly, questions are asked about knowledge of the purpose of Pap smears, how they are performed, and how frequently they should be obtained.

2. *Educational Needs.* The answers to the questions are used to find out if an educational campaign is needed and, if so, what topics should be included. The survey's results reveal that nearly 60% of the women do not correctly answer the question about the purpose of the test. Only 20% know how often to have a Pap smear, using guidelines set by the American Cancer

Society or the American College of Obstetricians and Gynecologists (the two groups differ). Nearly 92% of women who say they had at least one Pap smear know how it is performed. Based on these findings, the surveyors recommend the preparation of educational brochures in English, Spanish, and Portuguese, the main languages spoken by patients. The survey team also recommends a media campaign to encourage women to seek Pap smears.

3. *Explaining Attitudes and Behavior.* One survey question asks about the convenience of clinic hours. The survey team compares the women who say they favor increased clinic hours for screening tests with those who do not. The team's analysis demonstrates that women who correctly answered the questions about the purpose of Pap tests are definitely more favorably disposed (margin of 10 to 1) toward increased hours of clinic operation.

The boundary between attitude and knowledge questions is sometimes blurred. Consider these questions:

1. Using your best guess, what percentage of people do not report some of their pay to the Internal Revenue Service?

2. In your view, what is the best way to prevent influenza in people over 75 years of age?

Are the above questions asking for attitudes or knowledge? The first question looks like a knowledge question because it asks for a fact or a percentage. Estimates do exist of the proportion of people earning money and not declaring it to the IRS, but because most of us probably do not know the percentage, we guess. For many, the guess is as much a reflection of how much cheating we think is going on as an attempt to come up with an accurate estimate.

The second question seems like an attitude question. In fact, it is a knowledge question because a correct answer is available: Give them flu shots.

Knowledge questions are sometimes disguised so as to reduce their threatening appearance. This is done with phrases like "in your opinion," "using your best guess," and "have you heard or have you read that . . . ?"

Knowledge questions can vary in their difficulty. The easiest questions are relatively general and ask for recall of current or significant information. The most difficult questions ask the respondent to recall, understand, interpret, and apply information in innovative ways. Consider this example:

> *Easier:* Have you heard or read about President Kennedy's assassination?
>
> *More difficult:* From this list, select the name of President Kennedy's probable assassin.
>
> *Even more difficult:* Five cities are circled on this map. Please show me the location of the city in which President Kennedy was assassinated.

The first question is the easiest because the significance of the assassination suggests that nearly everyone (not just Americans) will have heard or read about the assassination. The second question requires recall of a name. President Kennedy was assassinated in 1963, and for many, the assassin's name has faded from memory. Others may have never learned the name. The use of a list helps respondents remember. The third question requires knowledge of the name of the city and its location on a map, and because it involves recall and understanding of geography, it is the hardest of the three questions.

Most surveys of knowledge are not achievement tests in the classical sense. They are not used to grade or promote students or find out what they have learned. You may be more interested in finding out how many respondents do not know about something. Many surveys of knowledge include "do not know" or "no opinion" response choices. These choices also help remove some of the threat associated with knowledge questions. Suppose you were surveying respondents about the physical environment. You might ask a question like the following:

A fossil of an ocean fish was found in a rock outcrop on a mountain. Which of the following best describes the meaning of this finding? Select **one** choice only.

Fish once lived on the mountain.

The relative humidity was once very high.

The mountain was raised up after the fish died.

Fish used to be amphibians like toads and frogs.

The fossil fish was probably carried to the mountain by a great flood.

I don't know.

By providing an "I don't know" category, people who might otherwise just guess are given a place to put their response. But beware! "I don't know" is sometimes used by those who are too lazy or do not want to think about the question even when doing so could result in the correct answer.

Demographics: Who Are the Respondents?

Demographic information consists of facts about a respondent's age, race/ethnicity, education job, gender, whether married or not, geographic place of residence, type of residence, size of family, and so on.

Compare the two typical demographic questions about race and ethnicity in Example 4.5.

EXAMPLE 4.5
Two Questions About Race and Ethnicity

Question 1

4. **Race**

Fill ONE circle for the race that you consider youself to be.

o White
o Black or Negro
o Indian (Amer.) (Print the name of the enrolled or principal tribe) ↓

If **Indian (Amer.)**, print the name of the enrolled or principal tribe._____ →

o Eskimo
o Aleut

Asian or Pacific Islander (API)

o Chinese	o Japanese
o Filipino ■	o Asian Indian
o Hawaiian	o Samoan
o Korean	o Guamanian
o Vietnamese	o Other API ↓

If **Other Asian or Pacific Islander (API)**, print one group: for example, Hmong, Fijian, Laotian, Thai, Tongan, Pakistani, Cambodian, and so on. _____ →

If **Other race**, print race _____ →

o Other race (Print race) ↑

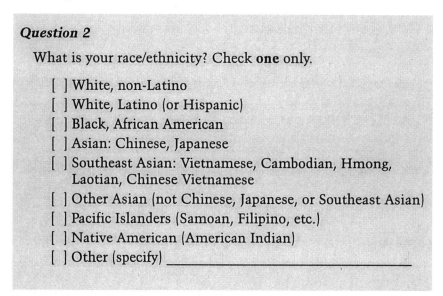

Question 2

What is your race/ethnicity? Check **one** only.

[ ] White, non-Latino
[ ] White, Latino (or Hispanic)
[ ] Black, African American
[ ] Asian: Chinese, Japanese
[ ] Southeast Asian: Vietnamese, Cambodian, Hmong, Laotian, Chinese Vietnamese
[ ] Other Asian (not Chinese, Japanese, or Southeast Asian)
[ ] Pacific Islanders (Samoan, Filipino, etc.)
[ ] Native American (American Indian)
[ ] Other (specify) _____

The aim of the two questions in Example 4.5 is to collect a vital statistic: the race or ethnicity of the respondents. The two questions differ in the following ways:

- Question 1 gives the choice of Black or Negro. Question 2 gives an open choice: Black, African American.

- Question 1 refers to American Indians and asks for the name of the enrolled or principal tribe. Question 2 gives the choice of Native American (American Indian) and does not ask for the name of the respondent's tribe.

- Question 1 includes as choices Hawaiian, Korean, Asian Indian, Guamanian, Eskimo, and Aleut. Question 2 does not mention these but does include Chinese Vietnamese.

Questions 1 and 2 differ because they were posed for surveys with entirely distinct purposes and groups of respondents. Question 1 comes from the U.S. Bureau of the Census official

1990 Census form. The question was asked of everyone in the United States in 1989. Question 2 comes from a 1991 survey of low-income women who participated in a federally funded project in California to improve maternal and infant outcomes through prenatal care.

Surveys differ in purpose and in target respondents. Before asking for demographic information, learn about the likely characteristics of the target group. Question 1 is concerned with the racial/ethnic characteristics of everyone in the United States. Question 2 addresses only low-income women in one state. If the Census Bureau had asked Question 2, many races would have been lumped into "other," necessitating a great deal of work to unscramble categories. If the prenatal study had asked Question 1, many categories might have remained unchecked; the study would not have obtained data on the number of respondents who were Chinese Vietnamese, a group that was important in the study of prenatal care.

Another difference between Questions 1 and 2 is use of language. In its 1990 census, the Census Bureau used the classification "Negro." By 1991, this term was no longer favored; it was therefore excluded from Question 2 and "African American" was used. At about the same time, "Native American" began to coexist with and even supplant "American Indian" as a category, and Question 2's response choices also reflect this.

Question 2 offers as one of the choices White, Latino (or Hispanic), but Question 1 does not include this choice. This group of people constitutes a large segment of the U.S. population. Strictly speaking, at least in 1990, Latinos were not considered a racial or ethnic group. The Census Bureau asked about Spanish *origin,* and the prenatal care study asked about country of birth, as shown in Example 4.6.

EXAMPLE 4.6
Asking About Origin or Country of Birth

1. Asked by the Bureau of the Census:

7. Is this person of Spanish/Hispanic origin?

Fill ONE circle for each person.

o No (not Spanish/Hispanic)
o Yes, Mexican, Mexican-Am., Chicano
o Yes, Puerto Rican
o Yes, Cuban ■
o Yes, other Spanish/Hispanic
(Print one group, for example:
Argentinean, Colombian,
Dominican, Nicaraguan, Salvadoran,
Spaniard, and so on.) ↓

If **Yes, other Spanish/Hispanic,**
print one group ————————→

2. Asked in a survey of low-income women receiving prenatal care in California:

If you are White, Latina (or Hispanic), then what is the country of your birth? Check **one** only.

[ ] United States
[ ] Mexico
[ ] Central America
[ ] Caribbean
[ ] South America
[ ] Spain or Portugal
[ ] Other: _____

An important distinction between the two questions is in the specificity of the responses. The Census Bureau's question provides data on the precise country of birth in South and Central America. The California question asks for less detailed information about these continents but singles out Mexico because of the large number of people of Mexican origin in the state. The two questions also differ in their use of Latino, a term commonly used in California by 1990.

Why do surveyors ask respondents demographic questions? A major reason is to tell who the respondents are. How old are they? Where do they live? What is their race/ethnicity? Demographic data are also useful in helping explain the results of surveys. In a survey of child-rearing practices, you might ask questions like these: Do differences exist among younger and older respondents? Among respondents from differing parts of the country? From differing countries of origin?

Demographic data are also needed to help explore the findings of research and of other surveys. Consider the survey team's task in Example 4.7.

EXAMPLE 4.7
Exploring With Demographics

The community is concerned that many people are not taking advantage of preventive health services like immunizations for children, influenza vaccinations for the elderly, prenatal care, and yearly mammograms for women over 50 years of age. A number of surveys are planned to help explore the barriers that deter people from using these services.

A team has designed the first survey to find out about barriers to the use of prenatal care. Their review of the published research reveals that currently unmarried women begin their care late and do not stay with it continuously. The also have poor birth outcomes. When compared to the babies of married women, the babies of unmarried mothers are more frequently of low weight and premature. The survey team is interested in exploring factors other than (or together with) marital status that may help explain inappropriate use of prenatal care.

The survey team reasons that currently unmarried women may be younger than other women. Births to very young mothers are riskier than other births, so age may be a contributing factor to the poor outcomes. The team also suggests that unmarried women may also be poorer than others, and that being poor is often associated with lack of access to and use of health services. They also consider that education may be a factor in the use of health services. If they find that the women in the community who are currently unmarried are also relatively young, then the surveyors will be especially interested in finding out about the extent of their completed education. Accordingly, the survey team includes demographic questions on women's birth date, income, and education.

Age, Income, and Education

To learn about age, ask for the precise date of birth. If you ask for age, some people will tell you their age that day, and others will tell you their age on their next birthday which happens to be next week. In a survey that takes, say, 6 months to complete, even the most accurate statements of age are difficult to interpret. Suppose you ask Respondent A his age today, Respondent B her age 2 weeks from today, and Respondent C his age 6 months from today. One year from today, you begin to summarize the data. Do you compute the ages on the basis of where the respondents were 12 months ago? Do you make any allowances for the fact that by the time you got around to Respondent C, Respondents A and B had aged? If you have the exact date of birth, you can much more easily compute exact frequencies and averages. You can pick one date, say, 6 months after the start of a 1-year survey, and compute everyone's exact age on that date.

Income questions are often considered "sensitive." In the United States, income is considered a private, even personal matter. Asking for income in surveys requires special handling. One way of protecting the respondent's privacy and yet giving you the data you need is to ask for income in terms of categories, such as between $40,000 and $50,000 or between $50,001 and $60,000. Remember to provide mutually exclusive categories:

Poor: Which best describes your personal income in 1994? Check **one** only.

> [ ] $35,000 or less
> [ ] $35,000 to $55,000
> [ ] $55,000 to $75,000
> [ ] $75,000 or more

Comment: The categories overlap so that a person whose income was $35,000 could correctly choose A or B. The categories for $55,000 and $75,000 overlap as well.

Better: Which best describes your personal income in 1994? Check **one** only.

> [ ] $35,000 or less
> [ ] $35,001 to $55,000
> [ ] $55,001 to $75,000
> [ ] $75,001 or more

When asking income questions with categorical choices, make sure the categories are meaningful. Wealthier people should be given many choices above the median income for the community, whereas poorer people should be given many choices below the median, as illustrated in Example 4.8.

EXAMPLE 4.8
Asking Questions About
Incomes in Two Settings

Setting 1

A survey is being conducted of all people who used Travelmore Travel Agency for three or more trips out of the country that lasted at least 2 weeks. One question asks about household income:

Which of the following best describes *your* income this
current year? Check **one** only.

[ ] $50,000 or less
[ ] $50,001 to $100,000
[ ] $100,001 to $200,000
[ ] $200,001 or more

Setting 2

A survey is being conducted to find out where low-income families obtain mental health services. People are approached outside schools, churches, and supermarkets. One question asks about income:

Which of the following best describes *your* income this
current year? Check **one** only.

[ ] $10,000 or less
[ ] $10,001 to $20,000
[ ] $20,001 to $30,000
[ ] $30,001 or more

Whenever possible, ask for precise information about income. The Census Bureau asks for total income. The respondent is asked to specify and add income from wages, salaries, commissions and tips; self-employment income from farms and other businesses; interest, dividends, rental income, incomes from estates and trusts; royalties, social security, or railroad retirement pay; Supplemental Security Income, Aid to Families with Dependent Children, or other public assistance or welfare; retirement, survivor, or disability pensions; and child support, unemployment benefits, and alimony.

When asking questions about income, you must specify a time period. Do you want to know about average income over 3 years? total income over the past year? You must also decide if you want a particular person's income or the household's. If you want the household income, you must define household as it pertains to income. An infant may be in the household but is not likely to be contributing income to it. Two or more unrelated adults may constitute a household if they contribute to some predefined proportion of the household's income.

Questions about education should be selected to meet the needs of the survey. A survey of physicians' education will have different choices from those given to a broader group of respondents, as illustrated in Example 4.9.

EXAMPLE 4.9
Two Questions About Education

Question 1

A survey of physicians in an academic medical center is interested in finding out how many of them have obtained academic degrees. The survey asks this question:

Do you have any of the following degrees? Circle yes **or** no for each degree listed.

	Yes (1)	No (2)
Master's degree in public health	1	2
Master's degree in business administration	1	2
PhD (specify field: _____)	1	2
Doctor of Dental Surgery	1	2
Juris Doctor	1	2
Doctor of Veterinary Medicine	1	2
Other (specify: _____)	1	2
Other (specify: _____)	1	2

Question 2

A survey of customers at Travelmore Travel Agency asks this question about their education:

How much school have you completed? Check **one** for the highest level completed or degree received. If currently enrolled in school, check the level of previous grade attended or highest degree received.

[ ] 12th grade or less
[ ] High school graduate or equivalent
[ ] Some college but no degree
[ ] Associate degree (academic or occupational)
[ ] Bachelor's degree
[ ] Master's degree
[ ] Professional school degree (such as MD, LLB, JD, DDS, DVM)
[ ] Doctorate (such as PhD, EdD, DrPH)

In a survey of teens' education, specify most categories before 12th grade (such as 9th grade, 8th grade, 7th grade, 6th grade, or lower); you may wish to include "Other" as a category. The following are guidelines for asking questions to get demographic information.

Guidelines for Asking Questions on Vital Statistics and Demographics

- *Learn the characteristics of the survey's targeted respondents.* You do this so that the response categories make sense. You can find out about respondents by checking census data, interviewing the respondents, asking others who know about the respondents, and reviewing recent literature.

- *Decide on appropriate level of specificity.* An appropriate level is one that will meet the needs of the survey but not be too cumbersome for the respondent. Remember, a self-administered survey and telephone interview should have no more than four or five response categories. An interviewer should use visual aids if more than five categories are used.

- *Ask for exact information in an open-ended format.* One way to avoid having many response categories is to ask the respondents to tell you in their own words the answers to demographic questions. Respondents can give their date of birth, age as of a specified date, income, ZIP code, area code, and so on.

- *Use current words and terms.* The words used to describe people's backgrounds change over time. Outmoded words are sometimes offensive. The world's geography changes, and people's affiliations and commitments alter. If you borrow questions from other sources, check to see that they use words in a contemporary way. Terms like "household" and definitions of concepts like wealth and poverty also change over time.

■ *Decide if you want comparability.* If you want to compare one group of respondents with another, consider borrowing questions and response choices from other surveys. For example, if you want to compare the education of people in your survey with the typical American's in 1990, then use the question that was asked in the census. If you borrow questions, check to see that the words and terms are still relevant and that the response choices are meaningful.

Exercises

EXERCISE 1: Read the description of the survey plan and then follow the directions given below it.

Description of Survey Plan

The Outdoors Mail Order Company is planning a mail survey of 150 customers who purchased goods within the past months. A Spanish-language version of the survey will be available upon request. The purpose of the survey is to find out to what extent a market exists for household and kitchen goods with an "outdoors" flavor. For example, many of the fabrics used by the company on furniture and for tablecloths and other linens have patterns of lakes, forests, and mountains. Pots and pans are fashioned after those used on camping trips.

The survey is expected to take no more than 10 minutes and will only use closed-ended questions. All responses will be confidential.

The survey has been designed to answer these questions:

1. How old is the average customer?
2. What proportion of customers live in differing geographic regions of the United States?
3. How many people are willing to purchase each of a selected list of household and kitchen goods sold by the company?
4. On average, how many purchases did customers make in the past 6 months?
5. How satisfied were customers with the service? with the quality of the products?
6. Are differences found in numbers and types of purchases that can be accounted for by age and satisfaction?

The following is an outline of the survey.

Outline for Survey of Market for Household and Kitchen Goods

Topic	Number of Questions	Information Collected
Age	1	Date of birth
Region of the country	1	Northeast, Middle Atlantic, Southeast, Midwest, Northwest, Southwest, West
Kitchen goods	5	Type of kitchen goods would purchase, if any (e.g., furniture, dishes, linens)
Household goods	5	Type of household goods would purchase, if any (e.g., furniture, pictures)
Frequency of past purchases from Outdoors	1	If ever, once before, twice, three or more times
Satisfaction	2	Satisfied with service, with purchase: extremely satisfied to extremely dissatisfied

Directions

Answer these questions using the description of the survey and the outline.

1. Describe the context in which the survey will take place by describing its purpose, respondents, surveyors, responses, timing, resources, and privacy requirements.

2. Write the questions for the survey using the above outline as your guide. (Do not worry about introducing the survey, the order the questions should take, or any special graphic requirements.)

3. For each question in the survey, tell whether you will be obtaining categorical, ordinal, or numerical data.

EXERCISE 2: Write a survey that answers these questions:

1. Does this book achieve each of its stated objectives?

2. On the whole, how helpful were the book's examples in assisting readers to learn?

3. How practical are each of this book's guidelines and checklists?

4. Do readers usually enjoy reading the text and doing the exercises?

5. Do readers who do and do not recommend this book to others have similar school- or job-related responsibilities?

6. Does a difference exist in younger and older readers in terms of their perceptions of the book's helpfulness and practicality?

ANSWERS

EXERCISE 1

1. The Survey's Context

Purpose. The purpose of the survey is to find out if a market exists for kitchen and household goods that are sold by Outdoors and, if so, to characterize it. The characteristics of concern are age, region of the country, willingness to purchase selected kitchen and household goods, frequency of purchases, and satisfaction with purchases and service.

Respondents. The respondents are 150 customers who ordered from the company within the past 6 months.

Surveyor. The mail survey

Responses. A variety of responses can be expected including ratings of satisfaction and categories to describe where people live geographically.

Timing. The survey is to take 10 minutes of each respondent's time.

Resources. A Spanish translation is needed

Privacy. The responses are to be confidential.

2. Questions for the Survey

What is your date of birth?

[   ] [   ] 19 [   ]
Month Day   Year

In which region of the country do you live? Check **one** answer only.

[ ] Northeast
[ ] Middle Atlantic
[ ] Southeast
[ ] Midwest
[ ] Northwest
[ ] Southwest
[ ] West

Check yes **or** no to indicate whether you would purchase each of the following if it had an outdoors theme. By outdoors theme, we mean fabrics that depict lakes, rivers, mountains, and so on and styles that are based on camping, fishing, and hiking gear.

Would you buy each of these kitchen goods if they were similar in appearance to those used when camping, fishing, or hiking and/or if they had an outdoors theme or design?

	Yes (1)	No (2)	Don't Know/ No Opinion (3)
Pots and pans	1	2	3
Flatware (knives, forks, spoons)	1	2	3
Dishes and glasses	1	2	3
Table linens (napkins, placemats, tablecloths)	1	2	3
Floor coverings	1	2	3

Would you buy each of these household goods if they were similar in appearance to those used when camping, fishing, or hiking and/or had an outdoors theme or design?

	Yes (1)	No (2)	Don't Know/ No Opinion (3)
Furniture for the living room	1	2	3
Floor coverings	1	2	3
Pictures and photographs	1	2	3
Bedroom furniture	1	2	3
Furniture for a study or den	1	2	3

In the past 6 months, how many items did you purchase from Outdoors? Select **one** best answer.

[ ] 1
[ ] 2 to 4
[ ] 5 to 10
[ ] More than 10

How satisfied are you with Outdoors' service and quality? Circle **one**.

	Extremely Satisfied (4)	Satisfied (3)	Dissatisfied (2)	Extremely Dissatisfied (1)	No Opinion (0)
Service	4	3	2	1	0
Quality	4	3	2	1	0

3. Types of Data Obtained From Each Question

Date of birth:	numerical
Region of the country:	categorical
Willingness to purchase kitchen goods:	categorical
Willingness to purchase household goods:	categorical
Frequency of purchases:	numerical
Satisfaction with service and quality:	ordinal

EXERCISE 2

1. Does this book achieve each of the following objectives? Answer yes **or** no for each objective.

Objectives for the Reader	Yes (1)	No (2)	Uncertain/ Don't Know (0)
Understand a survey's context (e.g., cultural, economic, political)	1	2	0
Ask valid survey questions	1	2	0
Compare the characteristics of open and closed questions	1	2	0
Distinguish between response formats that use categorical, ordinal, and numerical measurement	1	2	0
Identify questions that are written correctly	1	2	0
Apply techniques for asking questions to learn about behavior	1	2	0
Apply techniques for asking questions to learn about attitudes	1	2	0
Apply techniques for asking questions to learn about knowledge	1	2	0
Apply techniques for asking questions to learn about demographics	1	2	0

2. On the whole, did the book's examples assist you in learning? Please circle **one.**

Definitely yes	1
Probably yes	2
Probably no	3
Definitely no	4
Uncertain/no opinion	5

3. How practical are each of the following guidelines and check-lists for asking survey questions? Please rate the practicality of **each** guideline and checklist using this scale:

1 = Very impractical
2 = Impractical
3 = Practical
4 = Very practical
0 = Uncertain/no opinion

*Please make **one** rating for each*
of the listed guidelines and checklists.

Guidelines					
Guidelines for Asking Survey Questions	1	2	3	4	0
Guidelines for Using Conventional Language When Asking Survey Questions	1	2	3	4	0
Guidelines for Asking Closed Questions With Ordered Responses	1	2	3	4	0
Guidelines for Asking Questions on Vital Statistics and Demographics	1	2	3	4	0
Checklists					
Checklist for Deciding the Survey's Context	1	2	3	4	0
Checklist for Deciding Between Open and Closed Questions	1	2	3	4	0

4. Did you usually enjoy reading the text and doing the exercises? Please rate each.

	Almost Never (1)	Rarely (2)	Sometimes (3)	Frequently (4)	Almost Always (5)
Reading the text	1	2	3	4	5
Doing the exercises	1	2	3	4	5

5. Do you recommend this book to others who have similar responsibilities for asking survey questions? Please circle **one**.

Definitely yes	1
Probably yes	2
Definitely no	3
Probably no	4
Uncertain/no opinion	0

6. For which purposes do you plan to write survey questions? Check all that apply.

[ ] Evaluation/research

[ ] Policy

[ ] Program planning or development

[ ] Needs assessment/marketing

[ ] Other: _____

_____

_____

_____

7. In which settings do you plan to or are you actually asking survey questions? Check all that apply.

　　[　] School, college, or university
　　[　] Government
　　[　] Business
　　[　] Health professions
　　[　] Law
　　[　] Other: _____

　　_____

　　_____

　　_____

8. What is your date of birth? Write 01 for January, 02 for February, and so on. Write 01 for the first day of the month, 02 for the second, and so on.

　　[_ _] Month   [_ _] Date   [19 _ _] Year

Suggested Readings

Babbie, E. (1990). *Survey research methods.* Belmont, CA: Wadsworth.

A fundamental reference on how to conduct survey research. Good examples of survey questions with accompanying rules for asking questions.

Bradburn, N. M., & Sudman, S. (1992). The current status of questionnaire design. In P. N. Biemer, R. M. Groves, L. E. Lyberg, N. A. Mathiowetz, & S. Sudman (Eds.), *Measurement errors in surveys.* New York: John Wiley.

Addresses many of the major issues in designing questionnaires and asking questions.

Converse, J. (1987). *Survey research in the United States.* Berkeley: University of California Press.

An overview and good examples of the how surveys are used in the United States; helpful in understanding the context of survey research.

Fink, A. (1993). *Evaluation fundamentals: Guiding health programs, research and policy.* Newbury Park, CA: Sage.

Gives rules for asking questions and responses; provides a checklist for creating or adapting measures; and discusses the roles of categorical, ordinal, and numerical data in measurement and data analysis.

Fink, A., & Kosecoff, J. (1985). *How to conduct surveys: A step by step guide.* Beverly Hills, CA: Sage.

Gives many examples of survey questions and contains rules and guidelines for asking questions.

Fowler, F. J. (1993). *Survey research methods.* Newbury Park, CA: Sage.

Chapter 6 deals with designing and evaluating survey questions, including defining objectives.

Fowler, F. J., & Mangione, T. W. (1990). *Standardized survey interviewing: Minimizing interviewer related error.* Newbury Park, CA: Sage.

Contains good survey question examples and tells how to minimize error by standardizing the surveyor and the questionnaire.

Frey, J. H. (1989). *Survey research by telephone.* Newbury Park, CA: Sage.

Gives excellent examples of questions and how to get the information you need from telephone surveys.

Kosecoff, J., & Fink, A. (1982). *Evaluation basics: A practitioner's manual.* Beverly Hills, CA: Sage.

Tells how to write questions and how to use them appropriately in open and closed formats.

Lavrakas, P. J. (1987). *Telephone survey methods: Sampling, selection, and supervision.* Newbury Park, CA: Sage.

Discusses questions in the context of telephone surveys.

McDowell, I., & Newell, C. (1987). *Measuring health: A guide to rating scales.* New York: Oxford University Press.

Contains a very good compendium of scales to use in asking questions pertaining to health.

Miller, D. C. (1991). *Handbook of research design and social measurement.* Newbury Park, CA: Sage.

Discusses and defines all possible components of social research. Part 6 has selected sociometric scales and indexes and is a very good source of questions pertaining to social status, group structure, organizational structure, job satisfaction, community, family and marriage, and attitudes.

Schuman, H., & Presser, S. (1981). *Question and answers in attitude surveys.* New York: Academic Press.

Raises and addresses many of the important issues in designing questions about attitudes; contains good examples.

Stewart, A. L., & Ware, J. E. (1992). *Measuring functioning and well-being: The medical outcomes study approach.* Durham, NC: Duke University Press.

Tells of the design and validation of a wide range of self-reported functioning and well-being measures developed for a large U.S. study of health care; very good source of questions.

Sudman, S., & Bradburn, N. M. (1982). *Asking questions.* San Francisco: Jossey-Bass.

Very good source for examples of how to write questions pertaining to attitudes, knowledge, behavior, and demographics.

About the Author

ARLENE FINK, PhD, is Professor of Medicine and Public Health at the University of California, Los Angeles. She is on the Policy Advisory Board of UCLA's Robert Wood Johnson Clinical Scholars Program, a health research scientist at the Veterans Administration Medical Center in Sepulveda, California, and president of Arlene Fink Associates. She has conducted evaluations throughout the United States and abroad and has trained thousands of health professionals, social scientists, and educators in program evaluation. Her published works include nearly 100 monographs and articles on evaluation methods and research. She is coauthor of *How to Conduct Surveys* and author of *Evaluation Fundamentals: Guiding Health Programs, Research, and Policy* and *Evaluation for Education and Psychology.*

HOW TO CONDUCT
SELF-ADMINISTERED
AND
MAIL SURVEYS

THE SURVEY KIT

Purpose: The purposes of this 9-volume Kit are to enable readers to prepare and conduct surveys and become better users of survey results. Surveys are conducted to collect information by asking questions of people on the telephone, face-to-face, and by mail. The questions can be about attitudes, beliefs, and behavior as well as socioeconomic and health status. To do a good survey also means knowing how to ask questions, design the survey (research) project, sample respondents, collect reliable and valid information, and analyze and report the results. You also need to know how to plan and budget for your survey.

Users: The Kit is for students in undergraduate and graduate classes in the social and health sciences and for individuals in the public and private sectors who are responsible for conducting and using surveys. Its primary goal is to enable users to prepare surveys and collect data that are accurate and useful for primarily practical purposes. Sometimes, these practical purposes overlap the objectives of scientific research, and so survey researchers will also find the Kit useful.

Format of the Kit: All books in the series contain instructional objectives, exercises and answers, examples of surveys in use and illustrations of survey questions, guidelines for action, checklists of do's and don'ts, and annotated references.

Volumes in The Survey Kit:

1. **The Survey Handbook**
   Arlene Fink

2. **How to Ask Survey Questions**
   Arlene Fink

3. **How to Conduct Self-Administered and Mail Surveys**
   Linda B. Bourque and *Eve P. Fielder*

4. **How to Conduct Interviews by Telephone and in Person**
   James H. Frey and *Sabine Mertens Oishi*

5. **How to Design Surveys**
   Arlene Fink

6. **How to Sample in Surveys**
   Arlene Fink

7. **How to Measure Survey Reliability and Validity**
   Mark S. Litwin

8. **How to Analyze Survey Data**
   Arlene Fink

9. **How to Report on Surveys**
   Arlene Fink

THE SURVEY KIT
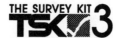
TSK 3

HOW TO CONDUCT SELF-ADMINISTERED AND MAIL SURVEYS

LINDA B. BOURQUE &
EVE P. FIELDER

SAGE Publications
International Educational and Professional Publisher
Thousand Oaks   London   New Delhi

For information address:

 SAGE Publications, Inc.
2455 Teller Road
Thousand Oaks, California 91320
E-mail: order@sagepub.com

SAGE Publications Ltd.
6 Bonhill Street
London EC2A 4PU
United Kingdom

SAGE Publications India Pvt. Ltd.
M-32 Market
Greater Kailash I
New Delhi 110 048 India

Printed in the United States of America

Library of Congress Cataloging-in-Publication Data

Main entry under title:

The survey kit.
    p. cm.
    Includes bibliographical references.
    Contents: v. 1. The survey handbook / Arlene Fink — v. 2. How to ask survey questions / Arlene Fink — v. 3. How to conduct self-administered and mail surveys / Linda B. Bourque, Eve P. Fielder — v. 4. How to conduct interviews by telephone and in person / James H. Frey, Sabine Mertens Oishi — v. 5. How to design surveys / Arlene Fink — v. 6. How to sample in surveys / Arlene Fink — v. 7. How to measure survey reliability and validity / Mark S. Litwin — v. 8. How to analyze survey data / Arlene Fink — v. 9. How to report on surveys / Arlene Fink.
    ISBN 0-8039-7388-8 (pbk. : The survey kit : alk. paper)
    1. Social surveys. 2. Health surveys. I. Fink, Arlene.
HN29.S724   1995
300'.723—dc20   95-12712

This book is printed on acid-free paper.

95 96 97 98 99 10 9 8 7 6 5 4 3 2 1

Sage Production Editor: Diane S. Foster
Sage Copy Editor: Joyce Kuhn
Sage Typesetter: Janelle LeMaster

Contents

Acknowledgments

We would like to thank Arlene Fink for her invitation to participate in this series and her helpful comments on earlier drafts of this manuscript; Tonya Hays, Terry Silberman, and Elizabeth Stephenson for their assistance in finding materials used in examples; Marilyn Hart and Christopher Corey for technical assistance; and Gloria Krauss for clerical and editing assistance. We particularly want to thank Deborah Riopelle, Project Coordinator for the Workplace Assault Study, for her assistance in putting together examples from that study; Maggie Robbins of the Service Employees International Union (SEIU), Bart Deiner of SEIU Local 660, and Wilma Cadorna of SEIU Local 535 who expedited the development and administration of the Workplace Assault Study.

The respondent letter used for the college student survey came from a study conducted by Jim Sidanius and Marilynn Brewer, funded by the Russell Sage Foundation (Attitudes About Cultural Diversity Among a College Population, Grant No. RSF 879.301). Data used in examples from the Prospective Evaluation for Radial Keratotomy (PERK) Study were collected and processed with funds from the National Eye Institute (Grant Nos. EY03752 and EY03761); data used in examples from the Workplace Assault Study were collected and processed with funds from the Southern California Injury Prevention Research Center under Grant No. R49-CCR903622 from the Centers for Disease Control.

How to Conduct Self-Administered and Mail Surveys: Learning Objectives

The aim of this book is to demonstrate how to develop and administer self-administered and mail surveys. Areas covered are the kinds of self-administered questionnaires, the circumstances under which they are appropriately used, and the skills needed in designing them, estimating their cost, selecting appropriate samples, and documenting the decisions made.

The specific objectives are to:

■ Describe the types of self-administered questionnaires

■ Identify the advantages and disadvantages of self-administered questionnaires

■ Decide whether a self-administered questionnaire is appropriate for your survey question

■ Determine the content of the questionnaire

■ Develop questions for a "user-friendly" questionnaire

■ Pretest, pilot-test, and revise questions

■ Format a "user-friendly" questionnaire

■ Write advance letters and cover letters that motivate and increase response rate

- Write specifications that describe the reasons for and sources of the questions on the questionnaire and the methodology used in administering the study

- Describe how to develop and produce a sample, identify potential resources for a sample, organize the sample, determine sample sizes, and increase response rate

- Inventory materials and procedures involved in mail and self-administered surveys

- Describe follow-up procedures for nonrespondents, methods of tracking a respondent, and number and timing of follow-up attempts

- Describe how returned questionnaires are processed, edited, and coded

- Describe data entry

- Describe how records are kept

- Estimate the costs of a self-administered or mailed survey

- Estimate personnel needs for a self-administered or mailed survey

- Fully document the development and administration of the questionnaire and the data collected with it

1

Overview of Self-Administered Questionnaires

Self-administered questionnaires are one of the most frequently used methods for collecting data in research studies. Furthermore, self-administered questionnaires appear in many areas of our lives. Think, for example, of the testing strategies used in most classrooms from kindergarten through graduate school. Classroom tests are a type of self-administered questionnaire. Similarly, we fill out forms or "questionnaires" to obtain everything from a driver's license to a death certificate.

Unfortunately, this very proliferation and familiarity of self-administered "questionnaires" in a wide variety of daily life settings results in neophyte surveyors often assuming that they can develop a self-administered questionnaire literally overnight and use it to collect data that will be available immediately. Like any research endeavor and the use of any procedure for collecting data, the development and administration of self-administered questionnaires takes time and thought. This book outlines the circumstances under which self-administered questionnaires provide a good or at least an adequate method for collecting information, what must be considered in designing such questionnaires, and the methods used in administering them while maximizing the collection of complete, reliable, and valid data.

Types of Self-Administered Questionnaires

A self-administered questionnaire is an instrument used to collect information from people who complete the instrument themselves. The stimulus is exclusively visual. As we noted at the outset, such instruments are not used exclusively for research purposes but can be used to collect information for a wide variety of purposes and in a wide variety of settings. To date, self-administered questionnaires have almost always been administered using paper-and-pencil techniques, but with the rapid proliferation of computers and the information superhighway it is likely that such procedures will increasingly be adapted to electronic mediums. To the extent that such developments occur, it is entirely possible that auditory stimuli could be added to the visual in soliciting information through such means in much the same way that sophisticated voice-mail systems now route telephone requests for information, service, or appointments. For the purposes of this book, however, we will stick with the traditional method by which such questionnaires have been historically administered—namely, each respondent receives a printed questionnaire, which is filled out using a pen or pencil.

There are two types of self-administered questionnaires, best described as the ends of a unidimensional continuum. At one end are questionnaires that people answer in the presence of the surveyor or other supervising personnel. At the opposite end of the continuum are questionnaires completed by the respondent outside the presence of the surveyor or other monitoring personnel.

Questionnaires sent through the mail provide the most common example of unsupervised administration. Such questionnaires—frequently called "mail questionnaires"—are the major focus of this book both because of their frequent use and because almost everything that applies to a mail questionnaire has equal applicability to self-administered questionnaires distributed through other means and administered in other environments. Before turning our attention to mail questionnaires, we briefly describe some of the different kinds of supervised or partially supervised environments in which self-administered questionnaires are distributed.

SUPERVISED ADMINISTRATION

One-to-One Supervision

In the most extreme form of group administration, the respondent is in a one-to-one situation with the surveyor and the surveyor is available to answer any questions that the respondent has about the questionnaire. This type of administration is rarely used because, as we discuss later, a major reason for using self-administered questionnaires is to reduce costs. The costs associated with one-to-one administration would more closely resemble those of telephone or personal interviewing than those of self-administration.

Nonetheless, one-to-one supervision is, on occasion, used—often within the context of a study where face-to-face interviewing provides the major method of data collection. For example, under the auspices of the National Institute for Drug Abuse (NIDA) self-administered questionnaires were developed for use in ascertaining respondents' current and historical use of drugs. The questionnaires were given to respondents as part of a face-to-face interview. Their format was such that the time taken to complete the questionnaire did not differ with current or past drug history. In other words, persons who had never used drugs took just as long to complete the questionnaire as did those who had used many drugs. Within the context of the face-to-face interview, elaborate procedures were developed to ensure that the interviewer did not see the questionnaire either while it was being completed or once it was completed. The purpose here was to maximize confidentiality, the assumption being that people generally underreport the use of drugs. At the same time, the interviewer was available to answer questions or to clarify concepts should it be necessary.

Group Administration

Far more common is the situation where questionnaires are passed out in a classroom, workplace, or other group setting. Each person is expected to complete the questionnaire without consulting other persons in the group, but the surveyor or other supervisory person is available to provide introductory instructions, answer questions, and monitor the extent to which questionnaires are completed and individual respondents communicate with each other during the period of administration. Depending on the purpose of the study, the administrator may be instructed to answer and clarify any and all questions that come up or may be instructed to defer or deflect all or most questions.

For example, when group self-administration is being used to develop a questionnaire, the surveyor will probably want to learn as much as possible about how the questionnaire "works," whether respondents understand the questions asked, whether the information requested is accessible to respondents, and whether the response categories provided are exhaustive, mutually exclusive, and readily understood. In such instances, the surveyor may invite respondents to raise questions as they move through the questionnaire, or, alternatively, the surveyor may ask the respondents to first complete the questionnaire and then solicit questions, comments, and problems as part of a general discussion following the administration of the questionnaire. In either case, the person supervising the group administration must keep careful notes of the issues raised by respondents because many of the questions and comments may necessitate changes in the questionnaire.

When, in contrast, a finalized questionnaire is being administered in a group setting, supervisory personnel often are instructed to deflect any questions or comments raised by respondents. Many of the instruments used to measure attitudes, opinions, physical health status, psychological distress, and a number of other things were developed to be administered as paper-and-pencil tests in either individual or group settings. Generally, these instruments have been developed over time and with substantial attention to establishing the validity and reliability of the measure. They also were developed to assess how a particular individual respondent compares with other groups of respondents.

When such instruments are administered, the surveyor wants to do everything possible to ensure that each respondent gets an identical stimulus and that the information obtained represents that individual's feelings, attitudes, or health status. In such cases, the administrator in a group setting will generally have a scripted set of instructions used to introduce the questionnaire. These instructions may or may not be repeated on the questionnaire itself. Included in the instructions will be a statement to the effect that there are no right or wrong answers to the questions being asked, that the purpose is to find out how this particular person feels about or experiences the topic under investigation, and, when pertinent, instructions are given on how to complete the questionnaire.

Semisupervised Administration

In group administrations, as described above, it is assumed for our purposes that everyone is in the same place—usually a room—for the duration of the administration period or at least for the beginning part of it. Everyone hears the same set of verbal instructions, and everyone's questions or comments are handled in a similar way. Self-administered questionnaires are also distributed in an almost infinite variety of semisupervised administrations. For example, questionnaires might be distributed in the waiting room of a well-baby clinic by a receptionist. In such a situation, no formal presentation of verbal instructions will be given to the potential group of respondents as a whole. Rather, the receptionist will give each respondent pertinent instructions when the questionnaire is passed out. Because personnel may change during the week and the activity level in the clinic will vary, the content and extent of instructions that a given respondent receives is also likely to vary. Respondents who arrive when the clinic is quiet may receive detailed instructions, whereas those who arrive when the patient load is heavy may receive no instructions. Clearly, the constancy of the stimulus provided in such situations, at least as indicated in instructions, has the potential to influence the validity and reliability of the data obtained. Nonetheless, someone—namely, the receptionist—is, at least titularly, available to answer questions about the questionnaire and monitor the data collection effort at some minimal level.

Questionnaires are also passed out in environments such as registration lines, auditoriums, amusement centers, and airplanes and as persons are entering or exiting a store or other site. Such questionnaires can also be considered "semisupervised" to the extent that the person who distributes and collects the questionnaires is available to answer questions or provide instructions. The amount of control the surveyor exerts in such an environment is, however, limited to the selection of who will receive a questionnaire, the ability to ensure that distributed questionnaires are completed and returned, and the consistency with which any verbal instructions beyond those printed on the hard copy of the questionnaire are, in fact, solicited by or available to respondents.

UNSUPERVISED ADMINISTRATION

To our knowledge, no statistics exist regarding the number of self-administered questionnaires that are used in research projects or how they distribute between supervised and unsupervised administration, but when people think of self-administered questionnaires within a research context, in all probability they are referring to questionnaires sent through the mail, which is the primary method by which unsupervised questionnaires are administered.

When a questionnaire is administered in a completely unsupervised administration, it is imperative that the questionnaire be completely self-sufficient, or able to "stand alone." When questionnaires are sent through the mail, no member of the research staff is available to answer questions or ensure that the correct person completes the questionnaire or, indeed, that anyone completes it. Even though the questionnaire's cover sheet can include a contact name and phone number for the potential respondent's use if clarification or information is needed, the respondent must initiate such contacts. Hence, the motivation to seek information must be high.

The remainder of this book focuses on the design of mail questionnaires because the requirement that they be able to stand alone places greater restrictions on what can be included in them and requires the surveyor to pay careful attention to how clearly the questionnaire is written and presented so as to maximize the response rate.

A summary of the advantages and disadvantages of using the aforementioned ways of administering questionnaires is provided in Example 1.1.

EXAMPLE 1.1
Four Ways of Administering
Respondent-Completed Questionnaires

Type of Administration	Advantages	Disadvantages
One-to-one	Interviewer available to answer questions Maximizes confidentiality in face-to-face interviews Provides in-depth data on the answerability of questions	Expensive
Group	Consistent instructions Simultaneous administration to all respondents Administrator can answer questions Provides some information on the answerability of questions Monitor communication between respondents Monitor completion by respondents Useful in pretesting	Not usable with general populations

Type of Administration	Advantages	Disadvantages
Semisupervised	Administrator can answer questions Efficient Some ability to monitor communication between respondent and others Some ability to monitor completion Useful in pretesting Inexpensive	Samples are frequently unrepresentative Inconsistent instructions
Unsupervised	Consistent stimulus to all respondents Possibility of more representative samples	No control over who responds No direct information on answerability of questions Questionnaire must stand alone

Advantages of Self-Administered Questionnaires

COST

The single greatest advantage of self-administered questionnaires is their lower cost compared to other methods (e.g., in-person and telephone interviews). Given the same-length questionnaire and same objective, a completed questionnaire administered by mail costs approximately 50% less than one administered by telephone and 75% less than one administered by personal interview.

SAMPLE RELATED

Mail questionnaires have three sample-related advantages: geographic coverage, larger samples, and wider coverage within a sample population. Although the three are interrelated, both with each other and with issues of cost, each advantage is briefly recognized.

Geographic Coverage

Mail questionnaires allow for wider geographic coverage. This is particularly true when mail questionnaires are compared to personal or face-to-face interviewing. A questionnaire can be mailed anywhere in the world, whereas face-to-face interviews tend to be restricted to a defined geographic area or areas where trained interviewers are available, can be monitored, and are able to physically contact intended respondents. Telephone interviewing also allows for a wider geographic coverage and, for all practical intents and purposes, can be conducted anywhere within the United States from a single site, assuming that funds are available for covering long-distance charges and the population under study has access to telephones. Telephone interviewing becomes problematic, however, if a substantial number of the designated respondents reside outside the United States.

For example, we used mail questionnaires to contact both undergraduate and graduate alumni of UCLA. Although most potential respondents lived in the United States (many of them in Southern California), a certain proportion of both groups resided in other countries. Because little money was available for either study, data collection using either telephone or face-to-face interviewing techniques would have prevented any attempt to obtain information from non-U.S. residents. In contrast, sending questionnaires through the mail allowed a substantial proportion of such respondents to be contacted and yielded response rates comparable to those of the sample as a whole.

Larger Samples

The lower unit cost of a mail questionnaire combined with its ability to cover a wider geographic area with little additional cost for respondents at a distance allows surveyors to study a larger sample of persons or groups. Thus, where available funds might allow for only 100 persons within a limited geographic area to be interviewed, they may allow for questionnaires to be mailed to 400-500 persons over a much larger geographic area.

Wider Coverage Within a Sample Population

Some people are reluctant to talk with people either in person or on the phone. This reluctance to talk with strangers has increased particularly in large urban areas. For example, it may be difficult or impossible to get residents of high-security buildings to agree to be interviewed—particularly if the interview is to be conducted in the home. These same persons may, however, be willing to respond to a mail questionnaire. Similarly, some persons do not have access to telephones or are reluctant to be interviewed by telephone. Again, some percentage of these persons may be willing and able to respond to a self-administered questionnaire.

In some cases, respondents are much more willing to complete a self-administered questionnaire when it can be done at their convenience rather than having to make a commitment to an interviewer to be available at an appointed time for a specific length of time to do an interview.

IMPLEMENTATION

Mail and other self-administered questionnaires are much easier to implement than other kinds of questionnaires. First, the number of personnel needed is substantially less because interviewers and those who hire, train, and supervise them are not needed. As is discussed in Chapter 2, self-administered questionnaires are shorter and simpler in structure, so fewer personnel and less complicated procedures are required for processing data once obtained. In contrast to telephone interviewing and particularly computer-assisted telephone interviewing (CATI), minimal equipment is needed to conduct a study by mail. In the simplest case, a single person can conduct an entire mail survey from start to finish.

TIMING

Unlike almost all other methods of data collection, it can be assumed that when a questionnaire is sent through the mail all members of the sample receive it simultaneously. Thus, the potential influence of events outside or unrelated to the study that might influence a potential respondent's experiences, opinions, or attitudes are reduced and can be assumed to be equal for all recipients of the questionnaire. For example, in our study of assault in the workplace, all questionnaires were mailed on the same day and were received by all respondents within the same 2- or 3-day period. Imagine telephone interviews being conducted with the same group of respondents. It is generally not possible to conduct 1,000 telephone interviews within a 2- or 3-day period—more likely, it would take weeks or even months.

Suppose that during that period of time an employee of the Los Angeles County Health Department is assaulted on the job and this assault is prominently featured in the *Los Angeles*

Times. Clearly, persons interviewed *after* the assault are likely to have different attitudes and opinions about assault in the workplace than those interviewed *before* the assault. The questionnaire that the two groups of respondents received cannot be assumed to have had an identical impact on their responses. In contrast, had the questionnaires been mailed on the same day, they can be assumed to have created a similar stimulus for all potential respondents. That is not to say that an event cannot occur at some point during the conduct of a mailed survey; however, the "window of opportunity" is greatly lessened.

SENSITIVE TOPICS

Earlier, we discussed the use of self-administered questionnaires to collect information about drug use within the context of an interview. Many surveyors believe that people are more likely to give complete and truthful information on sensitive topics if a self-administered questionnaire rather than an interview is used. Early methodological studies tended to support this perception on the part of surveyors, but more recent studies suggest that sensitive information may be collected as effectively or with even greater accuracy through telephone and face-to-face interviews.

The reason for the variation in findings across time and studies probably relates to the overall objectives of studies, the environments in which they are conducted, the ability of interviewers to establish rapport, the extent to which respondents believe that the data provided is both anonymous and confidential, and the ways in which both the overall questionnaire and individual questions are structured. We are of the opinion that sensitive topics can be effectively studied using all kinds of questionnaires.

Disadvantages of Self-Administered Questionnaires

Mail and self-administered questionnaires have a number of disadvantages that limit or prohibit their use in many research projects. These disadvantages can be grouped under three general headings: sample related, questionnaire construction, and administration.

SAMPLE RELATED

Availability of Lists

Although self-administered questionnaires are administered to admittedly nonrepresentative convenience samples, many surveyors want to use self-administered questionnaires and particularly mail questionnaires to collect data from samples that can be considered representative of the population from which they were drawn. The ability to do this—particularly when questionnaires are sent through the mail—is dependent on having a complete and accurate list of the population. To the extent that lists are unavailable, incomplete, or inaccurate, the data obtained cannot be assumed to represent the population to which the surveyor wishes to generalize.

In the worst-case scenario, the surveyor must either resort to other methods of sample generation and data collection (e.g., random digit dialing and telephone interviewing), conduct a census to establish the population from which the sample is to be drawn, or resort to convenience sampling techniques.

Response Rates

One of the greatest and most studied disadvantages to mail questionnaires is their low response rate. When a single mailing that incorporates no incentives is made to a sample of the general community, the surveyor can probably expect no better than a 20% response rate. The use of premailings, follow-up contacts, incentives, targeted populations, and a variety of other procedures combine to increase response rates, but even in the best case, response rates for mail questionnaires will be lower than those for telephone and face-to-face interviews.

Literacy and Language

One of the reasons why response rates are poor—particularly in studies targeted at general community samples—is because persons who are illiterate or who have difficulty reading simply are unable to respond even if they want to. The rate of adult illiteracy in the United States is estimated to be 20%. Obviously, persons who are functionally illiterate will be unable to complete a self-administered questionnaire and will be missed in *any* study in which they are part of the target population.

Visual acuity of the respondent can have an effect on response. Individuals who have problems with reading, such as the elderly, the visually impaired, or the dyslexic, may find the effort required to read the questionnaire too great and may not complete and return it to the surveyor. Obviously, if the target population tends to overrepresent any of these groups, it may be wise to consider an alternative method for collecting the data.

An additional problem—particularly in large urban areas on the East and West Coast—is the wide range of languages spoken in the home. For example, in Los Angeles County, 13% of the population is linguistically isolated—meaning that they speak no English—and an additional 28% report that a language other than English is the primary or only language spoken in the home. Obviously, when target populations include substantial proportions of respondents who are non-

English speakers, self-administered questionnaires must be translated and some mechanism devised for ensuring that each respondent receives a questionnaire in the correct language. As a result, data from multiple-language populations generally cannot be adequately or accurately collected using self-administered questionnaires.

QUESTIONNAIRE CONSTRUCTION

Objective

Self-administered questionnaires can be used only when the objective of the study is clear and not complex. For example, you would not want to use a mail questionnaire if you needed to collect an entire occupational history on respondents and wanted to investigate their satisfaction with their current worksite, job, employment benefits, and co-workers, and how these factors correlated with or interacted with lifestyle.

Obviously, surveyors hope to have motivated subjects in any research study, but motivation is particularly important when self-administered questionnaires are used for data collection. In the case of the workplace assault study, we decided that mail questionnaires could be used because union representatives informed us that many of their members had expressed concern about the physical safety of the environments where they worked. Thus, we believed that the topic under study would be considered important by potential respondents and that this heightened salience of the topic would increase respondents' motivation to participate in the study and hence increase our response rate.

Format

The need for a clear and noncomplex data-collection objective has ramifications for how the questionnaire is constructed and precludes the use of many strategies typically used in designing questionnaires. Chapters 2 through 4 discuss this issue in detail, so only some of these limitations are briefly noted here.

First, self-administered questionnaires must be shorter than questionnaires administered in other ways. If the questionnaire must be shorter, then obviously the number of questions asked and topics covered is reduced.

Second, the questions on self-administered questionnaires must be closed-ended ones. Although highly motivated respondents may be willing to answer a few open-ended questions, the surveyor who writes a self-administered questionnaire dominated by open-ended questions will find that few questionnaires will be returned and that those that are returned will frequently have substantial amounts of missing or irrelevant data.

Third, the questionnaire must "stand alone." In other words, all the information that the potential respondent needs to answer the questions must be provided on the questionnaire itself, as there is no interviewer available to clarify instructions or provide additional information to eliminate confusion. The objective is to make the questionnaire as easy as possible for the respondent to complete without assistance from others. This restriction means that cue cards or other visual aids cannot be used with self-administered questionnaires. It also means that the number of possible responses to a question must be limited to a number that can be readily assimilated by respondents and from which they can reasonably select those that apply to them. Thus, the need to create exhaustive lists of mutually exclusive responses may be impossible if the list becomes excessively long. Nor is it reasonable to expect respondents to rank order large numbers of alternatives. Not only are such lists burdensome for respondents to read, assimilate, and select from, but the issue of *primacy effect* becomes relevant. By primacy effect we mean respondents' tendency to select the *first* response they come to that reflects how they feel or behave even if it is not the best or most representative response available. Once a response is selected, the respondent ignores the rest of the list and goes to the next question. The necessity that the questionnaire be totally self-explanatory is probably one of the most difficult objectives to achieve in designing self-administered questionnaires.

Fourth, as part of the objective of simplifying the task for respondents, the surveyor needs to create a questionnaire without branches or skips. In other words, every question asked in the questionnaire should contain a response category that each respondent can comfortably use to describe his or her attitudes, behavior, knowledge, or characteristics. In some instances, this means that a "not applicable" alternative must be included among the responses provided for a question or series of questions.

Order Effects

When questionnaires are administered by telephone or face-to-face interviewer, the interviewer controls the order in which the questions are asked and controls whether or not the answer alternatives are made available to respondents—either by reading aloud the alternatives or by presenting them in written form on a cue card. In a self-administered questionnaire, everything is simultaneously available to the respondent. As a result, respondents can complete sections of the questionnaire in any order they choose, can refer to other sections in providing answers, and can complete the questionnaire over a series of days or even weeks. Thus, the surveyor cannot use self-administered questionnaires when one set of questions is likely to "contaminate," "bias," or "influence" answers to another section of the questionnaire.

For example, political scientists and politicians often are interested in knowing what the members of a community perceive to be the greatest problems facing their community today. What is typically asked next in the interview is a series of questions to ascertain respondents' concern over specific problems the surveyor assumes face that community. When respondents have the ability to look ahead in an interview and see the topics the surveyor selects as problems for their community, they are more likely to respond by selecting the topics that are specifically selected out later in the interview.

Similarly, it is not possible to build validity checks into a self-administered questionnaire. If, for example, the surveyor is suspicious that respondents are more likely to underreport their age when asked "How old were you on your last birthday?" than when they are asked "When were you born?", a self-administered questionnaire would not be a good way to check the "match" between the answers given to the two questions because respondents can compare their answers and change them to be consistent, if necessary. Opportunities to change answers are significantly reduced or even eliminated when interviewers control the order in which questions are asked and have been given instructions regarding the legitimacy of letting a respondent "change" an answer to a question.

ADMINISTRATION

No Control Over Who Responds

The single biggest administrative disadvantage to mail questionnaires is the fact that once the questionnaire leaves the surveyor's office, he or she has no control over who, in fact, fills it out and whether that person "consults" with others when completing it. Thus, in the Workplace Assault Study, we had a list of persons and addresses that was provided by the union. We addressed our cover letter and envelope to one union person. Once we sent the questionnaires out, however, we had no way to be sure that the designated respondent, who was a member of the union, completed the questionnaire and, furthermore, completed it without talking about it with other members of his or her household, workplace, or social group.

We know of one study conducted many years ago where questionnaires were passed out by a receptionist in a clinic waiting room. One day, the surveyor happened to walk through the waiting room just as one waiting patient was reading the questions to the rest of the waiting patients, who were then essentially "voting" on what answer should be selected. The resultant answers essentially represented a consensus of those available in the waiting room at that time rather than the opinions or behaviors of the person completing the questionnaire. Needless to say, the surveyor quickly changed his mode of administering questionnaires to a system that allowed for greater control over the number and identity of the persons completing the questionnaire. Unfortunately, when questionnaires are mailed, the surveyor has no way of checking up on these issues and must accept completed questionnaires "on faith."

Quick Turnaround

Earlier, we said that one of the advantages of mail questionnaires is that it can be assumed that all of them were administered on the same date and that all respondents received the questionnaire on the same date. In general, this means that data collected by mail will be more quickly completed than data collected by telephone or in face-to-face interviews.

There are exceptions to this. Generally, it takes a minimum of 2 weeks after each mailing for completed questionnaires to be returned to the surveyor. To the extent that the surveyor tries to maximize a good response rate by using follow-up mailings and telephone calls, the data collection period may extend to 2 or 3 months. In contrast, it is possible to conduct a telephone survey literally "overnight" if the surveyor has the resources necessary to hire a large number of interviewers and the necessary number of telephones *and if* the surveyor is willing to sacrifice a certain representativeness of the sample obtained. If, for example, all data are collected in one night from a sample of 500 persons, it clearly means that persons not at home that night have no chance of being in the sample. Also, persons whose lines were busy at the time of the attempted call will likely not be in the sample because, unlike regular telephone surveys, little or no redialing is done.

However, for interviews about fast-breaking events such as the Oklahoma City bombing on April 19, 1995, a quick telephone survey is the only way to measure rapidly changing opinions.

Self-Administered Questionnaires by Example: Assault and Vision Studies

The remainder of this book explains and describes how self-administered questionnaires are developed and administered. Two ongoing studies are used as examples.

The questionnaire used in the first study examined the extent to which members of two locals of the Service Employees International Union (SEIU) perceived their workplace sites as safe, the incidence of physical assaults experienced while at work during the preceding year, and the incidence of threats of assault within the past month. Questionnaires were sent by mail to the homes of a stratified random sample of 1,744 potential respondents on January 17, 1995 (for more information on stratified random sampling, see **How to Design Surveys** and **How to Sample in Surveys,** Vols. 5 and 6, respectively, in this series).

The questionnaire used in the second study examined the visual functioning, satisfaction, and experiences with side effects following radial keratotomy. Radial keratotomy is a surgical procedure that reduces myopia, or nearsightedness, by making slices in the patient's cornea. The questionnaire used here was administered as part of the 10-year follow-up examination in the Prospective Evaluation of Radial Keratotomy (PERK) Study, a multisite clinical trial of the 435 respondents who entered the study. In this study, questionnaires were administered at one of the nine clinical sites by clinic coordinators (for more information on clinical trials and other survey designs, see **How to Design Surveys** and **How to Sample in Surveys,** Vols. 5 and 6, respectively, in this series).

To reflect the normal progress and problems often associated with the design of data collection instruments, we discuss what worked, what did not work, and what could have been improved in our two questionnaires. Although most of our examples are drawn from these two studies, examples are also drawn from other studies where appropriate.

2 Content of the Questionnaire

This chapter begins by describing the types of data that can be collected using a questionnaire and how decisions are made regarding whether a mail questionnaire is an appropriate means of collecting data. The remainder of the chapter focuses on developing the content of the questionnaire.

Information Included in Questionnaires and Deciding Whether a Mail Questionnaire Is Appropriate

Studies of people generally collect data in one or more of five areas: personal information about the respondents, their environment, behaviors, experiences or status, and thoughts or feelings. We also sometimes think of studies focusing on people's knowledge, attitudes, and behaviors. One of the worst things that can happen to surveyors when getting ready to analyze their data is to discover that they failed to collect an essential piece of information. The first type of data is frequently referred to as **demographic data** (see **How to Ask Survey Questions,** Vol. 2 in this series, for more information on demographic data). Demographic data include such things as gender, completed education, occupational status, ethnic or racial identification, religious affiliation, and marital status. Inexperienced surveyors often forget to collect data on one or more of these important demographic variables.

The other four types of data, alone or in combination, usually form the focus of the research question. In our study on workplace assault, people are asked about their experiences —namely, were they assaulted or threatened?—their work environment, and demographic information—namely, gender, age, and the type of job they do. We hypothesize that reports of assaults and threats will be associated with the workplace environment and possibly certain demographic characteristics.

Three kinds of information must be evaluated in assessing whether or not data can be collected by mail or self-administered questionnaire. These are the literacy level of the targeted population, the motivation level of the targeted population, and whether characteristics of the research question make it amenable to data collection using a mail questionnaire.

LITERACY

In Chapter 1, we pointed out that mail questionnaires can be used only with literate respondents who are assumed to be highly motivated about the topic being studied. We have used mail questionnaires to study undergraduate and graduate alumni of UCLA. Clearly, such respondents meet the criterion of being literate. In contrast, mail questionnaires would not be a good means of studying participants in the Women, Infants, and Children's (WIC) supplemental feeding programs. WIC participants must meet a "means test" to qualify for the program. In California in 1994, the cutoff for participation was 185% of the poverty level. This meant that the annual income for a family of four could not exceed $27,380. Because income is correlated with education, a substantial number of the women enrolled in the WIC program did not complete high school, and many must be assumed to be functionally illiterate. Thus, self-administered or mail questionnaires would not be a good way to collect information about WIC participants.

MOTIVATION

Much more difficult to determine is whether a target population is motivated to answer the questionnaire. Certainly, one indication of motivation is that a group decides it needs to find out something about itself. For example, in the study of assault in the workplace, union members expressed concern about their vulnerability to assault and sought out methods by which they could do a needs assessment.

Another indicator of motivation is the amount of loyalty that individuals have to the group being studied. Using the criterion of loyalty suggests that mail questionnaires can be more successfully administered to identifiable groups—for example, alumni of UCLA, members of a professional organization, and members of a church—than to general populations.

The strength of appeal conveyed in the cover letter of the mailing can serve to motivate compliance. Developing a cover letter is discussed in Chapter 4.

AMENABLE TO STUDY

Four characteristics of a research question make it amenable to study using a mail questionnaire. First, the topic must be "contained"—that is, it must be one that can be reasonably covered in a relatively short and focused questionnaire instrument. For example, the study has a single objective, and all the "sections" of the questionnaire interrelate and work together to achieve that objective. In the Workplace Assault Study, the focus is exclusively on that—assault in the workplace. We are not trying to find out about assaults in nonworkplace environments, nor are we trying to find out other things about the workplace—for example, whether the respondents consider their jobs boring or challenging, why they chose this particular job, or even how long they have worked at the job.

Second, self-administered questionnaires generally work best when the focus is in the present. What is the respondent doing *now*? What do they know *now*? How do they feel *now*? In the Workplace Assault Study, we are not trying to find out the respondents' employment history or how and why they selected this particular career path. Rather, we *are* asking respondents about what happened to them in the past year (e.g., were they assaulted?) or in the past month (e.g., were they threatened?). Our hope is that our respondents' concerns about vulnerability to assault will result in them being highly motivated and therefore increase their willingness to complete a questionnaire that asks them to remember events that are somewhat in the past. In other words, we are assuming that the **salience** of the topic is sufficiently motivating to overcome certain other characteristics of the study that would usually argue against using a mail questionnaire.

Third, ideally the surveyor structures the questionnaire so that everyone answers every question. This can be done in one of two ways. The better of the two that the topic studied allows creation of closed-ended response lists for *every* question, thus enabling all members of the sample to describe themselves. This is sometimes accomplished by writing a question and including what is essentially a "not applicable" category as one of the response categories. For example, in our study of vision and how people use their eyes, we *failed* to allow for such a possibility in one question. The question read as follows:

When during the day do you usually read for pleasure?

> Morning 1
> Afternoon 2
> Evening 3

This question should have had a fourth alternative answer that read "Never read for pleasure" (coded 4). The inclusion of such a response would have allowed persons who never read for pleasure to describe themselves. The omission of such an alternative increases the risk that respondents get frustrated with the questionnaire, feel that their behavior or opinions are not sufficiently represented among the answer categories presented, and, as a result, do not complete the questionnaire or fail to return it.

Alternatively, "skips" or "branching" can be used to facilitate the questionnaire's applicability to all potential respondents, but their use must be minimized. Because assault is a "rare event," we do not expect many people in our study to say that they were assaulted within the past year, *even though many of them perceive themselves to be at risk of assault.* Consequently, branching or a "skip" instruction *must* be used in this questionnaire. The first question is therefore formatted as follows:

1. How many times have you been physically attacked or assaulted at work within the past year—that is, since October 1993?

RECORD NUMBER HERE

```
IF 0 ATTACKS IN PAST YEAR,
SKIP TO QUESTION 24 ON PAGE 7
```

Persons who had been attacked within the past year answered 22 questions that asked them to describe various things about the attack. Persons who had not been attacked—the majority of respondents—skipped over this set of questions.

Similarly, Question 24 asked about threats within the past month. Again, we did not expect many people to report threats, so these people were skipped to Question 43.

24. **Within the past month**—that is, in the past 30 days— how many times have you been physically threatened or harassed?

RECORD NUMBER HERE

```
IF 0 THREATS IN PAST YEAR,
SKIP TO QUESTION 43 ON PAGE 13
```

Those who had been threatened answered a series of questions; those who had not been threatened were skipped to questions about demographic characteristics.

In this particular study, the use of two skips or branchings appears to have worked. But note that the skip is of a single kind: A person either answers a set of questions or skips over a set of questions. Respondents are *not* asked to go to *different* sections of the questionnaire according to the answers given on a screening question. Furthermore, the number of skips included in the questionnaire was restricted to two and both were of the same kind. The general rule is this:

> SKIPS SHOULD BE AVOIDED IN
> SELF-ADMINISTERED QUESTIONNAIRES.

If skips *must* be used, their use should be minimal and should *not* result in multiple branching operations, with one group of respondents being directed to one part of the questionnaire, a second group directed to a second part, and a third group directed to a third part. Respondents generally will *not* follow such instructions and will be irritated by the effort expended in trying to follow them. Thus, a study of a general population's use of health services where respondents vary both in age and gender is *not* amenable to study using self-administered questionnaires because of the wide variety of types of services used and because the frequency of use by males and females and by different age groups varies substantially. Far too many skips or branching operations would be necessary to provide appropriate questions for the various subgroups in the population.

Fourth, self-administered questionnaires—and particularly mail questionnaires—should not be used in exploratory studies or when the surveyor is in the process of developing a research question and the procedures by which that question will be studied. Mail questionnaires should be used only when the surveyor has a clear idea of the research objective and the parameters of the study. During the developmental stages of a study, data should be collected in ways that maximize flexibility and the ability to pursue interesting topics that may or may not be central to the original question posed. The use of focus groups; semistructured face-to-face interviews that include a lot of open-ended questions; and the ability to probe a respondent's answer, observations, and even certain kinds of secondary data are far more productive methods of collecting data in the early stages of a research project. Once the boundaries of the research question are clearly delineated and assuming the question can be appropriately operationalized in a mail questionnaire (e.g., the sample is literate and motivated), then the decision is made about whether a mail questionnaire can be used to collect the data in the study.

Checklist: Deciding Whether to Use a Mail Questionnaire

✓ **Respondents are literate and can answer all questions.**

✓ **Respondents are motivated.**

   ■ They want to know the information.

   ■ They feel part of a group that has reason to want the information.

✓ **The topic is amenable to study.**

   ■ Objective is "contained" and focused.

   ■ Questions ask about the present rather than the past or future.

   ■ Questions are written so that they can be answered by everyone in the sample.

   ■ Skips or branchings are avoided.

   ■ The study is not exploratory or in the process of being developed.

Developing the Content
of the Questionnaire

Once the surveyor determines that it *is* appropriate to use a mail questionnaire to collect data, the first task is to conduct a thorough search of the relevant or related literature. This literature search has two major foci. First, it helps the surveyor refine the parameters of the data collection. What other studies have been done on this topic? How were the data collected in other studies? What was the content of other data collection instruments? How can the surveyor learn from or build on these other research efforts? In developing our study on assault in the workplace we reviewed studies on occupational injury. We found out three things:

1. Most studies on workplace injury focused on deaths that occur on the job, with particular attention to homicides.

2. Most studies completed to date used secondary data sets, such as coroners' or medical examiners' reports, death certificates, or official reports made to organizations such as the Occupational Safety and Health Administration (OSHA). Needless to say, studies based on such sources tend to concentrate on the most serious occupational injuries—those that result in death or injuries sufficient to be reported to medical or other authorities.

3. The few studies that had *not* depended on secondary data sources or focused on severe injury or death had studied injuries that occurred to staff (usually nurses, in institutional settings, usually psychiatric wards).

Knowledge of this literature and what it encompassed allowed us both to define how our study would build on or extend existent work in the area and to identify the data collection instruments that we should examine in deciding how to go about our study. Namely, our study extended earlier research by assessing the frequency with which assaults occur on the job *that never are recorded in official records* and by expanding the occupational groups studied *beyond those working in locked institutional psychiatric hospitals.* Once we had completed the literature review, we knew which studies had used questionnaires to collect data, and we knew that in most cases self-administered questionnaires had been used. We then made every effort to obtain copies of all the questionnaires *as they were actually administered to respondents.* We did *not* depend on descriptions of questionnaires as they appeared in published articles or project reports.

ADOPTING STANDARD QUESTIONNAIRE BATTERIES

Ideally, we would like to find sets of questions already developed and widely used and simply adopt those questions as written. There are multiple advantages to such a strategy, and the adoption of existent standard question batteries is particularly helpful in self-administered mail questionnaires.

First, such questionnaires are almost always closed ended. As we noted in Chapter 1, respondents are generally reluctant to answer open-ended questions in a self-administered questionnaire. Thus, the selection of possible answer categories has already been worked out and tested in prior studies. Second, instructions have been developed and tested. Third, using questions *exactly* as they were used in another study allows the data you collect to be compared to the data collected in those prior studies or to a standard population. For example, many surveyors choose to ask questions about ethnicity or race exactly as asked in the U.S. Census. This decision is not made because it is thought that the U.S. Census has the "perfect" method for asking such questions but because the surveyor wants to be able to compare his or her study sample to the 1990 population in the region. Questions 4 and 7 in Figure

2–1 show how the 1990 U.S. Census determined race and ethnicity. Using questions exactly as they were worded in the 1990 Census allows the race and ethnic distribution of the study sample to be compared to a "standard" population— namely, the U.S. Census.

In other situations, we "adopt" a question or set of questions because we want to compare respondents across samples. The Prospective Evaluation of Radial Keratotomy (PERK) Study is a clinical trial for which people volunteered because they were myopic (nearsighted) and wanted radial keratotomy, which surgically reduces myopia. Because study participants were "volunteers," we were interested in finding ways to compare these myopic volunteers to a more representative sample of myopes. A series of questions that asked people about their vision was included in RAND's Health Insurance Experiment (HIE).[1] Because the HIE was done on a more representative sample and data had been collected by self-administered questionnaire, we "replicated," or adopted, some of the vision questions exactly as used by RAND. For example,

43. During the **past 3 months,** how much pain have your eyes caused you? Would you say:

    A great deal of pain 1
    Some pain. 2
    A little pain 3
    No pain at all 4

44. During the **past 3 months,** how much have eyesight problems worried or concerned you? Would you say:

    A great deal 1
    Somewhat. 2
    A little 3
    Not at all 4

	PERSON 1	PERSON 2
Please fill one column ➡ for each person listed in Question 1a on page 1.	Last name / First name / Middle initial	Last name / First name / Middle initial
2. How is this person related to PERSON 1? Fill ONE circle for each person. If Other relative of person in column 1, fill circle and print exact relationship, such as mother-in-law, grandparent, son-in-law, niece, cousin, and so on.	START in this column with the household member (or one of the members) in whose name the home is owned, being bought, or rented. If there is no such person, start in this column with any adult household member.	**If a RELATIVE of Person 1:** ○ Husband/wife ○ Brother/sister ○ Natural-born or adopted son/daughter ○ Father/mother ○ Grandchild ○ Stepson/ stepdaughter ○ Other relative ⌐ **If NOT RELATED to Person 1:** ○ Roomer, boarder, or foster child ○ Unmarried partner ○ Housemate, roommate ○ Other nonrelative
3. Sex Fill ONE circle for each person.	○ Male ○ Female	○ Male ○ Female
4. Race Fill ONE circle for the race that the person considers himself/herself to be. If Indian (Amer.), print the name of the enrolled or principal tribe. _____ If Other Asian or Pacific Islander (API), print one group, for example: Hmong, Fijian, Laotian, Thai, Tongan, Pakistani, Cambodian, and so on. _____ If Other race, print race. _____	○ White ○ Black or Negro ○ Indian (Amer.) (Print the name of the enrolled or principal tribe.)⌐ ○ Eskimo ○ Aleut *Asian or Pacific Islander (API)* ○ Chinese ○ Japanese ○ Filipino ■ ○ Asian Indian ○ Hawaiian ○ Samoan ○ Korean ○ Guamanian ○ Vietnamese ○ Other API ⌐ ○ Other race (Print race) ⌐	○ White ○ Black or Negro ○ Indian (Amer.) (Print the name of the enrolled or principal tribe.)⌐ ○ Eskimo ○ Aleut *Asian or Pacific Islander (API)* ○ Chinese ○ Japanese ○ Filipino ■ ○ Asian Indian ○ Hawaiian ○ Samoan ○ Korean ○ Guamanian ○ Vietnamese ○ Other API ⌐ ○ Other race (Print race) ⌐
5. Age and year of birth a. Print each person's age at last birthday. Fill in the matching circle below each box. b. Print each person's year of birth and fill the matching circle below each box.	**a. Age** 0 0 0 0 0 / 1 0 1 0 1 0 / 2 0 2 0 / 3 0 3 0 / 4 0 4 0 / 5 0 5 0 / 6 0 6 0 / 7 0 7 0 / 8 0 8 0 / 9 0 9 0 **b. Year of birth** / 1 ● 8 0 0 0 0 0 / 9 0 1 0 1 0 / 2 0 2 0 / 3 0 3 0 / 4 0 4 0 / 5 0 5 0 / 6 0 6 0 / 7 0 7 0 / 8 0 8 0 / 9 0 9 0	**a. Age** 0 0 0 0 0 / 1 0 1 0 1 0 / 2 0 2 0 / 3 0 3 0 / 4 0 4 0 / 5 0 5 0 / 6 0 6 0 / 7 0 7 0 / 8 0 8 0 / 9 0 9 0 **b. Year of birth** / 1 ● 8 0 0 0 0 0 / 9 0 1 0 1 0 / 2 0 2 0 / 3 0 3 0 / 4 0 4 0 / 5 0 5 0 / 6 0 6 0 / 7 0 7 0 / 8 0 8 0 / 9 0 9 0
6. Marital status Fill ONE circle for each person.	○ Now married ○ Separated ○ Widowed ○ Never married ○ Divorced	○ Now married ○ Separated ○ Widowed ○ Never married ○ Divorced
7. Is this person of Spanish/Hispanic origin? Fill ONE circle for each person. If Yes, other Spanish/Hispanic, print one group. _____	○ No (not Spanish/Hispanic) ○ Yes, Mexican, Mexican-Am., Chicano ○ Yes, Puerto Rican ■ ○ Yes, Cuban ○ Yes, other Spanish/Hispanic (Print one group, for example: Argentinean, Colombian, Dominican, Nicaraguan, Salvadoran, Spaniard, and so on.) ⌐	○ No (not Spanish/Hispanic) ○ Yes, Mexican, Mexican-Am., Chicano ○ Yes, Puerto Rican ○ Yes, Cuban ○ Yes, other Spanish/Hispanic (Print one group, for example: Argentinean, Colombian, Dominican, Nicaraguan, Salvadoran, Spaniard, and so on.) ⌐
FOR CENSUS USE ➡	○ ○ □	○ ○

Figure 2–1.   1990 U.S. Census Form

45. During the **past 3 months,** how much of the time have eyesight problems kept you from doing the kinds of things other people your age do?

All of the time 1
Most of the time 2
Some of the time 3
A little of the time 4
None of the time 5

The inclusion of these three questions in the PERK questionnaire allowed us to compare the PERK volunteers' perceptions of their eyes to those of a more representative group of myopes. What we discovered was that PERK volunteers did *not* perceive themselves as having had more pain than RAND myopes but *did* perceive themselves as being more disabled by their vision than RAND myopes. To that extent, the PERK volunteers "differed from" a more representative group of myopes.

Existent sets of questions are also adopted exactly as developed for two other reasons. First, many questionnaires—particularly those developed in the psychological literature—are under copyright. A copyright assures the author(s) of the questionnaire that it cannot be used or changed without permission. In the PERK studies, we used the SF-36 to measure the physical and mental health status of our subjects. The SF-36 was developed over a number of years under the auspices of RAND's Health Insurance Experiment. It therefore has the second characteristic that encourages the use of questionnaires exactly as written—namely, the validity and reliability of the items have been extensively tested over time and with different sample populations.

In our opinion, the SF-36 was the best measure available for assessing the concept of health status. Furthermore, it had the advantage that most of the development work on the instrument was done within the context of self-administered questionnaires. As a result, it was particularly relevant for use in the PERK Study where subjects were asked to complete questionnaires at clinical sites. The existence of the copyright assures the author(s) of the SF-36 that we will not make changes in the instrument without informing the author(s). In some instances, royalties must be paid for copyrighted questionnaires, and in all instances, appropriate citation must be made to the person(s) who developed and tested the questions.

ADAPTING SETS OF QUESTIONS

Unfortunately, many surveyors think that it is "OK" to simply select "some" questions from an instrument. Neophyte surveyors and persons developing self-administered questionnaires are particularly prone to this problem and often fall into this trap because of their eagerness to be able to say to potential respondents that "it will only take 5 minutes to fill out this questionnaire." Occasionally, a questionnaire that obtains valid and reliable data *can* be completed in 5 minutes, but it usually means that the questions have gone through extensive development and pretesting and that the topic under study is very tightly defined and presented. It usually takes respondents more than 5 minutes to provide thoughtful and complete information.

There *are* occasions when instruments are changed or adapted for use in a questionnaire. But surveyors must be aware that *when* this is done, they can no longer reference prior psychometric testing of the instrument, nor can they make direct comparisons between their sample and those to whom the original instrument was administered.

Adaptation usually occurs for one of four reasons:

- Some instruments are too long to be used in their entirety.
- A population other than the original population is being studied.
- Instruments may need to be translated into other languages.
- Surveyors may need to expand, reorder, or otherwise elaborate on items or change the procedure by which data are collected —for instance, an item written for an in-person interview may be modified for a mail questionnaire.

If modifications are made in an instrument, pilot testing should be repeated, and the instrument's reliability and validity must be reevaluated.

For example, if after due consideration a surveyor decides to use a measure of health status, but he or she simply cannot afford the time it takes to fill out the complete health status measure, because the questionnaire being developed must operationalize multiple concepts and health status is not the major focus of the study. The surveyor should not come to this conclusion without pretesting the questionnaire and clearly demonstrating that (a) the questionnaire is too long in its original version and must be shortened and (b) health status is a concept that is *not* of primary importance to testing the research question. How does the surveyor now proceed?

The first step is to contact the author(s) of the instrument and request permission to select only certain items and ask for advice on which items might best be suited to the proposed study. If the instrument is under copyright and the surveyor learns that items cannot be selected out of the battery and used in subsets, then the surveyor must find another measure of health status. Even if the questionnaire is not under copyright, the surveyor has a responsibility to respect the advice of the author(s) of the original instrument. If it is agreed that modifications can be made, then the surveyor has a responsibility to carefully document the changes made and state the reasons for the changes and to acknowledge the source of the original questionnaire. The surveyor must also retest the validity and reliability of the questions.

EXAMPLE 2.1
Adapting the SF-36 in the PERK Study

In the PERK Study, we faced a different problem. Volunteers for the PERK Study were originally enrolled in the study in the early 1980s. Upon entry to the study they were asked to complete a questionnaire. We wanted to include a measure of health status in that questionnaire and talked to surveyors at RAND about using items from the Health Insurance Experiment's questionnaire. Because data from the HIE were being analyzed at the time, they suggested a subset of items that seemed to be "best" at that stage of their analyses. Subsequent analyses of the HIE data and other data sets ultimately resulted in the development of the SF-36 as a short form of the HIE's original measure of health status. Only some of the items in the original PERK questionnaire ended up in the SF-36.

As a result, when we designed the 10-year follow-up questionnaire for PERK patients we decided that it was necessary to incorporate *both* the complete SF-36 *and* the items not included in the final SF-36 but that had been used in PERK's baseline and subsequent questionnaires. The inclusion of both sets of items meant that we could make two sets of comparisons. First, we could compare the health status of PERK volunteers at 10 years with other, more representative samples of the U.S. population, and second, we could compare the health status of PERK volunteers at 10 years with themselves at baseline and earlier follow-up periods.

We adapted both sets of items and lengthened the self-administered questionnaire. Thus, at the analysis stage, new psychometric
analyses had to be completed, and during data collection, we ran
the risk of having lengthened the questionnaire either unnecessarily or detrimentally.

DESIGNING YOUR OWN QUESTIONS

We recommend that, whenever possible, questions be either
adopted or adapted from other studies. We think this is particularly important in self-administered questionnaires where
the surveyor wants to maximize the clarity of the questionnaire. Others have developed and tested questions that can be
used to operationalize concepts important to your research
question. When questions are adapted or adopted from other
sources, research ethics demand that you document where you
obtained the instrument and give credit to the original de-
signer(s). The following guidelines describe what needs to be
considered if you must design your own questions. Some of
these guidelines should also be used in evaluating whether and
how questions developed by others can be adopted or adapted
for your use.

Guidelines for Deciding on
the Content of the Questionnaire

- Conduct a literature review to define the parameters of the
  study, learn what others have done, and learn what others
  recommend.

■ Adopt standard questionnaires to maximize closed-ended questions, because questions and instructions have already undergone development and testing, and allow for comparison with other studies. Give proper credit to persons who developed questions, and pay royalties, if required.

■ Adapt questions from other studies because either the original questionnaire is too long, the mode of administration has changed, a different population is being studied, or translations must be made. Pilot testing must be repeated and reliability and validity reassessed. Also, document the source of questions adapted and the reasons for adaptation.

■ Develop questions when no existent sets of questions can be adopted or adapted for the purposes of your study.

Note

1. RAND is a nonprofit institute located in Santa Monica, California, that seeks to improve public policy through research and analysis. Begun in 1971, the Health Insurance Experiment (HIE) was one of the largest controlled experiments ever attempted. Over a 15-year period, 2,700 families were randomly enrolled in health insurance plans that ranged from free care to 95% co-insurance. The objectives of the experiment were to determine which medical services to cover and the extent of coverage, to develop techniques for measuring health incomes, and to assess quality of care and the fairness and feasibility of different cost-sharing plans.

3 "User-Friendly" Questionnaires and Response Categories

Mail questionnaires more than any other type of questionnaire must maximize "user friendliness." Areas that should be considered in designing a user-friendly questionnaire are the following:

1. The way in which questions are actually written
2. How answer categories are created
3. Minimum use of open-ended questions
4. Instructions that are both clear and sufficient
5. Every effort made to avoid projecting personal biases into the wording of questions and answer categories

41

Construction of Questions

SHORT-AND-SPECIFIC FORMAT

Questions must be as short as possible and specific rather than general in what they reference. The creation of short, specific questions in part necessitates following the rules developed for the construction of any kind of questionnaire—for example, being careful to avoid double-barreled questions that ask two things at once, such as "How would you rate your local police on courtesy and effectiveness?" or "How often do you see or hear from your children and grandchildren?" Another rule is avoiding long run-on sentences—examples of which follow.

> When you think about the traveling you might do in the next year or so, do you think you will make arrangements to travel in the next year if you decide to go by cruise ship?

> Some people like to go out to the movies; others like to rent movies on video, others like to watch movies on cable TV, and others do not like to watch movies in a theatre, on video, or on TV at all. How do you feel?

Creating short, specific questions may mean asking multiple questions rather than a single question. In the Workplace Assault Study, we needed to find out about the respondent's work environment—including the hours that he or she worked. We originally designed a question that read as follows:

When do you work? _____
RECORD HOURS WORKED

During pretesting of the questionnaire, we discovered that this question was not precise enough for a variety of reasons. Some respondents in our sample worked different work shifts, others had rotating shifts, not every respondent worked the same days of the week, and so on. In responding to this question, some respondents gave us both days of the week and hours worked, others simply gave us the time that they normally arrived at work, and others simply skipped the question apparently because they found it too vague. We revised the question into a series of questions as follows:

1. What time do you usually arrive at work?

   _____ AM PM
   RECORD TIME OF DAY

2. What time do you usually leave work?

   _____ AM PM
   RECORD TIME OF DAY

3. What days of the week do you usually work?

   _____
   RECORD DAYS OF THE WEEK

4. How many hours a week do you usually work?

   _____
   RECORD NUMBER OF HOURS/WEEK

In creating this set of questions, we did two things that we generally recommend *not* doing: The answers to these questions are all open ended, and we used the adverb "usually," which is considered a vague qualifier.

There are two reasons for creating open-ended questions in this situation. First, the answers requested of respondents were not judged as burdensome, nor did they require respondents to write down a lot of information. Second, even in self-administered questionnaires, surveyors sometimes create open-ended questions because they provide better data and take up less space. Questions 1, 2, and 4 request information that can be considered "continuous" or "interval" in nature. In the case of Questions 1 and 2, the responses can be coded using a 24-hour clock; in Question 4, responses can be entered into the data set exactly as given by the respondent.

In contrast, creating closed-ended questions that included all the possible alternative responses would be difficult and would take up a lot of space that could be better used to ask additional questions. The one possible exception is Question 3, where it might have been preferable to format it as follows:

3. What days of the week do you usually work?

                    CIRCLE ALL THAT APPLY

        Sunday 1
        Monday 2
        Tuesday. 3
        Wednesday 4
        Thursday 5
        Friday 6
        Saturday 7

Clearly, this list of responses is exhaustive and mutually exclusive. Furthermore, it allows the respondent to circle any combination of the seven responses and, quite frankly, makes future data entry easier. However, making lists for any of the other three questions would have required far more than seven mutually exclusive alternatives. Because Question 3 was part of a set of four questions, it could be argued that it is easier for the respondent to use the same kind of answer format for all four questions rather than changing to a different strategy in the middle of the set. Nonetheless, this is a judgment call on the part of the surveyor.

The word "usually" was inserted in this set of questions because of the wide variety of work schedules and sites represented in this study. Included among others surveyed were nurses, probation officers, sheriff's department employees, employees of the department of parks and recreation, and employees of the municipal courts. Many of these employees worked a standard 40-hour week, but others worked unusual hours and shifts. Nonetheless, most respondents did have a "usual" time of starting work and a "usual" time of leaving work. Inclusion of the word "usually" allowed us to communicate to respondents that there might be variation in their work days and hours without taking up further space with this set of questions.

To summarize, the original question—although short—was not sufficiently precise. It did not give us a complete picture of the days and hours that the respondent worked. In this case, the solution was to develop multiple, more specific questions. In other cases, it may be necessary to add qualifications onto the question. An example of the latter situation occurred in the PERK Study. In a follow-up questionnaire at 6 years, respondents were asked "What proportion of the time do you wear glasses or contact lenses?" Respondents frequently reacted in two ways regarding this question: First, they wrote on the questionnaire "Do you mean when we are awake?" or some other similar comment, and second, because many respondents either did not wear lenses at all **or** only needed lenses for one eye, they either provided us with that infor- mation or simply skipped the question. Once we realized that the question did not allow some of our respondents to adequately and accurately describe themselves, we were in a position of not knowing how to interpret the data for respondents who skipped the question or who did *not* write in further information.

We attempted to clarify and correct this question in two ways when we wrote the questionnaire administered at 10 years. First, we elaborated the question to read as follows:

24. What proportion of the time that you are **awake** do you wear contact lenses in **either or both** eyes or glasses?

Second, we developed a much more elaborate set of questions that asked respondents about the extent to which and the reasons for which they wore lenses and the type of lenses worn. Thus, in this instance, we had to lengthen the question to make it sufficiently specific and precise. Obviously, when it is necessary to lengthen a question, the surveyor must be clear about *why* this is being done and take care to avoid constructing an overly long question.

CAUTIONARY USE OF VAGUE QUALIFIERS

In the preceding section, we showed an example of adding the word "usually" to a question. Surveyors generally try to avoid adverbs like "usually" when they write questions because such words mean different things to different people. For example, we could have asked Question 24 as follows:

24. When you are awake do you **usually** wear glasses or contact lenses in **either or both eyes?**

Yes 1
No. 2

The problem with using "usually" in this instance is that, for some people, "usually" would equate with wearing glasses all or most of the time; for others, it may mean that they wear glasses less than 50% of the time when they are awake, but, in their opinion, 50% of the time is too much. In other words, "usually" works as a vague qualifier in this example and, when combined with the answer categories provided, gives us imprecise information about our respondents and particularly about those who answer "yes" to this question. Our solution here was to ask respondents about the proportion of time they wore lenses. The word "proportion" could also create difficulty for some respondents who may be unfamiliar with the word or not understand it. Because this study's sample was literate and highly educated, respondents appeared to understand the term and to have no difficulty in providing an appropriate answer.

Unless the surveyor remains vigilant, all adverbs are likely candidates for vague qualifiers. Whenever an adverb shows up in a question or in a series of response alternatives, the surveyor should carefully evaluate whether the question precisely measures the concept under study.

CAUTIONARY USE OF
ABSTRACT TERMS AND JARGON

Surveyors must be particularly careful to minimize the use of abstract terms or jargon in mail questionnaires or, when used, to carefully assess that respondents understand it. This is a caveat in all questionnaire construction, but it is particularly important in mail questionnaires where there is no interviewer available to clarify or provide a definition of the abstract term if a respondent appears confused or hesitant in answering the question that contains the term.

For example, in the PERK Study, respondents were fairly sophisticated about their vision and about ophthalmology. Thus, terms like "myopia" and "radial keratotomy" would be easily understood. If, however, questions about vision were being directed to a general sample of the population, we could not assume that respondents would understand *either* term. Instead of asking if they were myopic, we would ask them if they were nearsighted or if they had difficulty seeing things at a distance. Even in the PERK questionnaire, we never used the term "myopia"; instead, we asked respondents about their ability to see at a distance.

We had a somewhat different problem in studying assaults in the workplace. The major objective of our study was to assess the prevalence of physical assaults in the workplace; we were not interested in emotional or verbal assaults. At the same time, we could not be sure that all of our respondents would understand the word "assault." So, in introducing the series of questions about physical assault, we provided respondents with a definition of physical assault. The reason for doing this was to maximize the number of respondents who understood the question in the way that we intended it. The introduction read as follows:

In the next set of questions we would like you to describe any physical assaults or attacks that you have experienced within the past calendar year (that is, since January 1994) while you were at work. By a physical assault or attack we mean a situation where one or more persons intentionally hit you or touched you with some part of their body or with a weapon or an object.

The data collected in both the pretest and the actual study suggested that respondents understood the term "physical assault" in the way we intended.

Far more problematic was a section of the questionnaire that asked about physical threats. We could find no formal definition of "physical threat" that is used consistently in collecting official statistics or other data. To the extent that threats have been studied, surveyors have tended to create their own definition of physical threat. After substantial discussion, we decided *not* to define the term for our respondents. Instead, we considered a secondary objective of the study as that of finding out inductively what people thought constituted a "physical threat" and whether reports and perceptions of threat varied with job category, frequency of reported threats or assaults, perceptions of the work environment, demographic factors, or other characteristics of our respondents.

In deciding not to define physical threats for our respondents we put an additional burden on them in that they had to generate their own definition. Some complained about this, and the fact that we did this may have reduced our response rate.

It also provides an example of an area of research where an interview with follow-up probes would probably work better than a mail questionnaire in finding out how people heard and used the term "physical threat." However, given that we did not have the resources for interviewing our respondents but considered this an important topic for study, we chose to keep it in the questionnaire. Of course, we could have provided our respondents with a definition of threat, but in so doing, we would likely have created a definition that was either too restrictive or too broad and which, in either case, represented our own perception of the word rather than the range of perceptions of threat represented across our respondents.

To better understand this range, we asked respondents who said they had been threatened in the past month to answer an open-ended question that asked them to describe ". . . **the most serious threat** . . .", the results of which might help us generate a definition of physical threat for use in future studies.

We considered asking *all* respondents in our study to describe what they thought the term "physical threat" meant, but we decided that that would be unnecessarily burdensome for those who had not, in their opinion, experienced recent threats. Furthermore, by restricting our request to those who reported actual threats, we felt the information we received would be more accurate. This decision does not, of course, allow for the possibility that persons who did *not* report threats have a higher threshold at which they perceive a verbal or physical action to *be* a threat. For example, Respondent A may tell us that he was threatened in the past month and describe an occasion when a frustrated client swore at him. In contrast, Respondent B, who was similarly sworn at within the past month, may not remember the incident or may not consider it a threat. Hence, he does not report being threatened and, as a result, does not subsequently describe this incident to us.

In summary, abstract terms or jargon should be avoided in mail questionnaires as much as possible. If such a term must be used, the surveyor should provide a definition of it. This is possible if a standard definition is readily available in the literature but may be impossible in new areas of study. In the latter case, a mail questionnaire may not be the best way of collecting the data, but if it must be used, the respondents must be given an opportunity to tell the surveyor how they are using the term or what they understand it to mean. A decision may also have to be made as to whether all respondents will be asked to describe how they use the term or whether only those who respond in a certain way will be asked to define the term.

EASY-TO-DIFFICULT PROGRESSION

In designing all questionnaires, we try to start with the easiest questions and proceed to more complex or sensitive questions. Even though respondents can decide to answer a mail questionnaire's items in any order they choose, this rule still holds and is possibly even more important for mail questionnaires in that the surveyor wants the first few pages of the questionnaire to look inviting and to encourage the respondent to participate in the study and answer all the questions asked.

In the 10-year follow-up for the PERK Study, we were particularly interested in the extent to which and the occasions on which respondents used glasses or contact lenses to see well. Thus, a substantial part of the questionnaire focused on this topic. Figure 3-1 shows part of the sequence of questions asked.

Notice that the first question asks whether the respondent currently wears glasses or contact lenses in either eye. We then go on to ask a general question about the *amount* of time that lenses are worn. (Remember that eventually we ask respondents for more detailed information about the actual *proportion* of time they wear their lenses.) Questions 4 through 8, which are excluded from Figure 3-1, ask further general questions about respondents' vision now and prior to having radial keratotomy.

Starting with Question 9, the questions become more complex and require more thought. Because it has been hypothesized that persons who had radial keratotomy might have to wear reading glasses sooner and for a greater number of activities than would comparably aged persons who did *not* have surgery, it was important for us to obtain detailed information about the circumstances under which respondents had to wear glasses or contact lenses to see. It was also important to find out whether or not they remembered ever being told that they might have to wear lenses for close work.

Questions 9 and 10 are more difficult than Questions 2 and 3 in that they ask respondents about use of lenses for particular activities—namely, close work and reading. But Questions 9 and 10 are significantly easier to answer than Questions 11 and 12. Question 11 requires respondents to use "retrospective

Since your last examination in the PERK Study, some patients have had a lot of changes in their lenses and the extent to which they need to wear lenses. Others have had no changes. The next set of questions asks about **your** experience with corrective lenses. (CIRCLE THE NUMBER THAT CORRESPONDS TO YOUR ANSWER.)

2. Do you currently wear glasses or contact lenses in **either** eye to improve your eyesight?

    Yes . . . . GO TO Q3 1
    No . . . . GO TO Q3 2
    No, but should wear lenses. . . . ANSWER A. 3

    A. Why don't you wear lenses and why should you wear lenses?

    _____

    _____

3. Do you wear these all the time or only sometimes?

    All the time . . . . ANSWER A. 1
    Only sometimes . . . . ANSWER A. 2
    Do not wear lenses . . . . GO TO Q4 3

    A. What are your **main** reasons for wearing corrective lenses?

    _____

    _____

9. Did anyone in the PERK Study ever tell you that **after** you had surgery you might have to wear glasses or other lenses for **reading** and other **close work**?

    Yes. 1
    No. 2

10. Has that happened to you? Do you **currently** wear reading glasses or lenses for:

    CIRCLE ALL THAT APPLY

    Left eye, ... 1
    Right eye, or 2
    Neither eye? 3

11. **Following surgery** for radial keratotomy, when did you **first** start wearing reading glasses or lenses for one or both eyes?

CIRCLE ALL THAT APPLY

First started wearing reading lenses
in my right eye in: _____/_____ 1
YEAR   MONTH

First started wearing reading lenses
in my left eye in: _____/_____ 2
YEAR   MONTH

Do not wear reading glasses or lenses. 3

12. Some people have reading glasses or lenses but do not need to wear them for all near tasks. Others need reading lenses for only one of their eyes. Please use the following list to describe your use of lenses for **near vision** on **each eye**.

I must use glasses or some other visual aid on my **RIGHT EYE** to:

	YES	NO
Read newspaper headlines	1	2
Read newspaper articles	1	2
Read telephone books	1	2
Read numbers on a microwave	1	2
Read my watch	1	2
Read a computer screen	1	2
Read in dim light	1	2
Read in bright light	1	2
When my right eye is tired	1	2
Read a book in the morning when I get up	1	2
Read a book in the evening	1	2
Thread a needle	1	2
Other	1	2
SPECIFY: _____		
I use my right eye **without** a lens for near vision	1	2
I **never** use a lens on my right eye for near vision	1	2

(continued)

I must use glasses or some other visual aid on my **LEFT EYE** to:

	YES	NO
Read newspaper headlines	1	2
Read newspaper articles	1	2
Read telephone books	1	2
Read numbers on a microwave	1	2
Read my watch	1	2
Read a computer screen	1	2
Read in dim light	1	2
Read in bright light	1	2
When my left eye is tired	1	2
Read a book in the morning when I get up	1	2
Read a book in the evening	1	2
Thread a needle	1	2
Other	1	2
SPECIFY: _____		
I use my left eye **without** a lens for near vision	1	2
I **never** use a lens on my left eye for near vision	1	2

Figure 3–1.   Constructing and Ordering Questions From Easy to Difficult

memory"—in other words, to think back in time. If they are now wearing reading glasses, when did they start? In Question 12, respondents are provided with a list of tasks that may require the use of glasses and asked whether or not they wear lenses for this task.

Furthermore, respondents are asked to *differentiate between* their two eyes. Generally, we would not expect respondents to be able to make such detailed distinctions between their eyes without help from an interviewer. However, because these particular respondents have been enrolled in a vision study for more than 10 years, they are substantially more sophisticated about their eyes than the average person is, and so we were able to obtain this information. Yet even with this sample we began with general questions and gradually progressed to more complex ones.

LOGICAL ORDER

Questions should be asked in logical order. One common error that beginning surveyors make is to order questions according to when they think about them instead of ordering them logically. In the most extreme case, respondents may be asked to flip back and forth between topics. Figure 3-2 provides an example of this kind of error. Here we have two demographic questions (Questions 1 and 3), two questions about physical activity (Questions 2 and 5), and one question about health (Question 4). Related questions should be grouped together. In other words, Questions 1 and 3 should be in sequence and placed with other demographic questions, Questions 2 and 5 should be together and placed with other questions about physical activities, and Question 4 should be placed with other questions about health status.

Figure 3-1 also provides an example of putting questions in logical order. It makes no sense to ask respondents about the circumstances under which they wear glasses or contact lenses *before* asking them if they wear lenses at all. As we see here, questions work better when general ones are asked before more specific ones.

DEMOGRAPHIC QUESTIONS PLACEMENT

In the preceding section we advised that questions be grouped by topic area. This applies to demographic questions, which ask for information about respondents (e.g., their age, gender, employment status, income, and marital status).

The question arises as to *where* in the questionnaire they should be located. Surveyors differ on this. We are of the opinion that demographic questions should be placed at the

1. Are you currently employed at a regular job?

    Yes . . . . ANSWER A-B 1

    No . . . . GO TO Q2 2

  A. What days of the week do you usually work?

    _____

  B. What hours do you usually work?

    _____

2. About how often do you participate in sports or physical activities? Would you say:

    At least once a day. 1

    Less than once a day but several times a week 2

    2-3 times a week 3

    Once a week 4

    Less than once a week. 5

    Never 6

3. How old were you on your last birthday? _____

                                           RECORD AGE

4. In general, would you say your health is:

    Excellent. 1

    Very good 2

    Good 3

    Fair 4

    Poor. 5

5. When you participate in physical activities, about how long do you participate each time?

    _____

    RECORD # OF MINUTES

    DO NOT PARTICIPATE 999

Figure 3-2. Example of an Illogical and Poorly Ordered Questionnaire

end of the questionnaire. We recommend this for three reasons. First, mail questionnaires are almost always preceded by an introductory letter or statement that describes the subject matter of the study and encourages respondent participation. Whether such a letter is sent in advance or included with the questionnaire itself, its purpose is to intrigue respondents and encourage their participation in the study. If the first questions in the questionnaire are demographic ones, they tend to negate the purpose of the introductory letter.

Second, many people find demographic questions boring. By beginning with boring questions, the surveyor increases the probability that respondents will become disinterested in the study and never complete the questionnaire. Finally, some demographic questions, such as age and income, are considered sensitive by respondents. To start a questionnaire with questions that respondents are reluctant to answer again reduces the probability that the questionnaire will be completed and returned to the surveyor.

Although it is true that respondents can read an entire mail questionnaire before answering any of its questions, we still believe that starting a questionnaire with easy questions that immediately engage the respondent in the topic of a study will increase response rates and reduce the amount of missing data.

Other surveyors disagree with this position and believe that demographic questions should be asked at the beginning of a questionnaire. Their reasons for this position are twofold: first, that demographic questions are easier for respondents to answer because the information sought is well known to them, and second, that those respondents who return an incomplete questionnaire tend to leave the last part of the questionnaire unanswered. Thus, by putting the demographic questions at the beginning of the instrument the surveyor maximizes getting complete demographic information about the respondent.

In our opinion, this latter argument—if operative—has more salience for face-to-face or telephone interviews, where the interviewer controls the order in which questions are asked, than it does for self-administered questionnaires, where the order in which questions are answered ultimately rests with the respondent. Also, we suspect that if respondents are not going to answer a substantial number of the questions in a questionnaire they will very likely not even return the questionnaire to the surveyor.

Checklist for Constructing Questions

✓ **Keep questions short.**

✓ **Make questions specific.**

✓ **Avoid vague qualifiers.**

✓ **Avoid abstract terms.**

✓ **Avoid jargon.**

✓ **Start with easier questions and move to more difficult ones.**

✓ **Ask questions in a logical order.**

✓ **Decide WHERE to place demographic questions and WHY you are choosing that location.**

Open- Versus Closed-Ended Questions

Items in questionnaires can be either open ended or closed ended. Questions 2, 3, 10, 11, and 12 in Figure 3-1 and Questions 1, 2, and 4 in Figure 3-2 are examples of closed-ended questions. Questions 2A, 3A, and the dates in Figure 3-1 and Questions 1A, 1B, and 5 in Figure 3-2 are examples of open-ended questions. Open-ended questions have no lists of possible answers; closed-ended questions, however, contain lists of possible answers from which respondents select the answer or answers that best represent their view or situation.

Although open-ended questions are much easier to write than closed-ended items, they generally are more difficult to answer, code, and analyze because surveyors must develop code frames or categories to organize and summarize the collected data. This process is sometimes referred to as *content analysis.* In contrast, closed-ended questions are much more difficult to design but, if designed carefully and with sufficient pretesting, result in much more efficient data collection, processing, and analysis. Instead of having to write out an answer to the question, the interviewer or respondent selects the word, phrase, or statement from the list of answers that best matches the respondent's answer.

We noted in Chapter 1 that open-ended questions do not work well in self-administered or mail questionnaires. Although the neophyte surveyor may think that an open-ended question allows respondents to express themselves in greater detail and with greater accuracy without being "forced" to put themselves into a category, in fact, respondents do not like to answer open-ended questions partly because the physical process of writing out an answer is tiring. It also requires respondents to generate their own answers without any prompting from the surveyor. In general, then, open-ended questions should be avoided or used only sparingly in mail and other self-administered questionnaires.

Note in Figures 3-1 and 3-2 that open-ended questions are asked only in situations where the amount of writing demanded of a respondent is minimal, where it was not possible for the surveyor to generate a complete list of possible responses in advance (e.g., Question 2A in Figure 3-1), and where dependent questions are used. By dependent questions we mean questions that are asked of only some respondents. For example, in Figure 3-2, only those respondents who told us they are currently employed at a regular job are asked to answer Questions 1A and 1B; unemployed respondents skip these two open-ended questions.

Construction of Response Categories

Clearly, if mail questionnaires are dominated by closed-ended questions, the task of developing the response categories for such questions is particularly important. Four issues must be considered in developing response categories:

- Response categories must be exhaustive while simultaneously not being too long.
- Response categories must be mutually exclusive and the boundaries between them easily determined by respondents.
- Response categories must be set up to allow the respondent to provide multiple answers when relevant.
- When appropriate, surveyors must provide for a "residual other" category.

Generally, the number of response categories provided for each question in a mail questionnaire must be smaller than the number provided in an interviewer-administered questionnaire. The surveyor must also remember that the number and range of responses provided are always seen by the respondent, whereas in an interviewer-administered questionnaire, responses may be provided for the interviewer to use but *not* read to the respondent.

The advantage of having respondents see the response categories is that they are less likely to be influenced by either a primacy or a latency effect. In other words, instead of tending to hear the first or the last response provided and selecting one of those at the expense of all other alternatives, the respondent is more likely to "see" the entire list of responses. In general, people recognize and retain visual cues better than they do auditory cues. So if they see the list of responses, they are more likely to select the one that best represents them rather than the one that they best or most recently recall hearing.

The disadvantage is that respondents are less likely to volunteer answers that are not on the list even if the available responses do not provide an adequate description of their behavior or feelings. If response alternatives are persistently too restrictive or too vague, respondents become frustrated by their inability to accurately describe themselves. To the extent that frustration increases, response rates decrease. Thus, it is extremely important that surveyors spend sufficient time developing and pretesting the response alternatives provided for each question in a mail questionnaire.

EASILY USED CATEGORIES

In the 10-year follow-up on the PERK Study, we wanted to find out about some of the common activities for which people use their eyes (e.g., reading, driving, and watching television). We wanted to know both the extent to which they used their eyes in such activities, whether or not the amount of time they spent in such activities had changed over the past year, and when during the day they engaged in such activities. At the same time, we did not want to ask a large number of questions about these activities. Figure 3-3 shows the series of questions that was designed.

In the next set of questions we need to find out about some of your daily activities and how you spend your time.

54. Do you currently read magazines, books, and newspapers as much as you ever did, more than you did a year ago, less than you did a year ago, or don't you read for pleasure at all?

I read for pleasure:

Much more than a year ago 1
Somewhat more than a year ago 2
About the same as a year ago............................ 3
Somewhat less than a year ago.......................... 4
Do not read for pleasure at all 5
Never read for pleasure.................................. 6

55. About how often do you read for pleasure?
Several times a day....................................... 1
At least once a day 2
Less than once a day but several times a week 3
2-3 times a week.. 4
Once a week 5
Less than once a week 6
Never... 7

56. When during the day do you usually read for pleasure?
Morning 1
Afternoon 2
Evening.................. 3

57. When you read for pleasure, about how long do you read each time?

RECORD # OF MINUTES

DO NOT READ FOR PLEASURE 999

---

58. How often did you drive a car in the past week?

I never drove a car.................................. 1
I no longer drive a car 2
I did not drive in the past week 3
I drove 2-3 times.................................. 4
I drove several times 5
I drove every day 6

59. How often did you watch television in the past week?

I never have watched television 1
I no longer watch television 2
I did not watch TV in the past week 3
I watched TV 2-3 times 4
I watched TV several times......................... 5
I watched TV every day............................ 6

60. When, during the day, do you usually watch television?

Morning.................. 1
Afternoon 2
Evening 3

61. When you watch television, about how long do you watch each time?

_____

RECORD # OF MINUTES

NEVER WATCH TELEVISION 999

Figure 3-3. Exhaustive and Mutually Exclusive Answer Categories

Notice that neither Question 56 nor 60 provides an exhaustive list of categories. To accomplish that, we should have done two things; first, added a category that allowed for persons to state that they "never read for pleasure," and second, provided instructions that allowed for persons to circle "all that apply." Question 56 provides a good example of how vague qualifiers (which frequently are adverbs) can get a surveyor into trouble. Here, the use of the word "usually" was intended to indicate "when you mainly read for pleasure" or "when you do your major pleasure reading." Many of our respondents either circled multiple alternatives or wrote along the side of the question that they read for pleasure, for example, in both the morning and the evening.

If a self-administered or mail questionnaire contains too many questions with these kinds of problems, the average respondent eventually will get irritated and, as a result, may refuse to complete the questionnaire.

MUTUALLY EXCLUSIVE CATEGORIES

Notice that Questions 54 and 55, which ask about reading for pleasure, attempt to incorporate answers that allowed us to assess both the current frequency with which people read and the extent to which reading patterns might have changed in the past year while *simultaneously* allowing response categories that differentiated persons who no longer read for pleasure from those who never read for pleasure.

Questions 58 and 59 were similarly set up to find out about driving and watching television. Unfortunately, however, the wording of the last two alternatives in Question 54 was neither clear nor mutually exclusive. In part, the confusion resulted from the fact that the present tense and past tense of the word for "read" is spelled the same way. Had we seen the confusion during pretesting, we could have rewritten the response categories in Question 54 to be analogous to those used in 58 and 59—for example, "I no longer read for pleasure" and "I have never read for pleasure."

MULTIPLE ANSWERS

Surveyors use two techniques in making response categories more flexible and exhaustive. The first of these techniques is to set up response categories so that respondents can select more than one answer to describe themselves. In Figure 3-4, Questions 25 and 26 both allow for multiple answers to be selected. Although most physical attacks are usually committed by a single person with a single weapon, Question 25 asks respondents how many people were involved in the attack, and Question 26 provides an opportunity for respondents to describe multiple attackers in terms of the kind and variety of roles that they had relative to the respondent. Thus, if in Question 25 a respondent reported having been attacked by three persons, these three persons might be described in Question 26 as a "patient/client with whom I had worked," a "patient/client whom I did not know," and "friends/relatives of a patient/client." Similarly in Question 27, the respondent might report that both a chair and fists were used in the attack.

When provisions are made for multiple answers to be given, the data set similarly must be set up to allow for the multiple answers to be efficiently and completely coded into the data set for analysis. The easiest way to do that is to create a separate variable for each answer response provided and to set up consistent codes for whether a given response is or is not selected or circled by the respondent. In the current example (Figure 3-4), we might decide that circled responses would be coded 1 for "mentioned" and those not circled would be coded 2 for "not mentioned." The responses for Question 26 would generate 10 different variables—one for each of the possible available categories provided. Similarly, the responses for Question 27 would generate six different variables.

For the respondent described above, the codes corresponding to the 10 variables created in response to Question 26 would

22. Please describe the <u>**most serious attack you had in the last year:**</u>

_____

_____

23. When did this attack occur? _____ / _____ / _____
                                  MONTH   DAY   YEAR

24. What time of day did this attack occur? _____
                                             RECORD TIME OF DAY

25. Were you attacked by one person or more than one person?

        One person 1
        More than one person 2
        How many? _____

26. Who was the person(s) who attacked you?

                                              CIRCLE ALL THAT APPLY

        Patient/client with whom I had worked 1
        Patient/client whom I did not know 2
        Friends/relatives of a patient/client 3
        Co-worker/other employee 4
        Supervisor or boss 5
        Subordinate or person who works for me 6
        Former employee 7
        Person in legal custody 8
        General public/someone "off the street" 9
        Other 10
        Who? _____

be 1 for each of the variables that coordinate with "patient/ client with whom I had worked," "patient/client whom I did not know," and "friends/relatives of a patient/client" and 2 for each of the other 7 variables. For Question 27, a code of 1

27. Did the person(s) who attacked you have a weapon?

CIRCLE ALL THAT APPLY

Yes, a gun. 1

Yes, a knife. 2

Yes, an object. 3

    What was the object? _____

Yes, a chair or other piece of furniture 4

They used their fists or body 5

Other. 6

    Please describe: _____

Figure 3–4. Examples of Residual "Other" and Use of Multiple Response Categories

would be recorded for each of the variables that correspond to "Yes, a chair or other piece of furniture" and "They used their fists or body" and 2 for each of the variables that correspond to "Yes, a gun," "Yes, a knife," "Yes, an object," and "other."

RESIDUAL "OTHER"

Residual "other" is another technique used to increase flexibility in answer categories. Both Questions 26 and 27 in Figure 3-4 include a residual "other." We consulted the literature and used information provided by focus groups and pretests in creating the list of answer categories provided in Questions 26 and 27. In Question 26, we tried to create an exhaustive list of the different kinds of people that might attack a member of Locals 535 and 660 of the Service Employees International Union. Because a wide variety of jobs are represented by the two locals, we needed to create a list that would be as exhaustive as possible and allow for the fact that, for example, psychiatric nurses and employees of the Department of Parks and Recreation interact with different types of people and different mixes of people. A psychiatric nurse who works on a locked ward will spend a substantial part of her work time interacting with incarcerated persons. In contrast, an employee of the parks department will interact primarily with fellow workers.

In creating an exhaustive list, we did not want to create too long a list or one that was *too* detailed. For example, in Question 26, we combined "patients" with "clients." Once we had finished our pretest and felt that our list was fairly exhaustive, we could not be exactly sure, so we added a residual "other." Thus, if a person was attacked by someone we failed to include in our list of categories—for example, a member of the union staff—the respondent can circle 10, which corresponds to "other," and describe this person in the space provided.

Sometimes, respondents are unsure about which category to use. For example, if a female respondent works in the tax office and is attacked by someone who works down the hall for the courts, she may not consider the person who attacked her a "co-worker or other employee." As a result, she would not circle 4, which corresponds to "co-worker/other employee," but would circle 10 for "other" and describe the person in the space provided.

Once all the questionnaires have been returned, the surveyor must decide how to handle the residual "other" answers in data analysis. There are two choices: either move the volunteered answer into one of the existent variable categories or create a new—in this case, 11th—variable that represents this new answer to Question 26. In the two examples above, we would create a new variable for the union employee but would consider the court worker a co-worker or other employee and so would recode both as 4.

Two general rules are used in deciding whether or not a new category or variable is created from answers recorded in the residual "other" category. First, we need to determine how closely the answer given in the residual "other" category relates to answer categories already specified. In the above example, we suggest that a person who works in an office down the hall is appropriately considered a co-worker but that a union employee constitutes a "different" category of person and thus necessitates the creation of a new answer category or variable. Second, we need to examine the number of times or number of respondents that put the answer into the residual "other" answer. If, for example, we had a substantial number of respondents tell us that co-workers from offices down the hall had attacked them, we might well decide that the number of responses justifies the creation of two categories of co-workers: those who work within the same office and those who work in adjacent offices. The decision as to whether or not new categories and variables should be created is made during data entry.

In developing answer categories, the surveyor tries to minimize the use of residual "other." If more than 10% of your sample has to use this category to describe its attackers, you have probably done insufficient thinking before creating your list of answer possibilities. When large numbers of respondents have to use the residual "other" category, the surveyor will have to postcode these data if they are to be meaningful. Furthermore, when respondents find that the list of responses provided for questions consistently do *not* allow them to describe themselves accurately, they will likely do one of two things. They will arbitrarily put themselves into a category simply because it is there but not because it accurately represents them, or they will become so frustrated by the questionnaire that they neither complete it nor return it.

Checklist for
Constructing Response Categories

✓ **Avoid open-ended questions.**

✓ **Create an exhaustive list of responses.**

✓ **Keep answer alternatives short and precise.**

✓ **Create mutually exclusive answer categories.**

✓ **Decide whether respondents should be restricted to a single response or allowed to provide multiple responses.**

✓ **Consider the need for a residual "other" answer category.**

Clear and Sufficient Instructions

Instructions are important in any questionnaire, but they are particularly important in a mail questionnaire where there is no interviewer who can help the respondent understand the questions or what is to be done in completing the questionnaire. Three kinds of instructions are necessary: general, transitional, and question answering.

TEN-YEAR FOLLOW-UP QUESTIONNAIRE
Prospective Evaluation of Radial Keratotomy (PERK) Study
Psychosocial and Visual Characteristics

As part of the Prospective Evaluation of Radial Keratotomy (PERK) Study, we are interested in finding out about your current vision and some of your experiences since you were last examined in the PERK Study. This questionnaire includes questions about your current vision, your general health, your use of corrective lenses, and about any problems you might have had since we last examined you. Although we know that you may find some of the questions repetitive, please answer all of them. Questions are repeated so that we can compare your experiences and opinions now—10 years after your first surgery—with your experiences before surgery, immediately after surgery, and 6 years after surgery.

We are interested in **your** opinions, ideas, and experiences. All the information you provide is confidential and will be published **only** in summary, statistical form. You will not be identified in any way. In order to get accurate information about radial keratotomy and how it affects people's vision, we need information from **all** PERK patients. So please help us by answering the questions to the best of your ability.

Please fill out the entire questionnaire now. We have arranged for you to have enough time to finish the questionnaire before we start your vision testing. When you are **finished** with the questionnaire, **seal** the questionnaire in the attached envelope and **leave it with** the clinical coordinator for the PERK Study.

Figure 3–5.   Example of Instructions Used at the Beginning of a
Questionnaire

GENERAL

It is usually necessary to have some set of general instructions that introduces the questionnaire itself. Figure 3–5 shows the instructions that introduced the PERK questionnaire.

Notice that the instructions provide information about the kinds of questions that will be asked. Because respondents may find some of the questions repetitive, a brief explanation of *why* repetition occurs is given. The instructions emphasize the fact that the surveyors are interested in the respondents' opinions, ideas, and experiences. This kind of instruction is particularly important when questionnaires are being distributed within an institutional site, such as a school, health clinic, or workplace, or when respondents may consciously or unconsciously think that the answers they give will be used in providing them with access to services, jobs, or goods.

The instructions also state what the respondents are supposed to do with the questionnaire when they finish it—namely, "**seal** the questionnaire in the attached envelope and **leave it with** the clinical coordinator." This procedure was developed because of our concern that respondents might think that, because they were filling out this questionnaire in a clinic, the ophthalmologist or other health personnel might have access to the questionnaire and thus know who completed it and that this access might in some way influence their health care—especially if they said something negative about the surgery or the clinical site. Surveyors can never be completely sure that such instructions eliminate "acquiescence bias," or the need to please the surveyor, but such procedures provide a method for attempting to address and reverse such processes.

Finally, this set of instructions assures respondents that they will have sufficient time to complete the questionnaire. This was added to the instructions because we discovered that earlier questionnaires had sometimes been given to patients after dilating drops were put in their eyes, which made the questionnaires difficult for them to read, or that some patients were asked to complete questionnaires as they progressed through the various ophthalmic tests.

Some questionnaires do not demand such elaborate introductory instructions. This is particularly true if cover letters are provided with the questionnaire or if advance letters have been sent to the respondents. For example, the questionnaire for the study on workplace assault did not provide lengthy introductory instructions because both advance letters and cover letters were included in the study design.

TRANSITIONAL

The second kind of instructions are those that introduce a section or provide a transition between sections of a questionnaire. Examples are the introductory statements in Figures 3–1 and 3–2. In Figure 3–3, the instructions are primarily provided so that the respondent knows that the topic of the questions is changing. The questions that preceded this instruction asked the respondents about their experiences with radial keratotomy; now they are going to be asked about daily activities. The respondents are also told that there will be multiple questions about daily activities. Such instructions give respondents a chance to "catch their breath" and help them change the focus of their thinking.

The instructions in Figure 3–1 are more elaborate. Here, the instructions are not given simply for purposes of transition; rather, they provide a context. Respondents are told that they are going to be asked questions about their experience with corrective lenses. The instructions recognize that the lens-wearing patterns of some respondents have changed since they had surgery; others have experienced little change. The purpose here is to inform respondents that the surveyor expects to find a variety of experiences reported. The respondents are also given a brief instruction about how to answer the questions, namely, "Circle the number that corresponds to your answer."

QUESTION ANSWERING

In some cases, it is necessary to provide more elaborate instructions about filling out a questionnaire. This constitutes a third kind of instructions: those whose major purpose is to provide respondents with instructions for answering the questions. The first set of questions in the PERK Study needed this kind of instructions. Respondents were asked to read and answer 63 questions that assessed both their vision and their opinions about their vision. The answer categories were the same for all 63 questions and used a 7-point Likert-type scale. The instructions read as follows:

The first set of questions asks about your overall vision **right now** during the past week. In answering these questions, answer in terms of your **usual** lens-wearing pattern during the past week.

In answering each question, use a range from one (1) to seven (7) where "1" stands for "strongly agree" and "7" stands for "strongly disagree." If you "strongly agree" with the statement, circle 1; if you agree less strongly, circle 2, which stands for "agree pretty strongly," etc.

For some populations, the surveyor would be wise to provide a verbal interpretation of what **each** of the seven numbers stands for. In this case, we knew that this sample of respondents had successfully answered similarly formatted questions in the past, so we did not spell out what each number represented. There is a fine line between giving a respondent enough instructions and giving too many. If the surveyor is going to err, however, it is probably better to give too many instructions rather than too few.

Checklist for Writing Instructions

✓ **Decide whether general instructions will be given in a cover letter, the questionnaire, or both.**

✓ Tell respondents what the questionnaire is about, what they are asked to do, and why.

✓ Tell respondents what to do with the completed questionnaire.

✓ Identify places where transitions are needed (e.g., change of topic, context for questions that follow).

✓ Determine whether detailed instructions need to be provided for a subset of questions.

Projecting the Surveyor's Ideas
Onto the Respondents

Surveyors in all substantive areas are concerned with being as objective as possible in how they develop research questions and collect data to test those questions. Because human beings conduct research, it is probably impossible to eliminate all aspects of subjectivity from a research project. The task is to minimize bias and subjectivity as much as possible. The various suggestions that we have made regarding how to (a) decide on a research question, (b) write the questions, and (c) create the response categories all have as their ultimate objective maximizing the objectivity of the data collected. In collecting data from and about people, one of the most difficult things that surveyors must do is to minimize the extent to which they project their ideas about how people behave or what they think about onto the survey respondents.

Surveyors must be particularly sensitive to this problem and vigilant when they design mail questionnaires. The *way* we ask the question, the *number* of questions asked, the *order* in which we ask them, the range and type of *response categories* we provide, and the *instructions* given all provide an opportunity for making the data come out the way *we think* the world is organized. If, for example, we are convinced that there are a lot of workplace assaults, and that they occur because there are too many handguns available and because employers provide insufficient security, we can construct a questionnaire that will tend to confirm our perceptions by ignoring many of the things we recommended doing in this chapter.

In the questionnaire we designed to study workplace assaults, we asked only about assaults or threats that happened to the respondent within a specific time period. While we were designing our questionnaire, we conducted focus groups with union members. In the focus groups, most of the members reported that they had not been attacked but that they knew someone who had been attacked or that they knew someone who knew someone else who had been attacked.

One of the simplest ways to bias the estimates of attacks that we get would be to ask respondents about the number of attacks they have heard about rather than restricting our questions to attacks that they themselves experienced. This would undoubtedly raise the number of attacks reported, but the increase would be an artificial one because it is likely that multiple respondents will have heard about the *same* attack. If both Respondent A and Respondent B tell us they know someone who was attacked and we fail to find out who that person was, when the attack occurred, and so on, we are likely to conclude that *two* attacks occurred when, in fact, both respondents may be reporting the same attack.

Similarly, because we are biased toward thinking that guns are used in most attacks, we might create answer categories for Question 27 in Figure 3–4 that simply consisted of "gun" and "other." The fact that no other kind of weapon is listed may well result in respondents overreporting the use of guns simply because it is easier to circle the number associated with "gun" than it is to fill in the blank associated with "other."

Figure 3–6 shows two of the five questions that were actually used in the Workplace Assault Study. Given the bias suggested above, there are many things that we could have done in designing these questions to maximize that the data supported our biases. First, we could have restricted our questions to simply asking about the presence of security personnel and not bothered to ask Question 31 about security features and devices other than personnel.

Second, we could have constructed the questions so that a respondent circled only one answer. Because "security personnel" is only one of eight security devices listed in response to Question 31, it is likely that the restriction to a single answer would have resulted in fewer security personnel being reported.

Third, in Question 32, we similarly could have restricted our respondents to one answer, or we could have provided fewer options. For example, we might have provided only Option 1 —"Security personnel are always present in the same place" and Option 5—"There are no security personnel at my worksite."

In this chapter, we have demonstrated just a few of the ways in which the construction of self-administered questionnaires can restrict or bias the information obtained about people. Improperly designed and tested questionnaires always present a risk. Consequently, surveyors who use questionnaires to collect data must always remain aware of what their biases are and be vigilant about developing techniques that keep those biases from creeping into their questionnaires.

31. Which of the following security features/devices are available where you work:

CIRCLE ALL THAT APPLY

Locked doors to outside of building 1

Locked office doors 2

Limited public access to work areas
(counter, locked door, or other barrier) 3

Door alarms 4

Video cameras—monitored 5

Video cameras—unmonitored 6

Electronic key cards 7

Security personnel 8

Other. 9

     Please describe: _____

No security devices. 10

32. To what extent are security personnel present at your worksite:

CIRCLE ALL THAT APPLY

Security personnel are always present in the same place 1
     Please describe where they are located:

_____

Security personnel rove/roam. 2

Security personnel are on call 3

Security personnel monitor alarms and/or video monitors . . . 4

There are no security personnel at my worksite 5

Figure 3–6.   Assessing the Presence of Security Features in the Workplace

Checklist for Minimizing Bias

✓ **Be aware of what your bias is.**

✓ **Develop neutral questions.**

✓ **Ask enough questions to adequately cover the topic.**

✓ **Pay attention to the order of questions.**

✓ **Provide an exhaustive range of response categories.**

✓ **Write clear and unbiased instructions.**

✓ **Take sufficient time to develop questionnaires.**

Pretesting, Pilot-Testing, and Revising Questionnaires

The first draft of a questionnaire is never perfect and ready to administer. All questionnaires should be pretested or pilot tested.

PRETESTS

Pretests are used to test sections of a questionnaire. In some cases, pretests of mail questionnaires are conducted using interviewers or focus groups. For example, in the Workplace Assault Study, our first pretest was done in focus groups.[1] Union personnel helped us get three different groups of union members together. Each group was asked to do three things:

- Complete the questionnaire as it existed at that time
- Suggest what other items should be added to the questionnaire
- Discuss aspects of the existent questionnaire that might be changed

We mentioned earlier that one of the things that came out in the focus groups was union members' suggestion that we should ask about threats and attacks that occurred to persons other than the respondent. Although we did not adopt that suggestion, we did use some of the other suggestions that participants gave us.

We wanted to include questions that asked the respondents to describe their work location, but we were somewhat unsure about how many questions should be asked and how they should be structured. Information provided in the focus groups was particularly helpful in designing that section of the questionnaire. We also became aware of something that we did not act on at that point in the questionnaire development process but which, in retrospect, became particularly salient after we finished our pilot test. Focus group members made us aware of the fact that even though employees did not report actually having been attacked or threatened on the job, they clearly felt vulnerable to such events.

PILOT TESTS

In a pilot study, the complete questionnaire is tested using the administrative procedures that will be used in the study. In the Workplace Assault Study, the participants were to be members of two union locals. We asked each of the union locals to provide us with the names and addresses of 10 persons. We wrote a cover letter that was signed by both a union official and the senior author. The packet mailed to the 20 potential respondents contained the cover letter, the questionnaire, and a self-addressed, stamped envelope for returning the completed questionnaire to us. Two weeks later we sent a postcard to all 20 respondents. The postcard reminded people that they had been sent a questionnaire, thanked those who had already returned it, and asked those who had not to please do so (see Figure 3–7 for a copy of the postcard). The postcard included

---

January 24, 1995

About one week ago we sent you a questionnaire about workplace safety. Your name was randomly selected from a Local 660 membership list to participate in this survey.

If you have already returned the questionnaire, please accept our sincere thanks. If not, please do it today. Because it was sent to only a small number of Local 660 members, we very much need your questionnaire if the results are to accurately represent the opinion and experiences of Local 660 members.

If you did not receive the questionnaire, or it got misplaced, please call me at 300-855-5555 and I will get another one in the mail to you immediately.

Sincerely,

Linda Bourque, Ph.D.
UCLA School of Public Health

Figure 3–7. Example of a Follow-Up Postcard

---

a number to call for information. Two weeks later, or 4 weeks after the original mailing, a second complete mailing was sent to all persons from whom we had not received a questionnaire.

After all the mailings, we received 12 questionnaires, or 60% of those sent, with 6 of them being returned after the first mailing, 3 after the second mailing, and 3 after the third mailing. We considered this a good response rate *until* we realized that 9 of the 12 persons who returned questionnaires were members of one of the two locals. Thus, we had a 90% response rate for one local and only a 25% response rate for the other local. The question was, why the huge difference? It turned out that the major difference had to do with how union leaders selected persons for the pilot study.

The first local selected 20 people randomly, and we then sent questionnaires to 10 of the 20. The second local selected persons for the pilot study because the union leader knew them and knew that they were members of a committee concerned with workplace assault. Needless to say, this latter group was more aware of and concerned about workplace assault and, as a result, was more motivated to participate in the study. However, these individuals were not representative of the population of the local. Thus, our 25% response rate was probably a more realistic estimate of what we would get with the questionnaire as it was then designed.

We thought for some time about how to increase our response rate in the real study. We finally decided that we needed to do a number of different things to increase potential respondents' motivation to answer the questionnaire. The first thing we did was to talk with union leaders in the two locals. Because they were interested in the study and had, in fact, asked us to conduct it, they suggested some changes that we could make in both the questionnaire and the mailings and outlined what they could do to publicize the study.

We ended up changing the questionnaire and its administration in five ways. First, one union local had a monthly newsletter. They suggested that we publish a brief article in the issue that immediately preceded the mailing of the questionnaire. We also developed a flyer that was sent to union stewards and others to put on bulletin boards at the various work sites. Second, with the union's help, we mailed a letter to the 1,744 persons comprising our sample approximately 2 weeks before the questionnaire itself was sent (see Figure 3–8). This letter was on union letterhead and was signed by union leaders. The purpose of both activities was to raise awareness within the target population and encourage our sample to participate.

Third, again at the union's suggestion, we decided that the original cover letter was too imposing and that we needed to do three things to make it more "user friendly." First, we downplayed the topic of violence and assault in the cover letter and emphasized personal safety at work. This change in emphasis was also made in the questionnaire itself where we changed the title of the questionnaire from "Physical Assault in the Workplace" to "Personal Safety at Work." Second, we shortened the cover letter itself, shortened the sentences in it, and simplified the language (see Figures 3–9 and 3–10 for copies of the original and redesigned cover letter).

Finally, we added a flyer to the packet of materials. The flyer was designed to be eye-catching and to give the potential respondent some basic information that we hoped would increase their interest in reading the cover letter and completing the questionnaire (see Figure 3–11).

We made two changes in the questionnaire itself. First, as noted above, we de-emphasized violence and assault and emphasized workplace safety. We did this by changing the title, modifying the wording of some questions, and changing the order of the questionnaire. Originally, the questionnaire was divided into four parts and presented in the following order: questions about physical assaults experienced in the past year, questions about threats experienced in the past month, questions about the workplace, and demographic questions about the respondent.

We decided that this original order was problematic for two reasons. First, by starting with questions about assault and threat, the questionnaire emphasized violence and assault. Our pretest suggested that this topic might be too extreme for our respondents and needed to be introduced less abruptly and more gradually. Second, we realized that the majority of respondents would *not* have experienced an assault or a threat. Thus, they would be instructed to skip through the first half or two thirds of the questionnaire. In contrast, everyone in our sample had a work site to describe and, remembering back to our pretests with the focus groups, that some *felt* threatened

(text continues on page 88)

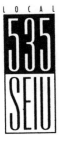

SOCIAL SERVICES
UNION

AMERICAN
FEDERATION
OF NURSES

309 So. RAYMOND
AVENUE
PASADENA
CALIFORNIA
91105
818-796-0051
FAX 818-796-2335

January 5, 1995

Dear Member,

You have been randomly selected from our membership list of Los Angeles County employees to take part in a survey about personal safety at the workplace. Your participation in the survey is very important. When you receive the questionnaire in the mail from UCLA, please fill it out and return it as soon as possible.

Our members who work for Los Angeles County are concerned about personal safety on the job. The union has raised this issue with management in contract negotiations and by filing grievances, but with only limited success. We need to do more. The SEIU Health & Safety Department and the Injury Prevention Research Center at UCLA's School of Public Health have worked with Local 535 members to develop a questionnaire addressing these issues. The questionnaire asks about concerns regarding personal safety at work as well experiences involving fear, verbal abuse, threats, and assaults on the job. Employers will not reveal this type of information. **It has to come from you!**

The results of this study will document the extent and nature of risks that our members encounter at work. Hopefully, future projects will address policies and practices intended to improve personal safety of Local 535's Los Angeles County workers.

Please fill out the survey from UCLA as soon as you receive it in the mail! If you have any questions or concerns about the survey, please feel free to call Wilma Cadorna at Local 535 or Deborah Riopelle, M.S.P.H. at UCLA at 310-825-4053.

Thanks for your help.

Sincerely,

Jerry L. Clyde   Linda Bourque, Ph.D.
President, Social Services Chapter   UCLA School of Public Health
SEIU Local 535

Figure 3-8.   Example of an Advance Letter

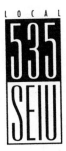

SOCIAL SERVICES
UNION

AMERICAN
FEDERATION
OF NURSES

309 SO. RAYMOND
AVENUE

PASADENA

CALIFORNIA

91105

818-796-0051

FAX 818-796-2335

October 7, 1994

Dear Member,

We need your help to stop workplace violence. Many people are worried that workplace violence has increased dramatically over the past several years. Studies have shown that homicide ranks as one of the leading causes of work-related injury deaths. However, little is really known about assaults and threats of violence in the workplace. The Service Employees International Union, AFL-CIO (Locals 660 and 535) is concerned about the violence its members may encounter on a day-to-day basis. Therefore, in cooperation with the Southern California Injury Prevention Research Center at the UCLA School of Public Health, SEIU is conducting a study of workplace violence. Results from this survey will help determine the extent and nature of threats and assaults that occur in the workplace and security measures which are already in place or which may be needed.

We need your help. Enclosed is a copy of the questionnaire that will be used in the study. This version of the questionnaire includes questions about:

    *   Your experience with workplace threats and assaults
    *   Security measures at your work site
    *   The type of work you do and the place where you work
    *   Your opinion about the content and format of the questionnaire

Based on your comments and suggestions, the questionnaire will be revised before a final copy is mailed out to other members of Locals 660 and 535 in Los Angeles County. Please take the time to complete the questionnaire and return it in the enclosed self-addressed stamped envelope. It would be very helpful to have your completed questionnaire returned to us by October 24, 1994. We would like to send out the final survey as soon as possible.

Your responses are confidential. No names or individual information will be used or released to your employer. If you have any questions or concerns, please feel free to call Deborah Riopelle, M.S.P.H. at UCLA, (310) 825-4053 or Wilma Cadorna at Local 535 (818) 796-0051.

Sincerely,

David Bullock
Southern Regional Director

Linda Bourque Ph.D.
UCLA School of Public Health

Figure 3–9. Example of an Original Cover Letter

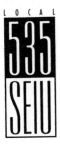

SOCIAL SERVICES

UNION

AMERICAN

FEDERATION

OF NURSES

309 SO. RAYMOND

AVENUE

PASADENA

CALIFORNIA

91105

818-796-0051

FAX 818-796-2335

January 17, 1995

Dear Member,

We need your help to improve personal safety on the job for Los Angeles County employees. Little is really known about personal safety and security while at work. The Service Employees International Union, Local 535 is concerned about the risks its members may encounter on a day-to-day basis. In cooperation with the Southern California Injury Prevention Research Center (SCIPRC) at the UCLA School of Public Health, we are conducting a study of workplace safety. Results from this survey will help determine measures that could be taken to protect our members.

You have been randomly selected from the membership list of Local 535's Los Angeles County employees to participate in this survey. Only a small proportion of Los Angeles County employees has been selected to participate, so your experiences and thoughts on the subject are very important. **You will be representing many employees who are similar to yourself.**

Enclosed is a copy of the questionnaire that includes questions about:

* **The type of work you do and the place where you work**
* **Personal safety measures at your work site**
* **How safe or unsafe you feel at work**
* **Your experience with workplace threats and assaults**

Please take the time to complete the questionnaire and return it in the enclosed self-addressed stamped envelope. It would be very helpful to have your completed questionnaire returned to us by **January 25, 1995.**

Your responses are confidential. No names or individual information will be used or released to your employer. If you have any questions or concerns, please feel free to call Deborah Riopelle, M.S.P.H. at UCLA, (310) 825-4053 or Wilma Cadorna at Local 535.

Sincerely,

Jerry L. Clyde   Linda Bourque, Ph.D.
President, Social Services Chapter   UCLA School of Public Health
SEIU Local 535

Figure 3–10.   Example of a Final Cover Letter

HOW SAFE IS YOUR WORKPLACE?

DO YOU FEEL UNSAFE OR INSECURE AT WORK?

HAVE YOU OR ANY OF YOUR CO-WORKERS
EVER BEEN THE
VICTIM OF THREATS, ASSAULTS,
OR VIOLENCE ON THE JOB?

LOCAL 660
IS WORKING TO CURB WORKPLACE VIOLENCE.

WE NEED YOUR HELP!

PLEASE TAKE A FEW MOMENTS TO COMPLETE THE
ENCLOSED CONFIDENTIAL SURVEY.

WORKING TOGETHER,
WE CAN MAKE OUR WORKPLACE SAFER.

Figure 3–11. Example of a Flyer Used for Motivation

in their work site even if they had not been assaulted or threatened. Thus, there was a perception of threat even if there was no objective evidence of it.

The two reasons in combination led us to reorder the questionnaire. Respondents were first asked to describe their work site and the security of their work site. They were then asked about threats they had experienced, followed by questions on assaults experienced and ending with the demographic questions. The changes made did increase our response rates somewhat. Of the original 1,744 questionnaires mailed, 38 had incorrect addresses and were returned to us. Of the remaining 1,706, 310, or 18%, were completed and returned after the first mailing. Another 258, or 15%, were completed and returned in response to the postcard. Thus, before sending out the second complete packet, 568, or 33%, of our sample had returned completed questionnaires. Another 285 completed questionnaires were returned in response to the mailing of a second questionnaire, bringing our total response rate after three mailings to 50%. This was considered insufficient for our purposes, so we turned to telephone follow-up. An attempt was made to conduct a telephone interview with each of the remaining 853 union members who had not responded to any of the three mailings.

VALUE OF PRETESTS AND PILOT TESTS

In this instance, both a pretest and a pilot test were conducted. Both provided us with valuable information, and both convinced us to change aspects of the questionnaire and the administrative procedures. They **also** made us aware of some biases that both we and the union leaders had about this study and this population of workers. We had assumed that union members were highly motivated to answer questions about assault in the workplace and that, in their eagerness to answer such questions, they would not be threatened by the topic. In fact, two things appeared to be going on. Although some proportion of these union members was concerned about workplace safety, when the questionnaire began by asking respondents to describe actual assaults, most had none to describe, and thus their motivation to answer the questions decreased. By changing the order of the questionnaire and increasing the publicity about the study, we were able to overcome some of this resistance.

Many things can be evaluated in pretests and pilot tests. Surveyors can learn how well their questions or instructions are understood and how comprehensive the response categories are. They may learn that they need to change the sequence of questions or modify the administrative procedures. Sometimes, it is necessary to ascertain how well a language translation works. Pilot tests can also help a surveyor estimate how much the data collection will cost in time and money. In this particular study, the pilot test made us realize that we had underestimated our mailing costs and the amount of personnel time it would take to set up four mailings (an advance letter, an original questionnaire, a follow-up postcard, and a second questionnaire mailing).

Pretests and pilot tests should always be conducted prior to the actual data collection, and the results should be carefully evaluated and used in making changes to the questionnaire and the study design. Such studies should always be conducted on representative members of the intended target population and, when serious or multiple problems are identified during a pretest or pilot test, revisions should be made and pretesting continued until the surveyor is confident that the data collection instrument is effectively and efficiently obtaining the data needed to validly and reliably test the research question.

Checklist for Conducting
Pretests and Pilot Tests

✓ **Decide whether pretests, pilot tests, or both are needed.**

✓ **Decide whether multiple pretests or pilot tests will be needed.**

✓ **How will pretests be conducted—in focus groups, by interview, in group administrations, or through the mail?**

✓ **Who is the sample for a pilot test or pretest—should it be representative?**

✓ **Pay careful attention to the results of pretests and pilot tests:**

   ■ Are questions understood?
   ■ Are instructions clear?
   ■ Is the order of questions appropriate?
   ■ Are the objectives of the study clearly understood by both surveyors and respondents?
   ■ Have costs been accurately projected?

Note

1. The use of focus groups to develop questions, item series, and/or concept areas has been increasing in recent years. A focus group usually consists of a trained moderator and 8 to 10 participants. The moderator is skilled in focus group techniques and either has some background in the topic under study or is briefed extensively on the topic. The participants are usually recruited at random from the community or may have responded to a survey in the past. If the topic area is one requiring particular knowledge or skills, recruiting will be directed exclusively toward individuals with those skills. A focus group session typically lasts 90 minutes, is led by the moderator using a guide of topic areas, and consists of an open discussion about the subject area. These discussions are audiotaped, sometimes transcribed, and used by the surveyor to develop questions for a survey. In this case, the focus groups were designed to test an existing questionnaire using cognitive questionnaire development techniques, which determine what respondents hear when asked a question and what they think the question is asking. The surveyor or moderator has the opportunity to determine how a question is processed in a one-on-one situation that closely resembles the interview process.

4 Format of the Questionnaire

Neophyte surveyors make two common errors in developing and formatting questionnaires: They indicate in instructions or cover letters that the questionnaire will "only take 5 minutes to fill out," and they format the questionnaire in ways to make it look shorter. Often, an unsophisticated surveyor will attempt to make the entire questionnaire fit on two sides of one page. The stated objective in both cases is "to increase response rates." Both are errors and, in fact, may *reduce* response rates for a number of reasons. If a research question is worth studying, data can rarely or never be collected from an individual in less than 5 minutes—regardless of how the data are collected. It takes 5 minutes to open the envelope and read the cover letter or introduction to the questionnaire!

If you have gone to all the trouble to develop a questionnaire, print it, and mail it, you want to make sure that you collect sufficient information to answer your research question. We know people who have eliminated demographic information from questionnaires because they wanted "to save space" only to discover during data analysis that their elimination of such information has made it impossible to answer certain important questions about their sample population.

Length

Surveyors squish all their questions onto two sides of one sheet of paper for the same reason. They want to make the questionnaire look shorter. But by doing this, they usually eliminate important information from their study, *or* they make the questionnaire unreadable. They leave no space between questions. Margins are small or nonexistent. The respondent needs a magnifying glass to see the print, and response categories are difficult to find or differentiate between.

In formatting a questionnaire, you want to "help" the respondent move through it. One of the most valuable things that can be done to help the respondent is to leave sufficient space between questions, between each question and the set of response categories, and between the alternative response categories. Space is as important as content in the presentation of a questionnaire. It has been suggested that mail questionnaires should be no longer than 12 pages; in general, most range between 4 and 12 pages. However, longer questionnaires can be used under two circumstances: when the respondents are highly motivated and when the reason for the additional number of pages is largely a function of increasing the questionnaire's readability.

Vertical Format

Notice in Figures 3–1 through 3–4 and 3–6 (Chapter 3) that we used a vertical format for our questions and answer categories. Other methods, such as shading, boxes, a newspaper column format, and arrows, exist for maximizing the clarity and order of a questionnaire. The 1990 Census, a page of which is reproduced in Figure 2–1 (Chapter 2), provides an example of a mail questionnaire where boxes and a newspaper column format are used to clarify how the respondent proceeds through the questionnaire.

We like a vertical format for two reasons. First, it simultaneously differentiates the question from the possible response categories and differentiates the response categories from each other. If, for example, we had used a horizontal format for Question 4 in Figure 3–2, we might have ended up with something like this:

In general, would you say your health is:
Excellent . . . 1 Very Good . . . 2 Good . . . 3 Fair . . . 4 or Poor . . . 5

or even this:

In general, would you say your health is:
____Excellent ____Very Good ____Good ____Fair or ____Poor

Many people think that respondents are unable to work with precoded questions such as those used in our examples. Instead, they have respondents put a check mark next to the appropriate answer category. Then, for reasons we have never been able to explain, they put the space for the check *in front of* the answer category *and*, to save space, use a horizontal format! What's wrong with this strategy?

First of all, we in the United States are used to filling out precoded questionnaires. We have no difficulty circling a number or filling in a box on a prescanned data form. Second, we read from left to right in English. Putting answer spaces or categories to the *left* of the word or phrase with which it corresponds is counterintuitive. Third, horizontal formatting of answer categories increases the errors made by respondents. In our preceding second example, a respondent can easily confuse the alternatives and put a check mark in the blank before "good" and that corresponds to an answer of "good" when what the respondent *really* intended to say was that his or her health was "very good." Similarly in the first example, even with the precoding and the dots linking the verbal response with the numeric code, the respondent may well select the number physically *closest* to the word rather than the code linked to it by dots.

Finally, a vertical format with codes already assigned and placed to the right of the response category makes data entry much easier and more error free. With most answers placed to the right of each page, the person doing data entry can simply go down the side of the page when entering the data.

The one exception to vertical format in our examples is shown in Questions 12 and 13 in Figure 3–1 (Chapter 3). Here, there are stem questions and then, instead of simply asking respondents to circle the numbers that correspond to the situations for which they use reading glasses, we ask them to select either "yes" or "no." We do it here because this is particularly important information in this study, and the inclusion of the yes/no column tends to increase the likelihood that the respondent will read each activity. A horizontal format similarly is used when a set of questions is all going to be answered using the same answer categories—for example, in a Likert-type format. Figure 4–1 provides an example.

1. The first set of questions asks about your overall vision **right now** during the past week. In answering these questions, answer in terms of your **usual** lens-wearing pattern during the past week.

In answering each question, use a range from one (1) to seven (7), where "1" stands for "strongly agree" and "7" stands for "strongly disagree." If you "strongly agree" with the statement, circle the "1"; if you agree less strongly, circle the "2," which stands for "agree pretty strongly," etc.

			Strongly Agree		Neutral			Strongly Disagree
V20	1)	I can see well far away **without** correction	1	2	3	4	5	6	7
V21	2)	When I drive at night, I have a lot of problems with glare from lights	1	2	3	4	5	6	7
V22	3)	If I drive in the morning I have to wear my lenses, but if I drive in the late afternoon (before dusk) I can drive without my lenses	1	2	3	4	5	6	7
V23	4)	I have a lot of trouble with glare in my operated eye(s).	1	2	3	4	5	6	7
V24	5)	When I read, I need more light than I used to.	1	2	3	4	5	6	7
V25	6)	I hate wearing reading glasses	1	2	3	4	5	6	7
V26	7)	Without my lenses, I use one eye to look at things that are close to me and the other eye to look at things that are far away	1	2	3	4	5	6	7
V27	8)	Even with my usual lenses (if worn), my visual acuity is not as good at night as it is during the day.	1	2	3	4	5	6	7

Figure 4-1. Example of a Likert-Type Scale With Variable Names

97

Grids

Both Figures 3–1 (Chapter 3) and 4–1 provide simple examples of what we call "grids." Grids enable a surveyor to save space on a questionnaire. They can be set up when a series of questions to be asked will use the same selection of answer categories. Grids are particularly popular for use in writing a series of questions to be used in developing a scale or index. They can also be used to format multiple sets of question sequences. Such grids are usually complicated and complex and, as such, difficult for a respondent to work through in a self-administered questionnaire. Thus, they are usually only used in interviewer-administered questionnaires.

Spacing

Notice that in our examples we have left substantial space between questions and response categories and used dots to clearly indicate which numeric code is associated with which answer. In these examples, we have used at least double-spacing between questions and between each question and its response categories. Within each set of answer categories we have used 1.5 spacing. Notice also that we have indented sets of answers under questions to help clarify where one question stops and the next begins. Where we have dependent questions—for example, 1A and 1B in Figure 3–2—these questions are similarly indented. This helps the respondent follow the skip instructions that correspond to the answer given to Question 1. Respondents who say "yes" are asked to answer Questions 1A and 1B, whereas those who say "no" are asked to go on to Question 2. The combination of indentation, spacing, and instructions that are set off—in this case, by capital letters—helps the respondent move expeditiously through the questionnaire.

Printing the questionnaire as a booklet, which consists of folding pages in the middle lengthwise and stapling them at the fold to form a "book," is a format we particularly like. When funds are available to do it, a questionnaire that is printed as a booklet looks more professional. We generally use 8½" × 17" paper for booklets because larger print can be used.

Often, the pages of a questionnaire are produced on a word processor and the size of the page then reduced during printing and production of the booklet. In the process, however, the print is also reduced. Small print or ornate print can be difficult for respondents to read, especially so for those over age 50 who need to wear reading glasses or who have difficulty seeing in poor light. We recommend using a 10-point pitch size and an easily read font with equal character spacing, such as Courier. Surveyors should avoid using italics, which are difficult to read, and fonts that use proportional spacing (i.e., the letter "m" takes up more space than "i"), as they can cause alignment problems (and can create extreme headaches) when setting up a questionnaire.

Print and Paper

There should be good contrast between the print and the paper. When in doubt, use black print on a white background. Some colors of paper, such as the currently fashionable neon colors, are difficult for respondents to look at for long periods of time. Also, colors that lower the contrast for color-blind persons should be avoided.

In our examples, we have used combinations of **bold**, <u>underlining,</u> and CAPITALS when we want to emphasize something in the text of a question or give an instruction about how to fill out the questionnaire. We consistently use capitals in providing instructions—for example, the instructions CIRCLE

ALL THAT APPLY, GO TO Q2, and ANSWER A. We use bold type and sometimes underlining to emphasize key words or phrases in a question—for example, **reading** and **close work** in Question 10 of Figure 3–1.

Other techniques, such as shading or boxing information, are also used. As we recommended earlier, italics should not be used because they are harder for a respondent to read, but other surveyors do use italics for emphasis or in instructions. We also find it problematic to put too much information in bold type. Some surveyors print all their instructions in bold. If a page contains a lot of instructions, the text of the question itself and the response categories tend to get lost, with the result that the respondent sees the instructions very well but tends to miss key phrases in the question or key answer alternatives.

Consistency

Whatever the size and format of print selected, the key is to be consistent. If the decision is that instructions contained within the body of the questionnaire are going to be under-lined, then make sure you underline *all* the instructions in the body of the questionnaire and do *not* use underlining to provide emphasis in the text of a question. Rather, use bold type for emphasis.

Similar consistency should be used in the spacing between questions and in the use of indentations. If you decide to have single spacing in the text of a question and double spacing between questions, then be sure that you are consistent throughout the questionnaire. Notice that our examples are consistent in the way we line up the answer categories. In Figure 3–1 (Chapter 3), the text of all questions is indented, and the answer categories for all questions are similarly indented, with the beginning of each answer lined up and the respective codes lined up.

Splitting Questions Between Pages

A common error that new surveyors often make is to split a question between pages, to split the instructions for a section from the questions that it is describing, or to split related and dependent questions across pages. This often occurs in the interests of saving space or simply because the surveyor doesn't think. Take a moment to look at Figure 3–1 in Chapter 3. Imagine that there was sufficient space on a prior page for the instructions that precede Question 2 but insufficient space for the question itself. Some surveyors will go ahead and put the instructions on the prior page and then wonder why respondents subsequently have difficulty understanding the questions that follow on the next page.

Another common error is to place the instructions and Question 2 on one page because there is sufficient room but then to place Question 2A on a subsequent page. Because Question 2A is logically dependent on Question 2, this practice increases the probability that respondents never see Question 2A or that they do not understand it.

Finally, look at Question 12. Here, the two parts of the question are followed by long lists of possible responses. Yet another common error is to split this list of possible responses between two pages—again to save space. What happens is that respondents fail to see the complete list and, as a result, never read or consider those responses found on the second page. This is particularly problematic when respondents are asked to select a *single* response to the question. Because they do not equally weigh the possible answers on the second page with those seen on the first page, the result is a significantly lower number of persons selecting the responses on the second page.

Occasionally, a list is too long to be printed on a single page even if the question (e.g., Question 12) starts at the top of the page. In general, we recommend against using such long lists in a mail questionnaire. However, sometimes it is unavoidable. If lists must continue onto a second page, then the questionnaire *must* be printed in a booklet form, with the question itself and the first part of the list of responses on an even-numbered page and the continuation of the list on the facing odd-numbered page.

Checklist for Formatting Questionnaires

✓ **Do not make unrealistic time estimates.**

✓ **Ask enough questions to obtain the information needed.**

✓ **Use space between questions.**

✓ **Use vertical format, space, boxes, arrows, shading, or other devices consistently to maximize the clarity and order of questions.**

✓ **Do not avoid precoded response categories, but clearly indicate the code that corresponds to each response.**

✓ **Consider the use of simple grids.**

✓ **Use a booklet format when possible.**

✓ Have good contrast between print and paper.

✓ Use 10-point pitch.

✓ Use an easily read, equally spaced font, such as Courier.

✓ Avoid italics.

✓ Use bold, <u>underlining,</u> or CAPITALS judiciously and consistently for emphasis and instructions.

✓ Do not split instructions, questions, and associated responses between pages.

Coordinating With Data Entry Personnel and Data Processors

As questionnaires are being developed, the surveyor needs to consider the needs of persons who will be doing the data entry and data processing. We have already recommended that closed-ended questions be precoded with clear indications of where and how answers are to be recorded. We also recommend setting up the protocol by which the data will be entered into the computer prior to actually finalizing the questionnaire and then providing either variable names or column information on the questionnaire itself at the time it is printed.

Figure 4–1 provides an example of a set of questions where the data entry program was preset and the variable names that corresponded to each question in the data set were included on the questionnaire when it was printed. Some people object to having such information on questionnaires given to respondents on the grounds that this information is not understood by respondents and confuses them. In our own research, we have not noticed that such information reduces response rates or confuses respondents. Regardless of whether or not surveyors include such information on the form, they must, at minimum, ensure that the data being collected can be efficiently transferred into machine-readable form.

Ending the Questionnaire

The questionnaire should be ended by inviting respondents to comment on its content, to make suggestions about what might have been missed by the surveyor, and even to complain about the questionnaire itself. Such questions are often referred to as "ventilation" questions because they allow respondents to "ventilate" their feelings about the topic or the questionnaire.

Next, respondents should be given instructions for mailing back or returning the questionnaire. Stamped envelopes pre-addressed to the surveyor often get lost or mislaid. If an address is not provided on the questionnaire itself, respondents who have lost the envelope have no way of knowing how to return the questionnaire. Letting respondents return completed questionnaires by fax is an option that surveyors might consider.

Finally, respondents should be thanked for their time and cooperation. This is a courtesy due any study participant.

Camera-Ready Copy

If all of the above points have been considered and solved and the content carefully proofread for possible errors, the questionnaire is "camera ready," or ready for duplication and production. Usually, questionnaires are either photocopied or set up for offset printing. The details and costs of such procedures are discussed in Chapter 5.

Checklist for Finalizing the Questionnaire

✓ **Format to facilitate data entry.**

✓ **Afford respondents the opportunity to comment on the questionnaire.**

✓ **Make sure the return address is printed on a mail questionnaire.**

✓ **Thank respondents.**

✓ **Carefully proofread the questionnaire one final time.**

✓ **Duplicate or print the questionnaire.**

Correspondence and the Motivation of Respondents

All self-administered questionnaires must be accompanied by an explanation of the purposes and sponsorship of the study. When questionnaires are distributed to respondents at a single site or on a one-to-one basis, this explanation may partially be provided verbally, with the written explanation appearing on the first page of the questionnaire itself. Earlier, we provided such an example for the PERK Study. Because that questionnaire represented a 10-year follow-up to a study in which respondents had been contacted repeatedly, we did not repeat information about sponsorship in the introductory statement. However, most questionnaires represent the first contact with a respondent and are *not* distributed as part of a multiyear follow-up. Surveyors should always reconfirm, elaborate on, or repeat information in writing, even when some of the information is provided verbally.

Mail questionnaires must *always* be accompanied by a cover letter. Including a well-written cover letter with the questionnaire mailing that explains the purpose of the study, how and why the respondent was selected, and cites meaningful reasons for why a respondent should reply will help increase compliance. Stress how important it is for the individual to respond and how important that person is to your research. It is also beneficial to have the cover letter signed or endorsed by someone with positive name recognition for the respondents. For example, if your sample is composed of individuals belonging to a particular professional organization, having the president of the organization endorse the study may be helpful, unless it is thought that members of the organization distrust the leadership.

Fourteen kinds of information should be included or considered for inclusion in a cover letter or for use in motivating respondents:

1. Use of letterhead
2. Information about sponsorship
3. Dates
4. Salutation
5. Purpose of the study

6. Reasons why an individual's participation is important
7. Incentives to encourage respondent participation
8. Use of advance letters
9. How material incentives will be provided or distributed
10. Realistic estimate of the time required to complete the questionnaire
11. How and why the respondent was chosen
12. Explanation of confidentiality and how the data will be handled
13. Provision of a name and phone number to call for information
14. When and how to return the questionnaire

Figures 3–8 through 3–11 (Chapter 3) provide examples of an advance letter, an original cover letter, a modified cover letter, and a motivational flyer that were used in the Workplace Assault Study.

USE OF LETTERHEAD

The quality of presentation is important for stimulating respondent interest. Materials sent to respondents should be as attractive and professional looking as possible. Earlier, we described how different colors of paper, style of print, and format of the questionnaire affect response rate. In Chapter 5, we discuss the relative advantages of hand-addressing envelopes versus typing them and the use of stamps versus metered mail. Although most of these treatments seem to have little effect on response rates, the number of returns do increase slightly with special materials.

The use of letterhead is advocated by all surveyors because it helps establish the importance of the study, gives information about study sponsorship, and serves indirectly as a means of personalizing the contact with the respondent. The fact that the respondent is being contacted by a recognized, reputable organization serves to legitimate the importance of the study and the uniqueness of this particular respondent's position as a source of information. All of the examples in Figures 3–8 through 3–11 were printed on the letterhead of the respective locals of the Service Employees International Union (SEIU): The example advance letter was printed on Local 535 letterhead, and the example cover letters were printed on Local 660 letterhead. Use of SEIU letterhead identified the study as a union-sponsored activity and helped establish its legitimacy.

INFORMATION ABOUT SPONSORSHIP

All three letters (Figures 3–8 through 3–10 in Chapter 3) specifically stated who was conducting the study or sponsoring it. Because this was a joint activity of SEIU Locals 535 and 660 and the Southern California Injury Prevention Research Center (SCIPRC) located in the School of Public Health at the University of California, Los Angeles, *both* groups were noted as sponsors, and representatives of both groups signed both letters. Note that mailings to Local 535 members were signed by the president of the Social Services Chapter of SEIU Local 535, and that mailings to Local 660 members were signed by the general manager of Local 660. All letters were also signed by the senior author as a representative of the SCIPRC at UCLA's School of Public Health.

DATES

The importance of dates on cover letters and other mailings cannot be emphasized enough. Many surveyors simply neglect to put a date on letters or, alternatively, do not fully think out the sequence of administrative procedures (see Chapter 5). As a consequence, the date that appears on a cover letter, advance letter, or follow-up materials differs substantially from the actual date of mailing. It is important that the dates are either identical with or shortly precede the postmarked date on the envelope.

SALUTATION

If you have the capability, personalizing the inside address and salutation rather than using global salutations, such as "Dear Respondent," "Dear Resident," or "Dear _____ Member," increases respondents' sense of their importance as a respondent. This was not possible in the Workplace Assault Study because of insufficient resources. We were, however, able to personalize the outside envelope with the respondent's name and home address.

PURPOSE OF THE STUDY

Notice that all three letters (Figures 3–8 through 3–10) explain the purpose of the study. In the advance letter (Figure 3–8), the purpose is specified in Paragraph 2. In the final version of the cover letter, the purpose is specified in the first paragraph:

> . . . Little is really known about personal safety and security while at work. The Service Employees International Union, Local [660/535] is concerned about the risks its members may encounter on a day-to-day basis. In cooperation with . . . , we are conducting a study of workplace safety.

In the original cover letter (Figure 3–9), the purpose was similarly specified in the first paragraph, but remember that during the pretest we discovered problems that led us to soften and modify the stated purpose of the letter.

We also decided to shorten the introductory information in response to union officials' suggestions that we were providing too much information and that respondents were unlikely to read and comprehend so much verbiage. Both versions of the cover letter have been presented so that readers can see for themselves the kinds of changes we made.

REASONS WHY AN INDIVIDUAL'S PARTICIPATION IS IMPORTANT

In the final cover letter (Figure 3–10), the first and last sentence of the first paragraph describe why an individual's participation is important:

> **We need your help to improve personal safety on the job for Los Angeles County employees. . . . Results from this survey will help determine measures that could be taken to protect our members.**

These sentences reiterate information provided in the advance letter (Figure 3–8) where we explain that " . . . **your participation in the survey is very important . . .**" and that this information "**. . . has to come from you!**"

In the cover letter used for the pretest, an additional reason given for the importance of an individual's participation was the fact that it *was* a pretest. In the second paragraph, we stated that "based on your comments and suggestions, the questionnaire will be revised . . ." and, as we have already noted, revisions were indeed made after the pretest.

INCENTIVES TO ENCOURAGE
RESPONDENT PARTICIPATION

Incentives used to encourage respondent participation often overlap with information about the purpose of the study and how the respondent was selected for the study. That was the case in the Workplace Assault Study. In the final cover letter (Figure 3–10), we explained that

> . . . only a small proportion of Los Angeles County employees has been selected to participate, so your experiences and thoughts on the subject are very important. You will be representing many employees who are similar to yourself.

We also noted that the information will be used to improve workplace safety. Similar information was included in the advance letter (Figure 3–8):

> The results of this study will document the extent and nature of risks that our members encounter at work. Hopefully, future projects will address policies and practices intended to improve personal safety of . . . Los Angeles County workers.

Respondents can be motivated to respond in many ways. Response is always best when the subject matter of the study is on a topic that has some personal relevance for the respondents, or when respondents believe that by participating they are contributing to some other, greater good. These are the techniques used in the Workplace Assault Study.

Monetary or Material Incentives

Providing a monetary or material incentive to respond is another method of increasing response rates. Incentives such as money, pencils or pens, notepads, calendars, raffle tickets, and the like can be used to increase participation. Some surveyors prefer to enclose a gift with the first mailing as an incentive to complete and return the questionnaire; others use it as an inducement to respond, promising to send the gift once the completed questionnaire is received. If a raffle or lottery is used, the winner or winners are chosen from among those who responded.

There is some controversy over the use of incentives, such as money or a small gift, to increase response rates. Some surveyors believe that the data collected from individuals who receive incentives is unreliable. Their reasoning is that the use of incentives "buys" responses from individuals who normally would not respond and who will pay little or no attention to the import of the study when filling out the questionnaire, merely putting down any answer.

Other surveyors feel that the use of incentives is entirely credible and in some circumstances is the only way to obtain a satisfactory response rate. These surveyors argue that the incentive merely indicates to individuals that their time is valuable and worth compensation.

Whether or not to use an incentive is up to the individual surveyor. Another decision that must be made when giving incentives is whether to give them with all first attempts or to only give them to those individuals who participate. If you have decided to use an incentive other than cash, consideration should be given as to the universality of the appropriateness of the gift.

Other Forms of Motivation

We are sure that other surveyors have utilized an infinite variety of other methods in an effort to motivate respondents and increase response rates. In the Workplace Assault Study, we added a cover flyer to the mailing of the questionnaire (see Figure 3–11). This was developed as a result of the pilot test and at the suggestion of union officials. Our reasoning was that many potential respondents were not taking sufficient time to read the cover letter. As a result, motivations included in the cover letter were not being received by the potential respondent. The purpose of the flyer was to "catch" the respondent's attention. Notice that the flyer was printed in large and varied print, contained an appeal to what we perceived were respondents' concerns—namely, workplace safety—briefly emphasized the purpose of the study, and referenced the union.

The flyer was printed on canary yellow paper to catch the potential respondent's eye. As noted earlier, we do not recommend using colors like canary yellow for a questionnaire or a cover letter because it is too difficult for a respondent to read for any period of time, *but* such colors can be used productively for occasional emphasis and to catch a respondent's attention.

Offering to supply the respondent with an abbreviated copy of the survey results is sometimes used as a motivator. Respondents enjoy being able to compare their answers to the results and being part of a research project. This is a relatively inexpensive means of increasing response rates. However, this "reward" for responding should not be offered if there is any chance that you might not be able to provide it or if sending the results would occur so far in the future that respondents won't remember the study.

USE OF ADVANCE LETTERS

Occasionally, the surveyor finds it profitable to send a letter or place a telephone call to the selected respondent in advance of the questionnaire being mailed. Although this usually is not possible in group self-administered situations, there are instances where the individuals can be informed that they will be part of a study at some future date. For example, employers can notify workers or teachers can tell students that they will be part of a study at a particular time and place and give them an idea of the study purpose. If you are using a letter or telephone call, it should introduce the study and give some brief information about it while alerting the respondent that he or she has been chosen as one of the special individuals who will receive the mailing within a few days.

An advance letter (Figure 3–8) was used in the Workplace Assault Study. The decision to have an advance letter was made as a result of the pilot study.

HOW MATERIAL INCENTIVES
WILL BE PROVIDED OR DISTRIBUTED

In the Workplace Assault Study, the question of whether or not to use monetary or material incentives was moot; we simply did not have sufficient resources to consider this option. If such incentives are to be used, the process by which and the circumstances under which the respondent will receive the incentive must be described in either the cover letter or an advance letter or both. In another study conducted by a UCLA professor, an award of $50 was provided by lottery to four students who returned a questionnaire that examined the social attitudes of American college students and compared them with those of peers in other countries. The cover letter was headed **WIN $50!!**, and the procedure was described in the body of the letter as follows:

As an added incentive, we will award $50 each to four students returning a completed questionnaire. The winning students will be chosen at random from the pool of those returning a fully completed questionnaire to us. In order to award the $50 prizes, we need to know which students returned the questionnaire and which students did not. To ensure confidentiality, this information will not be associated with the students' questionnaires. To accomplish this, you will place your completed questionnaire inside of the plain, unmarked envelope and mail this envelope to us. You will notice that the larger envelope has a number in the lower left-hand corner. This will tell us that you have returned a questionnaire. At this point your outer envelope will be destroyed and the inner envelope containing your completed questionnaire will be placed in a separate pile. Thus, it will not be possible to associate a given name with a given questionnaire. Your confidentiality will then be assured.

Notice that these instructions provide information on how confidentiality will be ensured while still allowing for provision of a cash incentive.

REALISTIC ESTIMATE
OF THE TIME REQUIRED TO
COMPLETE THE QUESTIONNAIRE

The surveyor should provide either a direct or an indirect estimate of the time required to complete the questionnaire. When the surveyor has determined just how long the questionnaire will take the *average respondent* to complete and the questionnaire is relatively short, then a direct estimate of the time needed can be provided. We stress "average respondent" because people differ in the amount of time they take and also differ as to whether they complete the questionnaire at one sitting or over multiple sittings. If an exact time estimate is given, the surveyor should clearly indicate that this represents only an average: Some respondents will take less time and some will take more time. An estimate of time needed should only be given after thorough pretesting and pilot work have been completed.

When surveyors anticipate that a questionnaire will take longer or may necessitate more thought on the part of respondents, it is better to indirectly indicate the probable time needed. This is what we chose to do in both the Workplace Assault Study and the PERK Study. In the cover letter for the assault study (Figure 3–10), we itemized the kinds of information we sought to collect—namely, the type of work they do and the place where they work, personal safety measures at their worksite, how safe or unsafe they feel at work, and their experience with workplace threats and assaults. We then went on to ask respondents to "please take the time to complete the questionnaire and return it in the enclosed self-addressed stamped envelope."

In the PERK Study (Figure 3–5), we similarly itemized the kinds of information to be collected and, in the third paragraph, assured respondents that "we have arranged for you to have enough time to finish the questionnaire before we start your vision testing."

The reason for using indirect methods to indicate the length of time needed in both of these studies was because we knew, for example, that in the Workplace Assault Study, those who had experienced assaults or threats would take significantly longer to complete the questionnaire but that the "average" respondent would not have had such experiences and would therefore not need a lengthy period of time. Thus, the range of time needed across the sample was broad but skewed toward less time.

In contrast, in the PERK Study, we knew from prior experience that respondents took about 25-30 minutes to complete the questionnaire; the respondents also knew that. Because we were careful to provide adequate time and resources for completing the questionnaire, we saw no reason to state a time in the introduction.

HOW AND WHY THE RESPONDENT WAS CHOSEN

Respondents are chosen in many different ways. In the Workplace Assault Study, respondents were selected randomly after union lists were prestratified according to job classification. Ten strata were created, and either 175 or 188 union members were selected from each stratum regardless of the number of persons in it. For purposes of the cover letter, it was not necessary to attempt to explain stratification to the respondents or exactly how randomization was achieved. It *was* important to emphasize that only some union members were being asked to complete the questionnaire, that these persons had been selected randomly, and that their responses were important because they represented others like themselves. This information appears in the first two sentences of the advance letter (Figure 3–8) and is described in more detail in the second paragraph of the cover letter (Figure 3–10) as follows:

> You have been randomly selected from the membership list of Local 660's Los Angeles County employees to participate in this survey. Only a small proportion of Los Angeles County employees has been selected to participate, so your experiences and thoughts on the subject are very important. **You will be representing many employees who are similar to yourself.**

In other studies, such as the PERK Study, everyone in a population receives the questionnaire. This is briefly referenced in the second paragraph of Figure 3–5 (Chapter 3) as follows:

> . . . In order to get accurate information about radial keratotomy and how it affects people's vision, we need information from **all** PERK patients. So please help us by answering the questions to the best of your ability.

EXPLANATION OF CONFIDENTIALITY AND HOW THE DATA WILL BE HANDLED

Both federal law and research ethics require that subjects of all research studies be provided with information about how the collected data will be used and how their privacy or the confidentiality of their data will be ensured. In self-administered questionnaires, advance letters, cover letters, and introductory instructions provide the best occasion for describing this information. In some studies, the collected data are truly anonymous in that no effort is made to log responses or contact nonrespondents. That was not the case in either of the two example studies.

As part of a long-term, ongoing study where questionnaires were filled out at a clinical site, PERK respondents clearly were identifiable. Furthermore, during analyses, questionnaire data were linked to ophthalmic measures of vision. At the same time, it was important that we provide as much confidentiality and anonymity to respondents as was possible within the requirements of the study. This was in our interests and in the interests of the respondents to maximize the probabilities that respondents' answers were honest and complete. As we noted earlier, one of the major issues was to assure respondents that the information collected would not be available to personnel at the clinical site and would not affect their health care. The last sentence in Figure 3–5 (Chapter 3) describes what respondents should do to ensure confidentiality: "When you are **finished** with the questionnaire, **seal** the questionnaire in the attached envelope." . . .

In the Workplace Assault Study, we had had no prior contact with the respondents, so we emphasized the confidentiality of the data and clearly specified that no information would be released to respondents' employers (see Figure 3–10). Furthermore, we increased confidence in our assurances of confidentiality by sending questionnaires to respondents' home addresses (not work) and by having questionnaires returned to UCLA rather than to the union offices. We were unable to guarantee anonymity from the research staff because we did indeed plan to follow up on nonrespondents. We also included questions at the end of the questionnaire that asked persons to volunteer for follow-up interviews and included code numbers on the outside of each return envelope.

PROVISION OF A NAME AND PHONE NUMBER TO CALL FOR INFORMATION

Respondents always must be provided with a name and phone number of someone who will be available to answer questions about the questionnaire. This person should be accessible, be able to answer questions, send additional copies of the questionnaire, or respond to other requests the respondents may have. Often, this will be the person or persons who sign the cover letter. In the case of the Workplace Assault Study, we provided the name of Deborah Riopelle, the project manager who was located at UCLA, and that of a recognized member of the union staff.

There are always potential respondents who will call to verify the purpose or sponsorship of a study to assure themselves that the organization is legitimate or that confidentiality will be maintained. Other potential respondents will have questions about the content of the questionnaire or how their name was selected for the sample. If no name and number are listed to call, the respondent is unlikely to complete and return the questionnaire. Whenever possible, we recommend offering the respondent the option of calling the project collect. Unfortunately, this was not possible in the Workplace Assault Study because telephones within the University of California cannot be set up to accept collect calls, and we were unable to provide a non-University number for respondents to contact.

WHEN AND HOW TO RETURN THE QUESTIONNAIRE

Many surveyors include in the cover letter a deadline for returning the completed questionnaire. This can work either way: The respondent may be motivated to complete the form and return it immediately so as not to miss the deadline, or, if the packet is put aside and picked up close to the deadline or after the deadline, respondents may believe that it is too late to respond. In the Workplace Assault Study, we attempted to go between the horns of this dilemma by giving a deadline date but providing latitude in the way we stated it. For example, "It would be very helpful to have your completed questionnaire returned to us by January 25, 1995."

The cover letter asked respondents to return the questionnaire "in the enclosed self-addressed stamped envelope." Remember that earlier we also strongly recommended that the return address be placed at the end of the questionnaire itself in case the questionnaire gets separated from the envelope.

Checklist for Motivating
Respondents and Writing Cover Letters

✓ **Explain the purpose of the study.**

✓ **Describe who is sponsoring the study.**

✓ **Consider sending an advance letter.**

✓ **Consider using other methods such as newsletters or flyers to publicize the study.**

✓ **Include a cover letter with the questionnaire.**

- Use letterhead.
- Date the letter to be consistent with the actual date of mailing or administration.
- Provide a name and phone number for the respondent to contact for further information.
- Personalize the salutation, if feasible.
- Maximize the attractiveness and readability of the letter.

✓ **Explain how respondents were chosen and why their participation is important.**

✓ **Explain when and how to return the questionnaire.**

✓ **Describe incentives, if used.**

✓ **Directly or indirectly provide a realistic estimate of the time required by the average respondent to complete the questionnaire.**

✓ **Explain how the confidentiality of the respondents' data will be protected.**

✓ **Determine whether and how a deadline date will be provided for returning questionnaires.**

Writing Questionnaire Specifications

Once a questionnaire has been finalized, the surveyor should write questionnaire specifications. Questionnaire specifications provide the first major documentation about the study, what its objectives were, who the respondents were, how the questionnaire was administered, how follow-up was conducted, how completed questionnaires were processed, and the reason that each question or set of questions was included in the questionnaire. Surveyors frequently feel that once they have completed the design and administration of a study they cannot possibly forget any detail of its creation or the decisions made.

In fact, substantial amounts of time can pass before collected data are actually analyzed or written up. Sometimes, surveyors run out of money to complete the study in a timely fashion. Sometimes, other competing activities or research projects necessitate the postponement of the study's completion. Sometimes, the original people involved with the study leave the organization to take other jobs. We personally know of situations where it has taken as long as 10 years for a study to be completed! Even when such interruptions do not occur, it behooves the conscientious surveyor to document the decisions made in constructing and administering the questionnaire.

At minimum, questionnaire specifications should include information about the objective of the study, the selection and tracking of the sample, the number and timing of administrations and follow-up procedures, and the sources and reasons for each question.

When questionnaires are administered by interview, specifications are reduced to "interviewer specifications," which are used in training interviewers and for interviewers to use as reference in the field.

OBJECTIVE OF THE STUDY

The specifications should briefly summarize the purpose of the study. In the specifications for the PERK Study, the objective of its questionnaire was stated as follows:

Objective: The 10-year questionnaire has three objectives. First, it allows us to get systematic information from patients at all the nine sites about problems they might have had, their current vision, and the current lens-wearing patterns. Second, it allows us to compare patients with themselves at baseline and at 1, 2, and 6 years after radial keratotomy on their first eye. Third, it allows us to compare the health of PERK patients to other, more representative samples of the United States' population.

Notice that the questionnaire had three objectives. The first objective was one that necessitated the collection of "new" or original data from this questionnaire, but the second and third objectives imply that some of the questions on the questionnaire will be adopted or adapted from past PERK questionnaires or other sources that will enable the data collected to be compared with existent data sets. The specification of these three objectives already alerts the reader as to the kind of questions that will be asked and the fact that some of the questions on this questionnaire are not original but are drawn from other studies.

SELECTION AND TRACKING OF THE SAMPLE

In the PERK Study, the questionnaire was given to *all* participants in the clinical trial as soon as they entered the clinical center for their 10-year examination. No effort was made to administer to patients who did not come in for this follow-up examination.

In contrast, in the Workplace Assault Study, union personnel randomly selected between 175 and 188 members from each of 10 job categories in the two locals.[1] This resulted in 1,763 names. Insufficient addresses existed for 19 of these names so they were immediately eliminated from the sample.

On January 5 and 6, 1995, advance letters were sent to the remaining 1,744 persons. On January 17, 1995, packets containing the questionnaire, a cover letter, a flyer, and an envelope for returning the questionnaire were mailed to the same 1,744 persons, which we considered our sample. On January 24, 1995, reminder postcards were sent to these persons, regardless of whether or not they had returned the questionnaire (see Figure 3–7 in Chapter 3). Then, on March 4 through 6, 1995, a second questionnaire with a new cover letter was sent to the 1,143 persons who had failed to respond to our first two mailings but for whom addresses appeared to be correct. Note that the new cover letter repeated some of the same information given before but added a section that emphasized the importance of getting responses from people who were *not* assaulted or who did *not* perceive their workplaces to be unsafe (see Figure 4–2). Finally, in April 1995, we began contacting by telephone those who still had not responded.

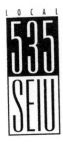

SOCIAL SERVICES
UNION

AMERICAN
FEDERATION
OF NURSES

309 So. RAYMOND
AVENUE
PASADENA
CALIFORNIA
91105
818-796-0051
FAX 818-796-2335

February 21, 1995

Dear Member,

　　About four weeks ago we sent you a questionnaire about personal safety and security while at work. As of today, we have not yet received your completed questionnaire.

　　The Service Employees International Union, Local 535 is conducting this study of workplace safety in cooperation with the Southern California Injury Prevention Research Center at UCLA because of concerns members have expressed about personal safety while at work. Results from this survey will help determine measures that could be taken to protect Local 535 members.

　　You may feel that because your safety at work has not been threatened you don't need to reply. This is not true. By hearing about the experiences of all Local 535 members we can develop a better idea of which situations are safer than others. We are writing to you again because of the importance **each** questionnaire has to the study. **We need your completed questionnaire.**

　　We recognize how busy you must be and greatly appreciate you taking the time to complete this questionnaire. If by chance you did not receive the first questionnaire or it got misplaced, we have enclosed a replacement. It would be very helpful to have your completed questionnaire returned to us by **March 3, 1995.**

　　<u>Your responses are confidential.</u> **No names or individual information will be used or released to your employer.** If you have any questions or concerns, please feel free to call Deborah Riopelle, M.S.P.H. at UCLA, (310) 555-4053 or Wilma Cadorna at Local 535 at 818-555-0051.

Sincerely,

Jerry L. Clyde   Linda Bourque, Ph.D.
President, Social Services Chapter   UCLA School of Public Health
SEIU Local 535

Figure 4–2.　Example of Cover Letter Directed to Respondents as Part of Second Full Mailing (Nonresponders)

All of the above information, starting with how the sample was selected and why it was selected that way and ending with response rates by time of contact and job category, is documented in the questionnaire specifications. Thus, when we get ready to analyze and write up our findings, we can quickly go to the Questionnaire Specifications to refresh our memory about how and why we selected the sample we did, the kind of response we obtained at each stage of the mailing, and the extent to which response rates differed by job stratum.

TIMING OF ADMINISTRATION

The above section also documents the *timing* of contacts with the sample. In the PERK Study, the questionnaire was given out only once, and every effort was made to ensure that clinic personnel obtained a completed questionnaire from each respondent.

In contrast, in the Workplace Assault Study, respondents were contacted a minimum of three times (advance letter, first mailing of questionnaire, and follow-up postcard) and a maximum of five or more times (advance letter, first mailing of questionnaire, follow-up postcard, second mailing of questionnaire, and one or more phone calls).

By keeping track of *when* a respondent responded relative to the timing and number of the contact, the surveyor can assess various things about the sample—for example, whether responsiveness varies with job category, gender, age, perceptions of vulnerability in the workplace, or actual experiences of physical assault.

INSTRUCTIONS FOR ADMINISTERING QUESTIONS

Once the timing and method of contacting respondents had been specified for the Workplace Assault Study, no further administrative requirements had to be outlined in the specifications.

In contrast, in the PERK Study, the specifications contained instructions to the clinical coordinator for administering the questionnaire as follows:

ADMINISTRATION
OF THE QUESTIONNAIRE

TIME: Allow at least 30 minutes for the patient to fill out the questionnaire. If you interview any patients over the phone, make sure that they have the time to do it. You may want to call them and arrange a special time for you to conduct the interview.

SITE: Provide each patient with a quiet room or secluded area in the general waiting room. Provide them with a pencil or pen, table or clipboard, and the envelope in which to put the completed questionnaire.

OTHER PEOPLE: Discourage other people from "helping" the patient fill out the questionnaire. If you interview them, try to do it at a time when they will not be interrupted by family or colleagues and at a time when they have no other things to do.

EMPHASIZE: We want to know about **their experiences** with radial keratotomy and how they feel about things. There are no "right" or "wrong" answers, and patients should not try to please you with the answer they give. We **expect** to find variations in opinions and experiences.

In general, remember that **we need their opinions** of their vision, not our observations about what we think their vision is. Please give them enough time to think about their answers and avoid hurrying them through the questionnaire. If patients do not like our alternatives, encourage them to write down their feelings or experiences and we will evaluate the information they provide.

COVER PAGE:	The cover page provides the patient with a brief description of the information that the questionnaire is designed to collect. As you give the questionnaire to the patient, direct his or her attention to the second and third paragraphs in particular. These describe how the data will be used and tell the patient what to do when he or she has completed the questionnaire.
COORDINATOR:	Before giving the questionnaire to the patient, please make sure that the patient's identification number is on every page of the questionnaire and that the date of administration is filled out on the cover page.

Notice that the above instructions are formatted in a way to make it easier for the survey administrator to find information on a particular subject, and that every effort is made to encourage the clinic coordinator *not* to interfere with the patient while he or she is filling out the questionnaire. This is particularly important when the persons administering a questionnaire are not professional interviewers. In the same way that surveyors must try to recognize and compensate for their own biases, they also need to try to anticipate the biases of others who may be involved in the collection of data.

QUESTIONS RAISED BY RESPONDENTS

In the same way that questionnaire specifications attempt to anticipate the attitudes and behaviors of data collectors, surveyors need to try to anticipate questions or challenges that respondents may direct to a data collector. Whenever possible, data collectors should be given information that helps them answer such questions or handle such challenges. The following information was included in the specifications for the PERK Study:

QUESTIONS RAISED
BY THE PATIENT

Questions asked about the questionnaire will probably be of two types: a question of clarification or a question designed to have **you** provide the information or **your** opinion about their vision.

CLARIFICATION:	If a patient does not understand a question, try to find out what it is that he or she does not understand and try to find a synonym or another way to say it. Please make a note of the question asked and let Portia Griffin at Emory know about it.
NO APPROPRIATE ANSWER AVAILABLE:	If a patient cannot represent him/herself with the answers available, tell him or her to write down an answer that **does** represent his or her feelings or experiences.
CHALLENGES:	If a subject starts to challenge the objective of the questionnaire or a particular item in it, or says that it is repetitive, etc., please listen, be polite, and be noncommittal. **Do not give** patients the answers or indicate that you will let them stop answering the questions.

Source and Reason for Questions

The major historical purpose of questionnaire specifications has been to document the source and reason for including a question or set of questions in an instrument. Figure 4–3 provides an example of the specifications from the PERK Study, which describes Questions 2 through 12 (see Figure 3–1, Chapter 3), Questions 43 through 45, and Questions 54 through 61 (see Figure 3–3).

Notice that specifications may be provided for sets of questions (e.g., Q2-25), subsets of questions (Q2-7, Q9-13, Q43-45, and Q54-65), or for individual questions (e.g., Q9, Q10, Q11, and Q12). Each specification describes what the purpose of the question or questions is and whether it replicates or revises an earlier question or, by implication, indicates that it is a new question. For example, Questions 2 through 7 replicate questions that were asked in earlier PERK questionnaires and the RAND Health Insurance Experiment. In contrast, Questions 9 through 13 are new to this questionnaire because this is the first time that we are assessing presbyopia, or a person's increased inability to see things that are close as he or she ages.

Questions 43 through 45 also replicate questions that were used in other PERK questionnaires and in the HIE. In the case of these questions, however, data collected were reported in an earlier article. The fact that this occurred is documented as part of the specification, and complete citations are provided for those articles. This reminds the surveyor at a later time that these earlier analyses had occurred and provides a quick reference as to where to find information about them.

In general, if a specification cannot be written for *why* a question exists, then there probably is no reason to have the question on the questionnaire.

PERK 10-Year Questionnaire
August 17, 1992

LENS-WEARING PATTERNS:

Q2-25   Questions 2-25 ask patients to tell us about their current lens-wearing patterns.

Q2-7   Questions 2-7 were used in both the baseline and 6-year questionnaires to measure patients' functional vision. These questions are similar to questions used in RAND's Health Insurance Experiment and a wide range of other studies where vision has been assessed. We are repeating them so that we can see what kind of effect radial keratotomy has had on their functional vision. The questions on presbyopia and distant vision that were added to Question 1 above represent an effort to improve the precision of information traditionally collected exclusively with Questions 6 and 7.

Q8   In evaluating how presbyopia affects the eyes of persons who have had radial keratotomy, we realized that we have no way of identifying patients who might have been presbyopic at baseline. Question 8 provides an opportunity to get a rough estimate of this.

Q9-13   Questions 9-13 assess whether patients have become or are becoming presbyopic and how presbyopia is affecting both their vision and their use of lenses. These questions can also be used in assessing how severe over-correction affects the daily vision of PERK patients.

Q9   Ascertains whether the patient was told about presbyopia in the context of the PERK Study.

Q10   Ascertains whether the patient is presbyopic and whether presbyopia has necessitated the use of spectacles for near vision.

Q11   Ascertains when presbyopia resulted in the use of spectacles.

Q12   A number of situations are listed in Question 12. Patients are asked to respond for **each eye.** By looking at the pattern of responses to Question 12, we will be able to assess to what degree patients are disabled by presbyopia or severe overcorrection of their vision.

.
.
.
.

(continued)

Q43-45   These three questions were in both the baseline and 6-year questionnaires. Originally included in RAND's Health Insurance Experiment, data obtained with these questions were reported in Borque, Rubenstein, Cosand et al., Psychological characteristics of candidates for the Prospective Evaluation of Radial Keratotomy, Archives of Ophthalmology 1984; 102:1187-1192. Inclusion of these questions will allow us to compare the patients both to themselves at earlier points in time and to RAND myopes.

.
.
.
.
.

Q54-65   Questions 54-65 provide us with information about how and when PERK patients use their eyes to read, drive, watch television, and participate in sports and other physical activities. The number and type of activities done as well as the time of day at which they are done may influence their need for and use of lenses.

Figure 4–3.   Example of Questionnaire Specification

Checklist for Writing Questionnaire Specifications

✓ **Briefly describe the objective of the study.**

✓ **Describe the study sample and response rates.**

✓ **Describe any tracking done of the sample.**

✓ **Describe timing of data collection and tracking.**

✓ **Provide instructions for administering questionnaires.**

✓ **Provide answers for data collectors to use in response to anticipated questions.**

✓ **Index specifications for easy reference.**

✓ **Describe why a question is asked.**

✓ **If questions are adopted or adapted from other studies, explain the reasons for such decisions and provide complete citations to the other studies.**

Note

1. Nine strata were selected from Local 660, the largest local, and 175 names were randomly selected within each stratum. The population of each group at the time of the sample draw was as follows: Public Social Services, 6,208; Public Health Department, 1,336; Public Library, 309; Probation, 578; Sheriff's Department, 908; Parks and Recreation, Animal Care and Control, and Public Works, 922; Assessor's Office, Children's Services, and Treasurer and Tax Collector Offices, 1,625; Municipal and Superior Courts, 1,067; and Hospitals, 3,501. Only 3,221 members of Local 535 work in Los Angeles County, with the largest group being the 2,090 in the Department of Social Services; 188 persons were randomly selected from this stratum.

5 Implementation

The implementation of self-administered and mailed surveys requires considerable coordination and attention to detail. This multistage process begins with sample selection and ends with the processing of the last of the returned and completed questionnaires.

In this chapter, we discuss issues associated with the identification and selection of the sample as well as the material costs and staffing needs associated with self-administered and mailed surveys. We elaborate on the processes involved in coordinating self-administered surveys, or in the case of mailed surveys, preparing packets for mailing, posting these packets, subsequent follow-up and return of packets, and procedures typically used for the tracking of envelopes returned

135

due to unknown addressee or no such address. Actual examples of expected expenditures and person hours are provided.

Developing and Producing the Sample

Typically, a self-administered or mailed survey is considered only when the investigator is confident that the desired sample population is accessible at a designated location. This survey methodology is often the only efficient means of obtaining data from a somewhat rare population. When the goal of a survey is to collect data about individuals with a characteristic that is not common in the population, this is known as a rare population. For example, say a major motorcycle manufacturer wanted to test the acceptance of a new concept in handle bars by the motorcycle-riding public. The easiest approach might be to mail a survey to members of motorcycle clubs or to hand out questionnaires at large motorcycle distributorships or motorcycle repair shops.

These characteristics of groups sampled for self-administered questionnaires can be further refined by even greater selectivity of the location of administration. For example, if the purpose of the study is to determine the types of baby products used by mothers of infants, a quick and easy sample source would be to conduct self-administered surveys with parents in the waiting rooms of well-baby clinics. In short, samples can be gathered from many sources such as waiting rooms, a line in a place of business, a classroom, a home address, a place of employment, or a temporary residence, such as a school dormitory or a hospital room. Self-administered surveys conducted in this manner are known as convenience samples and are generally used as a means of getting data easily and quickly from highly specialized populations. In many instances, a self-administered survey eliminates what would otherwise be an overwhelming effort and cost to locate at random particular types of individuals within the general population.

Mail surveys are often sent to members of professional, political, religious, or social organizations; employees within a particular institution or job classification; students; subscribers to newsletters and magazines; and consumers of particular products or services. Again, a major consideration in favor of using a mailed survey is the appreciably lower cost of locating appropriate populations.

Not all self-administered or mailed surveys are conducted because of the ease of finding a rare population, however. Frequently, this method is chosen because it is far less expensive to conduct than is a telephone or face-to-face survey. Additionally, mailed surveys can sometimes be more successful at getting data from hard-to-reach populations such as doctors, business executives, and politicians.

There are certain caveats to consider when evaluating a mailed survey coming from certain sources. For example, if you are considering using addresses and/or names and addresses obtained from telephone directories, you should first consider the approximate mobility of the population under consideration and the rate of unlisted households in the area. If you are mailing to specific names in the telephone book, you should determine the rate of turnover in telephone number ownership, that is, how many people are likely to change their telephone number by the time you use the directory for a sample. Obviously, this will result in undelivered or unanswered mail.

It is also wise to determine from your local telephone company the proportion of households with unlisted numbers. If the number is not listed, that household will have no opportunity to be included in the survey and will therefore be underrepresented in the population. If having an unlisted telephone number is typical of particular population types, such as the elderly, those with a high income, or single females, your sample will be biased away from that portion of the population. In some cities, such as Los Angeles, the unlisted rate is around 60% of the households, whereas in less urban areas, it can drop below 20%. A different twist on this problem is households with the telephone number listed in the directory but with the street address suppressed. Regardless of the source, you should always try to determine how your sample might be biased due to lack of inclusion.

SAMPLE AVAILABILITY

When a self-administered survey is to be conducted in a group setting, permission to access this population must be obtained from the institution where these individuals are. In the case of the well-baby clinic, we would need permission from the hospital or medical director of the establishment to approach the patients. Likewise with the motorcycle club members, we would need to be granted access to these individuals by the executive level of the club or clubs. For dealerships or repair shops, we would also need owner permission to approach customers on the premises.

In some instances, it may be necessary for the organization granting the access to obtain informed consent from the individuals to be studied, prior to allowing you access. In most cases, with mailed surveys, the name and address of the sampled individual is recorded and available in some electronic medium. Obviously, access to these files is not possible without proper authorization. Permission to access the data banks or lists must be obtained from the organization.

The fees for samples can vary considerably. When working with groups or organizations who are either sponsoring the research or are interested in the results, you may simply be asked to cover the cost of materials (i.e., labels and machine time), or you may have to pay for both the labor and materials required to program and process your request.

In some instances, the cooperating organization may provide the labels free of charge and, not uncommonly, will help defray part or all of the mailing costs. Typically, the association should be able to provide either addressed mailing labels or raw data on some compatible computer medium. There are publishing companies who specialize in the compilation and production of directories of government officials and employees, corporate officials, business firms within professions, and the like.

In other instances, the focal point of the research may be on types of individuals with particular sociodemographic or socioeconomic characteristics. The addressee may be known, or the survey may have to be sent to an anonymous "resident" or "occupant." In a situation such as this, a sample may be purchased from a directory publisher, commercial bulk-mailing establishment, or specialized marketing firm. These organizations have compiled mailing addresses within certain demographic domains. Often, U.S. Census data are linked to ZIP codes so that samples can be focused on neighborhoods where households with particular characteristics are more likely to exist, such as married senior citizens with annual incomes over $30,000. Many organizations involved in providing address samples supplement the data with information they have gathered from other sources, such as sales profiles from department or grocery stores, newspaper readership, and other surveys conducted in the area.

In today's computer-based environment, the amount of information available about each of us is at times very disconcerting. When using purchased samples, keep in mind that they are not necessarily representative of the general population and may be subject to innumerable biases.

List samples can often be unreliable. They may be out-of-date—that is, they do not have current address and/or telephone number information on an individual—or they may not contain all the candidates possible for inclusion in the study. Lists can be up-to-date and inclusive and still contain clerical errors that will cause problems reaching the respondent. It is always a good idea to spot-check your sample before using it—for example, mailing to a few addresses, making some telephone calls, or comparing list information to another source, such as the telephone directory.

SELECTING THE SAMPLE

When administrating a questionnaire at a site such as a grocery store, you may want to ask all individuals encountered to fill out the form, or you may want to select a subsample of these individuals. If you decide on a subsample, you need to determine a means of representatively selecting respondents rather than taking only the first group to appear. Ideally, you want to spread your sample out evenly over times of day, days of the week, or types of individuals. A commonly used means of selecting respondents is to determine a sampling interval.

For example, assume that 1,000 parents of infants come into the well-baby clinics in our sample in any given week. We have decided that we want to interview only 200 of them. To spread the sample across the entire week's population, we would approach every fifth client who comes for well-baby care. This is known as a sampling interval. This method of selection provides a systematically selected sample within a given time period and place.

If a subgroup within the general sample population is of interest, such as people between 35 and 55 years of age or African Americans, you will want to select the respondents at different sampling intervals to ensure that you obtain data from a sufficient number of individuals for each group you want to compare. This is called stratified systematic sampling.

In some group settings, such as clinics or classrooms, you may be able to preselect respondents from patient charts or class rosters. Again, you will need permission to gain access to these records. If a list is not available, you will have to determine another means of selecting respondents, such as the order in which they signed in or entered the room.

Selecting a mailing sample uses essentially the same process. If not using the whole list (or universe), you will want to give instructions to the processor as to how to select the sample using a sampling interval. When selecting or drawing samples it is a common practice to start at a random starting point in the list and, using a constant interval, rotate from the bottom around to the top of the list and down to the initial starting point. If, for example, we have a list of 1,000 mothers who bring their babies to a clinic and we want to send questionnaires to 200, we select a random start point—say, woman #322 on the list—and then take every fifth woman on the list (e.g., 327, 332, 337, etc.). Again, if the data file contains individual data on characteristics of particular interest, you want to draw the sample with different sampling intervals for different types of individuals.

ADDRESSING THE MAILING

There are three methods for putting the sample address on the mailing packet. Addresses can be handwritten on the envelopes, typed or printed directly on them, or labels affixed to them. There has been some research indicating a nonsignificant increase in the rate of returns with hand-addressed envelopes. Similarly, machine-printed envelopes are received a bit more favorably than those with labels affixed. Unless the sample size is extremely small, say, a few hundred, the intensive labor involved in hand-addressing envelopes does not warrant this approach. Similarly, if the sample file must be created by hand-typing, it would be wiser to spend this clerical time entering the information into a computer file so that it is available for subsequent mailings.

As a final precaution, with much of the mail being optically scanned today, it is wise to check with your local post office to determine if there are any specific layout restrictions on bulk mailing. As an example, we discovered that if more than four spaces occurred between the last number of the street address and the street name, the post office scanner stopped reading at the unit number and found the address "incomplete." When you lay out your data field for addressing, be sure that the address length and width conforms to the size of your mailing labels.

PLANNING THE SAMPLE FILE

When providing specifications for the sample format or label layout, consider how many mailings you plan to send to each respondent. If the sample file is not easily accessible, you will want to have all the necessary materials run at the same time. For example, if you plan an initial mailing and two follow-ups, ask for three copies of the labels to be run along with a hard-copy printout of the sample. This will eliminate the need to return to the supplier and ask for additional label runs and will give you a master copy of the sample against which you can log in your returns.

This can save costs in the long run because typically a substantial part of the cost in running address labels is in the initial set-up time or programming. Thus, requesting additional sets of labels on the initial run adds only to the cost of materials and not to the cost of labor. If for some reason you cannot obtain more than one set of address labels, most copying machines can generate label sheets if the original label format is a standard three addresses across.

If you are running the address labels from within your own organization and there is no problem with access, you probably will not want to run all the sets at one time. If you are going to have the postal service send back address corrections, or you plan to do tracking on bad addresses, you will want to make these changes or corrections to your master file before you produce the next batch of labels. Additionally, if you are logging in the completed returns, you will have eliminated labels for these respondents and for those who are lost to follow-up (deceased, no useable address, etc.).

Another consideration for label production is whether to use self-adhesive versus Cheshire labels.[1] If you are putting labels on by hand, only self-adhesive labels are possible. If the labels are to be machine affixed, consult with your mailing coordinator to determine the type of machine to be used for your mailing.

The final consideration for label production is how the materials are to be delivered. If your mailing is to be delivered using the U.S. Postal Service, specify that the sample address labels be run in ZIP code order. This is especially important if your mailing is large, say, 500 pieces or more. The Postal Service will discount postage on large mailings if your addresses are presorted by ZIP code.

If on the odd chance you are dealing with a sample that is not computerized—that is, it does not exist in a machine-readable file—it may well be cost- and time-effective to enter it into a computerized medium.

When entering the address data or setting up the sample file, it is advisable to have the final file accessible to some type of spreadsheet program or other software that will enable you to call up individual respondents on request. If you are going to log in your returns by individual, you will want to be able to call up the identification number of the case and preestablish entry locations for the date of return and the type of outcome. By outcome we mean keeping track of the undeliverables as well as the completes. Examples of outcomes are moved and left no address, no such address, insufficient address, respondent deceased, refused to complete, and completed questionnaire received.

You will want to run sample progress reports at some designated interval, such as once a week. This report should compile the information in your file to document the total number of completed questionnaires, the number of undeliverables, and the number yet to be resolved. These files can be very extensive and can include information on tracking progress variables such as telephone directory search initiated, Department of Motor Vehicles search initiated, search outcome, date of initiation or outcome, and possibly the individual responsible for the search.

In the case of group administration where a sample list is not likely to exist, you will minimally want to keep daily records of number of completes and, if special populations are being sampled, the numbers within each subgroup that have been completed. You should also keep a count of the number of individuals who have declined to participate.

ETHICS AND RESPONSIBILITIES

Always keep respondent confidentiality foremost in your planning. The maintenance and storage of your sample should never provide the opportunity for anyone outside your survey staff to see who, what, and where potential respondents are, nor whether or not they have returned the survey. As is often the case, you may have individuals working on some aspect of your study who have never been exposed to survey research. It is incumbent on you to educate these employees on the protection of subjects and any information that may have been gathered about them.

In some work settings, such as hospitals, clinics, or schools, there may already be established a human subjects protection committee whose mandate is to review all research protocols and ensure that no harm can come to respondents if they participate in any research. Protecting the respondents and doing them no harm are the primary responsibilities of anyone who conducts a survey.

Another "standard" adopted by the sincere surveyor is to be honest about your intent in the survey. It is dishonest to solicit participation in any type of survey under one pretext and then use the survey to promote something else. Some surveyors will claim that they are not trying to solicit a product or money and then turn around and try to sell a product or solicit funds later in the interview. Sometimes, information is solicited in the interview that is later used for a follow-up for solicitation. This is not only deceitful but gives the entire profession of survey research a bad name.

SAMPLE SIZE

Several factors must be taken into account when considering the size or number of individuals or institutions to whom you will administer or send the questionnaire. The first concern should be to determine how many completed responses will be required to demonstrate that your research hypothesis is correct. There are several easy-to-use publications available that provide basic survey sampling guidelines (see **How to Design Surveys** and **How to Sample in Surveys,** Vols. 5 and 6, respectively, in this series). In situations where the number of individuals qualified to respond to your survey is limited, you may need to survey the entire universe of individuals or institutions.

Once the minimally acceptable completed sample size (the number of filled-out, returned questionnaires) has been determined, the total sample size, or the number of individuals or addresses required to produce the desired number of usable returns, can be estimated. With self-administered questionnaires in group settings, sample loss occurs because individuals decline to participate, group turnout is lower than expected, or the materials have not been distributed as directed. In mailed surveys, there are two main causes of respondent loss that need to be compensated for: bad addresses and nonresponse.

If an initial purpose of the mailing is to screen a population for particular characteristics, it will be necessary to factor in the proportion of your overall population that you estimate will qualify and increase your mailing sample size accordingly. For example, you have a list of all homeowners in a particular area, but your primary focus is on homeowners with minor children in the household. You will need to obtain an estimate of the proportion of owner-occupied homes with children under 18 in residence and adjust your overall mailing size upward to account for the loss of owner-occupied homes without minor children.

All address lists are subject to attrition and error. Often, these lists are at least a year old. In some population types, residential or occupational mobility is extremely high. Also, many address files are based on information that is handwritten; therefore, the entry is subject to the interpretation of the individual typing in the data as well as the completeness of the information provided. Typing or entry errors are a final source of address error. It takes only one error in street address or ZIP code to render a mailing undeliverable.

Due to these sources of error, the next item for consideration in determining sample size is an estimate of the proportion of names and/or addresses in your sample file that will be unusable. By unusable we mean those mailings that the post office has deemed undeliverable. Some of the reasons for postal nondelivery are addressee unknown, moved and left no for-warding address, forwarding order has expired, incomplete address, no such address, and refused delivery. The post office will maintain forwarding address orders for one year and no longer. You will need an estimate of the proportion of the sample you will lose for these reasons.

It may be possible for the supplier to estimate the loss based on prior experience, or you may have to conduct a pretest to arrive at this figure. A pretest would involve mailing a packet to a small representative group from the sample to determine the rate of bad returns. Ideally, you will have conducted at least one pilot pretest of your questionnaire and methodology (see Chapter 3). A pilot test of the methods and questionnaire to be used in your final study can provide the rate of bad returns while assessing questionnaire performance.

There are two approaches to compensating for bad ad-dresses. You may decide not to pursue the bad addresses and simply provide enough overage in the sample draw to compen-sate for these returns, or you may try to track the correct addresses. Usually, no matter how good your tracking efforts, some respondents can never be found. Be aware that by simple replacement of good addresses for bad ones (e.g., not tracking new information on the original sample), you may introduce a level of bias into your results by including only those respon-dents who are easy to reach or who are either residentially or occupationally less mobile. This can have major conse-quences, depending on the focus of the research.

The next consideration for estimating sample size is the anticipated response rate, or the number of subjects from the sample population who will complete and return the question-naire within the study time period. The proportion of respon-dents who do not participate compared to the number who could have is referred to as the nonresponse rate. Response rates for mailed surveys can vary widely, depending on the accuracy of the sampled addresses, the rigor of the follow-up procedures, the quality of presentation of the study materials, and respondent incentive or interest in the study topic.

Another consideration for the success of a survey, self-administered or mailed, is timing. If at all possible do not initiate surveys around the time of major holidays. Generally, these are times when postal volume increases, and you do not want your survey to risk being delayed or lost in delivery because of the extra load being handled by the postal service at this time. Also, many households and businesses are inundated at these times with charity appeals, mail-order catalogues, and other "pulp" materials. Your survey runs a greater risk of being discarded or put aside during these peak periods. Finally, you will not want your survey conducted at a time when individuals are already overloaded with preparations for a holiday. Depending on the type of individuals being surveyed, summer months when people tend to go on vacation can also be deadly times for response rates.

Other Factors Affecting Response Rates

Mailing experiments have tested hand-addressed envelopes versus typed addresses, typed versus affixed labels, and affixed postage versus postal metering. Some of these treatments have a positive but nonsignificant effect on response rates, but special treatment of the mailing does have a beneficial effect. Accuracy of the sampled addresses has already been discussed; follow-up procedures and respondent motivation are covered later in this chapter. Response rates for mailed surveys can be 30% or lower when follow-up is minimal and the sample is composed of disinterested, nonmotivated respondents. Conversely, when there is repeated contact with respondents by mail and by telephone and a large portion of the respondents are interested and motivated, response rates up to 70% or more have been achieved.

Components of the Field or Mailing Packet

Successfully completing self-administered surveys, especially mailed surveys, requires good coordination and great attention to detail because of the numerous steps involved. The best way to impose organization on a self-administered study is to make a checklist of all the major steps involved. The best way to anticipate the steps involved is to make a checklist of the components of the group administration or mailing packet.

Group Administration Packet Checklist

✓ **Sample: Access and means of selection?**

✓ **Schedule: Calendar of date/time/place**

✓ **Informed consent: If necessary, quantity?**

✓ **Cover letter: Print quantity?**

✓ **Questionnaire: Print quantity?**

✓ **Incentive: If used, quantity?**

✓ **Other handouts: If any, quantity?**

✓ **Means of retrieval: Collect/box/mail back?**

Mailing Packet Checklist

✓ **Sample labels/addresses: Quantity?
Number of follow-ups?**

✓ **Outgoing mail envelopes: Quantity?
Size of questionnaire? Additional materials?
Number of follow-ups?**

✓ **Outgoing postage: Metered or stamped?**

✓ **Cover letter: Print quantity? Initial letter?
Follow-up letter(s)?**

✓ **Questionnaire: Print quantity?
Number of remailings?**

✓ **Incentive: If used, quantity?**

✓ **Other inserts: If any, quantity?**

✓ **Return mail envelope: Postage-paid business reply/
metered/stamps? Number of remailings?**

Follow-Up Procedures

The surest method for increasing response rates is through follow-ups. By follow-ups we mean recontacting respondents to remind them to complete the questionnaire and mail it back. These follow-ups can be in the form of a postcard, a letter, a telephone call, and/or a complete remailing. Some studies use mailgrams or telegrams or overnight, registered, or certified mail to draw attention to the study and to stress the importance of each return. Minimally, you will want to send a follow-up postcard or letter to either your nonrespondents or the entire sample approximately 10 days after you posted your initial mailing. This postcard or letter should remind respondents that they have been sent a questionnaire to fill out and return, restate the importance of their participation, and encourage them to take a few minutes to do so now if they have not already done so. Include the name and telephone number of someone on the project staff to call collect if the respondent has misplaced the questionnaire and wishes a replacement to be sent, as is shown on the postcard used in the Workplace Assault Study (see Figure 3–7 in Chapter 3).

In this letter or postcard, indicate that you are aware of the possibility that the respondent has already completed and mailed the materials and apologize for any nuisance this follow-up mailing may have caused. Sometimes, offering the respondent an excuse for not responding helps (e.g., "We recognize how busy your schedule must be . . ."; "Perhaps like many of us do when we are busy, you have put the questionnaire to one side and forgotten it . . ."; or "Perhaps someone else in your office/household has mistakenly thrown the questionnaire away"—then explain that all they need to do is call and another packet will be sent). Of course, if you are working with a postcard, the text will have to be brief and all you can accomplish is to ask the respondent to complete the questionnaire and send it back.

Another option is using facsimile (fax) machine transmission. If your respondents have a fax machine or access to one, you can fax them the questionnaire. Conversely, you can encourage respondents to fax their completed forms back to you if they have the means to do so. If the subject matter of the questionnaire is such that it would reveal confidential material, you would not want to suggest this method unless you are able to guarantee that no one outside the project team could possibly see the material.

Depending on the nature and confidentiality of your study, it is desirable to have assigned an unique identification number to each subject in the sample population prior to mailing. This number should be printed somewhere on the questionnaire itself or on the return mail envelope. The back or last page of the questionnaire is the least obtrusive. If you have been explicit about confidentiality in your cover letter that was sent with the questionnaire, few respondents will react negatively to seeing an identification number on their materials. There are always the few exceptions who will scratch out or tear off the identification number.

There are two major reasons for assigning identification numbers before mailing. First, you will be able to keep track of who has responded by logging the returns against a master sample list of the individuals to whom you sent the mailing. Knowing who has not responded allows you to limit your follow-up efforts to only that group of individuals rather than the entire sample. In a large study, you can realize significant savings in the time and cost involved in conducting follow-ups. Second, identifying the sample can sometimes provide you with a profile of the nonresponding group so that you may venture an estimate of how alike or different the two groups are (respondents vs. nonrespondents). Clearly, the more alike they are, the better your data will represent the sampled population.

TYPE, NUMBER, AND TIMING OF FOLLOW-UPS

There are several issues to consider when planning follow-ups for your survey: the type, the number to be conducted, and how frequently or at what critical times to administer them. Typically, these decisions are based on the resources available to you and the amount of time you have allotted for your study. If you are producing a sample status report, as discussed earlier, you will find these reports an invaluable aid in deciding what measures need to be taken for follow-ups.

For example, if from the sample status report you see that after the first follow-up you have received 80% of your expected returns, you may decide to conduct only one more follow-up. If you are collecting data in a group setting and your "completes" are coming in at a faster rate than expected, you may need to alter your sampling interval to collect respondents at a slower rate, or you may want to lower the number of days during which you collect data.

Conversely, if after your first follow-up you have only received 20% of your expected returns, you may decide to conduct more intensive follow-ups, such as telephone calls and priority mailings, sooner than originally anticipated. If, from these reports, you notice a particularly high rate of bad addresses—that is, the number of nondeliverables precludes your ability to obtain the minimally desired number of returns from your study—you may want to pursue the possibility of pulling another sample. In a group administration, if the number of "completes" is lower than anticipated, you may shorten the sampling interval, add more days to the administration, or add more sites of administration.

Mailed follow-ups require additional printing, postage, envelopes, and labor. Telephone follow-ups assume that you have valid telephone numbers for your respondents and require considerable labor and the space and equipment to conduct the telephone calls, which may involve toll or long-distance charges besides the monthly cost of the telephone. Depending on the type of sample you are seeking, numerous calls may be required to contact each respondent. This is particularly true with elite samples, such as doctors, public figures, and executives.

As mentioned earlier, conducting follow-ups is the best means of increasing response rate. At minimum, you will want to send a postcard reminder to each person in your sample who has not returned a completed questionnaire. Typically, this postcard is sent 10 days to 2 weeks after the initial mailing date, with subsequent follow-ups made at 2-week intervals or longer.

If you have the time and resources to conduct several follow-ups of various types, it is often best to begin with the least expensive method first—postcard or letter—and use more expensive methods later, such as a complete remailing of the packet, priority mailings (e.g., registered or certified letter, mailgrams, etc.), and telephone calls. If you have been able to keep a log of your sample returns and can identify who has not responded, you will be using the more expensive methods on increasingly smaller sample sizes. Although this is a more economical approach, the researcher does not always have the luxury of time to consider this.

The greatest efficiency for follow-ups seems to peak at about three or four. Obviously, if time and money are of no consequence you may make as many attempts as you wish. There does come a point, however, at which it makes no sense and is in fact no longer relevant to push for returns. This is a highly individual decision. If response has been particularly poor on a study, some researchers will continue to make follow-up attempts using every resource available. Remember, the credibility of the study rests in large part on the number of sampled individuals you have successfully represented.

When the telephone is used as a follow-up method, it is not uncommon for the call to be used as a means of gathering the data contained in the questionnaire rather than waiting for a mailed response. This assumes that the individuals making the calls are familiar with telephone interviewing and with the questionnaire and are capable of collecting the data in a competent manner. A telephone interview is only possible when the questionnaire you are using is relatively brief and does not require the respondent to have access to other information, such as files or records, to answer the questions. In studies where self-administration is the only desirable method due to study sensitivity or the perceived honesty of the respondent, you will not want to use the telephone to collect the data.

If you do collect some of your data using the telephone, it is wise to indicate in the data set which interviews have been self-administered and which were conducted by telephone. In survey jargon, this is known as using "mixed methodologies." It has been established that the various modes of administration—face-to-face, telephone, self-administered—have different effects on the respondent and hence on the data. When you begin analyzing your data you should compare the results found with each of the modes of administration to ensure that the distribution of answers across questions is not dramatically different. If gross differences are found, you may decide to report the information from the two methods separately or combine the two but report your findings with a caveat about possible unreliability of the data, or you may decide not to use the data obtained by a method different from that by which the majority was collected.

When using self-administered questionnaires in a group setting there is often little that can be done to follow up on those individuals who were not present at the time of administration. If the study is being conducted in a more structured setting, such as a classroom, clinic, or place of work, it is possible to keep track of all individuals in attendance at the time of administration. In this case, it is possible to approach these individuals either at another visit or through another individual (e.g., a teacher, supervisor, or nurse) who has contact with these people, or you may be able to contact them by telephone.

In deciding to make follow-up contacts, you want to consider whether there is a risk of "contaminating" the data in that the nonrespondents may have had the opportunity to discuss the contents of the survey with those who were present at the time of administration and therefore may respond to the survey differently from how they would have if they had answered without prior knowledge. In the situation where a self-administered questionnaire is being brought to the sampled individual, such as schoolchildren bringing a questionnaire home for a parent to complete, the same courier—in this case, the student—can take reminders to the respondent.

CONTENT OF THE FOLLOW-UP REMINDER

The wording of the follow-up communication is similar to the initial cover letter sent with the first mailing. If a postcard is being used, it could be worded as simply as this:

> A few weeks ago you received a questionnaire from (name of sponsor/researcher/organization) asking for your participation in a very important study about (topic). To date we have not received your response. It is very important that we be able to include your opinions in our study. If you have already responded, thank you for your help and excuse this card. If you have not responded, won't you please take a minute now to do so? If you require additional information, please call (contact person and telephone number) collect. Again, thank you.

If you are using a letter, you can expand on the importance of the study and its purpose or use. Make a point to explain how important the respondent is to the success of your study and mention that he or she is one of a select few who have been picked to represent hundreds or thousands of others, depending on the universe from which the sample was drawn. Reinforce that the data are confidential and that the individual will not be identified in any way. If you have the endorsement or sponsorship of an individual or organization known to the respondent, indicate their support of the study. Finally, provide a name and telephone number where the individual may call for more information or another packet to be sent.

If the telephone is being used to make follow-up calls, select the individuals making the calls carefully. Callers should have pleasant, friendly voices. Unless you are dealing with a non-English-speaking population, you will want callers with speaking patterns similar to those of your sample. If reminder calls are made by individuals with heavy accents, the respondent may become frustrated trying to understand the caller and possibly will become alienated from your study.

All callers should work from a script. A script is essentially a written structure not unlike the follow-up letter. Callers should identify themselves, their affiliation, and the purpose of the call. Again, the importance of the study and the respondent's participation should be the focus. This script should contain all the information the caller will need to answer any questions a respondent might have. Although each caller develops an individual style for effectiveness, a script helps prevent your caller from creating dialogue on the spot or giving information to the respondent that may be misleading or untrue. In some cases, it may be necessary for a higher-level supervisor or even the researcher to speak on the telephone with a reluctant respondent.

If you decide to use the telephone to gather data from the individuals you successfully contact, pretest the questionnaire a few times over the telephone to make sure that it will adapt well to telephone administration. There are some types of self-administered questions that do not lend themselves well to telephone interviewing and may need to be modified in some way. This is another reason to record which interviews were conducted via telephone versus self-administration. Changing the format of the question can produce dramatically different results.

If you are conducting multiple follow-ups, it is profitable to keep track of the response rate after each method is tried. For example, if your first follow-up is a postcard, note how many returns come in after the card is sent and before the next method is used. Say the next method you use is a remailing of all the study materials. You might mark the questionnaires that go out in this mailing with an identifiable mark so that when they are returned you can differentiate the returns between the first mailing and this follow-up. Keep track of the effect of each procedure. If you should happen to conduct another mailed survey in the future, you can better judge how many and which follow-ups give the best return for the investment. It is possible you will even have to use this information later in your first study. If your goal is to get as many returns as is humanly possible, you may want to evaluate which method or methods worked best with your sample population and try it or them again.

Whether postcards, letters, or telephone calls, follow-up attempts are extremely important to the overall success of the study. Because they are so important, do not treat these procedures casually. Method of delivery, content, and quality of presentation all leave an impression on the potential respondent. You will witness the rewards for your efforts by the level of response you receive.

Follow-Up Procedure Guidelines

- Ten days after original mailing, send follow-up.
- Follow-up can be a postcard, letter, or telephone call.
- Use a mailgram or telegram or overnight, registered, or certified mail to call more attention to the survey mailing.
- Use a facsimile machine for sending and/or receiving questionnaires.
- Content of follow-up message should stress the importance of response and purpose of study.
- Include in the text of letter the name and telephone number of a survey staff member who can be contacted for assistance in responding.
- Conduct additional follow-ups every 10 days.
- Keep track of the rate of return for each follow-up method used.

SAMPLE TRACKING

There are two basic types of mailing addresses: residential and commercial. In designing the study you will have decided whether the sample target is a particular individual, an address, or a position. In other words, do you want Jane Doe at 111 Main Street, or is any adult living at 111 Main Street appropriate?

Another example is whether you want John Smith, Employee Benefits Manager for Company XYZ, or whoever is filling the position of Employee Benefits Manager at XYZ. If your mailed packet is returned because the specific individual cited is no longer there, you do not need to track the address; simply change the name or make the addressee noncommittal, such as "Resident" or "Employee Benefits Manager." Ideally, you will have set the address file up this way at the onset of the work so that this becomes an issue only in a rare event.

When the focal point of a mailing is a specific individual, tracking becomes essential. In the case of bad addresses or unknown addressees, the Postal Service will not automatically notify you of such outcomes. If an addressee has moved and the mail forwarding order (which the post office retains for one year only and then destroys) is active, the mailing packet will automatically be sent to the new address without your being given the updated address. If a packet is undeliverable due to a bad address, no such person, or other condition, it often remains in a "dead letter" bin at the post office without your knowledge.

It is a wise idea to have made a rubber stamp saying "ADDRESS CORRECTION REQUESTED—DO NOT FORWARD" to stamp on each outgoing mailing packet or, if you use an envelope addressing system, to program this into the address. The Postal Service will charge you 50¢ for each address correction, but by using this procedure you will retain better control of the sample.

Bad addresses can also occur through human error. If an envelope is returned with a notation of "no such address," "no such number," or "no such street," some common sense and a quick check of a local street guide may clear up the problem. It could be that the street name was misspelled, that the street needs a direction such as north, south, east, or west, or that the ZIP code is wrong.

Changes of addresses should be corrected or updated and remailed. Updates of corrected or new addresses should be made to the sample files for future follow-up contact. If the new or correct address for an individual is not found, tracking of respondents can be initiated if time and budget allow.

There are numerous resources that can be used in attempting to obtain correct respondent addresses. The process of trying to find out where an individual has gone is sometimes referred to as tracking. The first place to look for updates is the sample supplier. It is possible that the provider may have new addresses or address corrections for sampled respondents that have not yet been changed in the main data file.

Typically, even if the supplier is able to provide some corrections, there will still be those addresses that are unresolved. Business addresses are typically easier to track than are those for individuals. If the business is local, it may be as simple as looking in the telephone directory, checking both residential and classified listings. Calling the local telephone company's directory information may be another resource, especially if the institution has recently moved. Reverse directories, also called cross-reference or criss-cross directories, are telephone directories that are referenced by city, street name and number, and telephone number. These are also useful for tracking. There are several major companies that publish these directories. Criss-cross directories may also be found in your public library or at your local telephone company headquarters.

Many marketing companies and/or directory publishers maintain address files for the majority of mailing addresses in the United States and often can provide certain types of samples. They can produce mailing labels, and some will fold, stuff, seal, and post your mailing for you for a price.

As the geographic area of the sample gets wider, the number of resources required to track sample addresses gets more complex. Typically, most institutions maintain only their local directories. It is not unusual for a major public library to keep telephone directories for other major metropolitan areas. Your local telephone company headquarters may maintain a reference library of all the telephone directories produced by the parent company. If the number of addresses to be checked is large, it may be worthwhile to pay a directory publishing company to run these checks for you against their computer database.

The ability to access information about a particular individual varies widely across areas in the United States. In some states, the Department of Motor Vehicles will allow a search of drivers' licenses, usually for a fee. Other states, like California, require special permission to search without permission from the individual license holder. In any case, having the name, date of birth, and last known address of the individual you are tracking can help narrow down the possibilities.

Another option involves local public utilities, such as gas, water, and electricity. Regulations on obtaining this type of information vary considerably from area to area. Public utilities and other resources in large metropolitan areas are less likely to provide information on individuals than are those located in less populated areas.

Sample Tracking Procedure Guidelines

- Check for typographical or clerical errors in address.
- Remail new packet to each corrected address.
- Stamp outgoing envelopes "ADDRESS CORRECTION REQUESTED" and correct address file based on corrected returns.
- Remail to corrected addresses.
- Check with sample provider for updates, if applicable.

- Check telephone directories, telephone directory information, and reverse directories.
- Check utilities/Department of Motor Vehicles.

Processing Returns

Having a plan for the handling of returns is as important as collecting the data. When we write of processing the returns we mean the methods used to record the receipt of the completed questionnaires and how the data from these instruments will be converted into numeric results ready for analysis. It is assumed that these returns will be entered into a computer file and read into some software that can be used to compile the results and hopefully calculate at least basic statistics on the findings. Some self-administered surveys are processed or analyzed by hand rather than on a computer, so most of the processing procedures discussed in this section pertain to both hand and computer tabulation.

SAMPLE STATUS REPORTS

Earlier in the section entitled "Preparing the Sample," we discussed the merits of maintaining a sample log or roster, either in paper-pencil form or computerized, to check-in your returns. Ideally, this log will reflect the identification number assigned to the respondent; number and types of follow-ups; tracking procedures used, if any; corrections to the mailing file, if any; and the date the completed questionnaire was received. In organizations that routinely conduct surveys, the next item in this file might be a date indicating when a questionnaire is turned over to data reduction. The ideal sample log is a means by which the location and status of any given questionnaire can be found upon request.

DATA REDUCTION

Data reduction may include the editing of the completed questionnaires, coding of any open-ended material, providing codes for missing data, eliminating incorrect responses, and entering the questionnaire responses into a machine-readable file. In some organizations, data may still be keypunched onto an 80-column card and read into a computer, but in most instances, the data are entered directly onto the hard drive or onto a diskette. In more technologically advanced settings, the data may be entered into the data file via scanning. Numerous software programs are available for setting up a data entry format that is analyzable by statistical software or spreadsheet programs.

Returned questionnaires should not go to data entry without prior editing. Respondents may have skipped questions or entire sections of the questionnaire. In questions asking for only one answer, respondents may have recorded several. Questions that were inappropriate for the respondent to answer, based on some prior information elicited, may have been answered. The respondent may have felt that the answer categories given were insufficient and decided to write an alternative answer on the page. Perhaps the handwriting is barely legible. The ways that individuals can find for not following instructions (no matter how straightforward the instructions nor how simple the questions) are as varied and numerous as are the differences between and among people. As a result, you should plan on having someone edit or look over each completed questionnaire prior to data entry.

How these inconsistencies or inaccuracies are handled is at the discretion of the researcher. If the correct response is obvious, the researcher may allow corrections to be made. In some cases, where respondent telephone numbers are available, the respondent may be called to clarify or obtain the response on the questionnaire. In other cases where a problem answer has occurred, no response may be taken. In any case, a plan will have to be developed whereby inconsistent, incorrect, or missing data are either assigned a numeric value or skipped altogether.

Who handles this varies. In some survey houses, the questionnaires are edited by field clerks in an area that specializes in the collection of data. In other places, the questionnaires are edited as part of the coding process. Coding is the process of converting written answers into numerics using an established coding scheme or plan. This plan is known as a codebook. A coding clerk may edit and code the instrument in one step. In some research houses, the editing, coding, and data entry are performed concomitantly. It is our opinion that this places too great a burden on the individual and invites error. If the same person is to perform all tasks it would be better to have editing and coding done in one step and the data entry done separately. (More in-depth instruction on the processing of data is found in Bourque and Clark's *Processing Data*, which is listed in the Suggested Readings section at the end of this book.)

Estimating Costs

Typically, you will be required to develop an estimate of costs to conduct a self-administered or mailed survey prior to the time you actually incur expenses. The first decision you must make prior to estimating costs is sample size. Specifically, you will need to know how many initial mailings you anticipate, an estimate of the number of completed returns you expect, and costs for address corrections if you plan to use this option.

In the following pages, we first cover expenses unique to a mailed survey, then costs that are unique to a self-administered study, and finally, costs that occur with either method.

There are two types of costs: out-of-pocket expenses and constant costs, or costs for labor that is expended whether or not the study is conducted. Out-of-pocket expenses are those that you must pay for; that is, they are costs for items not routinely paid for by your organization. Such costs might include postage, printing, envelopes, incentives, and any labor required for tasks that are not covered by employees already paid for. An example of a labor cost is the use of a mailing company to fold, stuff, and affix labels and postage to your mailing.

A word of caution: The expenditures itemized in the subsequent sections are approximate costs for January 1995. Certain costs listed may fluctuate considerably with geographic region. Labor charges that are inherent in certain items vary by location. Other overhead costs or markups similarly vary by the expense of doing business in different areas. Finally, the price of stock materials, such as envelopes or paper, may decrease, depending on the volume in which they are purchased. Generally, costs go down as volume increases. The dollar amounts presented here are meant as guidelines only—it is up to the individual surveyor to seek out the appropriate costs for these items in his or her market area.

OUTGOING POSTAGE

For a mailed study, you will need a postal scale that can accurately weigh ounces so you can estimate postage expense. Postal scales are commonly found in most office settings. Assemble a packet that mimics what you plan to send. For example, you will need an outgoing mail envelope, a return mail envelope, a sheet of paper to represent the cover letter, the questionnaire (use the number of pages you anticipate for the final copy), the incentive, if you plan to offer one, and other materials you plan to include in this mailing. Weighing all these materials together on the scale will tell you how many ounces the outgoing packet weighs.

Using the same packet, remove the cover letter, outgoing envelope, incentive, and any materials other than the return mail envelope and questionnaire and/or any other materials to be sent back by the respondent and then calculate the weight in ounces of the return mail packet. This will tell you the amount of postage required to return the packet to you. The cost of providing return-mail postage is discussed later in this section.

Always send materials at the first-class postage rate. Second-, third-, fourth-class, or other bulk-rate postage sends the message that the study and the respondent are not important to you. As of January 1, 1995 the typical outgoing postage is 32¢ for the first ounce and 23¢ for each additional ounce or fraction of an ounce. The post office offers discounts off this rate for mailings of 500 pieces or more that are presorted by ZIP code. To qualify for this discount, you must have at least 10 pieces outgoing to each ZIP code in your mailing. If you can meet these requirements, the discount rate is 27.4¢ per ounce. There are other cost breaks for mailings that use ZIP+4 or barcodes. It is wise to inquire about Postal Service rates and requirements before making a cost estimate and setting up your sample specifications.

You also need to include the cost of follow-up postage, if any, when preparing your estimate. Postcard postage is currently 20¢. The Postal Service sells sheets of 40 cards for $8.00 each. Again, there are discounts for presorting using ZIP+4 and barcoding. If a letter is to be sent as a reminder, assume it will be one ounce at 32¢. You can also buy personalized stamped envelopes from the Postal Service for $176.40 per 500 #10 envelopes. The decision to use stamped envelopes from the Postal Service should be based on resource availability.

If you work in a setting where there is a clerk to meter the postage, you may not need to buy prestamped envelopes. Similarly, if you can get a better volume discount on printing personalized envelopes or if such envelopes are freely available to you at your place of work, it makes no monetary sense to purchase prestamped envelopes. If you intend to remail the entire study packet at some point, the postage will be the same per-piece cost as in your original mailing.

INCOMING POSTAGE

You must include a self-addressed business reply envelope with the mailing. There are two options for providing return-mail postage: Affix sufficient postage in the form of stamps to the return envelope or open a postage-paid business reply mail account (BRM) with your post office. Affixing postage can be a waste of money in that not all respondents will complete and return the questionnaire. In these cases, you have spent the money for the postage but have not received a return. The postage-paid business reply option costs more than the regular per-ounce postal rate because there is an $85.00 12-month permit fee plus a surcharge for the handling. If the mailing is large enough the savings from using BRM more than offsets the loss of providing postage in the mailing.

There are two surcharge rates for BRM handling. If your expected return is fewer than 600 pieces, the post office will not require a deposit to open an account for handling returns, but the additional charge per piece over and above the postage is 44¢. If your expected return is more than 600 pieces, you can establish a BRM account with a minimum deposit of $205.00; then the handling surcharge is 10¢ per piece.

OPTIONAL MAILINGS

Charges for special handling by the postal service include Return Receipt Requested at the time of mailing, showing who signed for the packet and on what date, at $1.10, special delivery at $9.95, registered mail at $4.85, Express Mail next-day at $10.75, or certified mail at $1.10. Other delivery options are Federal Express, United Parcel Service, and other parcel delivery services. Although these options are more expensive, they do draw attention to the study and communicate its importance. Although budgetary constraints are always a consideration, the trade-off involved in paying for postage that enhances the quality presentation of the study materials versus saving a few dollars may not be worth the savings if a low response rate makes the study unusable.

PRINTED AND STOCK MATERIALS

The next budget item for consideration is the cost of printed materials used for the study. Some of these items may already be available to you without special purchasing, such as outgoing envelopes; others will not be. It is assumed that your materials for printing will be camera-ready. That is, you will have typed or word processed the final products as they will appear in print. Your printer will either film the originals and create a negative for printing or use a duplicating process, such as a photocopier. The quality of duplication today is such that on some machines you can barely tell a difference between the printer's page and a copier-generated one.

If your mailing is not bulky, you may be able to use a #11 (4½" × 10⅜") envelope for your outgoing packet and a #10 (4⅛" × 9½") envelope for returning the completed questionnaire. "Not bulky" means that your questionnaire is brief, no more than one 11″ × 17″ page folded and printed front and back, resulting in four printed sides, that your cover letter is one page, that you use a #10 reply envelope, and that there are no additional inserts to the mailing. The cost of 500 nonpersonalized #11 envelopes is approximately $27.00, and for similar #10s, $16.00.

Larger mailings will require the use of manilla-type envelopes. Not only can you put thicker materials into these envelopes, your materials do not have to be prefolded before being stuffed into the envelope. Heavy-duty 10″ × 13″, self-sealing, white first-class envelopes cost approximately $142.00 per 500. You will include in your mailing packet the same type of envelope for returning the questionnaire but it will be smaller (9″ × 12″) and costs about the same.

The outgoing envelopes should have your project name, organization name, and address imprinted in the upper left-hand corner or sender section of the incoming envelope. Incoming envelopes must have your business address in the addressee section in the middle of the front of the envelope. You may also want to repeat your address in the sender section of the envelope.

If a fairly high volume of mail is received at the return address you are using, you will want to identify your project on the face of the envelope either in the lower left-hand side or as a line in the addressee section. This will help the mail sorter identify your packets and deliver them in a timely fashion. If you are using barcoding, you will also need to print this on your return-mail envelope.

You should allow approximately 4¢ per piece for imprinting addresses. Due to high volume, it is possible that your printer will be able to bid the printing job, including the cost for envelopes, at a rate lower than you would get if you bought them separately. Again, when costing your study, remember to include the cost for additional follow-up mailing envelopes.

Other items that will be printed are the cover letter and the questionnaire. Printing costs for 500 letters on 20-pound bond paper will be approximately $25.00. Five hundred copies of a questionnaire printed on one piece of 11" × 17" paper on four sides and folded will cost about $125.00. The cost per printed side comes out to about 6.25¢ per printed side. Not only will these costs fluctuate from area to area due to varying labor and overhead costs, they will also vary depending on the weight and type of paper used for printing and the means by which the questionnaires are bound. When printing questionnaires on the front and back of the page, it is better to use 60-pound paper to eliminate the possibility of print "bleeding" through to the other side.

Always overprint the number of items you need. In other words, if you are mailing to 500 respondents, you should print 600 copies. These additional copies can be used to document the questionnaire in your archival files, to distribute to other workers or supervisors, to have on hand if some of the printing is unusable, and to replace any that might get lost or damaged.

Before you release materials for printing, decide whether or not you plan a second complete mailing to your sample. If so, it is more economical to print all the questionnaires at one time. Volume reduces cost per piece, plus you are not paying two separate job-setup fees. Always allow sufficient time before your mailing date for the printing to be done. If you are on an extremely tight time schedule, your printer will charge extra for "rush" printing. When estimating printing costs, remember to include the cost of printing follow-up letters or other materials you may use.

If you plan to use an incentive, the cost obviously will be dependent on the gift. Small key chains can be purchased for about 25¢ each, retractable ballpoint pens for around 50¢ each, or you may elect to enclose a $1 bill in the mailing (make sure that you send new, clean bills). You can estimate the most you would spend on an incentive and multiply that cost by the sample size to get a figure for your cost estimate. If you plan to include other materials in your mailing, you will need to add the cost for this into your budget.

Personnel Requirements

Material expenses are but one part of the cost to conduct a study. There is also a considerable amount of labor involved. Mailed studies generally require more labor than do self-administered studies simply because there are a great many tasks to be performed that require considerable coordination and management. Much of the labor needed to conduct these studies is at the skilled clerical level, but you will want the person coordinating the project to have the following characteristics: creative, detail oriented, good at managing tasks and individuals, good at problem solving, resourceful, skilled in communicating with vendors and other employees, and using good logic. It would be advantageous if the project manager had some degree of experience with word processing and spreadsheet programs on the personal computer. Ultimately, you will need at least one person with these skills so that you can produce your camera-ready copy of the questionnaire and set up a computerized record-keeping system for sample tracking. Also, prior experience obtaining bids for supplies and printing would be very helpful.

These same characteristics apply to the individual who manages a study requiring data collection by self-administration. It will be this person's responsibility to coordinate the printing and gathering of materials necessary to conduct the administration, to get cooperation from the sites to be included, to set up the logistics of date and time and availability of the desired population, to provide the trained individuals who will go to these sites to distribute and collect the forms if appropriate, and to see to the processing of the completed questionnaires as they are returned.

You may decide to contract out the labor-intensive aspects of your study: folding the study materials and stuffing them into the outgoing envelopes, affixing the address labels, opening up the returns as they come in, editing and coding the completed questionnaires, and entering the data into a computer file. Companies that provide mailing services—that is, they fold, stuff, label, and post your materials—can be found nearly everywhere as data processing companies that will open the envelopes, edit and code them according to your specifications, and then enter them into a file for you. If no tabulating experts or facilities are available within your organization, most data processing companies will also process your data, provide you with frequency distributions (the count and percentage of the number of responses to each answer category in a question) of your data, and cross-tabulate data to your specifications.

If you are able to perform this work within your organization, you will need to have one or more clerical workers, depending on the size of the study. The clerical workers needed on a mailed survey must be good with detail and work well with numbers. One or a few of the clerks, depending on the volume of work, should have some word processing and/or spreadsheet experience, and at least one should have 10-key experience for data entry.

For a self-administered study, you may need clerical-level help to carry out the survey administration. These will be the individuals who go to each study location and monitor and distribute the questionnaires to be completed. Depending on the complexity of the study, these individuals may have to

conduct on-the-spot sampling, make random respondent selections, make oral presentations regarding the purpose of the
study and its sponsorship, and finally, be able to answer
questions about any particular item in the questionnaire or
about the study in general. These individuals should be selected for their ability to interact with others and to present
themselves with a sense of competence and authority.

Unfortunately, the effort required to conduct either a mailed
or self-administered study is not constant over the duration of
the project. There are times of heavy labor intensity and then
times during which little or no effort is required. It is best if
the management personnel required for this project are already
in place and can allocate time to running the study.

The clerical time required is not as much of a problem. If
clerical personnel are not routinely available in your setting,
it is usually not difficult to find part-time, hourly workers from
temporary personnel agencies. If you are located near a college
or university, students can be a rich source of clerical help.
There is a wide variance in the hourly wage for clerical workers,
depending on geographic location and the level of skills required. Clerks who will fold, stuff, and affix labels need not be
as skilled as those who will edit, code, and use personal
computers. The hourly wage may be as low as $6.00 or as high
as $16.00 for these workers.

To determine the number of clerical hours necessary to
complete your project, use the following guidelines for a mailed
survey using a questionnaire with four open-ended questions
and the rest precoded—that is, one 11" × 17" sheet folded in
half (four printed sides), a #11 outgoing envelope, a #10
return-mail envelope, and a cover letter:

Task	Time
Folding survey materials, stuffing into envelopes, affixing labels to envelopes	100 packets/hour
Postal metering	500/hour
Open envelopes and log return	120 envelopes/hour
Edit a 4-page questionnaire	30 questionnaires/hour
Code 4 questions	12 questionnaires/hour
Enter into a computer file 4 pages/30 questions	30 questionnaires/hour

These figures are based on the assumption that the clerical personnel employed have a familiarity with some of their functions—for example, that data entry personnel are proficient on 10-key pads.

If this survey were to be mailed to 500 individuals, we would budget for 5 hours to fold the materials, stuff them into the envelope, and affix the mailing labels. If you need to add in the cost of metering the envelopes through the postal meter, add another hour to the clerical time.

For the purpose of this exercise, let us assume a response rate of 80%, or 400 returned, completed questionnaires. It would require approximately 4 hours to open the envelopes and check in each one by identification number against the master roster or log, 14 hours to edit these questionnaires, 34 hours to code them, and another 14 hours to enter them into the computer data file.

All told, 72 hours of clerical time are needed to ready the packets for mailing, meter them, log in the returns, edit and code the questionnaires, and enter them into a data file. In your time estimates, you will want to inflate these figures to account for break time, lunch time, and occasional pauses. Although the editing, coding, and data entry can be held and done together and the clerical functions are done all at one time, the logging in of returns must be done piecemeal as they come in so that you can keep track of your sample and response rate and, if necessary, take corrective measures.

The following budget illustrates how to use the costing estimates presented earlier and represents costs to date for the Workplace Assault Study cited throughout this book.

Development of Project	$ Cost
Writing proposal: 4 days @ $362.50/day (senior author's UCLA salary rate/outside consulting rate would double)	1,450.00
First draft of questionnaire and specifications: 2 days @ $362.50/day (senior author's UCLA salary rate)	725.00
Finalizing questionnaire: 8 hours @ $14.94 (project coordinator's hourly rate)	119.52
Establishing contacts and meeting with union personnel: 15 hours @ $14.94	224.10
Organizing and conducting focus groups: 24 hours @ $14.94/hour	358.56
Pretesting questionnaire: 8 hours @ $14.94/hour	119.52
Miscellaneous administrative tasks (arranging meetings, clerical, etc.): 4 hours @ $14.94	59.76
TOTAL DEVELOPMENT COSTS	3,056.46
Mailings	
Purchase and printing of 4 sets of mailing labels (labor contributed by Service Employees International Union [SEIU])	160.00
Purchase of envelopes for advance letter and first mailing of questionnaire	627.00

Development of Project	$ Cost
Advance Letter	
Duplication of 1,800 letters @ 4¢/letter	72.00
Postage for 1,800 letters @ 32¢/letter	576.00
Labor associated with mailing letters contributed by SEIU	
First Mailing of Questionnaire	
Duplication of 1,800 flyers @ 4¢/flyer	72.00
Duplication of 1,800 cover letters @ 4¢/letter	72.00
Duplication of 1,800 22-page questionnaires @ 5¢/page	1,980.00
Postage to mail first questionnaire to 1,744 SEIU members @ $1.01/packet (SEIU provided metering service, and labor to mail each packet)	1,761.44
Postage for 1,744 respondents to mail back first questionnaire @ 78¢/questionnaire (stamps placed on each return envelope)	1,360.32
Collation of 1,744 mailing packets: 54 hours @ $14.94/hour	806.76
TOTAL COST OF MAILING OF FIRST QUESTIONNAIRE	7,487.52
COST PER QUESTIONNAIRE MAILED	4.16
COST PER QUESTIONNAIRE RETURNED ($n = 310$)	24.15
Postcards	
Purchase of 1,800 postcards @ 20¢/card through UCLA + 20% per postcard	432.00
Labor to print postcards contributed by SEIU	
Labor to put labels on postcards: 4 hours @ $14.94/hour	59.76
TOTAL COST OF MAILING POSTCARDS	491.76
ADDITIONAL COST PER RESPONDENT	0.27
COST PER ADDITIONAL RESPONSE OBTAINED ($n = 258$)	1.91
COST PER TOTAL RESPONSE OBTAINED ([$7,487.52 + $491.76]/568)	14.05
Second Mailing of Questionnaire	
Duplication of 1,143 cover letters @ 4¢/letter	45.72
Duplication of 1,143 22-page questionnaires @ 5¢/page	1,257.30

→

Development of Project	$ Cost
Purchase of 3 boxes of 10 × 13 envelopes through UCLA: 500 envelopes/box @ $142.00/box	426.00
Printing of 1,500 envelopes @ 4¢/envelope	60.00
Postage for 1,143 packets through UCLA: 91¢ + 20% per packet	1,248.16
Postage paid on only those returned through UCLA business reply: 78¢ + 44¢ handling + 20% per questionnaire (estimated at n = 304)	445.06
Collation of 1,143 mailing packets: 36 hours @ $14.94/hour	537.84
TOTAL COST OF SECOND FULL MAILING	4,020.08
COST PER ADDITIONAL QUESTIONNAIRE OBTAINED (n = 304)	13.22
COST PER TOTAL RESPONSE OBTAINED ([$7,487.52 + $491.76 + $4,020.08]/872)	13.76
Logging In Returned Questionnaires	
Seven hours @ $14.94/hour for 872 returned questionnaires	104.72
Costs of telephone follow-up on remaining 871 respondents, data entry, and data analysis not available at time of writing	
Supervisory time by senior author over mailings and data entry contributed and not included in total costs	

Although some of the wage rates may not be applicable for your situation, this budget gives a general idea of the materials and personnel requirements needed to conduct a mailed survey. This budget also introduces the idea that some costs can be shared or eliminated by working with other individuals or groups who hold a common interest in the research. Obviously, the more you are able to offset costs within your organization, the less the out-of-pocket expense.

A common error made in first-time mail surveys is in not providing enough resources to cover additional follow-ups if they become necessary. Even though you may have conducted a reasonable pilot test of the procedures and sample, there is always the possibility, as we saw in the union employees sample cited in Chapter 2, that pilot-test returns will not accurately reflect the total population returns for reasons not obvious at the time of planning.

Always have a contingency plan for what you will do if completed returns fall significantly short of the necessary sample goal. It would be a terrible loss to go through all the work required to conduct a survey only to find out that you have insufficient numbers of returns to make use of the data.

Note

1. Cheshire labels are the forerunner to today's self-adhesive labels. Cheshires typically are printed on 8½″ × 11″ perforated sheets, such that labels are created when the perforations are ripped. The back of each sheet is preglued and requires moisture to affix. Typically, the sheets are run through a machine that chops and moistens each label and then affixes it to an envelope or other materials requiring labeling. Cheshire labels are less expensive than the more commonly used self-adhesive labels.

Exercises

1. A large corporation is considering changing the kinds of health insurance plans made available to their managerial and professional employees. They want to find out the kind of health insurance plans that employees currently have, both through the company and through other sources, and the extent to which employees express interest in three new plans currently under discussion by the corporation. Would a self-administered questionnaire be appropriate for this study, and if so, which type of self-administered questionnaire would you recommend using?

   One-to-one self-administered questionnaire 1
   Group-administered questionnaire 2
   Semisupervised questionnaire passed out in the
      workplace 3
   Questionnaire mailed to employees' homes 4
   Do not use a self-administered questionnaire 5

2. The Parent-Teacher Association (PTA) of an elementary school wants to find out the number of active PTA members who think it would be a good idea to hold a carnival to raise money for extra computer software for the school *and* would be willing to help organize the carnival. Would a self-administered questionnaire be appropriate for this study, and if so, which type of self-administered questionnaire would you recommend using?

One-to-one self-administered questionnaire 1
Group-administered questionnaire 2
Semisupervised questionnaire passed out as
    people come into a PTA meeting 3
Semisupervised questionnaire passed out as
    people leave a PTA meeting 4
Questionnaire mailed to students' homes 5
Do not use a self-administered questionnaire . . . 6

3. A neighborhood association is aware that a number of elderly Russian immigrants have moved into their community. It is their observation that many of these people are afraid to come out of their apartments. They want to find out what they can do to help these new residents of the community. Would a self-administered questionnaire be appropriate for this study, and if so, which type of self-administered questionnaire would you recommend using?

One-to-one self-administered questionnaire 1
Group-administered questionnaire 2
Semisupervised questionnaire distributed at
    community meetings 3
Questionnaire mailed to residents' homes 4
Do not use a self-administered questionnaire . . . 5

4. A dental clinic located in a university dental school wants to find out how satisfied patients are with their services. They have a draft questionnaire that they need to test to see if it is complete and to find out whether patients can fill it out. Would a self-administered questionnaire be appropriate for this study, and if so, which <u>type</u> of self-administered questionnaire would you recommend using?

> One-to-one self-administered questionnaire 1
> Group-administered questionnaire 2
> Semisupervised questionnaire 3
> Questionnaire mailed to patients' homes 4
> Do not use a self-administered questionnaire 5

5. The management of a factory that manufactures ball bearings has received a lot of complaints from employees about the homeless persons in the area around the factory. The managers have not seen many homeless in the area. They want to find out whether the complaints are representative of the total population of workers in the factory or simply represent the opinions of a few "squeaky wheels." Would a self-administered questionnaire be appropriate for this study, and if so, which <u>type</u> of self-administered questionnaire would you recommend using?

> One-to-one self-administered questionnaire 1
> Group-administered questionnaire 2
> Semisupervised questionnaire passed out as
>   workers punch in for work 3
> Semisupervised questionnaire passed out as
>   workers punch out from work 4
> Questionnaire mailed to workers' homes 5
> Do not use a self-administered questionnaire 6

6. The board of a regional symphony orchestra has received $20,000 from the county government to find out whether county residents know about the symphony, whether they have ever attended a concert, and the kind of music they prefer listening to. Would a self-administered questionnaire be appropriate for this study, and if so, which <u>type</u> of self-administered questionnaire would you recommend using?

One-to-one self-administered questionnaire 1
Questionnaires administered at various group
    meetings 2
Semisupervised questionnaire passed out as
    people come into community meetings 3
Semisupervised questionnaire passed out as
    people leave various community meetings . . . 4
Questionnaire mailed to a sample of 500 county
    residential addresses 5
Do not use a self-administered questionnaire . . . 6

7. A questionnaire contains the following two questions:

  1. What are the three most important problems in your community today?

_____

_____

_____

  2. People consider different things to be problems in their community. A list of 10 things that some people consider problems follows. Please rank order the list from 1 to 10, where 1 represents the problem <u>you</u> consider <u>most</u> important in your community and 10 represents the problem <u>you</u> consider <u>least</u> important in your community.

Problem	Rank Order
Street cleaning	_____
Corrupt officials	_____
Burglary and other crimes	_____
Mail delivery	_____
Telephone service	_____
Garbage and trash pickup	_____
Inadequate libraries	_____
Lack of up-to-date fire equipment . . .	_____
Low water pressure	_____
Public schools	_____
Other	_____

SPECIFY: _____

Would a self-administered questionnaire be appropriate for this study, and if so, which type of self-administered questionnaire would you recommend using?

One-to-one self-administered questionnaire 1
Questionnaires administered at various group
    meetings 2
Semisupervised questionnaire passed out as
    people come into community meetings 3
Semisupervised questionnaire passed out as
    people leave various community meetings . . . 4
Questionnaire mailed to county residents' homes . 5
Do not use a self-administered questionnaire 6

8. A study to be administered to high school juniors includes the following questions:

   1. Please give me the names of your five closest friends.

   _____
   _____
   _____
   _____
   _____

   2. For *each* person you named in Question 1, please tell whether that person is a male or female, how old, and whether s/he goes to this school.

PERSON #	SEX	AGE	SAME SCHOOL?

   3. Have any of these five people ever done anything illegal, like drink or take drugs or steal something?

   No . . . . SKIP TO Q4 1
   Yes . . . . ANSWER A 2

   A. Which of these five people have done something illegal?

   _____

   B. What did s/he do?

   _____

Would a self-administered questionnaire be appropriate for this study, and if so, which <u>type</u> of self-administered questionnaire would you recommend using?

One-to-one self-administered questionnaire 1
Questionnaires administered in classrooms 2
Semisupervised questionnaire passed out as
    adolescents come to school 3
Semisupervised questionnaire passed out as
    adolescents leave school 4
Questionnaire mailed to students' homes 5
Do not use a self-administered questionnaire 6

9. Identify whether or not a mail questionnaire would be a reasonable way to collect data in the following situations.

   a. The City Council wants to find out whether members of the Chamber of Commerce think a new parking structure should be built in the downtown area and the extent to which members would be willing to vote to pay higher taxes to construct it.

   b. The school board wants to find out why the number of high school dropouts has increased over the past 5 years.

   c. A health insurance company wants to find out how many childhood immunizations its members have had and when they had them.

   d. A college sorority wants to find out the current employment status of its alumni.

   e. The local newspaper published an article that suggested that county residents will not buy brown eggs. A local grocery store has recently placed an order for brown eggs because it can purchase them at a substantially lower price. After reading the article, the management becomes concerned that the store will lose business if they go ahead with their purchase of brown eggs.

10. Identify why the following questions would or would not work well in a self-administered questionnaire.

   a. How much water do you drink every day?

1 ounce	1
2 ounces	2
3 ounces	3
4 ounces	4
5 ounces	5
6 ounces	6
7 ounces	7
8 ounces	8
9 ounces	9
10 ounces	10
11 ounces	11
12 ounces	12
13 ounces	13
14 ounces	14

   b. Please describe all the jobs you have had for pay since you were 16 years old.

   _____

   _____

   _____

   c. How many times have you been hospitalized overnight?

Never	GO TO Q53	. . . .	1
Once	GO TO Q40	. . . .	2
Twice	GO TO Q27	. . . .	3
Three or more times	. . . . CONTINUE	. . . .	4

d. Do you rent or own your place of residence?

Own 1
Rent 2
Other 3
    SPECIFY: _____

e. What is your current marital status? Are you:

Married 1
Divorced 2
Separated 3
Widowed, or 4
Have you never been married? 5

f. How often do you see or hear from your children or grandchildren?

_____
_____
_____

g. When do you watch the most TV? Would you say:

    Monday 1
    Tuesday 2
    Wednesday 3
    Thursday 4
    Friday 5
    Saturday, or 6
    Sunday 7

h. Have you ever been audited by the IRS?

    Yes 1
    No 2

11. The State Department of Parks and Recreation wants to find out how residents of the state spend their leisure time. What steps should the department take in developing a questionnaire to survey residents?

12. Would the following set of questions make a good self-administered questionnaire? Why or why not?

1. How often do you vote? Would you say:

Every election, or 1
Something else? 2
    SPECIFY: _____

2. Do you drink milk every day?

Yes 1
No 2

3. What is your highest degree?

No degree 1
High school diploma 2
College degree 3
Postcollege degree 4
Something else 5
    SPECIFY: _____

4. Do you usually vote:

Republican 1
Democrat, or 2
Something else? 3

5. Are you on a special diet?

Yes 1
No 2

6. Are you registered to vote?

Yes 1
No 2

7. How many years of schooling have you completed and received credit for?

Less than 8 years . . . 1
9-11 years 2
12 years 3
More than 12 years . . 4

13. Two companies are considering starting a car pool program. Management has developed the following questionnaire. What kind of instructions will be needed, and where would you put them?

1. How did you get to work yesterday? Did you:

Drive alone in a car 1
Drive in a car pool 2
Take the bus 3
Ride a motorcycle 4
Ride a bicycle 5
Walk, or 6
Something else? 7
SPECIFY: _____

2. Was yesterday a typical day for you? Is that the way you usually get to work?

Yes . . . . . SKIP TO Q3 1
No . . . . . . ANSWER A 2

A. How do you usually get to work?

```
Drive alone in a car . . . . . . . . . . . . . . 1
Drive in a car pool . . . . . . . . . . . . . . 2
Take the bus . . . . . . . . . . . . . . . . . 3
Ride a motorcycle . . . . . . . . . . . . . . 4
Ride a bicycle . . . . . . . . . . . . . . . . 5
Walk . . . . . . . . . . . . . . . . . . . . . 6
Something else . . . . . . . . . . . . . . . 7
    SPECIFY: _____
```

3. Have you ever used the bus or other public transportation to get to work?

```
Yes, use public transportation now . . . . . . . 1
Yes, used public transportation in the past . . . 2
No, have never used public transportation . . . 3
```

4. Have you ever considered using public transportation to get to work?

```
Yes, and currently use it . . . . . . . . . . . . 1
Yes, but decided it was too expensive . . . . . 2
Yes, but decided it was too inconvenient . . . . 3
Yes, but decided against it for some other
    reason . . . . . . . . . . . . . . . . . . . . 4
    SPECIFY: _____
No, never considered using it . . . . . . . . . 5
```

5. Have you ever used car pools to get to work?

```
Yes, use a car pool now . . . . . . . . . . . . 1
Yes, used a car pool in the past . . . . . . . . 2
No, have never used a car pool . . . . . . . . 3
```

6. Have you ever considered using a car pool to get to work?

Yes, and currently use it 1
Yes, but decided it was too expensive 2
Yes, but decided it was too inconvenient 3
Yes, but decided against it for some other
     reason 4
     SPECIFY: _____
No, never considered using it 5

7. If the company started a car pool program, would you be interested in using it?

Yes 1
No 2

8. Which of the following incentives would encourage you to enroll in a car pool program?

CIRCLE ALL
THAT APPLY

Reduced fees for car pool parking 1
How long it took to get to work 2
How close to my house it came 3
How frequently it went 4
Extra time off for employees who used it 5
Other 6
     SPECIFY: _____

9. What is your job title?

_____

_____

10. What days of the week do you work?

CIRCLE ALL
THAT APPLY

Monday 1
Tuesday 2
Wednesday 3
Thursday 4
Friday 5
Saturday 6
Sunday 7

11. What time do you come to work?

_____
RECORD TIME COME TO WORK

12. What time do you leave work?

_____
RECORD TIME LEAVE WORK

13. How many miles do you live from work?

_____
RECORD MILES FROM WORK

14. What city or neighborhood do you live in?

_____
RECORD CITY/NEIGHBORHOOD

	Strongly Agree	Agree	Disagree	Strongly Disagree

15. Having people share transportation is a very good idea........ 1..... 2..... 3 4
16. The problem of air pollution is overrated... 1..... 2..... 3 4
17. Public transportation is a bigger cause of air pollution than cars. . 1..... 2..... 3 4
18. With the right incentives anyone will support car pooling. ... 1..... 2..... 3 4

19. What is your current marital status? Are you:

Married 1
Divorced 2
Separated 3
Widowed, or 4
Have you never been married? 5

20. Do you have children under 12 living with you?

Yes 1
No 2

21. Are you responsible for taking those children somewhere in the morning or picking them up in the evening?

CIRCLE ALL
THAT APPLY

Yes, taking them in the morning 1
Yes, picking them up in the evening 2
No, not responsible for children 3
No, have no children under 12 4
Other 5
SPECIFY: _____

14. A local health food store wants to find out about the lifestyles of community residents. The owners design the following questionnaire. What suggestions would you make to the owners?

We have designed the following questionnaire to find out about your healthy lifestyle. It will only take you three minutes to fill out and you will feel much better when you realize how healthy your lifestyle is!

1. Of course you exercise every day don't you?   Yes.....1 No.....2

2. When you exercise do you drink a lot of water? Yes, I drink a lot of water and then I run three miles.....1 Yes, I drink some water and run four miles.....2 Sometimes I drink some water before I run.....3 When I run I drink water but when I walk I don't.....4

3. How much do you *avoid* red meat? A lot_____ Some_____ Occasionally_____ When I think of it_____

4. How many people live in your household? Is it just you and one other person or are there more people there?

   Only me. 1

   Me plus one person 2

   Something else 3
   Who else is there?_____

5. When you finished school did you have a high school degree and a college degree or something else?

   High school degree and college degree 1
   Something else 2

6. *Rank order the following list of things that make for a healthy lifestyle from 1 to 10.*

List	Rank
Eating right	_____
Running at least 10 miles a week	_____
Doing meditation	_____
Getting 8 hours of sleep every night	_____
Eating leafy green vegetables every day	_____
Avoiding situations that make you angry	_____
Avoiding caffeine	_____
Never eating sugar	_____
Thinking good thoughts	_____
Lifting weights	_____

15. What kinds of specifications need to be written for the questionnaire included in Question 12?

16. What resources would you pursue if you were looking for a source for the following types of samples? What are the advantages and disadvantages of each source?

    a. A sample of residences in your local community?

    b. A sample of lawyers in your community?

    c. A national sample of physicians?

    d. A sample of local high school students?

17. You are the Director of Nursing Services at your local county hospital. You are responsible for a nursing staff of 300. You are contemplating a change in shift hours and want to know how your staff would react to this change. There are 10 service divisions within the department and two shifts on each service, with approximately 15 nurses per service per shift. You have decided that a survey of 100 nurses would be ample to determine what the overall reaction of the nursing staff would be. How would you select a sample, and what means of data collection would you use?

18. a. What are the components of a group self-administered study?

    b. What are the components of a mailed survey?

19. You are conducting a mailed survey of recipients of Aid to Families with Dependent Children (AFDC) who completed a job training program run by your department last year. You have mailed to 300 individuals who completed their training and have received only 50 completed returns. You have decide to select another 300 names to send the questionnaire to in order to increase the number of responses. Is this appropriate?

20. Make a list of standard sample tracking procedures.

21. From your mailed survey, the following envelopes have been returned by the Postal Service with the following reason for nondelivery. How would you go about trying to readdress them?

   a. Address:

      John Crawford
      1418 Ork Street
      Tree Town, OH 76024

   Reason for return: No such street

   b. Address:

      Mrs. Robert Adams
      907 River Ave. Apt. #
      Redbank, N.J. 85072

   Reason for return: Undeliverable as addressed

   c. Address:

      Julius Rosen
      247 B3 First Ave.
      New Bedford, MA 456023

   Reason for return: No such number

   d. Address:

      Doris Newhouse
      5201 Orange Grove Ave.
      Orange, CA 91204

   Reason for return: Not in this ZIP code

ANSWERS

1. Option 4:   The population should be sufficiently literate that they can respond to a mail questionnaire and the company should have sufficient money to send out a mail questionnaire. Respondents would also probably be more honest if they completed the questionnaires outside the workplace.

2. Option 3:   The PTA wants to solicit the support and participation of active members. Active members are more likely to come to meetings and they are more likely to be interested in enhancing the school's resources. Passing out questionnaires as members come into a meeting increases the likelihood that they will be completed during the meeting and returned at the end.

3. Option 5:   The fact that the group of interest is elderly and composed of recent immigrants who probably speak Russian rather than English argues against the use of a self-administered questionnaire and for the use of telephone or face-to-face interviews.

4. Options 1, 2, or 3:   The procedure used to test this questionnaire would vary with the amount of resources the clinic has available to develop the questionnaire and the extent to which it thinks that the questionnaire as drafted is incomplete or unclear. One-to-one self-administered questionnaires would allow the clinic to explore patients' responses in the most detail but would make it difficult to administer the questionnaire to large numbers of patients in a short period of time. Group administrations where patients were encouraged to discuss the questionnaire would probably provide more information than semisupervised questionnaires. Both techniques would allow for relatively rapid feedback on the questionnaire.

5. Option 4:   Questionnaires passed out as workers left the factory would probably provide a fairly representative and rapid assessment of the situation and allow the surveyor an opportunity for answering questions and encouraging returns. Questionnaires administered in groups at work or distributed as workers come in to work would increase the response rate but also probably increase the likelihood that workers would talk about the questionnaire and that the "squeaky wheels" would have undue influence over the responses. In general, factory workers are not going to respond at high rates to a mail questionnaire.

6. Option 5:   The board has sufficient money and the addresses needed to conduct a mail questionnaire but *not* enough money to conduct telephone interviews with 500 people. Although responses will probably be biased toward those with more education, the amount of money available would allow for a substantial amount of follow-up by mail and even by telephone. The responses to a mail questionnaire would be substantially more representative of the county population than would questionnaires distributed at various community meetings.

7. Option 6:   Two things argue against using a self-administered questionnaire for this study. First, an open-ended question is followed by a closed-ended question that contains a list of problems. In an interview, respondents will not have that list available when they are asked Question 1, but in a self-administered questionnaire they will. As a result, they are likely to select items from the list in responding to Question 1. Second, the list included in Question 2 is long, and respondents are asked to rank order it. This is a difficult task for respondents to do without assistance from an interviewer and argues against the inclusion of such a question in a self- administered questionnaire.

8. Option 6: This questionnaire has too many open-ended questions and is too complicated to expect students to complete by themselves. It is also subject to misreporting and bias if administered in a school setting, and parents are likely to insist on looking at the questionnaire if it is mailed to students' homes. Special procedures have to be followed when people under the age of 18 are used in *any* kind of research study. Generally, this involves obtaining permission from both the parent or guardian and the adolescent. Finally, this is not a very clearly written set of questions *even for* an interview.

9. a. Yes. The Chamber of Commerce is an identifiable group that should be motivated to respond and capable of responding to a mail questionnaire.

   b. No. It may take some exploratory work to find out how best to conduct this study. Furthermore, up-to-date lists and addresses are unlikely to exist for students who dropped out prior to the current year, and we cannot assume that dropouts would be either motivated to respond or capable of responding to a mail questionnaire.

   c. No. Data on childhood immunizations is difficult to get under any circumstances. It requires that people *either* have records *or* a parent available that can provide a complete listing of the type of immunizations they had as children and the dates of those immunizations. It is unlikely that respondents would be able to provide such information in response to a mail questionnaire.

   d. Yes. Sorority members can be expected to identify with the organization and be motivated to respond to its requests. Furthermore, the topic of the study is current and restricted.

   e. No. The management does not have a list of persons who regularly patronize their grocery store. They would be better advised to interview persons who come into the store over the period of a typical week to find out (a) how they feel about brown eggs, (b) whether they read the newspaper article, and (c) how regularly they buy groceries at this particular store.

10. a. No. The question is better than the response categories in that it is short and precise. It does contain an assumption that respondents drink the same amount of water every day. The answer categories are ridiculous. First, many people probably do not know what an "ounce" represents in volume. It is better to ask them about "typical cups" or "typical glasses" of water while simultaneously defining the number of ounces in a typical cup (6 ounces) or a typical glass (8 ounces). Second, the range of answers, while mutually exclusive, is *not* exhaustive; it does not allow for people who drink no water or those who drink more than 14 ounces. Third, the list of responses is unnecessarily long and skewed toward lesser amounts of water.

  b. No. This is a burdensome question for a respondent to answer validly without assistance from an interviewer. First, it is open-ended. Second, it asks older respondents in particular to provide a great deal of historical information without providing any guidance as to the *order* in which information should be provided or the *amount* of information that should be provided about each job.

  c. No. The question itself is all right, but the complicated skip pattern set up in the response alternatives argues against a self-administered questionnaire.

  d. Yes. This question is short and specific and the response categories are exhaustive and mutually exclusive. Furthermore, the residual other is unlikely to generate many responses but ensures that respondents who do not feel that the other two answers represent them can express themselves.

  e. Yes. This question is short and specific, and the response categories are mutually exclusive and exhaustive if we are interested in finding out about respondents' legal marital status. In some populations, the surveyor might want to add a second question that asked about unmarried co-habitation of either same-sex or different-sex couples.

f. No. This is even more than a double-barreled question! Also, it is open ended.

g. No. As written, the response categories are not exhaustive; they do not provide for respondents who watch no television or for those who watch equal amounts of television on multiple days. In the question itself, it would be better to say "television" instead of "TV." Although most persons probably understand the abbreviation, better safe than sorry!

h. No. The response categories are fine, and the question is short and precise, but it contains abstract terms (e.g., audited) and jargon (e.g., IRS) that may not be understood by some respondents.

11. The State Department of Parks and Recreation should (a) conduct a literature review to see what, if anything, has been published about leisure time; (b) consider adopting or adapting questionnaires developed by others; and (c) pretest one or more draft questionnaires to make sure that the questionnaire is understandable to a representative sample of the state's residents and to estimate the cost of conducting the survey. After pretesting, the department may find that it cannot obtain reliable and valid information through a mail questionnaire.

12. No, not as written. The questions are not logically ordered. Within any given topic, questions are not ordered from less complex to more complex. For example, respondents are asked if they vote before they are asked if they are registered. Question 3 is unlikely to be understood where it is and should be preceded by Question 7. There are no instructions to the respondent, nor are there any transitions between questions or topics. Question 1 was written by a lazy surveyor and is likely to result in many different answers in the "residual other" category that will have to be postcoded.

13. As written, this questionnaire needs four kinds of instructions. First, general instructions need to be provided and a decision made regarding whether these general instructions will be in a cover letter or on the first page of the questionnaire. The selection of procedure will probably vary with how management plans to administer the questionnaire. If the plan is to distribute it at the workplace or as employees come to or leave the workplace, instructions could be put on the questionnaire itself. If the plan is to send the questionnaire to employees' homes, a cover letter should be used. These general instructions need to explain the purpose of the questionnaire and who is conducting the study, describe how confidentiality will be protected, explain how respondents were chosen, provide motivation for employees to respond to the questionnaire, anticipate any problems or concerns that employees might have in responding to the questionnaire, provide a way for employees to get more information about the study or confirm its legitimacy, and tell employees how to return the completed questionnaire. If a cover letter is used, it should be printed on letterhead and, if possible, a personal salutation added.

Second, brief sets of instructions need to be provided before Question 1, between Questions 8 and 9, and before Question 19. These instructions "alert" respondents to the upcoming topic and to transitions between topics.

Third, detailed instructions need to be provided before Question 15 that explain to the respondent that these are questions about opinions or attitudes, that there are no right or wrong answers, and how to use the available answer categories.

Finally, an ending needs to be provided for the questionnaire that (a) encourages respondents to comment on the questionnaire or add additional information, (b) thanks respondents, and (c) repeats what the employee is supposed to do with the completed questionnaire.

14. This questionnaire breaks almost every rule of questionnaire construction. First, the print is too small. Second, italics are used, which are difficult to read. Third, the owners of the

health food store clearly have an "agenda." Their questions do not allow for the possibility that respondents might *not* do the things that the owners consider healthy. Fourth, the responses for Question 3 are all vague qualifiers. Fifth, there is no consistency in spacing or formatting. Some response categories are listed vertically while others are listed horizontally. Et cetera, et cetera.

15. Specifications should document the purpose of the study, how respondents were selected to participate, how the questionnaires were administered, the number and timing of follow-up contacts, and *why* each question or set of questions was included in the questionnaire. If questions were adopted or adapted from other studies, the source of those questions, the reason for their selection, and the reason for any changes should be explained.

16. a. SOURCE: The most ideal situation would be to have a 100% list of all residences in your sampled community. Short of going out and hand-listing every address on every street in the area, you will probably have to resort to less reliable resources. Check commercial mailing houses, which are the companies that mail fliers, ads, product samples, and the like to households in the area. Speak to the local telephone company to determine the rate of unlisted residential telephones in your study area. If the unlisted rate is low, the telephone directory may be an adequate resource. Also, check with the main depot of your local Postal Service, which may be able to recommend a source for addresses.

ADVANTAGES: Commercial sources usually provide quick, economical access to large numbers of addresses. Often, these resources will be able to provide many of the services required in a survey mailing. They most likely will have computerized lists and therefore will be able to pull a sample according to your sampling specifications, run your address labels for you, fold and stuff your survey materials mechanically, and mechanically post your mailing.

DISADVANTAGES: Using commercial sources such as mail order companies and postal addressing firms probably does not include more casual residences, such as garages converted to living space, unless these changes have been made according to local code and legally registered on the local housing rosters as a residential address. Telephone directories may have high household coverage; however, there will still be those residences with unlisted numbers that will be missed. Also, there may be a considerable number of listings where the address is suppressed. It is also unknown if one telephone covers more than one residence or if one residence has more than one telephone number and therefore has more than one chance of being included in the sample.

b. SOURCE: The commercial listings or "Yellow Pages" section of your local telephone directory is probably as good a resource as any. The State Bar Association would be another good source, but it may limit access to its files.

ADVANTAGES: The local telephone directory is an easily available and inexpensive resource. The State Bar Association would most likely have the names and addresses computerized so that accessing and producing a mailing sample would be considerably more time efficient and possibly cost efficient.

DISADVANTAGES: The local telephone directories will miss any lawyer or law group that has not paid for listing in the commercial pages, so there is the probability that you will miss some individuals in your sample. In the case of law firms, it may be difficult getting the name of each individual lawyer working within the firm. The State Bar Association may not have current addresses for all individuals.

c. SOURCE: Most practicing physicians are members of the American Medical Association (AMA). You can contact them to explore the possibility of obtaining a sample of physicians from them. If a sample is not available from the AMA, there are commercial companies that maintain lists of professionals such as physicians to sell to firms, say, pharmaceutical companies.

ADVANTAGES: Both resources will have computerized files, making it easy to select a sample and produce mailing labels.

DISADVANTAGES: Getting in touch with an appropriate and cooperative individual in the AMA may require extra effort. Neither resource is free. Neither resource will have 100% coverage, but the AMA probably has a more complete listing of practicing physicians. Both lists will not be 100% up-to-date on current addresses. Getting the names of individuals in group practices or health maintenance organizations (HMOs) may be a problem.

d. SOURCE: Contact the administrative offices of your local school district for public schools and individual administrative offices for private schools. You will have to obtain permission "systemwide" to be able to access any information. Once you have obtained this access, you will have to contact the high schools you have selected for inclusion in your sample. Schools may place different conditions upon your accessing students. If you are not taking a 100% sample in the classroom, an identification number may have to be used for sampling rather than a name because you may not be given access to individual names. You may be asked to distribute a letter requesting signed permission from a parent or guardian of each student to have him or her participate in your study. This will probably have to be coordinated through a "homeroom" teacher. If and when parental consent is obtained, you will probably have to also have consent from each student. If you are not allowed address access to students you may have to either arrange for group administration of your survey at some time when all students are in one place, like "homeroom" or assembly, or supply the student with a packet to be completed at some later time and either mailed back or returned to a designated location at the school.

If access is denied by the school board, you may have to resort to using a "convenience" sample by going to places in your community where high school students are accessible, such as church groups, fast food outlets, or other such attractions. You may find a situation where you can conduct a group administration or at least hand out forms to be completed at another time and returned by mail.

ADVANTAGES: A school-based sample of students essentially guarantees you that nearly every student in your area has the possibility of being selected. The group setting allows for group administration or distribution, maximizing the number of individuals you can survey in one contact. Although the time spent obtaining access may be considerable, there is virtually no cost in obtaining the sample.

Convenience samples are generally easy to access. The cost to obtain the sample is minimal. Data can be collected in a very short period of time.

DISADVANTAGES: School-based samples are fine if all you want to represent are students. If you are interested in representing teenagers, you will miss that portion of the population that has dropped out of school. If you use a school-based sample, any student who is not present at school on the day of your administration or distribution will not have an opportunity to participate in the study. Therefore, your sample has less chance of being truly representative.

Convenience samples can be extremely biased. The resource from which you obtain your sample will usually limit the representativeness of the sample. For example, if you go to video arcades, you will find only those students who go to these types of amusements. The return on this type of sample may be extremely low. There is little incentive for the student to comply with participation unless the topic is of overwhelming interest.

17. Each service/shift should be sampled for 5 respondents. 15 ÷ 5 = 3. Make an alphabetical list by service by shift of all nurses on the staff. Take every third name. To avoid possible influence from co-workers and to protect respondent anonymity, you would probably mail the questionnaire to the nurses at their home addresses and provide stamped, self-addressed envelopes for the return.

18. a. Group Administration Packet Checklist

✓ Sample
Access? Means of selection

✓ Schedule
Calendar of date/time/place

✓ Informed consent
If necessary. Quantity?

✓ Cover letter
Print quantity?

✓ Questionnaire
Print quantity?

✓ Incentive (if used)
Quantity?

✓ Other handouts (if any)
Quantity?

✓ Means of retrieval
Collect/box/mailback?

b. Mailing Packet Checklist

✓ Sample labels/addresses
Quantity?

✓ Outgoing mail envelopes
Sample size?

✓ Size of questionnaire?
  Additional materials?

✓ Outgoing postage
  Metered or stamped?

✓ Cover letter
  Print quantity?

✓ Questionnaire
  Print quantity?

✓ Incentive (if used)
  Quantity?

✓ Other inserts (if any)
  Quantity? ·

✓ Return mail envelope
  Postage-paid business reply/metered/stamps?

19. No. By not using a follow-up to increase response rates from the original sample nor tracking bad addresses, you may be missing important feedback about the success of your program. For example, the program may have been highly successful, and a significant number of individuals have obtained good jobs and moved on and are no longer at their original addresses. Conversely, the program may have had very little impact on most of the respondents' lives, and they are not motivated to respond. By replacement sampling you will probably never receive responses from either of these types of participants, and you will not have accurate information with which to evaluate your program.

20. SAMPLE TRACKING PROCEDURES GUIDELINE

✓ Check for typographical or clerical errors in address

✓ Remail new packet to each corrected address

✓ Stamp outgoing envelopes "ADDRESS CORRECTION REQUESTED" and correct address file based on corrected returns

✓ Remail to corrected addresses

✓ Check with sample provider for updates (if applicable)

✓ Check telephone directories, telephone directory information, and reverse directories

✓ Check utilities/Department of Motor Vehicles

21. a. If you have checked with your sample source and the results are the same, there is probably a typographical error in the street name. "Ork" would be a fairly unusual name for a street. Look for a likely name spelled similarly, such as "Oak." If Oak Street DOES exist in the sampled area, try readdressing it to that address.

b. Check with your sample source for the missing apartment number. If the result is the same, try to determine the correct apartment number through the appropriate telephone directory. If the name is listed with a telephone number, you can try calling the number, explaining your purpose, and asking for the correct address. If the building is accessible to you, you might look at mailboxes or the building directory to see if you can determine the apartment number. If the number cannot be found, try leaving "Apt. #" out of the address entirely and see if the postal person might know the name and deliver it without the apartment number on the address.

c. In this case, the apartment number appears to be a part of the street address. Never type the unit number next to the street address. Rather, put it after the street name or on the next line.

d. The wrong ZIP code was used on this address. There are often ZIP code directories available at main branches of public libraries, or you can call the post office and ask for the ZIP code that covers that address. In this case, the ZIP code was one number off on the final number of the code. It should have read 91203. It is sometimes the case that a ZIP code will change numbers in the middle of a street.

Suggested Readings

Aday, L. A. (1989). *Designing and conducting health surveys.* San Francisco: Jossey-Bass.

Basic textbook on the design and administration of all kinds of surveys. Draws on methodological work on surveys in general and health surveys in particular.

Aquilino, W. S. (1994). Interview mode effects in surveys of drug and alcohol use. *Public Opinion Quarterly, 58,* 210-240.

Reports the results of a field experiment designed to study respondents' willingness to admit use of illicit drugs and alcohol in three conditions: personal interviews that incorporated the use of a self-administered questionnaire to obtain the sensitive information, personal interviews without a self-administered questionnaire, and telephone interviews. The use of a self-administered questionnaire within a personal interview resulted in somewhat higher estimates of illicit substance use, and telephone interviews resulted in somewhat lower estimates.

213

Berry, S. H., & Kanouse, D. E. (1987). Physician response to a mailed survey: An experiment in timing of payment. *Public Opinion Quarterly, 51*, 102-114.

Compares the response rates of questionnaires mailed to physicians when $20 was included in the original mailing with those promised $20 upon receipt of the completed questionnaire. Prepayment was found to have significant positive effects on response rates.

Bourque, L. B., & Clark, V. A. (1992). *Processing data: The survey example.* Newbury Park, CA: Sage.

Systematic explanation of how to perform data processing using today's technology. The authors adopt a broad definition of data processing that starts with selecting a data collection strategy and ends when data transformations are complete. Much of the material covered has direct applicability to the design, administration, and processing of self-administered questionnaires.

Bourque, L. B., Cosand, B. B., Drews, C., Waring, G. O., Lynn, M., Cartwright, C., & PERK Study Group. (1986). Reported satisfaction, fluctuation of vision, and glare among patients one year after surgery in the Prospective Evaluation of Radial Keratotomy (PERK) Study. *Archives of Ophthalmology, 104*, 356-363.

Provides a description of the PERK Study population and how results of the surgery related to satisfaction and side effects 1 year after surgery on the first eye.

Bourque, L. B., Lynn, M. J., Waring, G. O., Cartwright, C., & PERK Study Group. (1994). Spectacle and contact lens wearing six years after radial keratotomy in the Prospective Evaluation of Radial Keratotomy Study. *Ophthalmology, 101*, 421-431.

Describes the PERK study population 6 years after surgery on the first eye and 5 years after surgery on the second eye. The questionnaire used in this study provided the basis for the questionnaire discussed in the examples in this book.

Bradburn, N. M. (1983). Response effects. In P. H. Rossi, J. D. Wright, & A. B. Anderson (Eds.), *Handbook of survey research* (pp. 289-328). New York: Academic Press.

Focuses primarily on questionnaires used in interviews. However, information presented on open versus closed questions, question order, question length and wording, and retrospective memory have relevance for the design of all questionnaires—including self-administered ones.

Brook, R. H., Ware, J. E., Rogers, W. H., Keeler, E. B., Davies, A. R., Donald, C. A., Goldberg, G. A., Lohr, K. N., Masthay, P. C., & Newhouse, J. P. (1983). Does free care improve adults' health? Results from a randomized controlled trial. *New England Journal of Medicine, 309,* 1426-1434.

One of the first major publications that reported the results of RAND's Health Insurance Experiment. Includes a description of the design of the study and the data collection techniques used.

California WIC Program manual (WIC No. 210-60). (1994). Washington, DC: Department of Health, Education, and Welfare (overseer of state programs).

Source of the information reported in Chapter 2 on the federal Women, Infants and Children (WIC) Program, which is administered at the state level.

Church, A. H. (1993). Estimating the effect of incentives on mail survey response rates: A meta-analysis. *Public Opinion Quarterly, 57,* 62-79.

Reports the results of a meta-analysis of 38 experimental and quasi-experimental studies that implemented some form of incentive so as to increase response rates in a mail survey. The use of prepaid monetary or nonmonetary rewards included with the initial mailing were compared with the use of monetary or nonmonetary rewards provided conditional upon return of the questionnaire. The effects of incentives were found to be modest, with those that included rewards in the initial mailing being more effective in increasing response rates.

Converse, J. M., & Presser, S. (1986). *Survey questions: Handcrafting the standardized questionnaire.* Newbury Park, CA: Sage.

Succinct overview of what is involved in designing questionnaires, with particular attention to questionnaires administered in interviews and studies that focus on attitudes and opinions. Much of the information provided has relevance, however, to self-administered questionnaires.

Council of Professional Associations on Federal Statistics. (1993). *Providing incentives to survey respondents: Final report.* Washington, DC: General Services Administration, Regulatory Information Service Center.

Newsletter dealing with statistical gathering and matters of confidentiality.

Dillman, D. A. (1978). *Mail and telephone surveys: The total design method.* New York: John Wiley.

Classic reference on the design of mail questionnaires. A "must" for those interested in developing expertise in this area.

Fink, A., & Kosecoff, J. (1985). *How to conduct surveys: A step-by-step guide.* Beverly Hills, CA: Sage.

A "how to" book good for both the novice and more experienced surveyor. Purpose, goals, and examples are realistic.

Fowler, F. J., Jr. (1993). *Survey research methods* (2nd ed.). Newbury Park, CA: Sage.

A comprehensive summary of the methods of survey research and the sources of error inherent in each. Provides a guide for calculating survey statistics and error measurement.

Fox, R. J., Crask, M. R., & Kim, J. (1988). Mail survey response rate: A meta-analysis of selected techniques for inducing response. *Public Opinion Quarterly, 52,* 467-491.

Reports the results of a meta-analysis of the experimental studies that have examined 10 different factors felt to influence response rates to mail surveys. Results indicate that such things as advance letters, sponsorship, color of paper, the type of postage used, and follow-ups increase response rates. Increases in the amount of a monetary incentive appear to have decreasing marginal gains on response rates.

Henry, G. T. (1990). *Practical sampling.* Newbury Park, CA: Sage.

A sampling textbook designed for the "common surveyor." Not overly technical but highly practical.

James, M. J., & Bolstein, R. (1990). The effect of monetary incentives and follow-up mailings on the response rate and response quality in mail surveys. *Public Opinion Quarterly, 54,* 346-361.

The separate and joint effect of monetary incentives and follow-up mailings were compared in increasing response rates. Four mailings without an incentive produced a higher response rate than a single mailing with an incentive, but a combination of follow-up mailings and a higher monetary incentive produced higher response rates than follow-up mailings without an incentive. There was, however, some evidence of response bias across the different treatment groups.

Jobe, J. B., & Loftus, E. F. (Eds.). (1991). Cognition and survey measurement [Special issue]. *Applied Cognitive Psychology, 5*(3).

The collaboration to which this issue is devoted represents a movement to blend, or merge, the scientific value embedded in both the laboratory and naturalistic research settings and to do this under conditions that make possible the emergence of a methodologically innovative, mutually supportive interdiscipline.

Kalton, G. (1983). *Introduction to survey sampling.* Beverly Hills, CA: Sage.

A good primer on sampling theory for the beginning surveyor. Provides good illustrations, practical considerations, and problems likely to be encountered in sampling.

Kraemer, H. C., & Thiemann, S. (1987). *How many subjects? Statistical power analysis in research.* Newbury Park, CA: Sage.

Introduces a simple technique of statistical power analysis to compute approximate sample sizes and power for a wide variety of research designs.

Kraus, J. F. (1990). Homicide while at work: Persons, industries, and occupations at high risk. *American Journal of Public Health, 77,* 1285-1312.

Represents one of the articles used in conducting a literature review in preparation for the Workplace Assault Study. A study of work-related homicides in California from 1979 to 1981 reported an average annual rate of 1.5 homicides per 100,000 workers with a male-to-female ratio of 4.2:1. Rates were highest for police (20.8), security guards (16.5), and taxi drivers (19.0) and were elevated for persons who worked at night in retail or service jobs, such as convenience store clerks, bartenders, and janitors.

Kruger, R. A. (1994). *Focus groups: A practical guide for applied research* (2nd ed.). Thousand Oaks, CA: Sage.

Provides a detailed discussion of the focus group technique. Describes characteristics, conditions of use, and implementation.

Krysan, M., Schuman, H., Scott, L. J., & Beatty, P. (1994). Response rates and response content in mail versus face-to-face surveys. *Public Opinion Quarterly, 58,* 381-399.

Compares response rates from an hour-long, face-to-face interview with those from a shorter mail questionnaire. Both surveys were administered in Detroit in 1992. Response rates did not differ for white respondents but were significantly lower for black respondents who received mail questionnaires; responses differed by administrative procedure, with respondents to the mail questionnaire expressing more negative attitudes toward racial integration and affirmative action.

Rasinski, K. A., Mingay, D., & Bradburn, N. M. (1994). Do respondents really "mark all that apply" on self-administered questions? *Public Opinion Quarterly, 58,* 400-408.

Instructions to "mark all that apply" were compared to questions where each of the applicable categories was asked in the form of "yes-no" questions. Fewer response options were selected with the "mark all that apply" format, but whether that means such formats result in underreporting or "yes-no" responses result in overreporting cannot be assessed in this data set.

Schuman, H., & Presser, S. (1981). *Questions and answers in attitude surveys.* San Diego: Academic Press.

Reports the findings from a series of experiments conducted to determine how the way in which questions about attitudes are asked influences the data obtained.

Sheatsley, P. B. (1983). Questionnaire construction and item writing. In P. H. Rossi, J. D. Wright, & A. B. Anderson (Eds.), *Handbook of survey research* (pp. 289-328). New York: Academic Press.

Basic reference on issues to consider in deciding whether questionnaires are an appropriate method for collecting data, the kind of administrative procedure that is appropriately used, and how to develop questions and questionnaires.

Sudman, S., & Bradburn, N. M. (1982). *Asking questions.* San Francisco: Jossey-Bass.

Describes the development of questions used in structured questionnaires or interview schedules used in social and market research. Covers general issues on questionnaire design; the development of questions on nonthreatening and threatening behaviors, attitudes, and demographic characteristics; the development of response categories; and question wording and context.

Tanur, J. (Ed.). (1992). *Questions about questions: Inquiries into the cognitive bases of surveys.* New York: Russell Sage Foundation.

Questions about the rigid standardization imposes on the survey interview receive a thorough airing as the authors show how traditional survey formats violate the usual norms of conversational behavior and potentially endanger the validity of the data collected.

U.S. Bureau of the Census. (1992). *Census of population and housing: 1990, United States. Summary Tape File B* [Computer file]. Washington, DC: U.S. Department of Commerce (producer); Ann Arbor, MI: Interuniversity Consortium for Political and Social Research (distributor).

Source of 1990 Census data reported in Chapter 2.

Ware, J. E., Jr., Snow, K. K., Dosinski, M., & Gandek, B. (1993). *SF-36 Health Survey: Manual and interpretation guide.* Boston: Health Institute, New England Medical Center.

Describes some of the scales developed out of RAND's Health Insurance Experiment and Medical Outcomes Study. Provides information about questions included in the PERK Study.

Washington State Department of Labor and Industries. (1993). *Study of assaults on state employees at eastern and western state hospitals.* Tacoma: Safety and Health Assessment and Research for Prevention.

Represents one of the studies examined in the literature review for the Workplace Assault Study. In a study of two Washington State psychiatric hospitals, questionnaire responses were compared with injuries reported in various official reports. The number of assaults reported was roughly comparable for incident reports and questionnaire responses. However, Workers' Compensation and OSHA logs substantially underestimated the total number of occurrences in a given period. Whereas 12.4 injuries per 100 nursing FTEs (full-time equivalents) were reported in OSHA logs, 21.6 to 28.7 workers' compensation claims were made, 63.4 to 70.9 assaults per 100 FTEs were reported in incident reports, and more than 70% of the ward staff completing questionnaires reported experiencing at least one physical assault leading to mild injury.

Weisberg, H. F., Krosnick, J. A., & Bowen, B. D. (1989). *An introduction to survey research and data analysis* (2nd ed.). Glenview, IL: HarperCollins College Division.

A more sophisticated presentation of survey research methods, with greater focus than most guides on data analysis, report writing, and the evaluation of completed surveys.

Wentland, E. J., & Smith, K. W. (1993). *Survey responses: An evaluation of their validity.* San Diego: Academic Press.

Thirty-seven studies conducted between 1944 and 1988 were included in a meta-analysis that assessed the accuracy of individuals' responses to questionnaires when compared to independent criteria. Discrepancies varied with the extent to which the requested information was accessible to respondents, subject matter, and characteristics of the questionnaire.

Yammarino, F. J., Skinner, S. J., & Childers, T. L. (1991). Understanding mail survey response behavior: A meta-analysis. *Public Opinion Quarterly, 55,* 613-639.

A meta-analysis of studies designed to induce mail survey response rates. Results indicated that repeated contacts in the form of preliminary notification and follow-ups, appeals, inclusion of a return envelope, postage, and monetary incentives effectively increased response rates.

About the Authors

LINDA B. BOURQUE, PhD, is a professor in the Department of Community Health Sciences in the School of Public Health at the University of California at Los Angeles, where she teaches courses in research design and survey methodology. Her research is in the areas of ophthalmic clinical trials and intentional and unintentional injury. She is author or coauthor of 50 scientific articles and the books *Defining Rape* and *Processing Data: The Survey Example* (with Virginia Clark).

EVE P. FIELDER, DrPH, has more than 30 years' experience in survey research. Since her beginnings in market research, she has had working experience in all phases of survey methods and has conducted hundreds of surveys, both commercial and academic. For the past 23 years, she has been with the Institute for Social Science Research at the University of California at Los Angeles, where she is Director of the Survey Research Center, and has taught survey research methods at UCLA and at the University of Southern California. She has consulted on studies for numerous organizations and community service agencies and has a strong background in cross-cultural research.

HOW TO CONDUCT INTERVIEWS BY TELEPHONE AND IN PERSON

THE SURVEY KIT

Purpose: The purposes of this 9-volume Kit are to enable readers to prepare and conduct surveys and become better users of survey results. Surveys are conducted to collect information by asking questions of people on the telephone, face-to-face, and by mail. The questions can be about attitudes, beliefs, and behavior as well as socioeconomic and health status. To do a good survey also means knowing how to ask questions, design the survey (research) project, sample respondents, collect reliable and valid information, and analyze and report the results. You also need to know how to plan and budget for your survey.

Users: The Kit is for students in undergraduate and graduate classes in the social and health sciences and for individuals in the public and private sectors who are responsible for conducting and using surveys. Its primary goal is to enable users to prepare surveys and collect data that are accurate and useful for primarily practical purposes. Sometimes, these practical purposes overlap the objectives of scientific research, and so survey researchers will also find the Kit useful.

Format of the Kit: All books in the series contain instructional objectives, exercises and answers, examples of surveys in use and illustrations of survey questions, guidelines for action, checklists of do's and don'ts, and annotated references.

Volumes in The Survey Kit:

1. **The Survey Handbook**
   Arlene Fink

2. **How to Ask Survey Questions**
   Arlene Fink

3. **How to Conduct Self-Administered and Mail Surveys**
   Linda B. Bourque and *Eve P. Fielder*

4. **How to Conduct Interviews by Telephone and in Person**
   James H. Frey and *Sabine Mertens Oishi*

5. **How to Design Surveys**
   Arlene Fink

6. **How to Sample in Surveys**
   Arlene Fink

7. **How to Measure Survey Reliability and Validity**
   Mark S. Litwin

8. **How to Analyze Survey Data**
   Arlene Fink

9. **How to Report on Surveys**
   Arlene Fink

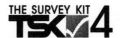
THE SURVEY KIT
TSK 4

HOW TO
CONDUCT
INTERVIEWS
BY TELEPHONE
AND
IN PERSON

JAMES H. FREY &
SABINE MERTENS OISHI

SAGE Publications
International Educational and Professional Publisher
Thousand Oaks   London   New Delhi

For information address:

SAGE Publications, Inc.
2455 Teller Road
Thousand Oaks, California 91320
E-mail: order@sagepub.com

SAGE Publications Ltd.
6 Bonhill Street
London EC2A 4PU
United Kingdom

SAGE Publications India Pvt. Ltd.
M-32 Market
Greater Kailash I
New Delhi 110 048 India

Printed in the United States of America

Library of Congress Cataloging-in-Publication Data

Main entry under title:

The survey kit.
    p. cm.
    Includes bibliographical references.
    Contents: v. 1. The survey handbook / Arlene Fink — v. 2. How to ask survey questions / Arlene Fink — v. 3. How to conduct self-administered and mail surveys / Linda B. Bourque, Eve P. Fielder — v. 4. How to conduct interviews by telephone and in person / James H. Frey, Sabine Mertens Oishi — v. 5. How to design surveys / Arlene Fink — v. 6. How to sample in surveys / Arlene Fink — v. 7. How to measure survey reliability and validity / Mark S. Litwin — v. 8. How to analyze survey data / Arlene Fink — v. 9. How to report on surveys / Arlene Fink.
    ISBN 0-8039-7388-8 (pbk. : The survey kit : alk. paper)
    1. Social surveys. 2. Health surveys. I. Fink, Arlene.
HN29.S724   1995
300'.723—dc20   95-12712

This book is printed on acid-free paper.

95 96 97 98 99 10 9 8 7 6 5 4 3 2 1

Sage Production Editor: Diane S. Foster
Sage Copy Editor: Joyce Kuhn
Sage Typesetter: Janelle LeMaster

Contents

Acknowledgments

The authors extend special thanks to Patricia Harmon for sharing her vast experience in supervising interview surveys, and for providing a multitude of "real-world" survey material from which many of the examples in this book were derived. Thanks are also extended to Robert Haile, Dr.Ph., for permission to include and adapt questionnaire and training materials from his projects, particularly the Kaiser/UCLA Sigmoidoscopy-Based Case-Conrol Study of Colon Polyps (Sigmoid Study), and to Barbara Vickrey, M.D., M.P.H. for permission to adapt material for study exercises related to epilepsy. Thanks also go to the Center For Survey Research of UNLV and the State of Nevada Nuclear Waste Office for materials that were used as illustrations and examples.

The authors would also like to express their appreciation to C. Deborah Laughton of Sage Publications and to Arlene Fink, Ph.D. for their patience and encouragement; several anonymous reviewers whose suggestions were very helpful in revisions of the manuscript; and Management Assistants, Veona Hunsinger and Susie LaFrentz, of the Sociology Department at UNLV, who were very helpful in the preparation phase of the manuscript.

How to Conduct Interviews by Telephone and In Person: Learning Objectives

The aim of this book is to guide the reader in the preparation and administration of survey interviews both by telephone and in person. Its specific objectives are to prepare the reader to:

- Choose the most appropriate interview mode (telephone or in person) for specific surveys

- Write interview questions with structured interviewer instructions

- Employ appropriate question-writing techniques based on whether the interview will be done by telephone or in person

- Construct useful visual aids

- Organize a flowing interview script that considers possible question order effects

- Write an informative introductory statement

- Write a preletter

- Write a script for a precall

- Design an eligibility screen

- Write and appropriately place transition statements

- Write a job description for an interviewer

- Develop an interviewer training manual

- Design an interviewer training session

- Describe the role of a supervisor

1

Overview
of Telephone
and In-Person
Interviews

A survey interview is a purposeful conversation in which one person asks prepared questions (the interviewer) and another answers them (the respondent). It is a directed conversation, the purpose of which is to gather information by means of administering the same set of questions in a consistent way to all selected respondents. These respondents presumably are representative of the population of interest, or **target population**.

The interview is a key data-collection tool for conducting surveys. A **data-collection tool** is a structured method of obtaining information about selected characteristics, or **variables**, in a target population. Depending on the topic of the survey, the variables may include specific knowledge, attitudes, and behaviors prevalent among the members of the population. The ultimate goal of the survey is to produce quantifiable measures of these variables that can be statistically analyzed to generate reliable observations. This is best done using a standardized questionnaire.

Standardized questionnaires are designed to reduce error that could be attributed to the interviewer. This is accomplished by scripting the question format and question order, defining in detail how the interviewer is to move through the questionnaire, and defining how the interviewer is to respond to questions or comments from the respondent. Standardization presumably leaves nothing to chance: Interviewers are instructed to be robotic when administering the instrument; however, they are also charged with the task of preventing the respondent from refusing to respond or prematurely terminating the interview. This is done by keeping the interview at a "conversational" level yet at the same time guiding the respondent along a prescribed path of questions and response alternatives.

Not many can fulfill this dual role of maintaining rapport through conversation while also performing a restricted, uniform, instrumental task. This makes interviewing a complex and demanding task. One can design the most technically proficient interview format, but if the interviewing is poorly done, the validity of the results can be severely compromised. The task of interviewing is made easier with properly designed questions (discussed in Chapter 2) and with adequate training and supervision (covered in Chapter 3).

Advantages and Disadvantages of Using Survey Interviews

Although surveys done by interview are usually more expensive, surveyors will choose them over self-administered questionnaires because of the role the interviewer can play in enhancing respondent participation, guiding the questioning, answering the respondent's questions, and clarifying the meaning of responses. In self-administered questionnaires, the respondent personally reads the questions and marks response options; the interviewer is not present to probe, clarify, and motivate the respondent to complete the questionnaire. Also, the surveyor loses control of the response pattern because the mailed questionnaire can be answered in any question sequence and by someone other than the selected respondent.

Another drawback of using self-administered questionnaires, whether mailed or distributed in a group setting, is their reliance on self-selected samples; that is, although the sample may be systematically determined, only those respondents personally motivated to complete and return the questionnaire will be heard from. Such samples often do not meet the criterion of representativeness—that is, the survey results obtained from the sample cannot be generalized to the target population. Interview samples are systematically determined and selected respondents are not in a position to "throw away" the questionnaire. Once contacted, they are more likely to participate in an interview survey (see **How to Sample in Surveys,** Vol. 6 in this series, for an in-depth discussion of sample selection).

IN-PERSON INTERVIEWING

One-on-one, in-person interviews have advantages over telephone interviews in terms of fewer limitations on the types and length of questioning and in the ability to use visual aids. Examples of locations for one-on-one interviews are the respondent's home, workplace, school, or the survey office, to name a few. Even though this form of interviewing is hampered by higher field costs, increased resistance on the part of respondents to invite strangers into their homes, and difficulty obtaining permission from management to conduct interviews in the workplace, it is regarded by researchers as one of the best ways to obtain detailed data. Other types of interview settings are possible:

- *Intercept interviews*, in which potential respondents are "intercepted" during an activity, such as shopping at a mall and questioned briefly on the spot
- *Group interviews*, in which formal techniques are used to question several people at the same time

This book discusses one-on-one, in-person interviews only. The reader is referred to Morgan (1993) and Frey and Fontana (1991) for a discussion of group interviewing.

TELEPHONE INTERVIEWING

Telephone interviewing is an increasingly popular means of conducting survey research because not only does almost everyone have a telephone but sampling techniques, such as **random digit dialing (RDD)**, make it easier to access unlisted and new numbers. Other reasons why telephone interviewing is being used more are its cost-efficiency and speed of data collection.

When used to survey the general population, as in national Gallup polls, telephone surveys also have the advantage of excellent sample coverage and generally high response rates. When telephone surveys are done for formal research, centralized calling units are often created. In such a unit, all interviewers contact respondents from specially equipped calling stations rather than calling from their own homes or private offices. The stations may employ special telephone equipment, such as listening devices and recording equipment.

Under such conditions, the telephone interview has its greatest advantage—the opportunity for quality control—because a supervisor (a person responsible for monitoring quality of interviewing) can observe interviews as they take place and give immediate feedback. In some **computer-assisted telephone interviewing (CATI)** operations, a supervisor can monitor an interview by listening from another station while the interview is being conducted. This is permissible if the interviewer informs the respondent that a supervisor may be listening to the interview for monitoring and quality control purposes. If the respondent agrees to continue the interview with full knowledge that a third party may possibly listen in on the conversation, then legal requirements of disclosure have been satisfied.

Of course, not all surveys are conducted as part of a sophisticated, well-funded research project. Smaller surveys (and many large ones) still use the paper-and-pencil method. Also, the creation of a central calling unit is not always possible. Other procedures can be developed. For example, an organization doing a small survey with limited resources can choose to have interviewers make calls from their homes and reimburse the charges. However, such a survey can also be able to imitate the central calling unit concept if office space with telephones can be made available so a supervisor can stand by.

Technological Advances in Interviewing

Recent technological developments have made interviewing, particularly by telephone, more feasible and more reliable.

The usual method for administering a questionnaire and recording responses is the "paper-and-pencil" method: Questions are read from a printed questionnaire in a prescribed sequence, and answers are recorded directly onto the questionnaire or code sheet. One of the problems associated with this method is human error on the part of the interviewer. For example, the interviewer may inadvertently overlook a question, ask questions in the wrong order, or accept an answer that is inconsistent with the range of response alternatives.

The integration of the computer into data gathering has improved the level of data quality for both telephone and in-person interviewing. For example, an organization with affiliates in several locations, such as the American Cancer Society, might find it worthwhile to equip each site with computers and software to standardize question asking for a large national survey. Computer-assisted telephone interviewing (CATI) and **computer-assisted personal interviewing (CAPI)** make it possible for the interview to be completed with fewer problems of interviewer error (for a fairly extensive discussion of computer-assisted survey techniques, see Frey, 1989).

The computer-assisted techniques direct the flow of each interview and automatically control the sequence of questions. Discrepancies in response can even be detected from one question to another. Also, these systems can be programmed to generate telephone numbers to call and to process data almost immediately. Although their use results in greater efficiency of administration, especially in larger surveys, and enhanced quality control, CATI and CAPI require considerable investment in hardware and presurvey programming and therefore may not lower a survey's overall cost. Which system to use is among the many decisions a surveyor must make when preparing an interview survey. The first and more basic decision required is whether to do the interviews by telephone or in person. Before delving into the specific issues associated with telephone and in-person interviewing, it is appropriate to discuss survey administration.

Survey Administration

Sometimes, surveyors pay little or no attention to the organizational or administrative details of the survey, assuming that these details will take care of themselves and that administration is not as important as data gathering. However, administration is a factor in **quality control** and therefore a factor in data quality. Quality control refers to procedures that organize and monitor survey activities for optimal results. For example, coordinating field operations, managing survey center operations, controlling sample selection, gaining productivity from interviewers, and properly implementing the survey according to plan are important administrative functions. If done properly, these procedures contribute to the overall quality of the data. Administrative procedures are developed in accordance with the **design** of the survey and its budget. Design refers to the overall plan for carrying out the following:

- How respondents will be sampled
- How many respondents need to be interviewed (see **How to Sample in Surveys,** Vol. 6 in this series)
- Complexity and length of questionnaire demanded by survey topic

- Interview mode
- How data will be analyzed (use of computer program or an outside consultant)

Once the design of the survey is determined and budgetary constraints are known, an administrative framework to handle implementation of this design can be conceptualized that includes the following:

- Number of interviewers needed and intensity of training required to meet sampling requirements
- Type and amount of supervision needed based on questionnaire complexity and interview mode
- Other personnel needed (clerks, data entry personnel, statistical experts) to handle data volume
- Facilities needed to house operations, including office equipment and storage space
- Amounts of supplies to stock (paper, pens, notepads, etc.)

After setting up the framework, administrative procedures that monitor and ensure the quality of the flow of data from interview through data analysis can be implemented. For example, a foundation that funds fellowships to support the development of academic researchers decides to do a survey to determine how many award recipients actually stay in academics (vs. going into industry). The foundation wishes to survey recipients over the past 10 years, or 150 fellows. The questionnaire will be simple (about five questions related to career development and current position) and administered by telephone. However, many addresses and phone numbers are outdated, but a complete list of names does exist. An appropriate administrative framework might include the following:

- Two part-time interviewers
- One part-time supervisor to stand by during interviews and do quality checks on completed surveys
- One part-time assistant to search for new telephone numbers of former fellows by calling the fellows' former institutions, scanning databases for recent publications (these list the author's affiliation), and using other location strategies. This duty could also be carried out by interviewers to keep personnel to a minimum.
- One or two calling stations, depending on whether both interviewers will be phoning at the same time
- A drawer in a filing cabinet to hold up to 150 interviews, even though not all fellows will be found and interviewed
- One part-time data enterer
- Several reams of paper, pencils, and notepads

ADMINISTRATIVE PLAN

The first step is to draft and implement an **administrative plan,** which defines the sequence of tasks, the timetable and person(s) having responsibility for these tasks, and all of the activities required as part of each larger task (e.g., sampling or questionnaire design). It is helpful to create a flowchart of major tasks in sequence, with the most important properly designated and singled out. That is, some tasks must be completed before any others can be carried out. For example, you cannot interview without the questionnaire. This technique is similar to the critical path method used in business and government for event planning.

ACTIVITY CHECKLIST

Another necessary administrative component is the **activity checklist.** This is an enumeration of all the major and minor tasks that must be completed. Each task is the assigned responsibility of a member of the research team and is given a scheduled completion date. All tasks should have a means of being monitored because many tasks are being carried out simultaneously. An activity checklist is especially helpful to survey administrators regarding distribution of the sample, determination of the status of each call or contact, and calculation of expense (i.e., budget).

An example of the activity checklist for a telephone survey follows. A similar format can be used for the in-person survey.

Activity Checklist

✓ Establish project timetable.

1. Interview training
2. Sample selection
3. Interviewing begins
4. Report due
5. Other _____

✓ Set up survey facility.

1. Reserved for calling
2. Equipment working
3. CATI system programmed

✓ Fill personnel requirements.

1. Operations supervisor(s)
2. Interviewers
3. Coder(s)/data entry
4. Programmer
5. Sample control person
6. CATI supervisor
7. Other _____

✓ Prepare budget.

1. Contract amount
2. Accounts and budget control procedure
3. Itemization
4. Other _____

✓ Select and train interviewers.

1. Recruiting
2. Training materials
3. Training scheduled
4. Employment contract
    − Employment referral form
    − Employee time card
    − W-4 form
    − Time sheet
5. Training completed

✓ Obtain supplies.

1. Phone books, if necessary
2. Pencils
3. Stapler
4. Other _____

✓ **Determine sampling and calling.**

1. Exchange/area proportions
2. Random selection of numbers
3. Number assignment forms
4. Call record form
5. Interviewer calling summary
6. Preletter, if necessary
7. Within-household selection procedure
8. Result codes
9. Codebook

✓ **Develop questionnaire.**

1. Pretest
2. Final draft
3. Printed and assembled
4. Assignment form
5. Probe instructions
6. Standardized responses to respondent questions

✓ **Analyze data.**

1. Codebook
2. Item codes
3. Coding form
4. Computer program
5. Computer accounts

✓ **Disseminate survey information.**

1. Formal report
2. Internal notification (e.g., department)
3. Press release or other publicity

Administration makes its major contribution to quality control and error reduction through continuous internal monitoring of the data collection process. This involves record keeping and close supervision. Interviewers must keep in continuous contact with their field supervisor, which means filing completed interviews or call summaries on a daily basis. This work is reviewed for accuracy and productivity. Every completed questionnaire must be edited and reviewed before being passed on to the data entry staff. Validation of at least 10% of completed interviews is implemented randomly; that is, all interviewers will have some of their interviews confirmed as to time and location.

Response rates, including refusals and partial completions, are monitored on a daily basis to assess the quality of the sample. Refusals and partial completions along with accuracy measures in the completion of the questionnaire become the basis on which to evaluate the performance of interviewers. Those who have the highest refusal rates or who seem to generate the same answer patterns (e.g., all respondents interviewed by "Jane" fall into the same category on most questions) or have a problem recording responses correctly and legibly may require additional training or should be terminated.

Replacement telephone numbers or field addresses are only assigned when the originally selected respondent has been determined to be ineligible or that respondent has been impossible to reach despite repeated callbacks because of a continuous no answer/answering machine or busy signal. In the latter case, that respondent remains "in sample" as a counted eligible respondent and becomes a part of the calculation of the actual response rate for the survey.

Attentive administration results in improved quality control, which means reduced systematic nonsampling and sampling error. Administration also means a careful and continuous assessment of the project's resource consumption. It is the rare project that is not limited by time, money, labor pool skills, and facilities. Tracking the budget is definitely a factor in quality control.

Determining the Sample

A **sample** is a portion or subset of the population the surveyor is interested in interviewing and is drawn when it is impractical to survey everyone in the population. A good sample is a miniature version of the population—just like it, only smaller.

Most surveys of special subpopulations use some kind of a list, or **sampling frame,** from which to draw a sample of potential interview respondents. For example, a school may use a roster of names and telephone numbers of first-graders' parents from which to randomly select respondents to call regarding their feelings about a new reading program. A research study may use medical records from the offices of selected lung specialists to identify asthma patients and record names and telephone numbers onto a list from which to sample.

However, lists are only one of the ways a sample can be obtained. A company wishing to survey employees regarding job satisfaction could randomly select office numbers and then randomly select desks within those offices without regard for who sits at them. The persons occupying the chosen desks comprise the sample. As long as everyone in the company has a desk, each person has an equal chance of being chosen.

Sampling is a complex topic worth understanding thoroughly when conducting any survey, whether by interview or otherwise. It is beyond the scope of this book to discuss sampling in detail, especially as the principles of sound sampling are not unique to interview surveys (see **How to Sample in Surveys,** Vol. 6 in this series, for a detailed discussion of sampling issues and techniques). There are, however, two sampling methods that are particularly relevant to telephone and in-person surveys of the general population: These are, respectively, random digit dialing (RDD) and area probability sampling. Both techniques eliminate the need for a list as possible respondents are chosen by randomly generating a telephone number or randomly choosing a housing unit within a geographic area. The person responding to the contact attempt is usually interviewed, if found eligible and willing, during that contact.

RANDOM DIGIT DIALING

For telephone surveys, access to the general population is enhanced by the use of *random digit dialing (RDD)*. This procedure is designed to overcome problems of sampling from telephone directories, which is the usual sampling frame for telephone surveys. Directories are often inaccurate and out-of-date. They are also incomplete because of unlisted numbers. As many as 60% or more of all telephone numbers are unlisted in some urban areas. RDD has overcome these flaws and thus made telephone interviewing a much more feasible option than it once was.

The first step in using RDD is to determine what three-digit exchanges (e.g., 458, 392) are in use in the target area (the geographic area within which the survey is to be conducted) and what blocks of 1000 or four-digit numbers are assigned. This information can be obtained by consulting the telephone directories that cover the target area or by contacting the local telephone company. If this information is not available from telephone directories or telephone companies, it is possible to purchase tapes from ITT listing central offices and numbers in use, but these are often out-of-date and inaccurate.

From this information, the surveyor can build unique seven-digit numbers efficiently. If the 739 exchange has residential numbers assigned between 2000 and 5000, the surveyor will draw a four-digit number randomly, within that range, usually via a computer program that generates listings of random numbers.

The four-digit number is then matched with the exchange. The combined number of 739-3467, for example, could be a number that one might have found in the directory, but it could also be a new number not yet listed or an unlisted number. That number is called. It is possible that the selected number will turn out to be a commercial setting or represent a household outside the target area. These possibilities mean that several calls may be made before an eligible respondent is reached. RDD and other improved telephone sampling techniques are reviewed in Frey (1989).

AREA PROBABILITY SAMPLING

A very useful strategy for household sampling because it can be applied to any population that can be defined geographically is what is termed **area probability sampling.** People living in a neighborhood, city, or country can be sampled this way. The basic concept is to divide the target area into exhaustive, mutually exclusive subareas with identifiable boundaries from which a sample is randomly drawn. Then, a list is made of housing units in each of these subareas, and a sample of these is drawn.

All of the people in selected housing units may be included in the sample, or they may be listed and sampled separately. This technique can be used both for sparsely populated rural areas and for downtown areas in large cities or any other geographic unit.

SAMPLE COVERAGE

When some of your target population cannot be reached by the interview mode you are using, data quality might be compromised by incomplete **sample coverage.** Any type of random sampling technique will overlook, for example, those who are homeless or live in cars or RVs, converted garages, or other nontraditional household settings. If these people are different from those you *can* reach in a way that is relevant to the survey objectives, your results will be biased (see Example 1.1). The incorrect conclusions you may draw are said to be due to "sampling error."

EXAMPLE 1.1
Compromised Sample Coverage

You are conducting a survey to determine levels of posttraumatic stress among survivors of a serious earthquake. Two weeks after the quake you can reach many survivors by telephone because lines have been restored and no longer need to be kept open for disaster procedures. However, the hardest hit victims are still living in tents and shelters without telephone service. If you survey by telephone only, you will lose their responses and hence will be omitting information about the stress manifestations of the hardest hit victims, which are likely to be different from those of victims still residing in their homes. Thus, your data will be incomplete and probably biased toward lower levels of posttraumatic stress than are actually being experienced in the population of earthquake survivors.

When interviewing special subpopulations, sample coverage must be considered in the context of the specific survey, its objectives, and target population. For surveys of the general population, however, random digit dialing and area probability sampling have overcome most sample coverage problems.

Deciding whether to interview by telephone or in person requires logistic and data quality considerations.

Logistics

It is not always obvious whether interviews should be done by telephone or in person for a particular survey. To decide which interview mode to use, start by considering three questions regarding the logistics of conducting the survey:

- What resources, including funding, personnel, time, and facilities, are available?
- What are the characteristics of the target population?
- What are the survey objectives?

AVAILABILITY OF RESOURCES

Funds

The availability of funds is often a powerful factor in determining how a survey will be conducted and may demand the less expensive interview mode from the start. When comparing telephone versus in-person interviews of the general public, the in-person mode is almost always more expensive. Because of the travel involved and because fewer interviews can be done in a given amount of time than by telephone, more and better-skilled interviewers and supervisors to monitor them are required. For these and other reasons, large-scale, in-person interviewing can be an extremely costly endeavor.

Surveys of smaller target groups using the in-person interview mode will usually also turn out to be more expensive but not always. Other resources, such as personnel, time for implementation, and facilities, need to be considered.

Personnel

Core personnel are interviewers to conduct interviews, supervisors to monitor the quality of interviewing, and any support staff (depending on the size of the survey) to handle administrative tasks, such as word processing, filing, and answering telephones. Depending on the nature and size of the survey, there may be an assortment of other personnel needed to run the survey, analyze findings, and locate difficult-to-reach respondents.

If the survey requires travel (as opposed to doing in-person interviews on-site, such as interviewing students at school), it is likely to require more personnel than a telephone survey. It may also be necessary to send more than one interviewer to a location where safety is a concern. This is true for some neighborhoods or locations where a potential threat exists. Also, because in-person interviews have more pitfalls for interviewers (discussed in a later chapter), more training will probably be required, and more supervisors may be needed.

Time

In-person interviewing will also usually take more time, again because of the travel factor. Using the telephone, a single interviewer can reach a large number of people over a wide geographic area in a short amount of time. Telephone interviews are often counted in numbers completed per hour. In-person interviews are more likely to be counted in numbers completed per day or per week, but if they are done on-site, as at a school, time is not as much of an issue.

Facilities

Facilities include space to house the survey's activities and equipment to carry out its functions. If you decide to set up a central calling unit so as to optimally supervise telephone interviewing, the cost of renting space and setting up calling stations with appropriate equipment may be more than sending interviewers to respondent's homes. If sufficient telephone equipment is available at your organization, say, during off hours (evenings and weekends), it will probably be cheaper to interview by telephone.

Inviting respondents to come to your facility for the interview is another possibility, although you might get a higher refusal rate if people have to go out of their way to participate in the survey. Sometimes, though, there is no other way to conduct the survey—for example, if respondents are asked to react to a nontransportable visual, like a museum display.

If a survey is large enough to consider implementing computer-assisted interviewing, facility costs (also personnel and training costs) go up.

CALCULATING THE COST OF INTERVIEWING

To determine which interview mode would cost you more to use, make a list of the resources you have available and those you would need to obtain for each interview mode and compare the costs.

EXAMPLE 1.2
Evaluating Resources to Compare Costs of Telephone Versus In-Person Interviewing

You work for a private women's college that is considering going coed to increase enrollment. You are afraid that enrollment could actually decline, however, if current students vehemently oppose going coed and drop out. You decide to interview a sample of current students to assess their views. No one currently on staff has ever conducted a survey before, but a reliable group of volunteer alumnae do regular telephone work for organizing campus events. You have very little money to conduct the study. You are also pressed for time because you need to know whether you are going to go coed in time for the print deadline of the application brochure.

You have an office available, equipped with several desks and telephones, where interviews could be done by telephone after 5 p.m. and on weekends. You also have access to a language lab that has private booths where you could conduct in-person interviews during the day. However, it is only available from 3 p.m. to 6 p.m. on weekdays, and your alumna volunteers are professionals who are not available during those hours. They also have no experience with in-person interviewing, so you would have to hire and train interviewers. You plan to design the questionnaire yourself and then hire a statistics student to do your analysis. You will get training to provide supervision yourself. You make a list of your resources:

Resource	By Telephone	In Person
Funding	Minimal funds available: Need to cover the cost of telephone bills (a few long-distance calls are expected), printing of questionnaires and training materials, and salary for the data analyst Alumnae will do interviews without compensation; however, a small stipend may be provided.	Minimal funds available: Need to cover interviewer salaries, printing of questionnaires and training materials, and data analyst salary; no travel costs if interviews are done in language lab
Personnel	Alumnae with telephoning experience are available to conduct telephone interviews evenings and weekends. They need to be trained in interviewing skills.	No existing personnel can do the job. Must recruit, screen, hire, and train interviewers
Time	Limited: If done by telephone, training can commence as soon as training materials are prepared.	Limited: More time will be needed than for the telephone interview to recruit and hire interviewers. Developing the training materials will take longer as will training.
Facilities	An office with telephones is available after hours and on weekends, which could constitute a calling unit where interviews could be listened to by a supervisor in the background.	The language lab provides a private setting for interviews from 3 p.m. to 6 p.m. each day.

Analysis of Survey Mode Options: Telephone Versus In Person

Telephone: Many of the resources to set up for telephone interviews are available. Costs can be kept low because most students live locally, avoiding the cost of long-distance calls, and a volunteer labor pool is available, except for the data analyst. There are essentially no costs for facilities, and setup would take very little time because interviewers need not be located. An up-to-date list of student names and telephone numbers should be available from the main office, making it easy to randomly select respondents and to use the telephone to reach them.

In Person: This survey is more expensive to do because of personnel costs for finding and training interviewers. It would also require more time to do the hiring and training. If you call students to arrange appointments at the language lab, more money and time will be required because recruiting and interviewing are separate, as opposed to immediate interviewing if done by phone. If you sample from classrooms (randomly choosing classes, and then students within classes), money, time, and personnel will be needed to make the selections and orchestrate the scheduling of interviews.

This survey is clearly more expensive to do in person. However, you have not yet considered whether doing the interviews by telephone will give you less useful data than doing them in person.

In a later section, a data quality checklist will help you focus on issues as they relate to interview mode. If money and time are so tight that you cannot do the interview in person, you still need to review the checklist. Otherwise, you will not understand the limitations within which to interpret your survey's results.

CHARACTERISTICS OF
THE TARGET POPULATION

The population of interest may dictate the mode of interview that is most likely to get results. Access to respondents in some target groups may be impossible by one mode or the other. If members of the target group are homeless, for example, logistically speaking, telephone interviews cannot even be considered. If the target group is widely dispersed geographically, in-person interviewing may be logistically impractical.

Other considerations in terms of target group characteristics are whether the overall education level and language skills are sufficient to allow comprehension of questions spoken over the telephone (which are easier to simplify in person) and whether fear for personal safety in a particular group (e.g., women living alone) would make it inappropriate to interview in the home. Many target group considerations will not rule out an interview mode completely but may have an impact on data quality, as when too many respondents refuse to participate because they are afraid to let an interviewer come to the home. The details of data quality considerations may be reviewed using the checklist provided later in this chapter.

SURVEY OBJECTIVES

The objectives of a particular survey may be more difficult to satisfy with one of the interview modes. For example, if the survey has objectives requiring direct observation of respondents' characteristics, it cannot be done by telephone. A psychological survey might have the following among its objectives: to compare consistency of body language cues with verbal responses to questions about drug use. Because body language cues must be observed, the survey has to be done in person.

To address the objective of finding out whether the local library is open at the right times for potential users to have access, the entire interview might consist of only three or four questions and take 5 minutes to complete. In this case, it would be logistically impractical to drive to respondents' homes for a 5-minute interview, so you would conduct your survey by telephone.

Data Quality

Logistic considerations will sometimes rule out an interview mode at the outset. Money or time availability may be severely restrictive, respondents may be absolutely inaccessible, or survey objectives may be impossible to meet by one mode or the other. Very often, however, the decision will require some thought. Logistic considerations must be weighed against a checklist of considerations concerning the quality of the data generated by one mode versus the other. Data quality involves the following:

- *Validity:* The accuracy with which the survey measures what it is supposed to
- *Reliability:* The precision, or consistency, of measurements from interview to interview of the data collected by each interview mode
- *Generalizability:* The extent to which conclusions about a sample are true about the entire population (also called external validity)

When logistics require choosing the less informative interview mode, the limitations of the data need to be understood for optimal interpretation. For example, if you were forced to do a survey by telephone knowing that generalizability might be compromised because some members of your target population were unreachable by telephone, you must qualify the conclusions you draw from your data. The checklist must therefore still be reviewed.

Data Quality Considerations Checklist

THE SAMPLE

✓ **Sample coverage:** Ability of a survey to reach all eligible respondents.

✓ **Response rate:** Degree to which the surveyor is successful in obtaining cooperation from all eligible respondents in a sample—that is, how often they are reached and agree to participate. The most informative way to calculate the response rate is to divide the number of completed interviews by the number of eligible respondents in the sample. When nonrespondents and respondents differ on important factors (e.g., education level), nonresponse bias is introduced. Also, if the response rate is low, the sample may become too small to produce precise and reliable findings.

✓ **Confidentiality:** Assurance given respondents that identifying information known about them (e.g., name, telephone number, and address) will not be revealed in any way. The issue with confidentiality is the ability to convince respondents that their identity can and will be kept secret. When respondents fear that confidentiality cannot be ensured, response rates may be lower.

  ■ *Comment:* Problems with sample coverage and response rates affect the generalizability of a survey's findings because those who are interviewed may be different from those who are not.

THE INTERVIEWER

✓ **Interviewer effects:** Interviewer behaviors and characteristics that bias the respondent's answers. Interviewers may interject their own opinions into the interview conversation, show approval or disapproval with tone of voice or facial expression, or present questions using their own words instead of those printed on the questionnaire.

✓ **Clarifications:** Done by interviewers when a respondent has not understood the question or the answer is not complete or is imprecise.

✓ **Ability to probe:** Technique used to get more information when a response is unclear or incomplete. Probes include simple gestures, such as nodding or saying "uh-huh," and neutral questions like "Could you tell me more about that?" to motivate the respondent to say more.

■ *Comment:* The interviewer can positively or negatively influence validity and reliability of questionnaire responses. Validity and reliability are compromised if the interviewer changes the meaning of questions or responses through biased interviewing technique, or insufficient skills in clarifying and probing. When the interviewer is skilled in these techniques, questioning is standardized, making responses more comparable from one respondent to the next. Data quality is thus enhanced.

THE QUESTIONS

✓ **Sensitive questions:** Ones that a respondent may be uncomfortable answering. Questions about finances, sexuality, illegal behavior (e.g., drug use), or embarrassing events (e.g., filing bankruptcy or being arrested) may be considered "sensitive" by respondents.

✓ **Complex questions:** Ones that require lengthy explanations or numerous response categories.

✓ **Open-ended questions:** Ones that do not offer response choices. Respondents are completely free to frame their answer.

✓ **Questions using visual aids:** Ones that involve visual tools to help respondents understand questions and answer them accurately. Visual aids, such as charts, maps, and lists, are rarely used for telephone interviews but are a valuable tool for in-person surveys.

■ *Comment:* Answers to sensitive, complex, and open-ended questions may compromise validity and reliability if not asked in a way that ensures respondent comprehension. Visual aids and certain question-writing techniques can simplify questions and response options to enhance comprehension.

THE RESPONSES

✓ **Item nonresponse:** Frequency with which a given item simply is not answered, or the answer is uninformative, such as "don't know" or "no opinion," or may not seem to make sense. Item nonresponse can be due to imprecise question wording, causing respondents difficulty in understanding, or they may refuse to answer because the question is sensitive or embarrassing. Alternatively, an item may be inadvertently skipped or incorrectly recorded by the interviewer.

✓ **Socially desirable responses:** Answers that respondents may give because of a belief that the response is what they "should" believe rather than what they actually do believe. For example, respondents who are smokers might respond favorably to limiting smoking in public places because smoking is viewed unfavorably among their peers. However, the respondents may actually find the restrictions annoying. Similarly, white respondents may give responses favorable to racial integration to an African American interviewer but actually resent integration measures. The latter is an example of a socially desirable response due to interviewer effect.

✓ **Questionnaire length:** Time required to ask all of the questions. Some topics can be covered in a few minutes with a small number of simple questions. Others require lengthy questioning using special procedures to present complex and sensitive items. Questionnaire length deserves consideration because lengthy interviews may result in respondent and interviewer fatigue. Fatigue can lead to less thoughtful responses or incomplete interviews.

■ *Comment:* Validity is compromised when respondents do not answer questions, give responses that do not reflect their true feelings to be "socially" acceptable, or stop answering thoughtfully because an interview is too long.

SAMPLE COVERAGE

Sample coverage is usually good with either interview mode, unless a specific target population as a whole or a certain group of people is difficult to reach by one mode or the other. This is discussed in detail in an earlier section of this chapter.

RESPONSE RATE

The degree to which cooperation is obtained from all eligible respondents in a sample is its **response rate.** The rate at which persons agree to be interviewed is influenced by many factors, including sampling technique, topic of survey, and how appealing the survey sounds during the introduction. No particular rate is accepted as standard, but if rates of 70% to 80% are achieved, one can feel comfortable with analyses based on the data. Every effort should be made to achieve this rate for the general population; lower rates may be acceptable for specialized, homogeneous populations.

Response rates are subject to significant variation in how they are calculated. The correct rate is generally a reflection of how successful the surveyor is in obtaining cooperation from all of the eligible respondents. It is the measure of the effectiveness of data collection and is determined as follows:

$$\text{Response Rate} = \text{Completed interviews} / \text{Number in sample eligible.}$$

Eligible respondents include completed interviews, refusals, partial completions, those with answering machines or who never answered, and numbers where a language barrier existed. Ineligible respondents are those who did not have a household member with the defining characteristic for inclusion, such as "adult over the age of 18" or "someone currently working full-time." Even if a household is never contacted, it is still considered eligible because there was no substantial evidence to eliminate it from the sampling pool.

Response is harder to get these days. Just contacting a potential respondent by phone is becoming increasingly difficult because of technological barriers, such as the answering machine and call waiting. Busy schedules, a desire for privacy, and fear for personal safety also make it difficult to obtain compliance. Surveyors must pay attention to these factors and address them.

At least five or six callbacks, or repeated attempts to reach a respondent, should be scheduled for telephone surveys—even more than that if it looks as if there is going to be some difficulty obtaining an adequate response rate. Field costs should include a budget for callbacks or return contacts with in-person respondents. Given the fact that respondents are harder to reach today than ever before, the surveyor could expect to make a callback or recontact in at least 50% of the sample cases. The denominator, or the definition of eligibility, is not consistently implemented in practice.

Often, survey research is reported with a response rate based on the ratio of completed interviews to refusals plus completions. This produces the "public relations" rate that makes the surveyor look good but is not an accurate record of response success. Response rates must be calculated at the end of each interview day and not at the end of the field phase of the survey.

The most revealing measure of a survey's success is the refusal rate or the number of eligible individuals who decide not to participate in the survey for one reason or another. Because refusals are known to be eligible, provisions must be made for refusal conversion. This is usually a task left to the most persuasive interviewers. When within-household selection techniques are used, the refusal could come at two points—with the person who is first contacted and with the selected eligible respondent.

In compiling the response summary for the study, each of these refusal points must be differentiated and included in the calculation. This will be important when refusal conversion, or convincing a person who previously refused to participate to do so, is attempted because the interviewer will need to know the exact status of the initial contact and who to try to contact when calling. Refusal rates are on the increase: 25% to 30% is not uncommon today. This, of course, creates concern about the representativeness of the sample. *With the use of sound sampling methods and systematic and persistent follow-up procedures, good response rates can be achieved for surveys using either telephone or in-person interviews.*

In some instances, the target group or survey content may lead to a poorer response rate by one interview mode or the other. Research has shown, for example, that so-called elite populations (people in socially elevated positions, such as lawyers and politicians) are more likely to participate in telephone interviews. Sensitive topics, however, are better approached in person.

CONFIDENTIALITY

Ensuring that respondents' **confidentiality** is protected is difficult in either interview mode but especially so with in-person interviews, where respondents are aware that the interviewer knows many of their identifying characteristics. These characteristics may include name, address, possibly telephone number, and personal appearance. Respondents' willingness to reveal information may hinge on their level of confidence that their identity will not be revealed.

Confidentiality can be compromised by validation callbacks ("checkup" calls to make sure the interview was actually done and not made up by the interviewer), which are often used in household and telephone surveys. These calls tell respondents that their name and telephone number have been passed on, even if only to the interviewer's supervisor.

It is not known how many respondents surveyed by telephone refuse to participate for privacy reasons. In surveys that employ RDD, the original identifying information is only a phone number as it is not necessary to have the respondent's name. The interviewer can assure respondents that their name is not known and will not be asked for. This may increase respondents' comfort level.

The possession of even the simplest of identifiers, such as a randomly generated telephone number, means that only **confidentiality**, not **anonymity**, can be ensured. Anonymity means that identifiers are not known; confidentiality means that no identifiers will be revealed. Confidentiality becomes a matter of trust—respondent of interviewer.

INTERVIEWER EFFECTS

The negative effects that an interviewer may have on the way a respondent answers a question are called **interviewer effects.** There are fewer negative effects for the telephone interview than for in-person questioning simply because visual cues, such as race or facial expressions, cannot be observed and so do not affect the response (Groves & Kahn, 1979). The interviewer can interject expectations and values into the interview exchange and can distort question wording, instruction guidelines, and probing guidelines, which can affect questionnaire completion.

Example 1.3 illustrates some instances of interviewer effects.

EXAMPLE 1.3
Interviewer Effects

1. *A question reads "What is your profession?"*

The interviewer ignores instructions to read questions verbatim and asks "What is your current job?" A teacher by profession might be currently working in a grocery store because of a teacher's strike and hence would answer the first question "teacher" and the second "grocery store clerk." The correct response is lost in this example, and what's worse, those who interpret the data will never know it unless the interview has been observed by a supervisor.

2. *A question reads "How did you find out about our program?" and has interviewer instructions "Do not read response options."*

The interviewer does not read the whole list of options out loud but begins offering some of them when the respondent hesitates. The respondent was about to say she was told about the program by a friend, but when the interviewer suggests a TV commercial, she says, "Oh, maybe I did see one." She does not go on to say that her friend's recommendation is what most motivated her to look into the program. The "correct" response has again been lost.

3. *A question reads "What is your opinion of how well the president is doing his job?"*

Although the interviewer's probing instructions are to remain neutral, say "uh-huh" and "please continue" to get a complete response, when the respondent says he is happy with the president's performance, the interviewer chuckles and asks, "Well, what about that illegal arms deal incident?" The chuckle tells the respondent that the interviewer disagrees with him, and the question about the arms deal takes the respondent in a direction he would not have chosen if left to respond on his own.

As previously stated, the centralized telephone interview can minimize biasing interviewer practices because of the close supervision that is possible. If, however, interviewers are allowed to make calls from their homes to save money, this advantage is lost. In-person interviews cannot be monitored constantly by a supervisor and are thus more vulnerable to interviewer effects. Interviewer body language, eye contact, and other nonverbal cues may influence respondents' answers. Standardized training of interviewers to follow the same protocol with each and every respondent is very important. The challenge is to follow the script but not to appear too mechanical about the questionnaire's administration because depersonalization contributes to nonresponse.

Clarifications and **probes** can be used most effectively in the in-person mode because of enhanced interviewer-respondent rapport and the ability to read a respondent's nonverbal cues indicating confusion or hesitation.

APPROPRIATE INTERVIEW MODE
FOR PARTICULAR QUESTIONS

Sensitive questions, or those that are potentially uncomfortable for the respondent to answer, can be asked in any type of survey because research shows no differences in response patterns by mode of inquiry (Frey, 1989). However, respondents are less likely to omit or give an incomplete answer to such items during the in-person interview simply because an interviewer is present to probe for a more complete response or to encourage respondents to answer the question despite its sensitive nature. Unfortunately, the potential for a socially desirable answer is also greater in the in-person interview. Telephone surveys show a higher rate of item nonresponse to sensitive questions (Frey, 1989).

Complex questions are also best asked in the in-person situation, mostly because visual aids can be used to help respondents understand the question or keep track of the response options. Respondents can get lost in the words over the telephone, losing track of multiple response categories or lengthy explanations. However, techniques such as funneling and split questions (described in Chapter 2) make it possible to ask more complex questions over the telephone. The advantage, however, still goes to the in-person interview, which also has the advantage when it comes to **open-ended questions.** Although these questions can be asked over the telephone, there is some evidence that they yield shorter, less detailed answers.

Visual aids are used almost exclusively with in-person interviews. They are difficult to use in telephone interviews because they need to be mailed in advance of the phone contact.

ITEM NONRESPONSE

Sources of **item nonresponse** include poorly worded or confusing questions and response categories, causing respondents difficulty in forming an opinion on the question. The expectations that an interviewer brings to the interview can also affect item nonresponse. For example, interviewers who believe that an item, such as a question on income or on abortion, is inappropriate or too difficult for a respondent will have higher item nonresponse rates. Interviewers who are less personable, more mechanical, and task oriented also will experience higher item nonresponse. In general, there is no appreciable difference in item nonresponse between telephone and in-person interviews, although nonresponse to the income question is higher for the telephone survey.

SOCIALLY DESIRABLE RESPONSES

Both types of interviews suffer from **socially desirable responses;** however, the problem is most prominent during in-person interviews. This is because the interviewer's sheer physical presence combined with visible characteristics, such as age or race, may influence the respondent's comments more than the removed voice on the telephone. The more personalized the interview, the greater the tendency for the respondent to answer in a manner perceived to be pleasing to the interviewer or to be generally expected within the social and political climate at the time.

QUESTIONNAIRE LENGTH

Questionnaire length is least restricted in the in-person interview. It is not uncommon to obtain interviews of 60 to 90 minutes in length. Over the longer interview time, interviewers can probe in greater depth, go further into establishing rapport, and thus be in a better position to ask sensitive questions. The development of new techniques in telephone questionnaire construction and interviewing procedure have made it possible to conduct somewhat lengthy interviews by telephone. Interviews of up to 50 minutes in length can be successfully conducted by telephone. Once the interviewer is past the introductory statements and into the first questions of the interview, length does not seem to be a problem. Respondents will complete the interview, apparently losing track of the time.

However, this does not mean that length is not an important consideration. After a certain time or number of questions, both interviewer and respondent fatigue affects the data quality. Answers may not be as thoughtful, and probing and clarifications on the part of the interviewer may be less thorough, causing data to be less complete.

Data Quality Summary

The weight given to the data quality considerations described in the preceding sections is influenced by the intended use of the data. Of course, high quality in terms of response accuracy and completeness and sample coverage is always a goal of any survey that is worth doing. However, the margin of error that can be tolerated will vary depending on how the data will be used.

If the study is only exploratory and the results are not a matter of "life and death," then the sampling/nonsampling error rate can be higher. For example, obtaining a population's general perception about social problems or community needs gives valuable information to politicians and policymakers, but sampling and interviewing technique may be compromised because a general sense is all that is required. However, if survey results will have a serious impact on jobs and appropriations, then these principles cannot be violated.

If the results of a knowledge, attitudes, and practices survey of smokers is going to be used to guide the planning of a larger-scale project, a certain margin of error may be tolerable. However, if data from such a survey will be used to determine national health education policy (which affects huge numbers of people and is hard to change once implemented), no detail of sampling, questionnaire construction, or questionnaire implementation (i.e., interviewing) can be left to chance.

There is no "right" way to conduct a survey. Modes other than the personal interview (e.g., mail surveys) can also be considered. Mode decisions will usually need to be made by weighing advantages and disadvantages of each mode in relation to the specific needs of the survey topic and target group. General advantages of telephone versus in-person interviews are summarized in the following table.

Data Quality Issue	Mode of Usual Advantage	Comments
Logistics		
Cost	Telephone	For most surveys, especially those of the general population, the telephone interview will be least expensive, requiring fewer personnel and less time.
Personnel	Telephone	
Time	Telephone	
The Sample		
Sample coverage	In person	Good sample coverage is usually possible with both modes. In-person interviewing provides better coverage with some special subpopulations.
Response rate	In person	Response rates are dropping for both modes. In-person interviews get somewhat higher rates.
Confidentiality	Telephone	Because a telephone interviewer usually knows less about the respondent, it is easier to ensure confidentiality. Neither mode can provide anonymity.
The Interviewer		
Interviewer effects	Telephone	Interviewer effects are lowest in the supervised centralized calling unit. They are also lower for telephone interviews in general because visible characteristics of the interviewer cannot influence respondent answers.
Clarifications	In person	Clarifications and probing are easier in person because the presence of the interviewer enhances rapport and allows observation of nonverbal cues indicating hesitation or confusion on the part of the respondent.
Ability to probe	In person	

$\rightarrow$

Data Quality Issue	Mode of Usual Advantage	Comments
Visual aids	In person	Visual aids enhance the in-person interview greatly. They are difficult to use in telephone interviews because they need to be mailed in advance and be available during the interview.
The Questions		
Sensitive questions	In person	In-person interviews get fewer omissions and incomplete responses for these. The reason is not known.
Open-ended questions	In person	More detailed answers may be given for these when asked in person.
The Responses		
Item nonresponse	Neither	Neither mode gets lower item nonresponse in general; nonresponse for the income question is higher by telephone.
Socially desirable responses	Telephone	These are more of a problem in person because the respondent may react to the interviewer's physical characteristics and may be more eager to please an interviewer who is physically present.
The Questionnaire		
Long questionnaires	In person	Longer interviews are possible in person because of increased rapport.

The most salient considerations for logistics and data quality in deciding interview mode will vary with the survey. Example 1.4 illustrates the decision process.

EXAMPLE 1.4
Survey Scenario

A survey of Los Angeles County (California) residents has the objective of describing the range of opinions on sensitive political issues, such as welfare reform, immigration laws, and health care policies. The nature of the questions is that they are complex and sensitive. The questionnaire is expected to be fairly long (at least 60 minutes). The county board of supervisors wants reliable data on which to base policy decisions and is providing reasonable funding.

The survey administrators realize that sensitive and complex questions are best asked in person using good visual aids, but they are worried that interviewer effects and social desirability will be a real problem. The political nature of the questions makes it likely that respondents will be looking for validation of their opinions from the interviewer, and their answers to the immigration questions may be influenced by the interviewer's race. The population of Los Angeles County is highly racially mixed, and the race match of the interviewer and respondent could have an effect. The length of the questionnaire favors doing it in person, although it is not impossible to do by telephone. There seems to be enough funding to do the interviews in person, but if done by telephone, a larger number of interviews can be done for the same amount of money. There is enough time to do the interview by either mode.

In weighing the considerations, the administrators decide that the validity of the more complex items will be compromised too much if they cannot use visual aids. There are too many complex items to address the problem with question-writing techniques that would allow the questions to be asked over the phone. Respondent fatigue would be inevitable. They also prefer the in-person mode because of the length of the questionnaire, which has not yet been developed. They prefer to leave open the option of a longer questionnaire, rather than having to cut items if the pilot test shows that the interview actually takes longer. They reason that only some of the questions might be affected by interviewer race and decide to assess the impact during a pretest.

They decide that a full week of training will be required to maximize interviewer skills. Special attention will be paid to providing practice in remaining neutral and reading questions as worded so as to minimize interviewer effects. Supervisors will accompany interviewers on occasional interviews to observe their techniques and give feedback.

Once preliminary decisions regarding the execution plan and interview mode of a survey have been made, the questionnaire can be designed. Questionnaire construction must take place with both the target group and the mode of interview in mind.

The next chapters discuss these issues.

2 Questionnaire Construction

The interview takes the form of a script. Its construction requires a marriage of art and science to achieve two primary goals: One is content that addresses the survey objectives; the other is smooth conversational flow. The interview script is composed of three important parts: introductory statement, eligibility screen, and questions. The introductory statement describes the survey and attempts to enlist participant cooperation, and the eligibility screen determines whether a potential respondent is suitable to be interviewed. Once respondents have been selected, the questions facilitate performing the real work of interviewing: data collection. A persuasive and informative introduction to the interview provides the means of obtaining the cooperation needed for successful data collection.

Introductory Statement

The crucial component of the interview for capturing the respondent's interest is the **introductory statement.** It must present information regarding the survey in conversational, nonthreatening language that convinces the respondent to participate. In the case of in-person interviewing, respondents have time to observe the interviewer and to listen to the introductory message. When a survey is presented by telephone, however, respondents have little time to make a decision. They must respond to an unanticipated, almost immediate request for an interview. In fact, prospective respondents for a telephone interview may not even hear the content of the introductory message or only hear selected components as they contemplate whether or not to agree to the interview. Thus, it is advisable to give each potential respondent as much time as possible to think about whether to participate.

The introductory statement, as short as it may be and with constraints of interviewer appearance and/or voice, has the major responsibility of building immediate rapport and trust with the respondent. A great deal of attention must be paid to the formulation of the introductory message. The following checklist can help guide the process.

Checklist for Preparing
Introductory Statements

✓ **Identify the person (use full name) making the contact.**

✓ **Identify the sponsor of the survey (e.g. foundation, university, marketing firm).**

✓ **Explain why the request is being made, including appropriate background on the survey, and what kind of information is sought.**

✓ **Verify that the right person, household, or telephone number has been reached.**

✓ **State any important conditions of the interview, such as level of confidentiality, voluntary nature of participation, approximate length of interview, and opportunity to ask questions.**

✓ **Describe any benefits of participation.**

✓ **Ask for permission to proceed with the questions.**

It is well documented that most terminations or refusals take place after the introduction but before the first question, so an interviewer will usually have an opportunity to describe the survey before the respondent decides whether or not to participate. The script for an introduction should first identify both the person making the contact and the sponsoring organization so as to establish the survey's credibility and then explain briefly why the request for an interview is being made. Respondents should not be wondering who is calling or what this is about when an identifying question using their name or phone number is asked. To avoid wasting both the respondent's and the interviewer's time, verification that the correct person or location has been reached should be made next. If the right person has been reached, brief details about the reason for the survey, its contents, and the conditions of the interview (e.g., confidentiality) and any benefits of participation should be given. These details offer the respondent the opportunity to make an informed decision about participation. Finally, a courteous request for permission to proceed makes the respondent feel respected and ensures voluntary participation.

There is some debate about just how much information should be given about the purpose of the survey. One view is that the respondent should be told as little as possible about the survey objectives to avoid biasing response patterns. For example, if respondents know that the survey is looking for the effects of alcohol in lowering the incidence of heart attacks, alcohol consumption might be reported differently than if they thought the subject was alcoholism.

Another view is that respondents should be well informed not only out of respect but to avoid possible accusations of malpractice or misconduct directed at the interviewer. The specific survey topic, its political context, the characteristics of the target population, and the cost in data quality (due to biased comments) must be considered in deciding how detailed the introductory statement can be.

Example 2.1 illustrates how introductory statements vary for telephone and in-person surveys.

EXAMPLE 2.1
Introductory Statements

Telephone

1. Hello. This is ___(full name of interviewer)___ calling from the Center for Survey Research at the University of Nevada, Las Vegas. We are conducting a survey of Clark County residents for their views on important issues facing the southern Nevada area. Is this the ___(respondent's last name)___ residence?

> (IF WRONG NUMBER OR INCORRECT LISTING, TERMINATE INTERVIEW BY SAYING SOMETHING LIKE "SORRY TO HAVE BOTHERED YOU"; IF CORRECT, PROCEED WITH REMAINDER OF INTRODUCTION)

Your number was selected at random from a local telephone directory, and your responses will be confidential.

> (INSERT SELECTION PROCEDURES FOR ELIGIBLE MEMBER OF HOUSEHOLD; REPEAT INTRODUCTION ABOUT PURPOSE OF STUDY)

May I begin asking some questions?

2. Hello. This is _____ calling from the Center for Survey Research at the University of Nevada, Las Vegas. We are conducting a survey of Clark County residents about community concerns. Before we continue, I need to know if I have dialed the correct number. Is this ___(number)___ ?

> (IF NO, END INTERVIEW BY SAYING "SORRY TO HAVE BOTHERED YOU"; IF YES, PROCEED WITH REMAINDER OF INTRODUCTION)

Your number was chosen for this survey by a random digit selection process. I would like to find out your opinions on some issues. May I proceed with the questions?

3.   Hello, my name is _____. I'm calling on behalf of Livingston Memorial Research Foundation. The Foundation is participating in a national study of the delivery of social services and their financing. Have I reached the Johnson residence? You should have received a brochure about the Livingston Social Services Programs within the past few days, and I'm calling to talk to you about your opinions of the programs. Your answers will be kept in the strictest confidence, and your name will not appear on the interview form. Do you have any questions? The interview will take about 5 minutes to complete. You may end the interview at any time. May I ask you questions?

The examples above illustrate how the components of the introductory statement might be synthesized for several different surveys. Although the flow is similar, the content and number of details (how names or phone numbers were acquired, whether length of interview is stated up front) varies with the nature of the survey and is a matter of the surveyor's judgment.

In Person

1.   Hello, my name is _____, and I represent the Democratic Party. We are doing a survey to get a feel for voter opinion on gun control legislation, and I am asking people in your neighborhood for their views. I will not ask your name or record any identifying characteristics about you on the survey form, except the neighborhood where the interview took place. Your participation will make your opinions heard in Washington. The survey takes about 7 minutes to complete. Do you have any questions? May I interview you?

(SHOW IDENTIFICATION IF NECESSARY)

2. My name is _____, and I am from UCLA. We are conducting a study of the health effects of environmental pollutants, funded by the National Institutes of Health. To learn about these effects we would like to ask you a number of questions about your health and daily activities. The information that you provide will be very important in helping us understand the relationship of the environment to health and will help to guide us in making decisions in these areas in the future. Your responses will be used for statistical purposes only and will not in any way be identified with you or members of your family. I'd like to begin by asking you some general questions about you and all other family members living in this house. May I continue?

Note that in both introductory statements the emphasis is on confidentiality information because the physical presence of the interviewer is more threatening to privacy than a request made over the phone.

These examples are intended as lead-in statements when the interview is to follow immediately. The respondent has been contacted either by telephone for an immediate interview or by a field interviewer who has knocked on the door or come to the workplace or similar setting. In the latter case, it is important that interviewers carry a letter of identification certifying that they represent a legitimate organization. Badges with the name of the interviewer and sponsoring organization clearly visible should be worn. Example 2.2 shows a letter of identification used in a survey on risk perception associated with the siting of a high-level nuclear waste repository.

EXAMPLE 2.2
Identification Letter

(LETTERHEAD - CENTER FOR SURVEY RESEARCH)

Date

Dear Clark County Resident:

This is to introduce _____ who is employed as an interviewer by the Center for Survey Research at the University of Nevada, Las Vegas. The interviewer will be asking several questions as part of a survey of Clark County residents on your attitudes and perceptions associated with various community issues and problems, including the proposed repository at Yucca Mountain. Your responses will be confidential. If you have questions or wish to verify the research, please feel free to call me or a field supervisor at 555-1234. Thank you for your help.

Sincerely,

James H. Frey, Ph.D.
Project Director

The message of this letter contains a statement of the survey purpose, an affirmation of confidentiality, and a telephone number the respondent can call to verify that the survey is genuine.

Advance Letters and Precalls

Interviews do not have to immediately follow the introduction. They can also be introduced by an **advance letter** (using a sampling list with addresses, if available) or a telephone **precall** (using either a calling list of known telephone numbers or RDD). Advance letters are also called "preletters." Introductory telephone calls describe and schedule an interview rather than administer it.

By reducing the surprise element and increasing the time that a potential respondent has to think about participating in the survey, advance letters and precalls can reduce refusal rates and increase data quality. These tools can also demonstrate the authenticity of the research so that the respondent does not assume that a sales pitch is coming.

Use of the following guidelines can help ensure that the introductory letter makes an appropriate impression on the respondent.

Guidelines for Preparing Advance Letters

- Use letterhead.
- For manageable sample sizes, use a personal salutation (e.g., Dear Mr. Jones), sign each letter individually in ink, and address each envelope individually rather than using labels.
- Date the letter to coincide with the mailing. A nondated letter gives it a less personal intrepretation.
- Provide an introductory statement regarding a future call or visit to conduct an interview, including timing of the contact, how the respondent was sampled and chosen, and whether someone else in the household might be ultimately interviewed.

- Describe the survey topic without being intimidating.
- Guarantee whatever level of confidentiality is possible.
- Give an honest estimate of the time required to complete the interview.
- Convey the importance of respondent views for valid results and potential impact.

It is important to convey an impression of legitimacy by having appropriate identification of the sponsor and source of the survey. Printed letterhead helps provide this identification. It is also crucial that respondents receive as personal an appeal as possible. They should feel that they were singled out for this interview and that *their* opinion is crucial to the study. Personalization through individualized salutations, original (not "rubber stamp") signatures, and individually typed envelopes have been shown to stimulate response, particularly from somewhat reluctant respondents (Frey, 1989). Of course, personalization is expensive to implement and cannot always be done for very large samples.

Information about the timing of a future contact helps respondents anticipate the call or visit and provides an opportunity to consider whether to participate in the survey. As with introductory statements in general, other details about sampling, survey topic, confidentiality, and so forth give respondents the necessary information on which to base their decision.

Advance letters may come directly from the survey group (see Examples 2.3 and 2.4) or may be an endorsement from a supporter or collaborator whom the person trusts (Example 2.5).

EXAMPLE 2.3
Advance Letter: Telephone Interview

(LETTERHEAD - CENTER FOR SURVEY RESEARCH)

Date

Mr. Bill Jones
2222 Elm Street
Las Vegas, NV 89000

Dear Mr. Jones:
During the week of June 3-10 an interviewer from the Center for Survey Research at the University of Nevada, Las Vegas, will be calling your home in connection with a survey of Clark County residents for their views on important community issues, such as transportation, growth, education, and the Yucca Mountain repository site.

Your name and number were selected at random from the local telephone directory. We are writing this letter because many people prefer to be informed in advance that a request for interview will be made in the near future. When the interviewer calls, he or she will request to speak to an adult, either you or another adult over the age of 18, in the household. This is done in order to be certain that all Clark County opinions are represented in the survey.

The interview should take approximately 10 minutes. Naturally, all of the responses will be confidential, and you can end the interview at any time.

Your participation will be greatly appreciated. This is a very important study for Clark County, and the results will be used by county officials in the formulating of policy for the area. If you have any questions, please feel free to call me at 555-1234. Thank you.

Sincerely,

James H. Frey, Ph.D.
Project Director

This advance letter is sent directly from the survey center using its letterhead.

EXAMPLE 2.4
Advance Letter: In-Home Interview

(LETTERHEAD - CENTER FOR SURVEY RESEARCH)

Date

Mr. Bill Jones
2222 Elm Street
Las Vegas, NV   89000

Dear Mr. Jones:

Recently you were called by the Center for Survey Research from the University of Nevada, Las Vegas, about participating in an extremely important study regarding issues facing the Clark County area (e.g., transportation, public safety, economic growth, and repository site). We need your opinions so we may help the county and the state prepare for the future. Your participation and cooperation are important so that the results of the research can be statistically valid. Please understand that you are one of 755 persons who have been scientifically selected from all adult residents of the Clark County urban area. Your responses will be treated with complete confidentiality.

We understand that you may have doubts about many appeals you receive for your opinion, particularly if that request is by telephone. We are not attempting to sell you anything; we only want your opinions. If you wish to verify this, or if you have any questions about the intent or purpose of this study, you can call me directly at the Center for Survey Research. The number is 555-1234.

When our interviewer calls you within the next few days, we would appreciate your making an appointment for an interview. We would like to conduct this interview in your home, and it will last approximately 45 minutes. Thank you for your consideration.

Sincerely,

James H. Frey, Ph.D.
Project Director
Center for Survey Research

P.S. We obtained your telephone number and address from the
Hill-Donnelly Criss-Cross Directory, which matches listed
telephone numbers and addresses.

This advance letter is sent from the survey center on its letterhead to inform a potential respondent that a request for an in-person interview is going to be made by telephone.

EXAMPLE 2.5
Advance Letter From a Trusted Collaborator
(PHYSICIAN'S LETTERHEAD)

Dear Ms. Smith:

I have been asked by the University of California to help them in a national study about the overall health of Americans. Many individuals from all parts of the country are being invited to help in this study.

In order to get correct information about the health of Americans I need your cooperation. Because this study is important I am asking my patients to take part in it. You can help me by answering a number of questions about your health. A study staff member will come to your home, or some other place if you prefer, to ask you some questions. The interview should take about an hour of your time.

The information you give will be kept strictly confidential. When your interview is finished, your name will be removed from the questionnaire. The answers you give will be combined with the answers given by all other persons interviewed and used for scientific study.

Please drop the enclosed postcard in the mail so that a member of the study staff may call you and answer any questions you may have and also arrange the best time and place for your interview. Or, if you prefer, the project staff or I would be glad to answer any questions. The staff can be reached at (310) 555-1234 (CALL COLLECT IF THIS IS OUT OF YOUR AREA).

I urge you to participate in this important study by the University of California conducted under the sponsorship of the National Institutes of Health.

Sincerely,

James Jones, M.D.

When confidentiality is of great concern, as in the case of having chosen a respondent from a medical records review in which sensitive information may be involved, the advance letter might come from a physician the respondent knows and trusts. If the physician is part of the survey team or clearly endorses the project, the letter serves to legitimize the study and make the respondent less uncomfortable about revealing personal information.

Similar to advance letters, precalls serve to inform respondents of their selection for interview and should include the same basic information about the survey. A future phone call (or visit) for an interview can be scheduled if the person consents. The precall can be referred to in the opening comments when the actual interview is done.

Advance letters, precalls, and introductory statements made immediately before the interview is administered all serve to entice the respondent into participating. One must be certain, however, that an *eligible* respondent has actually been contacted before the interview should proceed.

Eligibility Screen

In the course of the survey introduction it is important to determine whether the respondent is actually eligible to answer the questions. This is accomplished using an **eligibility screen.** In surveys of the general public, one is often interested in polling the views of individuals with specific characteristics, such as being registered voters or the person who most often does the grocery shopping for the family. If the survey respondents are grouped on a sampling list that was generated according to inclusion criteria (e.g., mothers of children with speech impairments who have received speech therapy at a local clinic), one presumably knows the name of the desired respondent and can ask for that person directly. This does not necessarily ensure eligibility, however, because there may be other criteria that need to be reviewed with the respondent directly (e.g., you may only be interested in mothers who also have at least one other child in the household). Interviewers must be trained in the importance of eligibility criteria and cautioned not to accept convenient substitutes.

The eligibility screen consists of one or more questions designed to determine whether the potential respondent has the characteristics the surveyor considers important. These questions should be asked after rapport has been established during the introductory phase and before the interview begins. Truthful answers to eligibility questions are more likely because the respondent trusts that the interviewer's purpose is legitimate, and resources are not wasted interviewing ineligible respondents whose data will have to be disregarded.

Example 2.6 illustrates both telephone and in-person eligibility screens.

EXAMPLE 2.6
Eligibility Screens

Telephone

1. Hello, my name is _____. I'm calling on behalf of Global Life Insurance Plan. We are speaking to persons who recently chose to terminate Global coverage to learn why they made that decision. Did you choose to leave Global, or did you have to leave because you were covered through your employer and you changed jobs or lost your job? (IF RESPONDENT CHOSE TO LEAVE, CONTINUE WITH INTERVIEW. IF RESPONDENT DID NOT CHOOSE TO LEAVE, THANK AND TERMINATE INTERVIEW.) Can I have a few minutes of your time to ask some questions about your opinions of Global? I can assure you that the information you give me will be confidential. It will be combined with information from several hundred other people and reported in statistical form only.

2. Good morning/evening. My name is _____,
and I'm calling from the Center for Survey Research at the University of Nevada, Las Vegas. We are conducting a survey of area residents on health issues. Today we are asking community residents 18 to 54 years old what they know about AIDS. Are you in this age group? (IF YES, CONTINUE. IF NO, ASK TO SPEAK TO SOMEONE ELSE IN THE HOUSEHOLD WHO IS THE SPECIFIED AGE. IF NO ONE IS AVAILABLE, THANK THEM FOR THEIR TIME AND TERMINATE THE INTERVIEW.) To assure you that your identity and responses will remain confidential, I want you to know that your telephone number was generated by a computer. I do not know your name or address, and I will not ask you for them. May I please have a few minutes of your time for this important survey? Thank you.

In Person

Hi. I'm with the Southern California Beaches Health Survey. We are here at the beach today asking families about their contact with the water. In about 10 days, another person from the survey or I will phone those who talk to us today. We will ask some follow-up questions about the water. We will also ask some health questions at that time. Are you willing to answer some questions today? Are you here with your family? (IF YES, PROCEED WITH SCREENING QUESTIONS.)

1. Have you or anyone in your household been swimming or playing in the water at this beach today?

      Yes   →   CONTINUE TO Q2
      No   →   THANK AND END INTERVIEW

2. Not including (3-day survey period), do you think you or anyone in your household will return to this beach in the next 10 days?

Yes, we will all return → THANK AND END INTERVIEW

Yes, some of us will return → CONTINUE **ONLY** FOR THOSE WHO WILL **NOT** RETURN BUT WHO **HAVE BEEN IN THE WATER**

No, none of us will return → CONTINUE INTERVIEW FOR ENTIRE HOUSEHOLD

SOURCE: Adapted from the *Santa Monica Beach Study Pilot.*

These examples are introductory scripts containing eligibility screens specific to the needs of the particular survey. In the first example, a respondent is eligible only if termination of insurance coverage was voluntary because the surveyor wants to know the reasons why people chose to discontinue coverage. In the second example, the respondents are eligible only if they fall into a specific age group in whose opinions the surveyor is interested. In the third example, which is a face-to-face encounter, the surveyor wants to limit findings to a single day of contact with the water during a specified period of time. Thus, anyone who may come back to the beach during that period is not eligible.

Often, it is necessary to sample within a household or living unit, particularly if an individual, not a household, is the unit of analysis. Because households can be clusters of eligible respondents, it is necessary to sample within the cluster to obtain a random probability sample. In some cases, it is only necessary to get responses from any member of the household who is familiar with the survey topic. It is also not necessary to implement a within-household selection procedure if the eligibility screen is directed at a very specific member, say, a female over the age of 55 or a member of the household who plays golf or has a disability. If such criteria are not defined, then one of several selection procedures is used. We discuss these only briefly here (for a more exhaustive review, see Dillman, 1978; Frey, 1989).

The selection of the *first eligible* respondent to come to the telephone or answer the door is often implemented when resources are limited and time may be a factor. In this case, the surveyor verifies that the potential respondent meets minimum qualification criteria (e.g., "Over the age of 18" or "Lived in household for more than 3 months" and then conducts the interview. This selection process produces a "convenience" sample that is not a probability design. Generalization to the larger population can be made only with some caution. This technique oversamples females, particularly in telephone surveys where women tend to answer the phone in a household. Some researchers implement a *male-female alternate* selection process, but this assumes that the distribution of gender is known and that substitution does not compromise the distribution of population characteristics.

Another type of selection procedure calls for the *enumeration of household members.* This technique asks for a listing of all members of a household by age, gender, and relation to head of household, and a respondent is then chosen from among them. This technique is time consuming and more demanding of interviewers. It produces higher-than-normal refusal rates because many households are headed by women who resist describing the composition of their home to strangers. This technique is more successful with in-person interviews than with those conducted by telephone.

One technique that is gaining in popularity with surveyors asks for the person in the household who has had the *last birthday* or will have the *next birthday*. The request for birthday information is not threatening to the respondent, and the probability of selection is preserved because it is assumed that the distribution of birthdays in a population is random, not systematic or patterned in any way. The interviewer simply asks,

---

"We need to be sure we give every adult a chance to be interviewed for this study. Thinking only of adults in your household, that is, persons over the age of 18, which one had the most recent birthday? (or will have the next birthday)? Would you be that person?"

IF YES, CONTINUE INTERVIEW
IF NO, "May I speak to that person?"
(REPEAT INTRODUCTION)

Very often, the person answering the telephone or initially responding to an in-person interview request is also the eligible respondent, that is, has the next or most recent birthday. In practice, the use of "last birthday" is preferable to using "next birthday" because it is easier to recall who had a birthday than to remember who will have one in the future.

Questions From Respondents

At some time during the introduction and the eligibility screen, potential respondents or other family members are very likely to ask questions regarding the survey to determine whether it is legitimate and to help them decide whether or not to participate. Although some of these questions might come up at the end of the interview or even during its administration, most will be asked near the beginning of the contact. Such questions must be answered in a consistent manner by all interviewers, with interviewers trained not to add information that could bias a respondent's answers. The questions most likely to be asked by respondents should have standardized responses (sometimes called "fallback statements") developed and made available to the interviewers.

Interviewers need to be very familiar with these standardized responses and keep them readily available as a memory backup during the interview. They should be instructed to call on a supervisor to respond to questions they cannot answer. In the case of telephone interviews done in a survey center, supervisors are immediately available to answer the question. However, in both small-scale phone interviews done from interviewers' homes and in-person interviews, no supervisors are present, so interviewers should tell respondents that a supervisor will call them soon to answer their questions (remember to write down the telephone number).

Some of the questions frequently asked by respondents are the following:

"How did you get my name (telephone number, address)?"
"Whom do you represent?"
"Who is sponsoring this survey?"
"Will you use my name?"
"How will you use my answers?"
"Will this cost me anything, or will I be paid for my participation?"
"What will happen if I don't participate?"

A few other questions will probably come to mind related to the specific survey being conducted (e.g., in a survey of satisfaction with health care, respondents might want to know whether their doctor will have access to their responses or name).

Example 2.7 lists possible questions that respondents might have regarding a nuclear power survey and the prepared answers supplied to interviewers.

EXAMPLE 2.7
Standardized Responses to Respondent Questions About a Nuclear Power Survey

What is the Center for Survey Research?

This is a research unit of the University of Nevada, Las Vegas, designed for the purpose of conducting public opinion polls and surveys on various social, political, and economic issues. The director is Dr. James Frey, also a member of the Sociology Department. If you have any questions or concerns about participating in this study, you can contact him at 555-1234.

Who is paying for this research?

This is a cooperative project funded by the Sagebrush Alliance and the Department of Sociology at UNLV.

Who or what is the Sagebrush Alliance?

The Sagebrush Alliance is a community group concerned with the evaluation of the impact of environmental changes on the quality of life of residents of the state of Nevada.

How did you get my name?

We do not have or need your name. Your number was dialed at random using a technique called random digit dialing. We did not use a list, such as the telephone directory, to get your name.

How do I know that this is confidential?

We do not have your name. We are interested only in combining the responses of the 400 or so persons who will be called. Individual responses will not be singled out. All of us working on this project are required to follow certain procedures and guidelines developed to protect the identity of persons who respond to the survey.

How will the results be used?

The information generated by this survey will be used by students in research methods classes. The results will also be made available to policymakers in the community to help them know and understand what county residents think about the nature and use of nuclear energy and about other issues.

What is the purpose of the survey?

This is a general survey of the public on a number of community issues including nuclear power. The study is designed to learn more about the public's opinions and perceptions.

How long will this take?

The interview should take about 10 minutes. You can end the interview at any time, but we hope you will not.

WARNING

 Do not provide any additional information to the standardized responses. If there are questions that you cannot answer or if your answer does not satisfy the respondent, call the supervisor.

Dealing with questions about conditions and intent of the survey is an important part of interviewer training, especially for field interviewers who cannot be monitored closely. Telephone interviewers in a centralized location can be easily monitored for responses, and corrections can be made immediately, if necessary.

Interview Questions

Once eligible respondents have agreed to participate, the real substance of the interview, the questioning, can begin. The design of questions for interviews is a complex process involving many considerations. The basic task is twofold: Write the questions and organize them into a coherent document, the questionnaire. The goals of question writing are to encompass content relevant to the survey objectives, use language that is meaningful to the target group, and use a presentation style that maximizes valid and reliable responses. The goals of questionnaire organization are to create smooth conversational flow for both the respondent and the interviewer and to provide structure for those who prepare the data for analysis—the coder who translates the answers into numeric codes and the data-entry person who enters the codes into a computer for analysis (for more information regarding coding and data entry, see **How to Analyze Survey Data,** Vol. 8 in this series).

CONTENT

The primary purpose of the questions is to meet the objectives of the survey. Deciding on the content of survey questions requires operationalizing the problems the survey is expected to address. This can be done by listing topic areas, or variables, that must be covered in an interview and/or ideas about the relationships among variables. Once these variables have been defined, decisions can be made about how they will be measured. The basic steps are listed in the following checklist.

Checklist for Determining Question Content

✓ **List the survey objectives.**

✓ **Conceptualize the components of each objective by listing relevant topics.**

✓ **Frame questions for each topic.**

Example 2.8 illustrates how the surveyor goes about capturing the survey objectives in the questions.

EXAMPLE 2.8
Operationalizing the Survey Problem

A survey has the following objective: To assess satisfaction among participants of a perinatal outreach program for low-income women in Los Angeles County.

The surveyor first operationalizes satisfaction by listing relevant topics:

1. Levels of satisfaction with specific program services

2. Reasons for dissatisfaction with program services

3. Perceived impact of program services on quality of life

4. Suggestions for program improvement

Then the questions are developed to measure satisfaction:

1. The first question set asks about satisfaction with each program service (referrals to prenatal care, transportation to prenatal visits, baby-sitting during prenatal visits, and housing assistance) is developed. The respondent is asked if she needed each service, and if so, whether the service was provided by the program. If yes, she is asked how satisfied she was with the service, using a scale from extremely satisfied to extremely dissatisfied.

2. The next set of questions refers the respondent back to every service with which she said she was dissatisfied. She is then asked why she was dissatisfied. No response options are offered because the surveyor does not want to influence what might be said. Possible responses are anticipated, however, and listed for easy check-off by the interviewer. Space for unanticipated responses is also provided.

3. Because the surveyor conceptualizes satisfaction to include a sense that quality of life has been improved by program participation, a third set of questions is developed asking whether program participation improved the respondent's quality of life. For purposes of this survey, quality of life is defined as: lowered daily stress level, improved sense of overall well-being, improved sense of personal health, and increased expectation of a healthy delivery. The respondent is asked to what degree program participation improved her quality of life in each area (very much to not at all).

4. The questionnaire ends with an open-ended question (one without possible answers for the respondent to choose from) asking for suggestions for program improvement.

Items for a survey may be written entirely from scratch, or items shown to collect valid data may be borrowed from other surveys. For example, the surveyor in Example 2.8 may postulate (form a hypothesis) that there is a relationship between depression levels among respondents and satisfaction with services. Depression may be common in this population of socially disadvantaged women. It may be a barrier to meaningful program participation and thus cause a respondent to be more likely to be dissatisfied. A known depression scale could be found in the literature and used in the survey to distinguish "depressed" from "nondepressed" respondents. (Some wording of items might need to be adapted to the target population.) In the analysis, the satisfaction level of depressed versus nondepressed respondents could be compared to see if there is a difference. If there is, a program modification could be planned to address this need, perhaps by adding social workers or psychologists to the outreach team.

To write the questions described in Example 2.8, the surveyor must take into account the characteristics, such as age and education level, of the respondents. In the example, respondents are to be asked whether program participation improved their overall sense of well-being. The women in the target group have low incomes, low expected levels of education, and possibly poor English-language skills because of the large Hispanic population in Los Angeles County. A question such as "How much did participation in this program improve your overall sense of well-being?" might not be very meaningful to these respondents. A more appropriate question might read as follows:

"Since this program has been helping you, have you been
   feeling better in your everyday life?"
IF YES, "Would you say you are feeling a lot, some, or a little
   better than before you found the program?"

Putting the question into simpler language better communicates the intent of the surveyor and is more consistent with the education and language-skill levels of the population.

WORDING

Wording questions is not as simple a task as it might seem. Stanley Payne (1951), in his classic book *The Art of Asking Questions,* enumerates 100 different factors that affect the form and content of each question appearing on the survey questionnaire. The survey problem and its theoretical or practical rationale, of course, should be the prominent factor in determining the questions that will be asked and the form that each question will take. Each question represents an "operationalization" of some component of the survey problem and a measurement, or quantifiable assessment, of that component. Thus, the question must be structured in a neutral fashion so that the respondent is not predisposed to a certain answer pattern. It must be justifiable in terms of its relation to previous and subsequent questions.

All questions must mean the same to both the respondent and the surveyor (Frey, 1989). This is a difficult task to accomplish.

The use of a **questionnaire map,** or explicit review of the justification for each question, which is covered in interviewer training, helps the interviewer understand the question and consequently communicate properly with the respondent. Pretests will help determine if respondents generally understand the question. There are several criteria to apply when selecting questions and their subsequent wording:

- The topic of each question is relevant to the research goal.
- The comprehensibility of the question has been established at a level consistent with the characteristics of the population.

- The question is consistent with previous and subsequent questions. Transition facilitates this connection.
- The question phrasing is neutral.
- The question pertains to only one concept or issue.
- The question is considered a valid measure of the concept of interest.
- Questions produce a minimum of nonsubstantive responses (e.g., "Don't Know" or "No Answer").
- Response categories on closed items are exhaustive and mutually exclusive.
- Pretest responses to the question produce sufficient variation rather than finding all responses in one category, such as "None."
- Interviewers experience no difficulty administering the question.
- Respondents do not have to ask the interviewer to rephrase or repeat the question.
- Coders have no difficulty coding responses for data entry.

There are many excellent discussions of question wording—for example, Payne (1951), Dillman (1978), Oppenheim (1992), and Schuman and Presser (1981). Specific guidelines for formulating survey objectives and determining variables of interest together with the mechanics of question wording, question types, formatting, and use of scales are described in **How to Ask Survey Questions** (Vol. 2 in this series).

Knowledge and behavior questions are the easiest to write because they generally are straightforward. "How often have you attended religious services or events in the past month?" and "Have you heard about the proposal to locate a nuclear waste repository at Yucca Mountain?" are examples. Often, they serve as filter questions, where one response (e.g., not heard of repository) leads to a sequence of questions that is different from the sequence asked of those who have heard of the repository.

The most difficult questions to ask concern attitude; they present the greatest problems with reliability and validity because of their focus on subjective dimensions (e.g., attitudes, beliefs, values, and opinions). Attitude items are indirect measures of these factors and therefore more difficult to construct because these dimensions vary in intensity, primacy, importance, and concern to respondents. Sometimes, respondents' difficulty understanding such questions can be lessened using visual aids, but this is, of course, possible only with in-person surveys.

Guidelines for Question Wording

- Avoid "loaded" questions that suggest to the respondent that one answer is preferable to another.
- Avoid the use of inflammatory words, such as "communist," "racist," or "exploitation."
- Be natural in wording but not folksy. Questions should have a conversational tone, written in much the same way as people talk.
- Avoid the use of slang terms or colloquialisms that may be understood by only a small subset of the population.
- Avoid the use of technical terms or abbreviations that might be misinterpreted. Not everyone knows that AMA stands for the American Medical Association.
- Be specific in the use of terms and concepts (e.g., government —which level? Federal, state, or local?).
- Be specific when using a time period as a referent for recall or a time limit on behavior.

- Make sure that facts contained within the question are accurate. Nothing can make an interviewer look more foolish than to present incorrect information, particularly to a knowledgeable respondent.

- Be careful not to *assume behavior* or *assume knowledge* on the part of the respondent.

- Use correct grammar and sentence structure (e.g., verb tense, no double negatives).

- Avoid double questions where two or more issues are mentioned. Split the question. It is difficult to determine the meaning of a response to a question like "Are you satisfied with the university and the Sociology Department?"

- Response categories should match the dimension addressed in the question. For example, do not list "Yes" and "No" as response categories when you ask for the extent to which respondents agree or disagree.

- Response categories should be mutually exclusive, thus limiting the respondent to one alternative.

- Ask questions about past or present behavior rather than about future behavior. A person's predictions of future behavior are very unreliable.

- Avoid all-inclusive terms, such as "never" or "always."

- Questions should include the response categories of "Don't Know" or "Refuse to Answer," but these are only read to the respondent when appropriate.

- Clearly communicate to respondents just how they are to answer the question. That is, make sure they know how to answer by reading the response in the context of the question. For example, "Do you strongly agree, agree, disagree, or strongly disagree that the benefits of the nuclear repository will outweigh the costs?"

- Avoid list that includes more than five items. Respondents will not be able to recall the list unless it is provided in the form of a visual aid.

- Be as concrete, specific, and simple as possible in phrasing and wording. Write questions for the respondent, not you. Never assume that a respondent is anywhere near as familiar with a topic as you are.
- Prepare a list of neutral probes that interviewers may use with open-ended questions.

Although the questions that are asked in the course of a survey are mainly a function of the survey topic, the interview mode should also be considered in deciding what can be asked and how the questions should be worded. The interview mode plays a major role in determining questioning styles.

Styles of Questioning

The in-person interview makes possible a wide range of questioning styles because of the greater opportunity to probe, to read nonverbal cues, and to use visual aids. The telephone interview places some limitations on question wording because of the inability to use visual cues to assist the respondent in retaining the contents of lengthy and/or complex questions. Respondents must understand questions and choose responses or rank items based on what can be kept in memory after the information is conveyed verbally by the interviewer. The respondent may not be able to remember all details of the question to voice an accurate opinion or may forget the first response option by the time the fourth is read. Also, the telephone interviewer has no ability to use facial expression or body language feedback to determine whether the respondent is following and comprehending and whether the pace of the questioning is appropriate. The overall goal to keep in mind when constructing questions for a telephone interview is to decrease complexity without compromising the depth and detail of the data to the point of meaninglessness.

Whenever possible, it is best to keep questions and response lists short and simple for both kinds of interviews. However, if a complex question is simplified too much, it may generate a large number of "no opinion" responses because the respondent doesn't have enough information to formulate an opinion. Detailed background information may be necessary prior to asking the question. Limiting response categories can be a problem if the options provided do not provide the detail needed for meaningfulness. The in-person interview can deal with these problems by using visual aids. In Example 2.9, lists of response options matching those that the interviewer sees on the questionnaire are handed to the respondent for reference when answering the question.

EXAMPLE 2.9
Visual Aids

Complex Response Options

QUESTION

31. Regarding **physical** activity, compared to others of your age and sex, when you were *(read age group below)*, were you *(read choices)?*

   (Show Flashcard H)

	Much Less Active	Less Active	Average	More Active	Much More Active
Teens and early 20's	1	2	3	4	5
Late 20's and 30's	1	2	3	4	5
40's	1	2	3	4	5
50's	1	2	3	4	5
60's	1	2	3	4	5
70's	1	3	3	4	5

FLASHCARD H

	MUCH LESS ACTIVE	LESS ACTIVE	AVERAGE	MORE ACTIVE	MUCH MORE ACTIVE
TEENS AND EARLY 20'S	1	2	3	4	5
LATE 20'S AND 30'S	1	2	3	4	5
40'S	1	2	3	4	5
50'S	1	2	3	4	5
60'S	1	2	3	4	5
70'S	1	2	3	4	5

SOURCE: From the Kaiser/UCLA Sigmoid Study.

This flashcard allows the respondent to study the list of complex response options without forgetting any of the choices in determining the answer for each relevant age.

Long List of Complex Responses

QUESTION

What is your natural adult hair color?

(Show Flashcard I)

Bright red	1
Red	2
Light blonde	3
Blonde (whole life)	4
Light brown (blonde as child)	5
Light brown (whole life)	6
Medium brown	7
Auburn (dark red-brown)	8
Dark brown/black	9
Jet black	10

FLASHCARD I

BRIGHT RED

RED

LIGHT BLONDE

BLONDE (WHOLE LIFE)

LIGHT BROWN
  (BLONDE AS CHILD)

LIGHT BROWN (WHOLE LIFE)

MEDIUM BROWN

AUBURN (DARK RED-BROWN)

DARK BROWN/BLACK

JET BLACK

SOURCE: From the Kaiser/UCLA Sigmoid Study.

This list not only involves complexity (different shades of hair color at different times of life), it is also rather long. This list would be very difficult to retain in memory if given over the phone but can be reviewed at the respondent's own pace during in-person interviews using a visual aid.

Another way of dealing with complexity is to use a variety of question-writing techniques. The techniques usually involve some method of reducing the complexity either by separating the question into components or by summarizing key components. The question is thereby simplified, and the numbers of response categories required for an individual question are reduced. The telephone interview relies much more heavily on these techniques than does the in-person interview. Techniques discussed here are the split, the funnel, the inverted funnel, the keyword summary, and recall.

SPLIT QUESTION TECHNIQUE

This technique reduces the complexity of a question area. It is similar to what is called the "unfolding" technique. The first question is general; a person may be asked to choose an answer from a list of options. Then, depending on the response to the first question, a clarifying question is asked, as shown in Example 2.10.

EXAMPLE 2.10
Split Question Technique for
Numerous Response Categories

Version Possible With Visual Aid Showing Responses

1. What was the highest level you finished in your education?

6th grade or less	1
Grade school through 6th	2
Some high school	3
Completed high school	4
Some college	5
Completed college (associate degree)	6
Completed college (bachelor's degree)	7
Advanced degree	8

Version Possible for Use in a Telephone Interview

1. What was the highest level you finished in your education?

Grade school	1
High school	2
College	3

IF THE RESPONDENT ANSWERS "COLLEGE"

1a. What is the highest degree you received?

Associate degree	1
Bachelor's degree	2
Master's degree	3
Doctorate	4

The split question technique reduces the number of responses that have to be considered at one time by separating the question so that some responses apply to the first question and some to the second. In this example, instead of listing eight education levels, the question is split so that respondents must only report their highest generic level of education for the first question. If the response is "college," a second question is asked to determine what level of college was completed.

The split question technique can also be used for ranking items. Ranking means putting items in order according to a criterion—for example, most important to least important. In the in-person interview, ranking is easily accomplished by handing the respondent a list of the items to be ranked, as in Example 2.11, or a set of cards showing one item on each card, which can simply be placed in rank order.

EXAMPLE 2.11
Visual Aid to List Response Options
for Priority Choice

QUESTION

Now, thinking about the chance of property damage, injuries, public health problems, and the loss of life, please rank the following hazards in order from most to least threatening to your community today.

HAND CARD TO RESPONDENT.
RECORD RANK ORDER IN RIGHT COLUMN.

Hazard	Ranking
Tornadoes	
Floods	
Earthquakes	
Water pollution	
Nuclear/radiation accident	
Hazardous chemical spill	
Don't know	

SOURCE: From the Kaiser/UCLA Sigmoid Study.

VISUAL AID

RESPONSE CARD

HAZARDS

Tornadoes
Floods
Earthquakes
Water Pollution
Nuclear/Radiation Accident
Hazardous Chemical Spill

Using this visual aid, respondents simply name the responses in the order they consider to be most to least threatening. The interviewer writes the ranking in the appropriate box on the interview form; the first hazard named is ranked 1, the second 2, and so on.

Without a visual aid, ranking is very difficult. However, the split technique reduces the difficulty. The respondent is read each item and asked for a general rating of priority or importance (e.g., very important, somewhat important, not important). The next question asks the respondent to state which item on the list is *most* important, which is second, and which is third, as illustrated in Example 2.12.

EXAMPLE 2.12
Split Question for Ranking

5. When choosing day care for their children, parents consider certain criteria in making a decision. Would you say each of the following criteria is very important, somewhat important, or not important to your own choice of day care for your children?

	Very Important	Somewhat Important	Not Important
Facility location	1	2	3
Cost	1	2	3
Staff training in child development	1	2	3
Hours of operation	1	2	3
Child/caregiver ratio	1	2	3
Lunch program	1	2	3

5a. Of the criteria listed (READ THEM AGAIN), which is the most important to you?

_____

5b. Which is the second most important?

_____

5c. Which is the third most important?

_____

Although not all items are ranked in order with this technique, a sense of the general importance of each item is achieved using a 3-point scale (very important to not important). Then, the top three items are ranked in order, telling the surveyor what is most important to the respondent.

FUNNEL TECHNIQUE

This technique guides the respondent through a complex concept using a series of questions that progressively narrows the field of interest. The series progresses from the general to the specific and usually begins with an open-ended question (one without response options), followed by several closed-ended or forced-choice items (items that provide a list of answers to choose from), as shown in Example 2.13.

EXAMPLE 2.13
Funnel Technique

7. What criteria do you think the media should use in determining what should be made public about the personal lives of political candidates?

_____

_____

_____

7a. If the media suspects that a political candidate has committed a crime, when do you believe the information should be revealed to the public? (READ OPTIONS)

Immediately	1
Not until some evidence has been uncovered	2
Not unless the person is actually proven guilty	3

7b. How much of a candidate's personal life do you believe
the public has a right to know about? Would you say
(READ OPTIONS):

Everything is relevant to the candidate's character
and should therefore be known   1
Limited information relevant to the person's
policies (such as family life, military experience,
education) should be revealed   2
The person's personal life is private and should
not be publicized   3

The first question allows respondents to introduce any
concepts, some of which the surveyor may not have anticipated. Now that the respondents are thinking in the right
context, Questions 7a and 7b focus them on specific aspects
that the surveyor has chosen to emphasize.

INVERTED FUNNEL TECHNIQUE

When a respondent is not expected to be knowledgeable
about a content area or have an articulated opinion on a
topic, the funnel technique may be reversed. Specific questions on components of the larger issue that one is interested in studying are asked first to focus and educate the
respondent. The general question follows. Example 2.14
illustrates this technique.

EXAMPLE 2.14
Inverted Funnel Technique

1. Over the past years, how often would you say you have gambled for money?

   > Not at all
   > 1 - 3 times
   > 4 - 6 times
   > More than 6 times
   > No answer

2. What versions of gambling are legal in your community?

   Nothing is legal
   Specify: _____

3. What is your view of the expanding legalization of many forms of gambling in America today?

   _____

   _____

   _____

This series begins with specific questions to focus the respondent on gambling and then asks a broad question about expanding the legalization of gambling.

KEYWORD SUMMARY

After reading the background information that precedes a question on a complex issue, keywords can be summarized in a brief repeat statement, followed by the question itself. For example, respondents might not be able to render an opinion regarding a proposed new law without first hearing a detailed description of the law and its enforcement. A description of the law (using unbiased terms) followed by a keyword summary can help respondents grasp the issues well enough to state an opinion when subsequently asked "Would you be in favor of the passage of such a law?" Example 2.15 shows how this technique is used to gather respondents' views on a proposed nuclear waste repository.

EXAMPLE 2.15
Keyword Summary

The federal government is making plans to locate a high-level nuclear waste repository on Yucca Mountain, 120 miles northwest of Las Vegas. This waste would be stored in cast-iron containers 1,500 feet below ground, and the repository would be filled within 30 years, at which time the site would be sealed.

Some people in the state of Nevada think that Nevadans should stop fighting the repository and try, instead, to make a deal with the federal government to get as many benefits (e.g., cash for roads, tax rebates) as possible for the state if the site is located there. Others believe that Yucca Mountain is a poor choice and that the waste cannot be stored safely. Thus, the state should continue to resist locating the repository and not compromise its position by making a deal for benefits.

Keyword Summary

OK. Some people support the location of a repository in Nevada in order to get benefits from the federal government; others say it is not safe and the state should continue to resist.

How do you feel? Should the state stop its opposition and make a deal, or should the state continue to resist even if it means the loss of benefits?

> Stop resisting and make a deal
> Continue opposition to repository
> Don't know
> No answer

The detailed background information is necessary because not all respondents will have heard all relevant information through the media. It is too much, however, to keep in mind long enough to answer questions thoughtfully. The keyword summary reminds respondents of the key points to consider when answering the question.

RECALL TECHNIQUES

Special techniques to enhance response accuracy are used when designing questions requiring recall. Two of these are aided recall and bounded recall. The use of visual aids is also discussed.

Aided Recall

The problem of *omission,* or forgetting an event entirely, can be addressed using a form of **aided recall.** For example, recall can be stimulated by presenting a list of events or behaviors and asking if the respondent has taken part. Instead of asking the open-ended question "What leisure activities have you participated in during the past year?", a list of activities is presented, and the respondent is asked to choose all that apply. For a telephone interview, the lists must be short, although several sets can be presented separately. This is not a problem in the in-person interview because lists can simply be handed to the respondent for review to make sure nothing is omitted.

Another technique is to ask respondents to recall a reference point and then guide them through time. One might ask respondents to recall a major event, such as a first job. A career progression across time could then be reconstructed with reference to the first job. Example 2.16 shows how aided recall using a reference point is applied to a question on weight.

EXAMPLE 2.16
Aided Recall Using a Reference Point: Weight at 18 Years of Age

63. Approximately how much did you weigh when you were 18 years old?

_____ pounds

RECORD THIS WEIGHT IN COLUMN B OF AGE/WEIGHT CHART

Prompt: **This is around the age people graduate from high school.**

64a. Until what age did you continue to weigh between
      (plus or minus 10 pounds of the last weight given)?

      RECORD THE AGE AT WHICH RESPONDENT'S
      WEIGHT CHANGED ON THE NEXT LINE, COLUMN
      A, OF THE AGE/WEIGHT CHART. IF RESPONDENT IS
      UNABLE TO GIVE ACCURATE INFORMATION IN
      10-POUND INTERVALS, ACCEPT RESPONDENT'S
      BEST ESTIMATE.

64b. How much did you weigh when you were
      (age last entered in the chart)?

      CONTINUE TO ASK Q64 UNTIL YOU HAVE
      REACHED RESPONDENT'S CURRENT AGE AND
      WEIGHT. IF RESPONDENT IS A FEMALE, DO *NOT*
      RECORD WEIGHT CHANGES DUE TO PREGNANCY
      BUT DO RECORD A WEIGHT CHANGE THAT IS
      MAINTAINED 6 MONTHS AFTER DELIVERY.

65.   **AGE/WEIGHT CHART**

                   A   B

AGE	WEIGHT
1. 18	
2.	
3.	
4.	
5.	
6.	
7.	
8.	
9.	
10.	

Another problem of recall questions, **telescoping,** or the tendency to report an event as having taken place more recently than it actually did, can be lessened if responses can be verified with a record. For example, a respondent might consult a weekly planner to verify the actual date of the last home-owner's association meeting attended. Depending on the record required, this can be very hard to do over the telephone, although a letter sent in advance could instruct the respondent to have a particular record available at the time of the interview. During the in-person interview, the interviewer can wait while documents are located and can even help interpret them.

Another approach is to use **landmark events** as a reference. For example, a respondent could be asked if a behavior occurred before or after the last election. Holidays and celebrations, major disasters, noteworthy international events like the Olympics, and high-profile media publicity of events like the O. J. Simpson trial are examples of landmark occurrences that can serve as adequate time referents because they are generally known to everyone. The in-person interviewer can use a calendar or timeline showing landmark events to visually assist a respondent in reconstructing the timing of events.

Bounded Recall

If sufficient funds are available, a technique called **bounded recall** can be used. Here, two interviews are conducted where questions in the second interview are phrased in reference to the time elapsed since the first interview. That is, during the second interview the surveyor can ask the respondent about certain behaviors/activities (e.g., played golf, absent from work, went to church) that have taken place since the first interview was conducted. This technique is more feasibly used in telephone interviewing because reinterviewing each respondent in person is very costly. Bounded recall can be implemented if a panel study is being conducted and the surveyor wants to prevent what is known as "forward telescoping," or the tendency to include more and earlier events in the time frame specified by the interviewer (see Converse & Presser, 1986).

Visual Aids

The in-person interview can use all of the questioning techniques described in preceding sections, including the use of visual aids. Besides helping respondents cope with complex or long lists of response options and questions requiring recall, visual aids can also help respondents deal with scales that require estimations, as illustrated in Example 2.17.

EXAMPLE 2.17
Use of Visual Aid for Rating Scale
Requiring a Visual Estimate

QUESTION

I'm going to ask you how *you* feel about various government agencies and institutions. Please tell me how much you trust . . .

	NO TRUST									COMPLETE TRUST
The President 0	1	2	3	4	5	6	7	8	9	10

VISUAL AID

RATING SCALE—TRUST

NO										COMPLETE
TRUST										TRUST
0	1	2	3	4	5	6	7	8	9	10

Using this visual rating scale, respondents estimate the amount of their trust in the President by looking at the scale and specifying a point that corresponds to that amount.

The uses and types of visual aids are virtually limitless. Some of the more common ones (including those previously described) are the following:

- List of response options (if complex or numerous)
- List of items to aid recall
- Rating scale requiring a visual estimate
- Information summary relevant to forming opinions for a question or question sequence
- Lists of information to educate the respondent
- Lists from which to make priority choices
- Photographs (e.g., pictures of medications) to aid recall
- Cards containing one item each for ranking
- Calendars to aid recall of timing of events
- Maps to clarify geographic relationships

Many other kinds of visual aids may be developed. Their design is part of the task of question writing. The next task is the organization of those questions.

Organization and Format

Once the questions and any visual aids have been developed, they must be organized into a questionnaire. Organization refers not only to the order in which the questions are presented but also the instructional guidelines for the interviewer and coder that hold all of the parts of the questionnaire together. The task of organizing the interview questions should be guided by two primary criteria: "flow" of the questionnaire and the potential question order effects. The transition from question to question and from question group to question group needs to consider the expectations and tasks of the interviewer, the respondent, and the data-entry person. Minimizing the effect of question order on response patterns requires careful consideration of how a respondent's exposure to one question might influence how a subsequent question is answered.

The following guidelines are helpful in maintaining the conversational flow of the interview while also providing clarity and logic for the respondent and the coder. Smooth question sequencing makes both the respondent's and the interviewer's task easier; disorganized interviewing increases error from inaccurate responses and results in lower response rates.

Guidelines for Questionnaire Flow

- Use a smooth conversational tone in all portions of the interview that are read to the respondent. This includes instructions, probes, and prompts.

- Set up the page so that interviewer instructions and coding guidelines are clearly distinguishable from the portions to be read aloud to the respondent; this may be accomplished using different fonts, typefaces, and graphics, such as instruction boxes. One of the best ways to distinguish instructions from questions is to put the instructions to interviewers in CAPS.

- Use directions and arrows to guide the interviewer through the form.

- Avoid organizing items in a way that requires the interviewer to page back and forth in the questionnaire; if reference to previous information needs to be made, repeat it.

The questionnaire items shown in Example 2.18 illustrate interviewer instructions that enhance flow.

EXAMPLE 2.18
Instructions to Enhance Flow

1. FIRST, I'D LIKE TO START BY ASKING YOU SOME GENERAL QUESTIONS ABOUT YOURSLF.

   What is your date of birth?

   _____ / _____ / _____
   Month   Day   Year

(Compute current age here: _____ years; also code age on p. 27)

2. What is your current marital status?

   Married 1

   Widowed . . . . 2 → SKIP TO Q4

   Separated or divorced . . . . 3 → SKIP TO Q4

   Never married . . . . 4 → SKIP TO Q4

3. Do you live with your wife/husband?

   Yes . . . . 1 → SKIP TO Q6

   No 2

4. Do you live alone?

   Yes . . . . 1 → SKIP TO Q6

   No 2

5. Do you live with other family members or with someone else?

   *(Circle only one; if respondent lives with other family members, circle 1 even if respondent **also** lives with someone else)*

   With other family members 1

   With someone else 2

6. NOW I WOULD LIKE TO LEARN MORE ABOUT MEMBERS OF YOUR FAMILY.

   (Go to the SUPPLEMENT for the questions to use with this section)

These instructions represent conventions to be used throughout this particular survey to tell the interviewer how to proceed.

SOURCE: From the Kaiser/UCLA Sigmoid Study.

In this example, transition statements (statements that introduce and separate sections) are given in capital letters, instructions to the interviewer are in italics, and skip patterns are designated with arrows followed by the number of the question to which the interviewer should skip. Although these conventions apply only to this particular questionnaire, every interview questionnaire should adopt standardized conventions to keep the interviewer from getting lost on the page or reading something aloud that is not intended for the respondent.

All of the anticipated answers already have a code assigned (in Question 2, married is coded 1, widowed is coded 2, etc.), making the task of recording responses very straightforward: The number of the answer given is simply circled. The coder then has no problem transferring responses to the database because they are already coded. Any time that responses could be coded in a variety of ways (as for open-ended questions), standardized coding instructions to the interviewer should be printed on the form to make coding, and therefore data entry, as clear as possible. Example 2.19 illustrates other forms of interviewer instructions.

EXAMPLE 2.19
Interviewer Instructions

Transit Survey

Hello. This is _____ calling from the Center for Survey Research at the University of Nevada, Las Vegas. We are conducting an opinion survey of Clark County residents about public transportation in the area. Your phone number was selected at random, and we do not need your name and address. All of your responses will be confidential, and the questions

I need to ask will take only a few minutes. OK? Before we continue, I need to know if you are 17 years of age or older.

IF YES, ASK: "What is your age?" _____ years. (CONTINUE INTERVIEW)

IF NO, ASK: "Is there anyone 17 years of age or older with whom we may talk?"

IF YES, REPEAT INTRODUCTION AND CONTINUE INTERVIEW.

IF NO, TERMINATE INTERVIEW: "Thank you. We need to talk with persons 17 years of age or older."

Baseline Survey for High-Level Nuclear Waste Repository Risks

INTRODUCTION: PART I

Hello, my name is _____. We're conducting a study of energy and the environmental issues. I'm calling from the JHF Corporation, a national survey research firm. As part of the study, I'd like to interview the male decision maker in the household over 18 years of age.

1. Would that be you?

Yes   1   → GO TO INTRODUCTION, PART II

No   2

↓

1a. May I speak with him now?

Yes   1   → REPEAT INTRODUCTION, PART I AND GO TO INTRODUCTION, PART II

No   2

INTRODUCTION: PART II

We're interested in learning your attitudes and opinions on issues about energy and the environment. You may choose not to answer a question or simply say "don't know" if that's appropriate. In all cases, your answers will be kept strictly confidential. (READ, IF NECESSARY: Because we have scientifically chosen the telephone numbers, your cooperation is especially important.)

A unique formatting challenge occurs when several household members need to be interviewed in the same survey. It would be cumbersome and wasteful to fill out a separate interview booklet on each household member. Instead, a format can be devised where the questions are on one side of the interview booklet and the answer columns on the facing side. Each answer column is labeled for the responses of one of the household members. Thus the responses of all household members are contained in one packet (see Example 2.20).

EXAMPLE 2.20
Multicolumn Format for Interviewing
Multiple Household Members

QUESTIONS (Page 1)	HOUSEHOLD MEMBERS (Page 2)			
	Respondent 1 (R1) Birth Date __ / __ / __	Respondent 2 Birth Date __ / __ / __ Relationship to R1:	Respondent 3 Birth Date __ / __ / __ Relationship to R1:	Respondent 4 Birth Date __ / __ / __ Relationship to R1:
1. Have you ever smoked cigarettes?	Y.....1 N.....2	Y.....1 N.....2	Y.....1 N.....2	Y.....1 N.....2
2. Have you ever smoked cigars?	Y.....1 N.....2	Y.....1 N.....2	Y.....1 N.....2	Y.....1 N.....2

The birth date of each respondent in the household is listed as an identifier in the response column. All answers given by that respondent are recorded in the same column. A great deal of paper is saved using this strategy.

Question Order

Formatting questions and instructions is one challenge; the order of placement of questions is another. Whether it is to be administered by telephone or in person, the first items in the questionnaire must maintain respondent interest and make responding easy. The questions should usually be related to the topic of the interview as expressed in the introductory statement. This means that background or demographic factors, such as age, income, or marital status, are not the first questions. When the questions flow logically from the introduction respondents are drawn into the interview rather than being distracted and perhaps annoyed by questions they consider irrelevant (but which the surveyor may need answered at some point for statistical purposes). A smooth start also sets the tone for the rest of the interview, establishing a "rapport effect" that builds trust and enhances willingness to participate fully in the interview. The first questions should be easy to understand and nonthreatening.

Once respondents have been drawn into the interview, complex or difficult-to-answer questions may be introduced. These should be asked before respondent fatigue becomes an issue, as responses will be less careful and likely less accurate if respondents are weary of the process. Easy-to-answer items, such as demographics, should be placed at the end of the interview. Such questions are least likely to be affected by fatigue, and because they are personal in nature are best answered after significant rapport has been established. The order of questions intended to reconstruct a history, such as a job history, should be chronological, either forward or backward, to assist respondent recall.

When ordering questions for optimal flow, one must consider the possibility of **question order effects,** or situations in which responses to certain questions may consciously or unconsciously influence how a respondent answers later items. This is a significant source of response error. Although not always easy to anticipate or avoid, three such effects are common: consistency, fatigue, and redundancy.

CONSISTENCY EFFECT

This effect occurs when a respondent feels that responses to an item must be brought into consistency with responses to earlier items. This might occur, for example, if questions about the personal life and character of a presidential candidate precede questions about competence for office. The respondent might feel that judgment about competence should be consistent with the responses given on the character questions. This context might not be present had the competence questions been asked first. The respondent might then have focused on intellectual competence, for example. The effect can be far more subtle than in this example and should always be kept in mind when ordering questions.

Dispersing items so they are farther apart in the questionnaire probably does not reduce the consistency effect much. One must use intuition and logic in deciding which sets of questions might influence responses to others.

FATIGUE EFFECT

This effect occurs if the respondent begins to grow weary or bored over the course of the interview. At the beginning, much thought may be given to answering informatively, but later, the respondent may begin to give incomplete answers or choose to omit difficult questions. Fatigue can set in after several related questions. It is useful to use transitions and variations of question or response form to recapture the respondent's attention. It also helps to put easy-to-answer questions at the end.

REDUNDANCY EFFECT

Respondents may not answer a question carefully, if at all, when it seems to repeat a previous question. When items are similar but distinct in the mind of the surveyor, differences need to be clearly pointed out. For example, questions regarding smoking history may begin with something general, such as "Have you ever smoked cigarettes?" A later question, designed in the mind of the surveyor to distinguish current smokers from past smokers, may read "Do you smoke cigarettes?" A respondent may not recognize the difference in meaning just from the context, especially if the second question does not immediately follow the first. The questions might be more clearly worded this way: "Have you **ever** smoked cigarettes (any time in your life)?" and "Do you **currently** (in the past 6 months) smoke cigarettes?"

Response Order

An issue similar to question order is the effect of **response** order on answers chosen by respondents. Response order is of greater concern with telephone interviews than with in-person ones. The answer given by the respondent can have more to do with the order of the options than their content. It is again the inability to use visual aids with lists of printed response options that makes this more of a concern in the telephone interview.

There are three sources of response order bias:

- Memory errors—The respondent loses track of all of the options and picks one that comes to mind easily rather than the most accurate one.

- "Primary" or "recency" effect—The tendency of the respondent to choose the first or last response regardless of content; this occurs with long lists and with rating scales (e.g., agree/disagree).
- Respondents' tendency with lists followed by rating scales (e.g., excellent/fair; approve/disapprove) to acquiesce or agree with the items regardless of their true feelings.

The latter phenomenon is referred to as **response set,** or the tendency to reply to attitude scale questions in the same manner regardless of the content of the question. For example, in a matrix question where respondents are asked to indicate the extent to which they agree or disagree with a series of statements, they tend to answer all consistently (e.g., "agree") without considering the content of each item or treating each item as an independent question.

It is advisable, especially for telephone interviews, to limit the number of response categories to four or five and to read them as part of the question to maintain continuity and a conversational tone. Lists with rating scales should be kept short (six or seven items) to reduce the likelihood of response set. When visual aids are used, longer lists can be tolerated better because it is easier to probe to make sure the respondent considered all the categories.

Question Grouping

For smooth reading and easy comprehension, questions should be grouped by topic, allowing the respondent to recognize relationships among questions. For example, questions about smoking behaviors should be grouped together, and questions about health problems should be grouped separately.

Although other groupings might seem logical to the surveyor who has analysis purposes in mind (a smoking question followed by a question about a health problem thought to be related to smoking), such groupings might seem illogical and confusing to the respondent and could have effects on response accuracy. It is better to group questions according to topic and reorder them later for analysis purposes.

When moving from one group of questions to the next, flow is maintained by the use of **transition statements.** These alert the respondent that a topic change is occurring and that the next set of questions is not dependent on the previous set. A good transition statement identifies the change of context for the respondent by giving information about the next set of questions. This information can reflect a change in the following:

- *Response pattern* (e.g., "Okay, the next set of questions has different possible answers from the one we just finished. Please answer the next set of questions with a simple yes or no.")
- *Conceptual level* (e.g., "The previous questions asked about what you know about gun control laws. Now I'd like to ask some questions about your **feelings** toward these laws.")
- *Level of complexity* (e.g., "Now that we have discussed these general issues, I'd like to ask you some more detailed questions on some specific topics.")

The statement may simply tell the respondent what topic the interviewer is going to address next. These statements should be used freely throughout the questionnaire to give the respondent a sense of movement through the interview and to provide an overall coherence among its parts. Example 2.21 shows the use of transition statements throughout an interview. Note that the statements are capitalized to catch the interviewer's attention.

EXAMPLE 2.21
Set of Transition Statements
Used in an Interview

1. FIRST, I'D LIKE TO START BY ASKING YOU SOME GENERAL QUESTIONS ABOUT YOURSELF.

2. NOW I WOULD LIKE TO LEARN MORE ABOUT MEMBERS OF YOUR FAMILY.

3. NOW I AM GOING TO ASK YOU SOME QUESTIONS ABOUT THE NONPRESCRIPTION MEDICATIONS THAT YOU MAY HAVE USED DURING THE PAST YEAR.

4. NEXT I WOULD LIKE TO ASK YOU SOME QUESTIONS ABOUT YOUR RECENT LEVEL OF PHYSICAL ACTIVITY, AND THEN I WILL ASK YOU SOME QUESTIONS ABOUT YOUR ACTIVITY 10 YEARS AGO.

5. NOW I WOULD LIKE TO ASK YOU SOME QUESTIONS ABOUT HOW OFTEN YOU ARE EXPOSED TO THE SUN AND HOW SENSITIVE YOUR SKIN IS TO SUN EXPOSURE.

6. NOW I AM GOING TO ASK YOU SOME QUESTIONS ABOUT YOUR TYPICAL EATING HABITS IN THE PAST YEAR.

7. NOW I AM GOING TO ASK YOU SOME QUESTIONS ABOUT SMOKING.

8. NOW I WOULD LIKE TO ASK YOU A FEW QUESTIONS ABOUT YOUR CURRENT AND PAST WEIGHT. THESE QUESTIONS ARE AN IMPORTANT PART OF THIS STUDY, SO PLEASE TRY TO ANSWER AS ACCURATELY AS YOU CAN.

9. WE ARE ALMOST FINISHED WITH THE INTERVIEW. I JUST HAVE A FEW STATISTICAL QUESTIONS THAT ARE USED TO GROUP YOUR ANSWERS WITH THOSE OF OTHER PEOPLE WHO ARE BEING INTERVIEWED.

10. THIS COMPLETES OUR INTERVIEW. THANK YOU FOR TAKING THE TIME TO ANSWER THESE QUESTIONS. DO YOU HAVE ANY COMMENTS YOU WOULD LIKE TO ADD?

Summary Guidelines

The following guidelines summarize some of the points about questionnaire construction made throughout this chapter.

Formatting Questions

- The needs of the interviewer, respondent, and coder should be considered in formatting questions.
- Treat all questions as part of a whole, not isolated or separate from other items.
- Arrange items and instructions for maximum readability by the interviewer. Do not break questions between pages. Provide adequate spacing in the text. Ensure that the interviewer does not have to page back and forth during questionnaire administration.
- Use different typefaces, graphics, and spacing to clearly distinguish questions from response categories and from instructions.
- Vary response patterns and group topics as often as practical. Response set and fatigue can affect responses after six or more items of similar interest or form.
- Get input from interviewers and coders on questionnaire design.
- Precode questions whenever possible.

Ordering Questions

- Reflect the focus of the research in the first question, as stated in the introduction to the interview. Choose easy items to start.

- Place any complex, difficult, or sensitive questions after rapport has been established but before respondent fatigue might set in.

- Place easy-to-answer questions, such as demographics, at the end of the interview to minimize inadequate responses due to respondent fatigue.

- Order questions in a logical way that makes sense to the respondent.

- Consider question order effects when arranging items. For the same topic, order items from general to specific, unless respondents are expected to be unknowledgeable about the subject matter. Consider using funneling techniques.

Grouping Questions

- Group questions according to topic. Arrange the groupings in an order that makes sense to the respondent.

- Use transition statements freely.

Pretests

The final step in preparing a questionnaire is to pretest it to determine if the parts of the questionnaire do not flow well and if there are unclear questions that need to be rewritten. Once the instrument is refined and finalized, the rest of the job of quality data collection is up to the interviewer.

Not only should pretesting be conducted on members of the relevant population, the instrument should also be pretested on interviewers and coders. These individuals can provide valuable feedback on the mechanics of the administration of the interview schedule, particularly on the quality of question flow, the accuracy and adequacy of instructions, the procedure for recording responses, the quality of the introduction, and the wording of questions. These individuals have a good idea of which question order and format will work or not work by virtue of their experience.

Pretests also give the surveyor a chance to experiment with sampling procedures, particularly the technique that will be used to select a member of a household. Of course, pretests provide an excellent training opportunity for all personnel involved in the survey.

One caveat is necessary here: It is possible to pretest too much. That is, seeking advice from others can be counterproductive, particularly when these individuals want to add some questions on their favorite topic or provide a very, very detailed critique. Because designing survey questionnaires is somewhat of an art, the perfect questionnaire will never exist, and all the pretests and consulting in the world will not produce perfection. Pretests are necessary, but sometime the line must be drawn and the questionnaire put into the field.

3 Interviewer Selection and Training

A well-designed questionnaire alone does not ensure valid data gathering for an interview survey. Interviewers who possess the right combination of abilities, knowledge, and skills must administer the questionnaire for optimal results. Data quality can be compromised by biased questioning styles, improper clarification techniques, inaccurate recording of responses, asking questions out of sequence or skipping questions, or failing to establish proper rapport with the respondent. As stated earlier, poor interviewing can compromise the quality of the best-designed questionnaire. A good interviewer uses unbiased questioning techniques, proper clarifications, and correct question order and establishes rapport with the respondent. Good interviewing is the result of quality training combined with an interviewer's natural abilities.

Roles

A skilled interviewer enhances the collection of reliable and valid data through artful application of standardized interviewing procedures. Successful interviewers use these procedures to perform three major roles:

- Maximize the number of completed interviews by keeping refusals and early terminations of interviews to a minimum
- Motivate respondents to participate thoughtfully by delivering the introductory statement, answering respondent questions, and engaging the respondent in the interview process
- Administer the questionnaire by asking questions, recording answers, and probing incomplete responses

To perform these roles well, interviewers must possess a combination of specific abilities, knowledge, and skills.

ABILITIES

Abilities are those underlying capacities that an interviewer must have to perform the basic tasks of the job without special training. An interviewer must, for example, be able to read and comprehend the interview, record the responses, work during hours when respondents can be reached, and, in the case of in-person interviewing, get to the interview site.

Abilities required of interviewers are the following:

- Speak clearly and use correct grammar in the language of the interview

- Read in the language of the interview to deliver written statements and question sequences without pauses and to understand written instructions

- Write in the language of the interview to record verbatim responses accurately with proper spelling

- Recall responses long enough to record them accurately

- Perform several tasks simultaneously: read questions, record answers, and follow instructions

- Work flexible hours, usually including evenings and weekends

- Travel to the interview site if conducting interviews in person

- Access a telephone for interviewing, unless the survey project has a central calling unit

- Participate in one or more formal training sessions to acquire specific knowledge and skills required for performing interviews

- Judge nonverbal and verbal cues of respondent so as to know when to administer reinforcement and clarification

- Exercise self-discipline and regulate verbal and nonverbal behavior so as not to improperly influence responses

KNOWLEDGE

Knowledge is the body of facts and principles that interviewers must internalize to perform the interview well. The requisite knowledge can be taught during formal training sessions, but above all, interviewers must understand that the interviewing role is a neutral one: The interviewer's task is to obtain information that is as truthful and accurate as possible. In other words, the interviewer should not be a source of error or inaccuracy.

Knowledge required by interviewers encompasses the following:

- Role of the interviewer in conducting surveys
- Understanding why maintaining neutrality is important during an interview
- Information about the survey project sufficient to answer respondent questions
- Objectives of the survey
- Techniques of minimizing refusal rates
- Principle of confidentiality as the most important means of protecting the identity of the respondent and the integrity of the data-collection enterprise
- Procedures for contacting respondents and introducing the survey
- Correct procedures for asking questions
- Techniques of probing during an interview
- Procedures for recording answers
- Rules for handling interpersonal aspects of the interview
- Administrative procedures related to project operation, such as filling out call sheets, mileage logs, reimbursement forms, and time sheets

SKILLS

Skills are capabilities to do specific tasks well. These capabilities may arise from talent, practice, or training (usually a combination thereof). A skilled interviewer *does* the tasks of the job well. A note of caution: Persons with telemarketing experience do not always make the best interviewers. They may have the skill to get a respondent to commit to the interview, but they often move through the questionnaire at an uncomfortable pace, skip questions, and treat respondents in a less than respectful manner. These persons need the training sessions despite their experience.

Skills required of interviewers are the following:

- Initiate and maintain a conversation with a stranger
- Respond professionally to unexpected questions and situations
- Remain neutral by keeping personal opinions out of the interview process
- Motivate reluctant respondents to participate in the interview
- Deliver the questionnaire in a flowing, conversational manner
- Probe incomplete responses in an unbiased manner for more useful results

Selection Process

Interviewing is a difficult job. Selecting interviewers for a particular survey involves recruiting applicants, evaluating their qualifications for becoming good interviewers (reviewing resumés and conducting job interviews), and offering positions to the most qualified candidates. A small survey with few resources may choose from among existing staff at the organization conducting the survey; a larger operation may formally recruit candidates from outside. In either case, it is important to select interviewers with the most promising characteristics and abilities because, as stated previously, not everyone has the potential to be a good interviewer.

Interviewer characteristics, such as gender, race, or age, apparently have no consistent effects on response. Nor is experience a factor in producing differential response rates. The voice of the telephone interviewer would seem crucial, but little is known about the impact of voice quality except that interviewers with slightly louder tones and the ability to pronounce distinctly have better response rates. An interviewer's personal appearance is more of a factor in interviews conducted in person, but just how much of an effect personal characteristics have on response rate is not known. There is some support for the practice of recruiting interviewers with the same characteristics as those of the population to be surveyed.

One factor that does seem to affect response rate is the expectation that an interviewer has of obtaining a completed questionnaire or being able to get a response to a difficult question or question sequence. Also, the higher the workload, the lower the response rates. Thus, allocating the workload in a reasonable and fair manner among interviewers who are optimistic about the prospect of obtaining responses should result in higher rates of completion for both telephone and in-person interviews.

JOB DESCRIPTION

The first step in identifying potential interviewers is to develop a **job description.** It describes the tasks and duties that an interviewer must perform on a specific survey project and lists the abilities, knowledge, and skills required to execute those tasks and duties. How detailed the job description is varies with the survey project. In general, a good job description contains four key sections:

> *Summary statement:* Brief description of the purpose of the survey and the role of the interviewer
>
> *Description of supervision provided:* How performance will be monitored and evaluated and what level of independence is expected

Duties and tasks: List of the components of the work the interviewer will be assigned (e.g., calling or visiting respondents, administering questionnaires, filling out forms)

Abilities, knowledge, and skills: List of the qualifications in specific terms of what a good interviewer must know and be able to do; the job description must specify which of these are required at the outset and which can be trained after hire

A sample job description is shown in Example 3.1.

EXAMPLE 3.1
Sample Job Description

Summary Statement
The Epilepsy Foundation of America® requires interviewers to administer a telephone survey of client quality of life. The survey will be administered under the auspices of selected Epilepsy Foundation affiliates to evaluate the effectiveness of a new quality-of-life assessment methodology. Affiliates will use this methodology to determine their effectiveness in improving the quality of life of their client populations and to assess continuing client needs.

Supervision
Under general supervision of an outside survey development team, interviewers will obtain questionnaire responses from selected clients by telephone. The survey team will train interviewers, monitor and evaluate completed interviews for accuracy and completeness, and provide feedback as necessary.

Duties and Tasks	Interviewer duties and tasks will include calling selected clients by telephone to enlist their cooperation in the survey and administering a structured questionnaire over the telephone, recording responses, and editing completed questionnaires for errors before submission to the survey team.
Abilities, Knowledge, and Skills	Interviewers must have good reading, writing, and speaking abilities to read questionnaire items according to skip patterns and record responses in English. They must also be available to conduct interviews during evening and weekend hours and to attend two half-day training sessions. Skills for maintaining confidentiality, administering questionnaires, and enlisting client cooperation will be trained.

The job description tells prospective interviewers what to expect of the job and what is expected of them if hired. It is used to advertise the availability of positions and recruit applicants. The required abilities, knowledge, and skills are matched to those listed on resumés in the process of screening applicants for job interviews. These qualifications are also used to formulate interview questions about an applicant's suitability for the job. Even if interviewers are being chosen from existing staff at an organization implementing its own survey, candidates should be screened and interviewed.

The best interviewers are those who have a certain intuition or talent for dealing with people in an engaging but professional manner. Intuition and talent are not measurable qualities. They will surface as trained interviewers begin testing their skills in practice sessions and on the job. Talented interviewers will likely stay on the job, whereas those lacking intuition will likely find the job unrewarding and drop out, although occasionally they may need to be removed from the job or reassigned to other tasks.

Training

Once interviewers have been selected and have accepted job offers, they must be trained. The depth and detail of the training materials will vary with the survey project. Training procedures will usually contain some combination of the following:

- Training Manual

  The training manual is an important document both for teaching interviewers how to do their jobs and as a reference on the job. The manual provides context for the interviewer, describes the interviewer's obligations, and outlines interviewing techniques. The next section of this chapter is devoted to a detailed discussion of the contents of the training manual.

- Lectures, Presentations, and Discussions

  Whenever possible, training procedures should include formal training sessions. During such sessions, the material in the training manual is presented orally by a trainer experienced in survey work and interviewing. Important skills and a model interview are demonstrated. A later section of this chapter focuses on the purpose and content of the training session.

- Practice

  The training sessions should provide trainees with ample opportunities for supervised practice. After seeing an interview demonstrated, trainees take turns role-playing the parts of both the interviewer and the respondent. Trainees also interview the trainer, who can ad lib difficult or unusual responses. The trainer observes the role-playing and gives direct feedback to trainees. If available, volunteer respondents (e.g., other survey staff members) may be brought in for trainees to interview after practicing among themselves. Trainees should be encouraged to perform as many simulated interviews (on friends, relatives, neighbors) as they can to become familiar with the interview. If the survey will be done by telephone, each trainee may be given an assignment to call the trainer on the telephone during the next week or two to conduct a mock interview. This gives the trainee the opportunity to get a sense of interviewing without eye contact and helps the trainer assess how the trainee comes across on the telephone. A mock in-person interview can also be set up for training and/or testing purposes.

- Observation

    If a new group of interviewers is being trained for an ongoing project, observation of veteran interviewers on the job can be useful for training. Listening in on telephone interviews is easily accomplished. Accompanying an interviewer on an in-person interview is also possible with the respondent's permission; however, survey administrators must weigh the possibility that the trainee's presence will influence the respondent's answers against the long-term advantages of well-trained interviewers. An alternative approach might be to have trainees listen to tape recordings of interviews.

Training Manual

Although many of the instructions given to interviewers are very similar from survey to survey, details and context will vary. Most surveys will require the development of a project-specific training manual. General topics to cover in a training manual are outlined in the following sample Table of Contents (Example 3.2). Each topic is then discussed briefly.

EXAMPLE 3.2
Sample Table of Contents of
an Interviewer Training Manual

Description of the Survey
Introduction to Survey Methods
Interviewing Techniques and Guidelines
    Preparing for the Interview
    Beginning the Interview
    Asking the Questions
    Probing
    Ending the Interview
The Interviewer's Responsibilities
    Contacting Respondents
    Confidentiality
    How to Use the Interview
    Editing the Interview
Item-by-Item Rationale for Interview Questions
Sample Interview
Forms and Administrative Procedures
    Interview Summary Form
    Control Sheet
    Call Record
    Time Sheets

SOURCE: Adapted from Kaiser/UCLA Sigmoid Study.

Description of the Survey: This section introduces the interviewer to the purpose of the survey in some detail, imparting the greater context within which interviews will be conducted. A description of the target population, sampling procedures used, and objectives of the survey is given. Key individuals, such as survey coordinators and collaborators, are named.

Introduction to Survey Methods: In this section, the basic steps of conducting surveys are outlined, emphasizing the interviewer's place in the process. The steps include data collection, coding, data entry, analysis, and reporting of results. The interviewer plays the key role in data collection and coding. The flow of data through the survey office, from interviewing through computer entry, and the nature of supervision to be provided for the project as a whole are described.

Interviewing Techniques and Guidelines: Statements about the following topics give the interviewer important information about how to conduct interviews.

Preparing for the Interview: Review of any materials and procedures the interviewer may still need practice with should precede the first phone call or field visit. Supplemental materials, such as introductory and fallback statements and visual aids, must be organized in advance for easy access.

Beginning the Interview: The initial stage of the interview conversation is about gaining cooperation. The interviewer and respondent need to establish good rapport at this stage. Cooperation can be gained by convincing the respondent that the survey is important and worthwhile. State the importance of a professional and friendly manner, well-delivered introductory statements, and successful answers to questions for engaging the respondent.

A discussion of the importance of the interviewer's own state of mind is appropriate here. The interviewer's personal conviction that the survey is worthwhile can help motivate respondents to participate. Tell the interviewer that success in engaging respondent interest at this point will minimize refusals, thus improving the chances of collecting unbiased data because more of the people initially chosen to participate contribute their views. Give interviewers suggested responses for dealing with refusal attempts (see Example 3.3).

EXAMPLE 3.3
Possible Responses to Refusal Attempts

Too busy	This should only take a few minutes. Sorry to have caught you at a bad time. I would be happy to call back. When would be a good time to call in the next day or two?
Bad health	I'm sorry to hear that. I would be happy to call back in a day or two. Would that be okay?
Too old	Older person's opinions are just as important in this survey as anyone else's. For the results to be representative, we have to be sure that older people have as much chance to give their opinion as anyone else does. We really want **your** opinion.
Feel inadequate	The questions are not at all difficult. There are no right or wrong answers. We are concerned about how you feel rather than how much you know about certain things. Some of the people we have already interviewed had the same concern you have, but once we got started they didn't have any difficulty answering the questions. Maybe I could read just a few questions to you so you can see what they are like.

Not interested	It's very important that we get the opinions of everyone in the sample. Otherwise, the results won't be very useful. So, I'd really like to talk with you.
No one's business	I can certainly understand. That's why all of our interviews are confidential. Protecting people's privacy is one of our major concerns, so we do not put people's names on the interview forms. All the results are reported in such a way that no individual can be linked with any answer.
Objects to surveys	The questions in this survey are ones that _(client)_ really needs answers to, and we think your opinions are important.
Objects to phone	We are doing this survey by telephone because we can reach a lot more people for a lot less cost.

Asking the Questions: Explain the importance of maintaining a neutral attitude when conducting interviews. A neutral manner is one that does not imply criticism, surprise, approval, or disapproval of anything the respondent says, or of anything contained in the questionnaire. The point is to refrain from any behaviors that could influence how the respondent answers the questions. Emphasize the need to ask all questions in the order presented and exactly as worded. The purpose of this is **standardization;** the less variation there is in the way interview questions are delivered from one interview to another and from one interviewer to another, the better the chances that answers will be comparable. Each respondent needs to **hear the same question** to ensure comparability of answers.

Tell the interviewer not to read response categories unless they are part of the question or the questionnaire instructs the interviewer to read them. During questionnaire preparation, thought was given to whether or not response options should be offered the respondent, depending on the nature of the question. It is the interviewer's job to make sure that the decisions made in question preparation are carried out to maximize data quality.

Explain the use of prompts if they are included in the questionnaire. Prompts are predetermined statements to be used when respondents seem confused or unclear about how to answer a question. For example, when asked how many cigarettes are smoked in a day, a hesitant respondent might be prompted with "A pack contains 20 cigarettes." Prompts are printed on the questionnaire near the item they support. They are read verbatim.

Probing: Probing is used to obtain more information if a respondent's answer is unclear, irrelevant, or incomplete. Probes may or may not be verbal. Remind the interviewer of the importance of keeping probes neutral, and give some examples (see Example 3.4).

EXAMPLE 3.4
Interview Probes

Show Interest. An expression of interest and understanding, such as "uh-huh," "I see," and "yes," conveys the message that the response has been heard and more is expected.

Pause. Silence can tell a respondent that you are waiting to hear more.

Repeat the Question. This can help a respondent who has not understood, misinterpreted, or strayed from the question to get back on track.

Repeat the Reply. This can stimulate the respondent to say more, or recognize an inaccuracy.

Ask a Neutral Question.

For Clarification:	"What do you mean exactly?"
	"Could you please explain that?"
For Specificity:	"Could you be more specific about that?"
	"Tell me about that. What, who, how, why?"
For Relevance:	"I see. Well, let me ask you again" (REPEAT QUESTION AS WRITTEN).
	"Would you tell me how you mean that?"
For Completeness:	"What else?"
	"Can you think of an example?"

SOURCE: Adapted from the Kaiser/UCLA Sigmiod Study.

Poor probes are those that make interpretations, as illustrated in Example 3.5.

EXAMPLE 3.5
Improper Probing

Question: "About how many hours of television would you say you watch in a 24-hour period?"

Answer: "Oh, I watch TV all day."

Improper Probe: "So you mean about 12 hours?"

Better Probe: "Could you be more specific? About how many **hours** would you say you watch in a 24-hour period?"

The improper probe puts words in the respondent's mouth. It is better to politely request a more specific answer without making any assumptions.

Ending the Interview: Let interviewers know the importance of thanking respondents and reinforcing the important role they have played by participating in the interview. Some time may be spent at this point answering questions the respondents may have and discussing concerns that may have come up regarding the content of the survey. In fact, depending on the content of the questionnaire, a short "debriefing" conversation may be a positive way to end the interview. The interview questions may have raised some emotional concerns for the respondent. For example, parents who have been questioned about their children's exposure to potentially toxic substances may have become fearful that their children are at risk for serious health problems. They may need to be reassured that no causative links between studied exposures and specific diseases are yet known to exist and that none may be found. A source of any information on what *is* known could be given at this time, if appropriate.

The Interviewer's Responsibilities: Tell the interviewer what he or she is expected to know and do.

Contacting Respondents: Give detailed instructions for how respondents are to be contacted. If this is done by telephone, describe when interviewers should make calls (days of the week and time of day), how interviewers will know what telephone numbers to call, and what to do in the case of no answers, busy signals, answering machines, wrong numbers, and unavailable respondents. Instructions might read as shown in Example 3.6.

EXAMPLE 3.6
Instructions for Contacting Respondents

Place calls to each telephone number listed on call sheets until you either reach a respondent or determine that the respondent cannot be reached at this number. Call at different times of the day and on different days of the week. The most productive times to call are weekday evenings after dinner and weekends, except Sunday morning. Time your last call so that it will end by 9 p.m., unless a respondent has asked you to call back late. If you get a busy signal or no answer, call back in 10 to 30 minutes. If you get an answering machine, leave a brief message about why you are calling and state that you will call back at another time. If you get a wrong number, verify that you dialed correctly. If a respondent is unavailable, politely ask when you might call back to catch the person at home. If someone agrees to an interview at a particular time, call back at that time.

If interviews will be done in person, tell the interviewer whether interviews will be conducted "cold" in the field after choosing a household according to a sampling procedure or will be scheduled in advance. If there is a sampling procedure, describe it. Make sure interviewers understand it well enough to implement it in the field. If advance contact is to be made, tell the interviewer how to go about it. For example, appointments may need to be made by telephone. Calls may need to be made at certain times of the day, as mentioned in Example 3.6. In-person interviewers also need to know what to do if no one is at home when they knock on a door—for example, how many times to return to the same household and whether to call to reschedule an appointment. "Stopping by" on the weekend to catch a respondent who previously agreed to an interview and then failed to be home at the appointed time is another option.

Be sure that interviewers understand internal procedures for tracking contact attempts. Tell interviewers how to identify interviews (usually using a numbering system) and how to record the outcome status of each interview. Forms should be prepared for this purpose and should include the time and date of the interview, its length, any problems encountered, and questions that a supervisor might need to answer. The interviewer can give an interpretation of the respondent's attitude toward surveys and reasons why a refusal or termination partway through the interview took place. This information is completed on a separate form but matched to the interview identification number. It is signed by the interviewer, and this document becomes the basis for determining the interviewer's productivity, or the number of completed interviews compared to hours worked. A sample of the summary form that interviewers complete is shown in Example 3.7.

EXAMPLE 3.7
Interview Summary Form

INTERVIEWER: Answer the following questions about the interview.

Interviewer _____ Date _____

Interview Start Time _____ End Time _____ Overtime _____

Which of the following best describes the respondent's attitude:

Very antagonistic	1
Somewhat antagonistic	2
Neutral	3
Somewhat helpful	4
Very helpful	5

How would you describe the respondent's interest in the interview?

Very *un*interested 1

Somewhat *un*interested 2

Neutral 3

Somewhat interested 4

Very interested 5

Did the respondent ask any questions about the survey?

Yes............................ 1

No............................. 2

Specify: _____

_____

ANSWER THE FOLLOWING *ONLY* IF THIS WAS A REFUSAL OR PARTIAL COMPLETION.

When did the respondent end the interview?
(Specify exact place—i.e., question number)

WHERE TERMINATED _____

Which best describes how the interview was terminated?

No warning or explanation 1

An explanation to which you were not given a
chance to respond 2

An explanation to which you *were* able to respond . 3

Please explain the exact situation under which the interview was terminated:

_____

_____

_____

Interviewer: _____
(signature)

Received and edited by: _____

Validation: _____

This form, along with the completed interview schedule, is turned in to someone at the survey center who will, in turn, edit the questionnaire for completeness, clarity in the recording of responses, and the status information. It may be necessary to have the original interviewer recontact the respondent to obtain responses to items that were either overlooked or answered unclearly.

Confidentiality: Devote a section of your training manual to the ethics of survey interviewing. It is extremely important that interviewers understand their ethical responsibility to maintain the confidentiality of the people interviewed. This means not only following protocol regarding not putting names on individual questionnaires but also conducting interviews in private settings and not sharing a person's responses with anyone.

The statements of confidentiality prepared for the introductory remarks of the interview should be reviewed thoroughly, and any internal procedures, such as keeping completed questionnaires in a locked cabinet, should be reviewed. Any identifier information, such as a name, address, or telephone number, should be removed from the completed interview. This is easily accomplished if this information is recorded on a separate cover sheet. Completed interviews should be stored in a secure location for a period of time following the survey until data entry is completed and the data files gleaned of improper codes. The interviews can then be destroyed.

Confidentiality is also protected when interviewers are admonished not to discuss any of the results during or after completion of the survey. Interviewers' assessment of the results of the survey is not representative because they interviewed only a small segment of the sample. As discussed previously, it is rare that the surveyor is not in possession of identifying information on the respondent (e.g., address, name, telephone number), so anonymity can almost never be granted. Thus, it

is more appropriate to state that confdentiality will be protected rather than anonymity.

In all surveys, especially in those funded by government
sources, it is necessary to provide for the conditions of **informed consent.** Informed consent is an absolute "must" if
the respondents are somehow "at risk" by participating in the
research. This is ordinarily not a problem in surveys, but it
could be if extremely sensitive information, such as participation in deviant acts, is questioned or there is a potential
invasion of privacy involved. Government criteria for informed
consent include "what a reasonable person would want to
know" (Frey, 1989, p. 248). The required items are as follows:

- Fair explanation of the procedures to be followed and their
  purpose
- Description of the discomfort or risk that might be experienced
- Description of the benefits that might be expected
- Offer to answer any inquiries concerning the procedure or
  intent of the research
- Instruction that respondents are free to withdraw their consent and to discontinue participation at any time

In telephone surveys, signed informed consent is almost
impossible to obtain unless the consent form can be mailed
and returned prior to commencement of the survey or is sent
to the respondent after completion of the interview. Neither is
done routinely because the respondent's identity is clearly
defined. Thus, a request like "May I proceed?" or "OK?" is
used, assuming the respondent is mature enough to make an
informed decision about participating. Obtaining a signed
consent form is not a problem with in-person surveys because
the interviewer can hand the respondent a form to sign before
the interview begins.

How to Use the Interview: Outline what the conventions in the interview format mean. The interviewer will need repeated exposure to these conventions to become comfortable using them. A set of possible conventions is described in Example 3.8.

EXAMPLE 3.8
Interview Format Conventions

Instructions to the interviewer are in italics. Italicized portions should not be read to the respondent. Skip patterns are identified using arrows followed by the number of the question you should move to next. Prompts are printed in bold face. Read them exactly as printed if the respondent seems unclear about answering the question.

Tell the interviewer how to record information (see Example 3.9).

EXAMPLE 3.9
Instructions for
Recording Information
on the Questionnaire

Write clearly, neatly, and legibly. Write "DK" when the respondent does not know the answer to a question. If you used a probe to get more information on a question, write "probed" in the margin. To record answers to precoded questions, circle the number of the response given. Answers to open-ended questions must be written verbatim. Do not paraphrase.

Editing the Interview: Editing is proofreading the completed questionnaire to find and correct errors, clarify handwriting, and add clarifying notes. Tell interviewers that they are expected to edit every questionnaire before turning it in and that a supervisor or other reviewer will do a second edit. If errors or incomplete sections are found, the interviewer will be asked to make corrections and possibly call the respondent back to fill in missing data.

Tell the interviewer how to record the status of the questionnaire in the process from interview completion through data entry. Many times, questionnaires will have a *control sheet* attached or incorporated into the cover sheet of the questionnaire. When a task is completed, the date of completion is recorded on the control sheet, and the questionnaire is routed to the next step. Example 3.10 illustrates the layout of a control sheet.

EXAMPLE 3.10
Control Sheet

STATUS	DATE	SIGNATURE
Interview Complete	_____	_____
Edit Complete	_____	_____
Corrections Complete	_____	_____
Data Entry Complete	_____	→ FILE

Once the interview is complete, the interviewer dates and signs the first line. When a reviewer has finished editing the questionnaire, the second line is dated and signed, and the questionnaire is routed back to the interviewer for corrections and callbacks, if necessary. On completion of corrections, the interviewer signs again and routes the questionnaire to data entry. Once data are entered, the questionnaire may be filed.

NOTE: Not every training manual will cover all of the described topics. There will be variations of what should be included and in what order depending on the survey, the experience level of the interviewers being trained, and the trainer's preferences. The following are some excerpts from a sample telephone interviewer's manual (Example 3.11).

EXAMPLE 3.11
Sample Training Manual
for Telephone Interviewers

General Interviewing Techniques Guidelines

A. NEUTRAL ROLE OF THE INTERVIEWER

The interviewer is a neutral medium through which questions and answers are transmitted. Therefore:

(1) Avoid interjecting your own opinions.

(2) Avoid being "clever."

(3) Avoid any unnecessary or overly enthusiastic reinforcement, such as "DY-NO-MITE!!"

(4) Be an "active" listener but only give the minimum of reinforcement, such as "OK," "I see," . . . [and] "uh-huh."

(5) Never suggest an answer.

. . . .

C. GENERAL TASKS OF THE INTERVIEWER

(1) Communicate questions accurately.

(2) Maximize the respondent's ability and willingness to answer.

(3) Listen actively to determine what is relevant.

(4) Probe to increase the validity, clarity, and completeness of the response.

Instructions to Interviewers

D. HOW MUCH INFORMATION TO GIVE

(1) Read questions precisely as written.

(2) I repeat, read them precisely as written. It is extremely important that everyone be asked the same question in the same way. Even a difference in one word could drastically change the meaning and thus the response.

(3) Information that you can provide to the respondent is listed below. . . . Do not go beyond this information to interpret questions from the respondent. Key phrases you might use to answer questions are:

"This is all the information available to us."

"We would like you to answer the question in terms of the way it is stated. Could I read it again for you?"

"I'm sorry, I don't have that information."

"I will write on the questionnaire the qualifications to your answer you have just mentioned."

(4) If the respondent still requires more information, call on the operations supervisor for assistance.

. . . .

E. WHOSE OPINION TO ACCEPT

Everything should be in terms of what the RESPONDENT thinks—not the respondent's kids, friends, boss, bartender, etc. Therefore, you might need to say:

"I see. Now, is that what you think?"

"It's your opinion that we really want."

ALSO, DON'T GIVE RESPONDENT YOUR OPINION.

F. RECORD EVERY CALL YOU MAKE, even though the number was not working, no answer was received, or the interview was not completed.

. . . .

K. DO NOT TAKE ANYTHING HOME WITH YOU. All questionnaires, code sheets, instruction sheets, etc. must be left in the survey center.

. . . .

L. AFTER YOU HAVE LEFT THE SURVEY CENTER

We are adamant about the following:

The only way we can be successful is to establish and maintain a reputation for confidentiality. Therefore, please:

(1) Do not tell anyone the names or locations of people you interviewed.

(2) Do not tell anyone the substance of an interview or part of an interview no matter how fascinating or interesting it was. We find it rather disturbing to hear from other faculty members or students details of an interview 2 weeks after a study is completed. Confidentiality is essential!

SOURCE: Excerpted from *Survey Research by Telephone* (pp. 222-227), by J. H. Frey, 1989, Newbury Park, CA: Sage. Copyright 1989 by Sage Publications, Inc. Adapted with permission.

What Not to Do as an Interviewer
(excerpts from a handout)

NEVER

Get involved in long explanations of the study

Try to explain sampling in detail

Deviate from the study introduction, sequence of questions, or question wording

Try to justify or defend what you are doing

Try to explain procedures or wording

Suggest an answer or agree or disagree with an answer

Interpret the meaning of a question

Try to ask questions from memory

Rush the respondent

Patronize respondents

Dominate the interview

Let another person answer for the intended respondent

Interview someone you know

Falsify interviews

Improvise

Add response categories

Turn in a questionnaire without checking it over to be sure every question has been asked and its answer recorded

Item-by-Item Rationale for Interview Questions: A written explanation of the purpose of each interview item is useful to have in a training manual. Understanding the rationale behind the inclusion of individual items helps the interviewer recognize whether a response actually answers the question or needs a probe (see Example 3.12).

EXAMPLE 3.12
Rationale for Specific Interview Questions

Question: What is your current marital status?

Explanation: We are interested in the respondent's current (meaning most recent) marital status. Those people who live with someone other than a spouse will be picked up in Question 5 (Do you live with other family members or with someone else?).

Question: Think about the walking you typically do each day. On average, how many miles do you walk each day? Count the distance you walk for exercise, to work, as part of your job, to the bus, to the store, and so on. Don't try to estimate the distance you walk while inside your home or office.

_____ miles OR _____ blocks

Prompt: **A mile is equal to 12 city blocks.**

Explanation: The intent of this question is to estimate any **active walking** the respondent may do during the course of a typical day. Do not ask the respondent to estimate incidental walking that may take place at home or at work, such as walking to the refrigerator to get water or moving from desk to filing cabinet.

SOURCE: Adapted from the Kaiser/UCLA Sigmoid Study.

Sample Interview: A copy of the actual interview questionnaire is important to have in the training manual. The interviewer needs to study the "real thing" in its entirety before practice interview attempts are made. If the questionnaire is not yet finished, use the most recent draft.

Forms and Administrative Procedures: Samples of forms, such as the Interview Summary Form (Example 3.7) and the Interview Control Sheet (Example 3.8), should be included in the training manual so the interviewer can learn how to fill them out. An especially important form is the call or contact record on which contact attempts are logged. By keeping track of interview contacts and outcomes, the surveyor gets a good idea of the level of response. These records also inform the surveyor of refusals that may have to be converted and callbacks that will have to be scheduled. The call records are analyzed every day to determine the progress of the survey, the response rate (which is calculated at the end of each interviewing day), the productivity of interviewers, and to note any other field problems that may arise.

In large surveys, someone should be assigned the specific task of monitoring the status of every interview and sample unit contact. This person would also be responsible for distributing new sample units. The call record is very important to quality control in surveys. A field contact record serves essentially the same purpose as a call record. It gives an account of field contact attempts and numbers of completed face-to-face interviews. Example 3.13 shows how a call record and a field contact record might be designed.

EXAMPLE 3.13
Call Record and Field Contact Record

Call Record

CALL RECORD				
Telephone Number: _____ Questionnaire ID: _____				
Contact Attempt	Date	Time of Call	Outcome Code	Interviewer
1				
2				
3				
4				
5				
6				
NOTES				

OUTCOME CODES:

CI	= Completed Interview	BZ	= Busy Signal
RF	= Refusal	AM	= Answering Machine
NA	= No Answer	DS	= Disconnected
CB	= Call Back	WN	= Wrong Number

A form like this one is used to keep track of call attempts for a particular phone number in a telephone survey. Each time the number is called, the date, time, and outcome of the attempt is recorded. Codes are used for each possible outcome. For example, if the line is busy, "BZ" is recorded in the Outcome Code column.

Field Contact Record

Period From: To:

Interviewer:

Date	Neighborhood Code	Interview Start Time	Interview End Time	Outcome

CI = Completed Interview   RF = Refusal
NH = Not Home   CB = Come Back

Mileage:

Date: Miles:

1.
2.
3.
4.
5.

Interviewer Signature: Total Hours:
Supervisor Signature: Total Miles:

This form may be used to document contact attempts in the field and how they turned out (e.g., respondent not home vs. interview completed) and the amount of time each interview took. In this example, the surveyor has chosen to include a mileage record on the same form for travel reimbursement purposes.

Other forms may also be used by survey interviewers, such as time sheets on which only the hours worked are recorded, and reimbursement forms for telephone bills (if calls are made from home) and any out-of-pocket expenses.

Training Session

Although some surveys may not require more than one day of training, in general, interviewers are much better prepared if they have had 2 to 5 days of instruction and practice. A sample training agenda is shown in Example 3.14.

EXAMPLE 3.14
Agenda for Interviewer Training Sessions

DAY 1

10:00 – 10:30	Introductions
	Review of the Training Manual: 1. Description of the Survey
10:30 – 11:30	2. Introduction to Survey Methods 3. Interviewing Techniques and Guidelines
11:30 – 12:30	4. The Interviewer's Responsibilities 5. Item-by-Item Rationale for Interview Questions

12:30 – 1:30	LUNCH
1:30 – 2:00	Interview Demonstration
2:00 – 4:00	Practice Interviewing (Role-Playing) Sample Interview Training Agenda
	DAY 2
10:00 – 11:00	Review of Interviewer's Responsibilities and Interviewing Techniques
11:00 – 12:30	Forms and Administrative Procedures
12:30 – 1:30	LUNCH
1:30 – 3:30	Practice Interviewing (Volunteer Respondents)
3:30 – 4:00	Wrap-Up and Practice Assignments

Training usually begins with a review of the training manual through presentation and discussion. The most important part of training, however, centers on interviewing techniques, which are demonstrated by skilled presenters who also give expert feedback to trainees during role-playing. It cannot be emphasized enough that repeated practice in both the training session(s) and as "home work" is essential for acquiring excellent interviewing skills.

Supervision

Training alone does not ensure maintenance of high-quality interviewing. Some mechanism of monitoring interviewer performance must be put in place. The importance of supervision has been mentioned many times in this book. There are four aspects of interviewer performance that require supervision:

- Cost
- Response Rate
- Quality of Completed Questionnaires
- Quality of Interviewing

COST

Interviewers can be "expensive" if the number of completed interviews for the time spent on the phone or in the field is low. This could be due to working at unproductive times, high refusal rates (a refusal can take as much time as an interview), or undisciplined work habits (i.e., finding other things to do). In the case of field interviewing, high mileage costs may be a problem if the interviewer lives far from the neighborhoods of the respondents. Supervisors need to look for these problems and give interviewers feedback, such as more productive times to work and review of procedures for minimizing refusals. Paying interviewers by the completed interview rather than by the hour can increase productivity, but could compromise quality if interviewers rush to get more interviews done. Quality checks need to be done.

RESPONSE RATE

High refusal rates should be investigated. If interviewers are assigned different samples of respondents, higher refusal rates in one group than another may not be due to the interviewer; the group being contacted may be harder to enlist. However, some interviewers will have problems engaging respondents adequately to get their cooperation. Supervisors can retrain interviewers in delivering introductory remarks. Some interviewers may never get the hang of it, however, and may need to be taken off the project. Those interviewers who *are* good at gaining respondent cooperation may be assigned by the supervisor to attempt "refusal conversions." Respondents who refused a first interview attempt are called back and a second attempt is made to convince them to participate. If done well, response rates can be raised somewhat with this practice.

QUALITY OF COMPLETED QUESTIONNAIRES

Supervisors should look for legible recording, correct following of skip patterns, answers complete enough for coding, and evidence that interviewers are recording responses to open-ended questions verbatim rather than paraphrasing.

Another task of the supervisor is validating that completed surveys were actually the result of an interview, rather than being made up by the interviewer. Although we would like to believe this never happens, the supervisor must do **validation callbacks** to a sample (about 10%) of respondents to make sure they recall having been interviewed, and to ask about the interviewer's conduct (see Example 3.15). A small sample of repeat questions can also be asked to see if they match the responses recorded by the interviewer. Knowing that periodic validation will be done helps motivate interviewers to do a good job.

EXAMPLE 3.15
Validation Callback Sheet

RESPONDENT'S NAME: _____

DATE OF INTERVIEW: _____

INTERVIEWER: _____

1. Was the interviewer on time? Courteous?

2. Did he/she hand you a map of your neighborhood at
   the beginning of the interview?

3. How long have you lived in that neighborhood?

4. Did you feel you had enough time to answer the questions?

5. Do you have any questions or comments regarding the
   interview?

QUALITY OF INTERVIEWING

To determine how well the interviewer conducted the interview, the supervisor must directly observe interviews. "Quality" means that appropriate introductions were made, questions were asked exactly as written, and probing was done appropriately and without bias. Telephone interviews may be observed with a supervisor listening in. In large telephone surveys, the supervisor may have listening equipment available for listening to entire interviews. In smaller surveys, the supervisor may simply be present in the room to listen to the interviewer, or interviews may be tape-recorded. For field interviews, the supervisor may randomly accompany the interviewer on a visit or may tape-record the interview. In this way, the supervisor can give feedback to interviewers to keep quality and standardization high.

Exercises

1. A school-based teen pregnancy prevention program plans a needs assessment to guide program improvements by interviewing students. It will be complicated to get necessary approvals to interview adolescents under the age of 18, so this process must be started as soon as a protocol is decided upon. Money is tight, but time is not limited by any particular deadlines. In developing the questionnaire the survey team will aim for an administration time of 20 minutes to be verified in a pretest. Interviews could be done by telephone, using a list of students and their telephone numbers obtained from each school. Interviews could also be done in person at each of the three schools the program serves. Students would be randomly selected from classrooms or in the cafeteria and invited to a private office or empty classroom to be interviewed. These are the survey's objectives:

   ▪ Describe the experiences of teenagers related to teen pregnancy, either from personal experience or from the experiences of peers.

   ▪ Describe student attitudes toward teen pregnancy and its consequences.

- Determine which program features students find useful and what improvements they recommend.

List the issues that should be considered in deciding whether to interview by telephone or in person.

2. The Epilepsy Foundation is planning a survey to describe the characteristics of persons with epilepsy in the United States. One of the characteristics is the types of seizures that people experience. Seizure types have different names, and individuals who have epilepsy may not know the medical names for the types of seizures they are having. One of the types is a *complex partial seizure.* During such seizures, a person may have an involuntary behavior, such as lip smacking, picking at one's clothes, saying something over and over again, staring ahead blankly, or not responding when spoken to. During a complex partial seizure, a person will always lose awareness and always lose touch with the environment but will not stiffen and jerk or have a convulsion.

   If you wanted to reliably ask respondents with epilepsy by telephone interview whether they have experienced this type of seizure in the past 12 months, how would you write the question? What technique would you use? If you were writing the question for an in-person interview, how would you do it?

3. For the following scenarios, name the question order effect that is operating and state how this problem might be overcome.

   a. About 20 minutes into a telephone interview, the interviewer asks the respondent to listen to a detailed paragraph about the welfare laws currently in effect in his or her state. The respondent is then asked for an opinion on these laws and is read four possible responses. He/she answers: "Uh, the last one, I guess." When the interviewer offers to repeat the question, the respondent says, "It's the last one. Let's keep going."

b. At the beginning of an interview, a respondent is asked what she/he has heard regarding allegations that a well-known actor was involved in a hit-and-run accident that injured a child. She/he answers that the details of the child's injuries were heartbreaking and the actor should be arrested. The respondent is later asked whether she/he would go to see the actor's soon-to-be-released next film. The respondent hesitates and finally says, "Well, I guess not."

c. At the beginning of an interview, the respondent is asked how often he/she exercises for leisure during a typical month. A later question is part of a series of questions about behaviors specifically engaged in to improve health. The question is fifth in a series of seven and reads "How often do you exercise during a typical month?" The respondent is irritated and says, "Like I said before, about three times."

4. You are a survey coordinator conducting a survey on changing knowledge, attitudes, and behavior regarding cigarette smoking for the California State Tobacco Control Program. The survey takes about 40 minutes and will be done by telephone interview of a large sample of California residents chosen by random digit dialing. You will set up a small calling unit with ordinary telephone equipment in an empty office at Tobacco Control headquarters. You will provide three half-days of interviewer training. The interview will be administered in English and in Spanish. Write a job description to guide your selection process.

5. In response to the open-ended question "How do you think drunk drivers should be dealt with by the law?", a respondent rambles uncomfortably about an incident in which a relative was arrested for drunk driving. The interviewer senses the respondent's discomfort and says, "I understand completely. I once had to bail my own son out of jail for drunk driving. Tell me, without worrying about this incident, how you think the law should deal with drunk drivers in general?" What is wrong with

this probe? Suggest a better probe the interviewer could have used.

6. Indicate how you would respond if the person you intended to interview said one or more of the following when you requested an interview:

   a. "I don't know. How did you get my name anyway?"

   b. "I am too busy now, but you can talk to my neighbor, Mrs. Jones. She likes to talk to people."

   c. "I'm sorry, but I never give my opinion to others. How I feel about things is my business."

   d. "Come in. We are having a little gabfest, but you can ask your questions anyway. I am sure my friends will not mind, and they can help out if there is a question I cannot answer."

   e. "I can't talk right now. Come back in 2 months when I have more time."

   f. "I don't know anything about the topic. You can talk to my wife. She is familiar with it."

   g. "I don't care about the topic. I want to tell you how I feel about another issue."

   h. "There is no need for you to come to my house. Can't we do this interview over the phone?"

   i. "I can't do this at my apartment. Let's meet at Joe's Tavern down the street."

   j. "Just how did you get my name, and what happens to the results?"

7. Assume that the following nine questions are to be part of a general population survey. Identify the flaw(s) in each question and rewrite the question into what you think is the correct format.

(1) I am going to read a list of recreation activities. Please tell me if you have regularly participated in these activities within the past 5 years.

(2) Do you feel that the public bus system operates in a timely manner?

Strongly Agree   Agree   Disagree   Strongly Disagree

(3) Currently, the United States spends $50-$75 billion on people on welfare who don't want to work. Do you think the amount should be:

a. Increased
b. Kept the same
c. Decreased somewhat
d. Decreased significantly
e. Decreased a great deal

(4) Do you favor or oppose the governor's stand on gaming taxes and the suggestions for raising property tax?

a. Favor   b. Oppose

(5) The city wants to build a football stadium on the university campus that will attract a professional team, create jobs, and bring national attention to the city. Do you favor or oppose the construction of such a stadium?

a. Favor   b. Oppose

(6) If a nuclear repository would be located in the next 5 years within 100 miles of your favorite vacation place, would you change your route even if it meant going 75-100 miles out of your way when going to that destination?

1 = Yes   2 = No

(7) The federal government plans to locate a nuclear repository 100 miles from Reno, Nevada. Would you be for or against locating the repository in the state?

$$1 = Yes \qquad 2 = No$$

(8) The DOE and NRC are concerned with cleaning up the environment. Do you trust these agencies to do a good job?

> 1 = No trust
> 2 = Some trust
> 3 = A great deal of trust
> 4 = Don't know

(9) What is your yearly family income after taxes?

> 1 = Under $25,000
> 2 = Between $25,000 and $100,000
> 3 = More than $100,000

Answers

1. *Funding.* Although money to do the survey is tight, in this case it is difficult to predict which interview mode would be more expensive. In-person interviews would all be done at the schools and thus require a minimum of driving around. Because teenagers may spend a great deal of time engaged in social activities away from home or may tie up the phone lines with long conversations, they might prove to be difficult to reach by telephone. Repeated callback attempts and fruitless calling sessions may make the telephone interview more expensive.

Time. Time is not restrictive, so it need not be considered very seriously, especially because it is difficult to predict which mode would take more time. For the same reasons that telephone interviewing might be more expensive, it could also be more time consuming.

Target population. There is no "logistic" reason why teenagers could not be interviewed by telephone or in person. However, adolescents cannot be expected to have telephone privacy in their homes, and their time at school is usually highly structured, making absences noticeable. As a group they are at a highly self-conscious phase of development and are significantly influenced by peer pressure. All of these characteristics may have an effect on data quality, depending on interview mode.

Survey objectives. Again, it is not logistically impossible to meet the survey objectives by either interview mode. However, because the objectives require asking sensitive questions about possible personal experiences with pregnancy, respondents' replies in a telephone interview may be less informative and thus affect data quality. In general, such questions are more likely to be answered honestly when teenagers are interviewed in person, especially if interviewers are very well trained and have excellent interpersonal skills.

Data quality. The response rate in this example is closely intertwined with confidentiality issues and the need to ask sensitive questions. Response rate may be compromised if interviews are done by telephone because of the lack of privacy; teenagers may refuse to participate rather than risk having a conversation about pregnancy overheard by their parents. If interviews are done at school, they may still refuse because they might be seen leaving class or being picked out in the lunchroom; however, the interviewer has more control over the environment in the in-person interview setting. This provides a somewhat better chance of ensuring privacy (a reluctant subject might be approached while sitting alone in the library, for example, or offered a private time slot after school). In either case, it is very difficult to ensure confidentiality in this survey.

Because adolescents are self-conscious and influenced by peer pressure, susceptibility to *interviewer effects* and *socially desirable responses* may be high. Teenagers as a group may be especially likely to try to please the interviewer or represent the views of their friends rather than their own. The age of the interviewer, even as estimated by voice quality over the phone, might influence responses and could be significant in the in-person interview. When interviewer effects and socially desirable responses are considered, the telephone interview has a slight advantage. If the in-person format is chosen, questions, prompts, and probes should be designed with these considerations in mind, and the effect of interviewer age should be estimated in a pretest.

2. One option for the telephone interview is to use the funnel technique, asking a general, open-ended question first, followed by a series of specific questions:

    1. For the seizures you have had in the past 12 months, what generally happens?

        =========================

    1a. For the seizures you have had in the past 12 months, please answer yes or no to whether you had each of the following involuntary behaviors:

Lip smacking	Y	N
Picking at your clothes	Y	N
Saying something over and over	Y	N
Staring ahead	Y	N
Not responding to people talking to you	Y	N

    1b. During the past 12 months, have you had seizures in which you *both* lost awareness and lost touch with your environment but did *not* stiffen and jerk?

           Yes   No

During the in-person interview, a description of a complex partial seizure may be given to a respondent to read, followed by the question "Have you had any complex partial seizures in the past 12 months?"

VISUAL AID:

COMPLEX PARTIAL SEIZURE - DESCRIPTION

During a COMPLEX PARTIAL SEIZURE you may:

smack your lips, OR
pick at your clothes, OR
say something over and over, OR
stare ahead, OR
not respond to people talking to you.

During a COMPLEX PARTIAL SEIZURE,

you will ALWAYS LOSE AWARENESS and
ALWAYS LOSE TOUCH WITH YOUR ENVIRONMENT,
but you will NOT STIFFEN AND JERK ALL OVER or have
a convulsion.

SOURCE: Adapted from *Quality of Life and Seizures after Epilepsy Survey: Executive Summary and Final Report to the Agency for Health Care Policy and Research, 1993.*

3a. This is the fatigue effect. The respondent is tired and no longer willing to give thought to a complex question. When possible, place complex questions early in the interview.

3b. This is the consistency effect. The respondent may be reluctant to admit an interest in seeing the movie after expressing disapproval of the actor. The problem might be solved by reversing the order of the questions.

3c. This is the redundancy effect. The respondent has not perceived the difference between exercise in the context of leisure activities versus exercise for the express purpose of promoting health. The difference should be pointed out in each question, and examples could be given to clarify the distinction. First question: "How often do you exercise for leisure, activities you do for fun like hiking, water skiing, or biking, during a typical month?"

Later question: "How often do you exercise to maintain your health, such as jogging, working out at a gym, or swimming laps?"

4. One suggested format is the following:

JOB DESCRIPTION

Summary Statement The California State Tobacco Control Program is sponsoring a survey on changing knowledge, attitudes, and behaviors related to cigarette smoking. Interviewers are sought to administer a 40-minute telephone questionnaire to English- and Spanish-speaking California residents.

Supervision The survey coordinator will provide ongoing observation of interviews conducted from a central calling unit at Tobacco Control headquarters. The coordinator will supervise all aspects of interviewing, including monitoring and evaluating completed interviews for accuracy and completeness.

Duties and Tasks Interviewer duties include telephoning potential respondents using a randomly generated list of telephone numbers, introducing and administering the survey to eligible respondents, and recording responses and editing completed interviews for errors before submission to the survey coordinator for review.

Abilities, Knowledge, and Skills Excellent reading, writing, and speaking abilities in English and/or Spanish are required. Bilingual interviewers are preferred. Availability to conduct interviews during evening and weekend hours and to attend three half-day training sessions is required. Skills needed for maintaining confidentiality, administering questionnaires in an unbiased manner, and encouraging respondent participation will be trained.

---

5. The interviewer's own values have been interjected ("It's OK because it happened to me too"), and so he/she has reframed the question by telling the respondent not to include this personal experience in formulating a response. A better prompt would be "Uh-huh. I'm unclear about what you mean. Let me repeat the question."

6. Suggested responses to respondents' concerns and queries are the following:

   6a. "Your name was drawn at random (describe process, such as RDD). We do not know anything else about you. Your responses will be treated confidentially."

   6b. "We need to get people from all walks of life, not just those who like to talk. We need your opinion."

   6c. "This is very important research. We need your opinion because it will be valuable for the larger study. The interviewer will keep your responses confidential. No one will know which views are yours."

   6d. "We only want *your* opinion, and it would be better if I could interview you without your friends present. Could I come back at a more convenient time?"

   6e. "Actually, 2 months is too late. The study will be completed before then. Could I make an appointment to come back for the interview within the next week?"

   6f. "I'm sure your wife is very knowledgeable, but we really need to talk to the persons selected for the sample. I need to get your opinion and no one else's. It doesn't matter how well informed you are as we don't expect you to know all there is to know about (topic)."

   6g. "I'm sorry, I need to get your views on (topic). Can I ask you some questions first, and then you can tell me your views on (other topic)?"

6h. "This interview needs to be done in your home because there are some things you will need to look at that can't be described over the phone."

6i. "I would prefer to conduct the interview somewhere, like your home, where there are fewer distractions. Besides, if we do the interview in your home, it will probably take less time."

6j. "Your name was selected randomly from (name the list used). The results will be used by city and county officials as they develop policy in the coming year."

7. You might find several things wrong with each question, so there will be more than one way to rephrase the question into an acceptable format. Some of the suggested corrections are as follows:

Question 1. The term "regularly" is imprecise. It could refer to once a year or twice a week. Five years is also too long a time period for a respondent to recall an activity. You need to specify the time frame, say, within the past year or 6 months, and ask the respondent to recall "on average" if a longer period of time is used or to state exact number of times if a specific, shorter time referent is used. Telescoping is a problem with this type of question.

"I am going to read a list of recreation activities. For each, please tell me how many times you have participated in that activity in the past 2 months. First, how often have you played golf?"

Question 2. This question assumes both knowledge and behavior by making the presumption that the respondent is familiar with the bus system and has ridden the system. The answer categories of "Agree-Disagree" do not match the manner in which the question was asked. "Do you feel" suggests a simple "Yes-No" response. A filter question to determine knowledge of the system and ridership experience is necessary before asking the question on timeliness.

"The city has been operating a public transit bus system for approximately 3 years. Have you ridden one of the city buses within the past 3 months?"

    1 = Yes (GO TO QUESTION #_____)
    2 = No (GO TO QUESTION # _____)

If YES, "To what extent do the public buses reach scheduled stops on time? Is it nearly all of the time, about half the time, or are they rarely on time?"

    1 = Nearly all of the time
    2 = Half of the time
    3 = Rarely on time
    8 = Don't know

Question 3. This is what is called a "loaded" question because it biases the response. The amount of money spent is inflammatory as is the term "welfare"; the phrase "do not want to work" is biasing and a false premise and suggests a research agenda; the answer categories are imbalanced in a manner that reinforces the bias of the researcher. The $50-$75 billion figure may not be accurate. It is also better to number the response categories rather than use letters of the alphabet.

"Currently, the United States supports a number of programs designed to support individuals and families in need. Do you think that the amount spent on these programs should be increased, remain the same, or be decreased?"

    1 = Increased
    2 = Remain the same
    3 = Decreased
    8 = Don't know

Question 4. This is what is called a double question or a "double barrel" question that is really two questions in one. It also assumes that the respondent has knowledge of the governor's proposals on gaming tax and property tax. A filter question or keyword summary question could be used to either determine the level of knowledge or inform the respondent before asking the question.

"The governor has proposed increasing the state's revenue by making changes in the tax on gaming operations. Are you familiar with this proposal?"

> 1 = Yes (GO TO QUESTION # _____)
> 2 = No (GO TO QUESTION # _____)

Question 5. This is a "loaded" question biasing the response to a position favoring the construction of the stadium. It is also a triple question in that it addresses issues of national attention, jobs, and securing a professional franchise. This is a topic on which many will not have an opinion so a "Don't Know" response is needed.

"The city is considering building a football stadium on the university campus in the near future. At this time, do you favor or oppose this project?"

> 1 = Favor
> 2 = Oppose
> 8 = Don't know

Question 6. This is a hypothetical question that asks the respondent to predict future behavior. It is also a wordy and confusing question. It is probably a question better not asked, although impact assessment studies often use such items.

"If a nuclear waste repository were located within 100 miles of your favorite vacation spot, what is the *likelihood* that you would change your travel route to avoid going near the site? Is it very likely, somewhat likely, or not likely at all that you would change routes?"

> 1 = Very likely
> 2 = Somewhat likely
> 3 = Not likely at all
> 8 = Don't know

Question 7. This question has many problems. First, the federal government plans to locate the site of the repository near Las Vegas, not Reno. The question assumes the respondent knows about these plans. The response categories of "Yes-No" do not match the response "Favor-Oppose" required by the question. Locating the repository next to a city is not the same question as locating it in the state.

"The federal government is investigating the possibility of locating a high-level nuclear waste repository within 100 miles of Las Vegas at Yucca Mountain. Have you heard of this possibility?"

> 1 = Yes (GO TO QUESTION # _____)
> 2 = No (GO TO QUESTION # _____)

Question 8. Do not use abbreviations or acronyms such as DOE or NRC because not everyone knows what they mean. It is also a double question, as trust could apply to either or both agencies. The answer categories do not match the response requirements of the question. The fact that the term "concern" is used is potentially biasing in favor of the DOE and NRC environmental activity. It would be better to ask two questions.

"The Department of Energy, or DOE, has as part of its mission to work on behalf of the environment. To what extent do you trust the DOE to properly work to protect the environment? Do you trust the DOE a great deal, to some extent, or not at all?"

> 1 = A great deal
> 2 = To some extent
> 3 = Not at all
> 8 = Don't know

Question 9. The income question is always a difficult one to ask. In this case, the answer categories are too broad to accurately reflect the actual distribution in the population. Respondents will have a better idea of their income if they are asked to estimate gross rather than net income.

"What is your yearly family income before taxes?"

> 1 = Less than $15,000
> 2 = $15,001 to $25,000
> 3 = $25,001 to $35,000
> 4 = $35,001 to $45,000
> 5 = $45,001 to $55,000
> 6 = More than $55,000
> 8 = Don't know
> 9 = Refuse to answer

Suggested Readings

Converse, J. M., & Presser, S. (1986). *Survey questions: Handcrafting the standardized questionnaire*. Beverly Hills, CA: Sage.

Brief but excellent discussion of question writing and administration.

Converse, J. M., & Sherman, H. (1974). *Conversations at random: Survey research as interviewers see it*. New York: John Wiley.

Classic account of how interviewers perceive the task of interviewing, especially how they overcome respondent resistance and how a standardized list of questions is administered in somewhat unstandardized contexts.

Dillman, D. A. (1978). *Mail and telephone surveys*. New York: John Wiley.

Considered the definitive statement on how to conduct mail and telephone surveys. The Total Design Method has generated a lineage of research on stimulating response and reducing all types of errors associated with survey research.

Fowler, F. J., & Mangione, T. W. (1990). *Standardized survey interviewing*. Newbury Park, CA: Sage.

This text discusses recruiting, training, and supervision of interviewers, techniques of asking questions, and strategies for establishing a working relationship with respondents. Major focus is on reducing errors that might be attributed to the interviewing process.

Frey, J. H. (1989). *Survey research by telephone* (2nd ed.). Newbury Park, CA: Sage.

A review of sampling, questionnaire construction, question writing, and interviewing associated with telephone interviews. Includes extensive chapter comparing telephone, mail, face-to-face, and intercept surveys on several dimensions, such as cost, response rates, and data quality.

Frey, J. H., & Fontana, A. (1991). The group interview in social research. *Social Science Journal, 28,* 175-187.

A review of the various formats for group interviews that have been used in research settings. Both casual, informal field situations and formal, controlled contexts are conducive to this type of interview.

Gorden, R. L. (1987). *Interviewing: Strategy, techniques, and tactics* (4th ed.). Homewood, IL: Dorsey.

Extensive discussion of the factors that influence the dynamics of face-to-face interviewing. Discusses the appropriate setting for interviews and how an interviewer must deal with verbal and nonverbal communication in the interview context.

Gorden, R. L. (1992). *Basic interviewing skills*. Itasca, IL: Peacock.

Excellent review of all stages of the interview from designing relevant questions to establishing a proper atmosphere for interviewing, listening to the respondent, probing responses, and properly recording information.

Groves, R. M., & Kahn, R. L. (1979). *Surveys by telephone: A national comparison with personal interviews.* New York: Academic Press.

One of the first studies to compare telephone and face-to-face interviews on a variety of dimensions, including sampling, response rates, item nonresponse, cost, and response error. The comparison of RDD sampling design with area probability designs is a very important contribution of this text.

Hyman, H., et al. (1955). *Interviewing in social research.* Chicago: University of Chicago Press.

Good review of interviewing principles. Particularly important discussion of the impact of interviewer expectations.

Lavrakas, P. J. (1993). *Telephone survey methods: Sampling, selection, and supervision.* Newbury Park, CA: Sage.

This text focuses on sampling for telephone interviews, but it also contains two useful chapters on structuring the interview and supervising those doing the interviewing.

Morgan, D. L. (Ed.). (1993). *Successful focus groups.* Newbury Park, CA: Sage.

This anthology includes contributions from leading authorities in the use of group interviewing, especially focus groups, in research. The advantages and disadvantages of this type of research are clearly delineated in this volume. There are several accounts of how the group interview can be used to augment survey implementation.

Oppenheim, A. N. (1992). *Questionnaire design, interviewing, and attitude measurement.* New York: St. Martin's.

Excellent discussion of the issues of survey design, with especially valuable chapters on pilot studies, attitude measurement, and the characteristics of standardized interviewing.

Rossi, P. H., Wright, J. D., & Anderson, A. B. (Eds.). (1983). *Handbook of survey research.* New York: Academic Press.

Comprehensive and detailed review of all aspects of survey design, including sampling theory, measurement issues, survey administration, computerization, and data analysis. Chapters by Bradburn on "Response Effects" and Sheatsley on "Questionnaire Construction and Item Writing" are excellent discussions.

Schuman, H., & Presser, S. (1981). *Questions and answers in attitude surveys: Experiments on question form, wording, and context.* New York: Academic Press.

The authors use more than 30 national surveys conducted over a 6-year period to experiment with the open versus closed format, wording strategies, question order effects, and response order variations.

About the Authors

JAMES H. FREY is Chair of the Department of Sociology and Director of the Center for Survey Research at the University of Nevada, Las Vegas. He is author of *An Organizational Analysis of University-Environment Relations* (1977), *Government and Sport: The Public Policy Issues* (1985), and *Survey Research by Telephone* (2nd ed., 1989) and of numerous articles on question order, group interviewing, and response rates. He has also published in the fields of the sociology of work, sport and leisure, and risk perception. He has been principal investigator on a number of telephone, mail, and intercept survey projects, including regional and national surveys of risk perception, community needs and issues, and leisure participation patterns. He is currently completing a textbook on the sociology of sport and conducting research on delinquency and the impact of gambling on communities.

SABINE MERTENS OISHI, who holds a MsPH degree in epidemiology from the University of California, Los Angeles, is an independent consultant to health projects and programs in the areas of survey development and grant proposal preparation and a senior researcher with Arlene Fink Associates, Pacific Palisades, California, where she is engaged in program evaluations of health and social services programs and health professional training programs. She has participated in a variety of research projects at UCLA and the RAND Corporation, been a health sciences specialist at the Veterans Administration Medical Center in Sepulveda, California, and managed a division of the Department of Medicine at UCLA. She designed and implemented in-person surveys in urban and rural Liberia, West Africa, with the Liberian Ministry of Health and Social Welfare, U.S. Peace Corps, and USAID.

HOW TO DESIGN SURVEYS

THE SURVEY KIT

Purpose. The purposes of this 9-volume Kit are to enable readers to prepare and conduct surveys and become better users of survey results. Surveys are conducted to collect information by asking questions of people on the telephone, face-to-face, and by mail. The questions can be about attitudes, beliefs, and behavior as well as socioeconomic and health status. To do a good survey also means knowing how to ask questions, design the survey (research) project, sample respondents, collect reliable and valid information, and analyze and report the results. You also need to know how to plan and budget for your survey.

Users. The Kit is for students in undergraduate and graduate classes in the social and health sciences and for individuals in the public and private sectors who are responsible for conducting and using surveys. Its primary goal is to enable users to prepare surveys and collect data that are accurate and useful for primarily practical purposes. Sometimes, these practical purposes overlap the objectives of scientific research, and so survey researchers will also find the Kit useful.

Format of the Kit. All books in the series contain instructional objectives, exercises and answers, examples of surveys in use and illustrations of survey questions, guidelines for action, checklists of do's and don'ts, and annotated references.

Volumes in the Survey Kit:

1. **The Survey Handbook**
   Arlene Fink

2. **How to Ask Survey Questions**
   Arlene Fink

3. **How to Conduct Self-Administered and Mail Surveys**
   Linda B. Bourque and *Eve P. Fielder*

4. **How to Conduct Interviews by Telephone and in Person**
   James H. Frey and *Sabine Mertens Oishi*

5. **How to Design Surveys**
   Arlene Fink

6. **How to Sample in Surveys**
   Arlene Fink

7. **How to Measure Survey Reliability and Validity**
   Mark S. Litwin

8. **How to Analyze Survey Data**
   Arlene Fink

9. **How to Report on Surveys**
   Arlene Fink

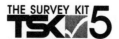

THE SURVEY KIT
TSK✓5

HOW TO
DESIGN
SURVEYS

ARLENE FINK

SAGE Publications
International Educational and Professional Publisher
Thousand Oaks   London   New Delhi

For information address:

SAGE Publications, Inc.
2455 Teller Road
Thousand Oaks, California 91320
E-mail: order@sagepub.com

SAGE Publications Ltd.
6 Bonhill Street
London EC2A 4PU
United Kingdom

SAGE Publications India Pvt. Ltd.
M-32 Market
Greater Kailash I
New Delhi 110 048 India

Printed in the United States of America

Library of Congress Cataloging-in-Publication Data

Main entry under title:

The survey kit.
    p. cm.
    Includes bibliographical references.
    Contents: v. 1. The survey handbook / Arlene Fink — v. 2. How to ask survey questions / Arlene Fink — v. 3. How to conduct self-administered and mail surveys / Linda B. Bourque, Eve P. Fielder — v. 4. How to conduct interviews by telephone and in person / James H. Frey, Sabine Mertens Oishi — v. 5. How to design surveys / Arlene Fink — v. 6. How to sample in surveys / Arlene Fink — v. 7. How to measure survey reliability and validity / Mark S. Litwin — v. 8. How to analyze survey data / Arlene Fink — v. 9. How to report on surveys / Arlene Fink.
    ISBN 0-8039-7388-8 (pbk. : The survey kit : alk. paper)
    1. Social surveys. 2. Health surveys. I. Fink, Arlene.
HN29.S724   1995
300′.723—dc20   95-12712

This book is printed on acid-free paper.

95 96 97 98 99   10 9 8 7 6 5 4 3 2 1

Sage Production Editor: Diane S. Foster
Sage Copy Editor: Joyce Kuhn
Sage Typesetter: Janelle LeMaster

Contents

How to Design Surveys:
Learning Objectives

The aim of this book is to guide the reader in selecting and using appropriate survey designs. The following specific objectives are stated in terms of aspirations for the reader.

- Describe the major features of high-quality survey systems

- Identify the questions that structure survey designs

- Distinguish between experimental and observational designs

- Explain the characteristics, benefits, and concerns of these designs:

    - Concurrent controls with random assignment

    - Concurrent controls without random assignment

    - Self-controls

    - Historical controls

    - Cross-sectional designs

    - Cohort designs

    - Case-control designs

- Identify the risks to a design's internal validity

- Identify the risks to a design's external validity

1 Useful Surveys

Surveys are systems for collecting information on a broad range of subjects of interest in fields as diverse as education, sociology, demography, health, psychology, economics, business, and law. The best survey information systems have these six features:

- Specific, measurable objectives
- Sound research design
- Sound choice of population or sample
- Reliable and valid instruments
- Appropriate analysis
- Accurate reporting of survey results

MEASURABLE SURVEY OBJECTIVES

A survey's objectives are measurable if two or more people can easily agree on all the words and terms used to describe its purposes. Measurable survey objectives are illustrated in Example 1.1.

EXAMPLE 1.1
Three Measurable Objectives

Objective 1: To determine the quality of UCLA's education in preparing students with important job-related skills. Quality is a combination of the skill's importance and the value of UCLA's education in teaching the skill.

> *Comment:* This objective becomes measurable by clarifying the term *quality* to mean importance and value. You can infer that some of the survey's questions will take forms like "Select the top three most important skills" and "Rate how valuable UCLA's education is, using a scale on which 1 = not very valuable, 3 = medium value, and 5 = extremely valuable."

Objective 2: To determine changes from 1984 to 1992 qualifications, such as advanced placement units, among entering students.

> *Comment:* Qualifications are made measurable by "advanced placement units."

Objective 3: To compare the effectiveness of three approaches to continuing mental health education in a workshop setting. The three approaches are (a) traditional lecture and small group dis-

---

cussion, (b) computerized cases and small group discussion, and (c) computerized cases and self-instruction. An effective approach is one that encourages participants to appropriately resolve important (as defined by experts) patient care issues in practice.

Comment: The effectiveness of an approach is defined to mean one that encourages workshop participants to appropriately resolve important patient care issues.

SOUND SURVEY DESIGN

A design is a way of arranging the environment in which a survey takes place. The environment consists of the individuals or groups of people, places, activities, or objects that are to be surveyed.

Some designs are relatively simple. A fairly uncomplicated survey might consist of a 10-minute interview on Wednesday with a group of 50 children to find out if they enjoyed a given film, and if so, why. This survey provides a cross-sectional portrait of one group's opinions at a particular time, and its design is called cross-sectional.

More complicated survey designs use environmental arrangements that are experiments, relying on two or more groups of participants or observations. When the views of randomly constituted groups of 50 children each are compared, for example, the survey design is experimental.

SOUND SURVEY SAMPLING

The participants in a survey may consist of all members of a given group, say, all 500 students in a school or all 70 patients who in the past 6 months have been diagnosed with diabetes. A subset of the population, say, 100 students and 25 patients, is a sample. The ideal sample has the same distribution of characteristics as the population. It has the same proportion of males and females, for example. To get a "representative" sample means using an unbiased method to choose survey participants, obtaining adequate numbers of participants, and collecting high-quality data by relying on valid and reliable survey instruments.

RELIABLE AND VALID SURVEY INSTRUMENTS

A reliable instrument is consistent; a valid one is accurate. Traditionally, survey instruments have been equated with mailed or self-administered questionnaires and telephone or face-to-face interviews. But the techniques for collecting and recording reliable and valid information perfected by survey researchers for these instruments also have been applied to other information-gathering techniques. These include forms for surveying the quality of medical care, the use of financial resources, and the content of the professional literature in business, health, and education.

One indication of the adaptation of these survey techniques to other instruments is the similarity of their purposes: to describe, compare, and predict. Another indication is how similar a questionnaire or interview form looks to, say, a record review form. Instead of asking questions of people, the questions are "asked" of records. As can be seen in the following examples, the two look identical:

Question from a self-administered questionnaire:

Which best describes your personal income last year? Circle *one* choice only.	
$25,000 or less	1
$25,001 - $40,000	2
$40,001 - $75,000	3
$75,001 or more	4

Question from a form for reviewing financial records:

Which best describes this person's income last year? Circle *one* choice only.	
$25,000 or less	1
$25,001 - $40,000	2
$40,001 - $75,000	3
$75,001 or more	4

All surveys, regardless of format, should only contain questions or items that are pertinent to the survey's objectives. The aim is to produce reliable and valid data. Reliable data are the results of consistent responses over time and between and among observers and respondents. Valid data come from surveys that measure what they purport to measure.

APPROPRIATE SURVEY ANALYSIS

Surveys use conventional statistical and other scholarly methods to analyze findings. The choice of method depends on whether the survey aims for description, comparison, association or correlation, or prediction, and also the size of the sample. The analysis must account also for the type of survey data available: nominal (categorical), ordinal, or numerical. Nominal or categorical data come from scales that have no numerical value such as gender and race. Ordinal data come from rating scales and may range, say, from most favored to least favored or from strongly agree to strongly disagree. Numerical data come from measures that ask for numbers like age, years living at present address, and height.

ACCURATE SURVEY REPORTS

Fair and accurate reporting means staying within the boundaries set by the survey's design, sampling methods, data collection quality, and choice of analysis. Accurate survey reports require knowledge of how to use tables and figures to present information.

Survey Design:
The Arranged Environment

To be useful and valid, surveys should be conducted in an arranged or designed environment. Consider these illustrations in Example 1.2.

EXAMPLE 1.2
Illustrative Survey Designs

Survey 1: College Students and Graduates

Background: Each year, UCLA prepares a student profile. Data for the profile come from records (including those maintained by the financial aid office and student loan services) and mailed student questionnaires.

Objective: To determine the quality of UCLA's education in preparing students with important job-related skills

Instrument: Self-administered questionnaire. Students were asked to indicate on a 3-point scale how important each of eight items was in preparing them for their job and then to rate on a 4-point scale the quality of UCLA's preparation in each of the eight areas.

Design: Descriptive (or observational), specifically, cross-sectional

Results: The responses for graduates who were employed full-time and not enrolled in graduate school are summarized in Figure 1.1.

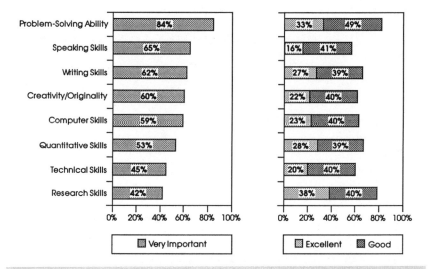

NOTE: Students were asked to indicate on a 3-point scale how important each of the eight items were in preparing them for their job and then to rate on a four-point scale the quality of UCLA's preparation in each of the eight areas. The responses for graduates who were employed full-time and not enrolled in graduate school are summarized in the chart above. *Problem-solving ability* was the skill most often considered by respondents to be very important for the work they were currently doing and it also received the highest combined rating of excellent or good. *Speaking skills* were second in terms of those who considered them very important for their job but last in the combined rating of excellent or good.

Figure 1-1   UCLA Preparation

Interpretation: Problem-solving ability was the skill most often considered by respondents to be very important for the work they were currently doing, and it also received the highest combined rating of excellent or good. Speaking skills were second in terms of those who considered them very important for their job but last in the combined rating of excellent or good.

Comment: This survey provides a cross section of descriptive information at one point in time. The survey collected its information directly from students by using a self-administered questionnaire.

Survey 2: *Entering Students*

Background: As part of its annual student profile, UCLA collects data on students who enter with advanced placement (AP) units.

Objective: To assess the extent of change in the proportion of students entering UCLA with AP credits

Instrument: Standardized record review (records from Undergraduate Admissions and Relations With Schools)

Design: Cross-sectional (to study trends)

Results: Figure 1.2 shows the percentages of entering students with AP credits in 1984 and 1992.

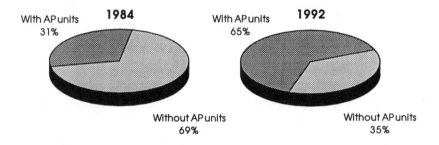

NOTE: The percentage of students entering with AP units has continued to increase from 31% in 1984 to 65% in 1992, and the average amount of college credit earned increased from 14 to 18 units.

Figure 1-2 First-Year Students Enter With One Quarter's College Credit

Interpretation: The percentage of students entering with AP units increased from 31% in 1984 to 65% in 1992. The average amount of college credit earned increased from 14 to 18 points.

Comment: The survey provided a description of trends in accumulating AP credits of two entering classes. Data came from surveying records, using the same form each time.

Survey 3: Comparing Educational Approaches

Background: The city is conducting a study to identify an effective approach to continuing education in mental health.

Purpose: To compare the effectiveness of three approaches to instruction in a workshop setting

Instrument: Self-administered questionnaires and standardized 10-item observation form used by two trained observers monitoring each workshop

Design: An experiment with concurrent controls in which survey participants are **not** randomly assigned to groups. Here, 200 eligible community mental health workers are assigned to three workshops, depending on their preference. The first workshop (Group 1) uses traditional lecture and small group discussion, the second (Group 2) relies on computerized cases and small group discussion, and the third (Group 3) employs computerized cases and self-instruction. Observations are made during each workshop session. Participants complete a questionnaire at the conclusion of the 3-hour workshop.

Results: Agreement between the two observers in each workshop was 81%, 76%, and 93% in Groups 1, 2, and 3, respectively. No differences were found in preference for type of instruction among participants in the three groups. Participants in the computerized cases and self-instruction group (Group 3) rated their experiences as "likely to carry over into their work" significantly more often than did the other two groups ($p < .05$.).

Interpretation: Participants in the computerized cases and self-instruction group stated that their learning is likely to carry over to their jobs significantly more often than the other groups stated. Their belief should now be tested in a controlled study.

Comment: This experimental study used a traditional survey method (a self-administered questionnaire) and an applied survey method (standardized observation) to collect data. Each type of survey information was collected just once: during the workshop (the observations) and at the conclusion of workshop participation (the questionnaire).

Survey 4: Comparing Educational Approaches

Background: The city is conducting a study to identify an effective approach to continuing education in mental health.

Purpose: To compare the effectiveness of three approaches to instruction by determining the number of important issues per topic (e.g., technical care, doctor-patient relationship, coordination of care) addressed in practice by participants. Important issues in patient care have been identified by a panel of experts.

Instrument: Self-administered questionnaires and case record review

Design: An experiment with concurrent controls in which survey participants are randomly assigned to groups. Here, 200 eligible community mental health workers are assigned at random to three workshops. The first work-

shop (Group 1) uses traditional lecture and small group
discussion, the second (Group 2) relies on computerized
cases and small group discussion, and the third (Group
3) employs computerized cases and self-instruction. Participants complete a questionnaire at the conclusion of
the 3-hour workshop. Before participation and 6 months
after, the case records of participants are reviewed, and
the number of important issues addressed is counted.

Results: The number of issues (e.g., improving the doctor-
patient relationship, fostering patient responsibility) addressed did not differ among the groups at baseline but
differed significantly after the intervention. The number
dropped significantly in Group 1 (2 to 0.5, $p < .05$); rose,
but not significantly, in Group 2 (0.5 to 1.5, *ns*, or not
significant), and increased substantially and significantly
in Group 3 (1 to 3.75, $p < .05$). [More information on
testing statistical significance and p values is given in
How to Analyze Survey Data, Vol. 8 in this series.] These
results are shown in Figure 1.3.

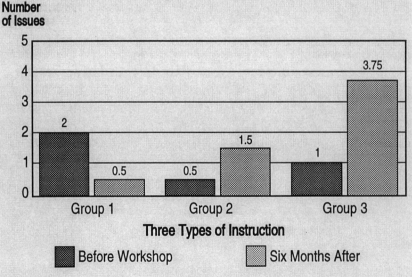

Figure 1-3   Number of Issues Per Topic Before and After Workshop

When Group 3 participants were asked to rate the likelihood that participation in the workshop contributed to their knowledge of important issues in caring for patients' mental health needs, nearly all (98%) chose ratings of 4 ("probably") or 5 ("definitely likely").

Interpretation: Computerized cases and self-instruction are an effective approach to continuing education for the city's mental health workers.

Comment: This study is experimental and randomly assigns participants to one of three groups. It uses questionnaires and record reviews to collect data.

The aim of Survey 1 is to find out if UCLA has done a good job in preparing its students with important job-related skills. The design used provides a one-time-only portrait of students' opinions as gathered from a self-administered questionnaire. The design is called cross-sectional and is discussed in much greater detail in Chapter 2. Survey 2 collects data from records in two cross-sectional studies.

Survey 3 uses an experimental design to compare the results of observations and self-administered questionnaires. Experimental designs involve arranging the environment so that comparisons can be made. A relatively simple experimental design, for example, would compare the reading ability of children who have participated in an innovative program with the reading ability of children who have not participated. Survey 4 also uses an experimental design, but in this case the three groups have been randomly assembled. Surveys 3 and 4 use self-administered questionnaires. Survey 3 also uses observations; Survey 4 also uses record reviews.

The four surveys use typical survey designs. These can be grouped into two general types: descriptive (also called observational) and experimental. How do you choose? Answer the following questions to select the right design.

Checklist of Questions to Ask
in Choosing a Survey Design

✓ **What is the survey's aim—describe, compare, predict?**

Surveys produce information to describe, compare, and predict attitudes, opinions, values, and behavior based on what people say or see and what is contained in records about them and their activities. Example 1.3 illustrates the three major survey aims.

EXAMPLE 1.3
Describing, Comparing, or Predicting

Describing

Objective: To *describe* the quality of life of men over and under 65 years of age with different health characteristics (e.g., the presence or absence of common conditions like hypertension and diabetes) and social characteristics (e.g., living alone or living with someone; employed or not), all of whom have had surgery within the past 2 years for prostate cancer

Target: Men of differing ages, health, and social characteristics who have had surgery for prostate cancer within the past 2 years

Number of times surveyed: Once, within 2 years of surgery

Comparing—Design 1

Objective: At the end of the school year, to *compare* a sample of boys and girls in Grades 1 through 6 in five schools regarding their views on their school's new dress code

Target: Boys and girls in Grades 1 through 6 in five elementary schools

Number of times surveyed: Once, at the end of the school year

Comparing—Design 2

Objective: Before and after participation in a safety course, to *compare* parents of children under 5 years of age, between 6 and 12, and 13 and over in terms of their opinions of their ability to cope with potential accidents and injuries in the home

Target: Parents who participate in a safety course

Number of times surveyed: Twice, before and after participation

Comparing—Design 3

Objective: To *compare* a sample of employees in three companies annually for 3 years about their views on uncompensated leave time

Target: Employees in three companies

Number of times surveyed: Three times, once each year

Predicting

Objective: In 1994 and 1995, to determine the extent to
which gender, education or income *predicts* preferences
for differing leisure activities, including reading, sports,
movies, and travel

Target: Male and female high school graduates, each of whom
earns an annual income of less than $30,000, between
$30,000 and $60,000, or more than $60,000

Number of times surveyed: Twice, in 1994 and in 1995

✓ Is a control group included?

The term "group" refers to an assembly of people, institutions, or units that is defined by participation in a program or
intervention or by shared personal, social, or health characteristics. Three illustrative groups are people who receive an
experimental medicine, employees who implement the terms
of a flexible work-hours policy for the first time, and schools
that try out an innovative adult literacy program. When a group
takes part in an untested intervention, such as those just
mentioned, it is called the **experimental** group. The experimental group is contrasted with the **control** group, which does
not participate in the experiment or innovation.

A basic survey design compares experimental and control
groups that have been created just for the survey. For example,
you can survey people trying out a new medicine (the experimental group) with a group of people using a traditional
medicine (the control group) and also with a second group not
taking any medicine (a second control group). Sometimes one
group serves as its own control. For example, you can survey

people just before they take a new medicine and again 1 year later. These two designs are **prospective** because the events of interest occur after the study begins. That is, the study begins and then the effects of the new medicine on people are surveyed over time, or **longitudinally.**

Another example of a longitudinal, prospective survey involves identifying a group whose members share important characteristics (e.g., severe headaches) and then surveying some or all of the members of the group at least once more. This group, called a **cohort,** can also be compared to a control group.

Retrospective designs are those for which the events have already occurred. For example, teens between 13 and 17 years of age who get headaches at least once a month and teens of the same age who rarely get headaches can be interviewed and the results compared. The teens with the headaches are called the **cases** and the teens without constitute the control group. This design is retrospective because the headaches were present before the study was initiated. A useful way to distinguish between prospective and retrospective designs is to focus on the direction of inquiry. If the direction is forward, the design is prospective. If the inquiry follows a path backward through time, the design is retrospective.

✓ Who is eligible?

The eligibility criteria separate those who are eligible for participation in the survey from those who are not. Those who are eligible are the target of the survey. The survey's findings can be applied only to the target.

In Example 1.3 under Describing, the target of the survey's findings is men of differing ages, health, and social characteristics who have had surgery for prostrate cancer within the past 2 years. Men who have had chemotherapy or observational treatment or who have had surgery more than 2 years ago are not eligible for inclusion in the survey. Because they are not eligible, the survey's findings about quality of life may not be applicable to these men. A survey's findings are only applicable or **generalizable** to the eligible participants—assuming they participate—because eligible nonparticipants may differ from participants. Nonparticipants' views are likely not as strong, for example; the survey results may only or primarily be based on the views of advocates.

In Example 1.3 under Comparing (Design 1), the target is schoolchildren in Grades 1 through 6. These children are the only ones who are eligible for the survey. Those in kindergarten or Grade 7 are not the target, and the findings may not apply to them.

The criteria for inclusion in a survey come from two sources: the survey's target population and geographic and temporal proximity. Consider the illustrative inclusion criteria in Example 1.4.

EXAMPLE 1.4
Illustrative Inclusion Criteria:
Target Population, Geography, and Time

Target Population

For a survey of quality of life after prostate cancer surgery:
- Men who have had surgery
- Men over the age of 65 years

For a survey of young children's attitudes toward school:
- Children in Grades 1 through 6

Geographic Proximity

For a survey of quality of life after prostate cancer surgery:

- Must live within 30 miles of the Survey Center

For a survey of young children's attitudes toward school:

- Must attend one of five elementary schools in the district

Temporal Proximity

For a survey of quality of life after prostate cancer surgery:

- Must have had surgery within the past 2 years

For a survey of young children's attitudes toward school:

- Must have participated in one of two current experimental reading programs

Practical inclusion criteria are often set simply to conserve resources. If the survey's participants live close by, then the costs of travel to and from face-to-face interviews is less than if relatively long distances must be crossed. Local calls (for telephone interviews) cost less than long-distance calls. Choosing sites with potentially large numbers of eligible respondents can simplify the logistics of the survey: Instead of surveying participants in many sites, surveys can be administered in relatively few.

Surveys sometimes have exclusion criteria. These are special criteria that apply to potential respondents whose inclusion is likely to impair the actual functioning of the survey or skew its data. Consider some exclusion criteria presented in Example 1.5.

EXAMPLE 1.5
Illustrative Exclusion Criteria

- Not likely to complete the survey (including people with memory deficits, major psychiatric illness, or severe vision impairment for written surveys and hearing impairment for interviews)

- Unable to read, understand, or write the language of the survey

- An event that happens rarely (e.g., infrequent occurrences of a social, educational, or medical event)

- The presence of only some of the inclusion criteria (e.g., a person is the right age and lives in the geographic area being surveyed but is unable to read English)

2 Classification of Designs for Surveys

Surveys are systems for collecting information to describe, compare, and predict attitudes, opinions, values, knowledge, and behavior. An essential component of the system is the design or environmental arrangement in which data are collected, analyzed, and interpreted. Designs can be categorized as experimental or descriptive (sometimes called observational), as depicted below.

■ Experimental

Experimental designs are characterized by arranging to compare two or more groups, at least one of which is experimental. The other is a control (or comparison) group. An experimental group is given a new or untested, innovative program, intervention, or treatment. The control is given an alternative. A group is any collective unit. Sometimes, the unit is made up of individuals with a common experience, such as men who have had surgery, children who are in a reading program, or victims of violence. At other times, the unit is naturally occurring: a classroom, business, or hospital.

Concurrent controls in which participants are randomly assigned to groups. **Concurrent** means that each group is assembled at the same time. For example, when 10 of 20 schools are randomly assigned to an experimental group while, at the same time, 10 are assigned to a control, you have a randomized controlled trial or true experiment.

Concurrent controls in which participants are not randomly assigned to groups. These are called nonrandomized controlled trials, quasi-experiments, or nonequivalent controls.

Self-controls. These require premeasures and postmeasures and are called longitudinal or before-after designs.

Historical controls. These make use of data collected for participants in other surveys.

Combinations. These can consist of concurrent controls with or without pre- and postmeasures.

■ Descriptive (Observational)

Descriptive designs produce information on groups and phenomena that already exist. No new groups are created. Descriptive designs are also called observational by some surveyors.

Cross sections. These provide descriptive data at one fixed point in time. A survey of American voters' current choices is a cross-sectional survey.

Cohorts. These forward-looking designs provide data about changes in a specific population. Suppose a survey of the aspirations of athletes participating in the 1996 Olympics is given in 1996, 2000, and 2004. This is a cohort design, and the cohort is 1996 Olympians.

Case controls. These retrospective studies go back in time to help explain a current phenomenon. At least two groups are included. When first you survey the medical records of a sample of smokers and nonsmokers of the same age, health, and socioeconomic status and then compare the findings, you have used a case-control design.

Experiments

Surveys in experimental studies can be conducted any number of times before, during, and after a program or intervention. Surveys conducted beforehand serve many important purposes—for example, to select groups to participate in a program, check the support for a program, ensure comparability of groups, and provide a basis for monitoring change. The uses of surveys as premeasures are illustrated in Example 2.1.

EXAMPLE 2.1
Surveys as Premeasures

To Select Participants

A self-administered questionnaire was given to all parents. They were asked to specify the number of years of formal education they had completed in this or any other country. They were also asked to rate whether they would be willing to participate in one of two experimental programs to improve literacy. All parents who stated that they had completed fewer than 10 years of schooling and indicated that they were definitely willing were eligible to participate in the program.

To Check the Support for a Program

A mailed questionnaire is sent to all residents to find out if they will participate in a program to teach home-based injury prevention. The questionnaire asks residents if they are willing to be in a control group, if randomly selected.

To Ensure Comparability of Groups

Students are assigned to the experimental and control groups. A survey is made to compare ages and reading levels before the start of the experiment to check that the two groups are similar with respect to these two important variables.

To Provide a Basis for Monitoring Change

Prisoners who have been selected to participate in either the experimental group or the control group are interviewed using a standardized measure of rage. A similar survey will be given after the experimental group completes 6 months of an art therapy program.

Surveys can also begin during an intervention to measure change and after to measure the outcomes and impact of programs and interventions. These uses are illustrated in Example 2.2.

EXAMPLE 2.2
Surveys as Interim and Postmeasures

To Measure Change

People over 65 years of age who have been to the emergency room for a fall are interviewed within 2 weeks and then 3, 6, and 12 months later. The experimental group has received a geriatric assessment; the control group has not. The interviews are used to compare the two groups with respect to their social, psychological, and physical functioning.

To Measure Outcomes

Prisoners in an art therapy program are interviewed by two psychiatrists within 3 months of completing their course of study. The results are compared with those obtained from interviews with the control group.

To Measure Impact

Elderly people receiving and not receiving special geriatric assessments after a fall are surveyed 1, 3, and 5 years later. The purpose of the surveys at 3 and 5 years is to assess and compare impact over time.

CONCURRENT CONTROLS
AND RANDOM ASSIGNMENT

The groups in this design are created by first setting up eligibility criteria and then randomly assigning eligible "units" to one or more experimental and control groups. The groups can be observed and measured periodically. If the experimental group is observed to differ from the control group in a positive way on important outcome variables (e.g., satisfaction, quality of life, health, and knowledge), the experiment is considered successful within certain predefined limits. The units that are randomly assigned may be individuals (e.g., Persons A, B, C, etc. or Teachers A, B, C, etc.) or clusters of individuals (e.g., schools, residential blocks, hospitals).

Random assignment (sometimes called randomization or random allocation) means that individuals or clusters of individuals are assigned by chance to the experimental group or the control group. With random assignment, the occurrence of previous events has no value in predicting future events. The alternative to randomization is regulation of the allocation process so that you can predict group assignment, such as assigning people admitted to a hospital on odd days of the month to the experimental group and those admitted on even days to the control group.

Example 2.3 shows one method of randomly assigning units to an experimental group and control group. The example makes use of a table of random numbers. Tables like these are available in most standard statistics texts. Random numbers can also be generated by computer; the principles underlying the use of a table or list of numbers are the same.

EXAMPLE 2.3
Using a Table of Random Numbers
in Random Assignment to Groups

Twenty schools are eligible to participate in a trial of a program to improve public speaking skills. Ten are to be in the experimental group and 10 in the control group. If the experimental program is more effective in improving skills and confidence, it will be offered to the control schools free of charge.

The names of all 20 schools are placed on a list and assigned a number from 1 to 20 (e.g., John Adams School = 1; Robert Burns School = 2; Joseph Zermatt School = 20). Then, using a table of random numbers, the first 10 numbers that appear are chosen for the experimental group. Here is how the selection is made.

1. *Randomly identify the row.* Place 10 slips of paper in a jar. Select a number. Place the slip back in the jar and make a second selection. Return the slip to the jar. Suppose the first number is 3 and the second is 5. Using the table below, and starting with the first column, this corresponds to the third block and the fifth row of that block, or number 1 4 5 7 5.

2. *Randomly identify the column.* Select two numbered slips from the jar. Suppose you get a 2 and a 1. Go to the second block of columns and the first column beginning with 1: 1 9 7 0 4.

3. *Choose the experimental group.* Follow down to where 1 4 5 7 5 and the column with 1 9 7 0 4 intersect at 3 5 4 9 0.

4. Ten schools are needed for the sample. You must therefore select 10 numbers between 01 and 20. Moving down column 2, and starting with the numbers below 3 5 4 9 0, the first double-digit number you come to is 70. The numbers you find that meet your needs from that point on are 12, 20, 09, 02, 01, 13, 18, 03, 04, and 16. These are the schools that constitute the experimental group.

1 8 2 8 3	1 9 7 0 4^2	4 5 3 8 7	2 3 4 7 6	1 2 3 2 3	3 4 8 6 5
4 6 4 5 3	2 1 5 4 7	3 9 2 4 6	9 3 1 9 8	9 8 0 0 5	6 5 9 8 8
1 9 0 7 6	2 3 4 5 3	3 2 7 6 0	2 7 1 6 6	7 5 0 3 2	9 9 9 4 5
3 6 7 4 3	8 9 5 6 3	1 2 3 7 8	9 8 2 2 3	2 3 4 6 5	2 5 4 0 8
2 2 1 2 5	1 9 7 8 6	2 3 4 9 8	7 6 5 7 5	7 6 4 3 5	6 3 4 4 2
7 6 0 0 9	7 7 0 9 9	4 3 7 8 8	3 6 6 5 9	7 4 3 9 9	**0 3 4 3 2**
0 9 8 7 8	7 6 5 4 9	8 8 8 7 7	2 6 5 8 7	4 4 6 3 3	7 7 6 5 9
3 4 5 3 4	4 4 4 7 5	5 6 6 3 2	3 4 3 5 0	**0 1 7 6 8**	2 9 0 2 7
8 3 1 0 9	7 5 8 9 9	3 4 8 7 7	2 1 3 5 7	2 4 3 0 0	0 0 8 6 9
8 9 0 6 3	4 3 5 5 5	3 2 7 0 0	7 6 4 9 7	3 6 0 9 9	9 7 9 5 6
				9 4 6 5 6	3 4 6 8 9
0 9 8 8 7	6 7 7 7 0	6 9 9 7 5	5 4 4 6 5	**1 3 8 9 6**	**0 4 6 4 5**
2 3 2 8 0	3 4 5 7 2	9 9 4 4 3	9 8 7 6 5	3 4 9 7 8	4 2 8 8 0
9 3 8 5 6	2 3 0 9 0	2 2 2 5 7	6 7 4 0 0	2 3 5 8 0	2 4 3 7 6
2 1 2 5 6	5 0 8 6 3	5 6 9 3 4	7 0 9 9 3	3 4 7 6 5	3 0 9 9 6
1 4 5 7 5^1	3 5 4 9 0^3	2 3 6 4 5	2 2 1 7 9	3 5 7 8 8	3 7 6 0 0
2 3 2 7 6	7 0^4 8 7 0	**2 0 0 8 7**	6 6 6 6 5	7 8 8 7 6	5 8 0 0 7
8 7 5 3 0	4 5 7 3 8	**0 9 9 9 8**	4 5 3 9 7	4 7 5 0 0	3 4 8 7 5
0 0 7 9 1	3 2 1 6 4	9 7 6 6 5	2 7 5 8 9	9 0 0 8 7	**1 6 0 0 4**
9 9 0 0 3	3 2 5 6 7	**0 2 8 7 8**	3 8 6 0 2	**1 8 7 0 0**	2 3 4 5 5
1 4 3 6 7	6 4 9 9 9	7 8 4 5 3	4 0 0 7 8	5 3 7 2 7	2 8 7 5 9

Explanations:

Numbers in **bold** = Sample of 10, consisting of numbers, between 01 and 20.
1 = Two random choices of numbers in a jar yield 1 (column) and 5 (block).
2 = Two random choices of numbers in a jar yield 2 (column) and 1 (row).
3 = Intersection of superscripts 1 and 2.
4 = Start here to get the sample.

Designs that use concurrent controls and random assignment are also called randomized trials, randomized controlled trials, and true experiments. Example 2.4 gives two illustrations of their use with random assignment of individuals and of groups or clusters of individuals.

EXAMPLE 2.4
Experimental Studies
With Concurrent Controls
and Random Assignment to Groups

1. Comparing Medical and Surgical Therapy

Medical and surgical therapy were compared for patients with stable ischemic heart disease. (Ischemia refers to an insufficient supply of blood to the heart.) Over 4 years, half of all eligible patients in each of 10 medical centers were assigned at random to either the medical group or the surgical therapy group. The design can be illustrated as follows:

	Intervention	
Medical Center	Surgical Therapy	Medical Therapy
1 (100 patients)	50	50
2 (60 patients)	30	30
3 (120 patients)	60	60
4 (90 patients)	45	45
5 (100 patients)	50	50

$\rightarrow$

	Intervention	
6 (90 patients)	45	45
7 (70 patients)	35	35
8 (150 patients)	75	75
9 (150 patients)	75	75
10 (100 patients)	50	50

To find out about length of survival, patients were compared across medical centers (e.g., patients in Medical Center 1 compared to 2, 3, and so on; those in Medical Center 2 compared to 3, 4, and so on). Comparisons were also made between patients in surgical versus medical therapy regardless of medical center.

No differences were found in survival between and across medical centers and type of therapy. The surgical group had a higher quality of life, as manifested by relief of chest pain, scores on a functional status questionnaire, and reduced need for drug therapy.

2. Changes in Physician Compliance
With Practice Guidelines

The investigators used a randomized controlled experimental design to measure changes in individual physician compliance with blood transfusion guidelines following an experimental education program.

Pairs of teaching and community hospitals were randomly selected from all hospitals who met entry criteria (including rates of transfusion for selected procedures and diagnoses) within three health service areas. After one teaching hospital and one community hospital had been randomly selected from the entire list, a second hospital of each type was randomly identified from one of the other two health service areas to minimize the risk of experimental contamination due to physicians' practicing at multiple sites within a health service area. One surgical service in each matched pair was then randomly assigned to the study group and the other to the control group; within each hospital the medical service was assigned to the treatment group opposite from surgery. To measure changes in physician practices, compliance with guidelines for transfusion were analyzed for control and study physicians for 6 months before and 6 months following the experimental intervention.

Random selection is different from random assignment. In the second illustration, hospitals are randomly selected from all that are eligible. In some surveys, the entire eligible population is used; in others, only a sample is chosen. In most instances, probability sampling methods (like random sampling) are preferred. Probability sampling methods are those in which all eligible units have a known chance of selection.

Experimental designs using randomly constituted concurrent controls enable you to pinpoint and isolate an intervention's outcomes. They are the gold standard or the preferred designs when doing scientific research. With a large enough sample, these designs can control nearly all errors or **biases** from extraneous factors, including those that you do not know about and do not measure. In fact, randomization helps ensure that all groups have, on average, the same distribution of extraneous factors if the sample is large enough.

What are these errors or biases that lead to false conclusions? One of the most potentially damaging biases comes from the method of "selection." Selection bias is present when people who are initially different from one another and have differing prior risks for the outcome of interest are compared. Suppose a survey is conducted after Schools A and B participate in a comparative test of two approaches to reading. The survey results reveal that children in School A's reading program—the control—score higher (better) on an attitude-to-reading inventory than do children in School B—the experiment. Although the results may suggest a failed experiment, the two groups may have been different to begin with, even if they appeared to be similar. For instance, both schools' children may be alike in socioeconomic background, reading ability, and the competence of their reading teachers, but they may differ in other important ways. School B, for example, may have a better library, a friendlier librarian, more resources to spend on extra program reading, a social system that reinforces reading, and so on. To avoid bias from the selection process, the survey team should have randomly assigned students into experimental and control groups regardless of school.

Biases can arise from unrecognized as well as recognized characteristics of the individuals compared. Randomization is the only known way to control for unknown biases and to distribute them fairly.

Designs using concurrent controls and random assignment are complex. One issue that often arises concerns the appropriate unit of randomization. Sometimes, for practical purposes, clusters (schools, companies) rather than individuals are chosen for random assignment. You cannot assume, however, that the individuals forming the groups are comparable in the same way as they would have been had they been randomized as individuals.

Other potential sources of bias include failure to adequately monitor the randomization process and to follow uniform procedures across all groups. Training people and monitoring the quality of the randomization process are essential.

In some randomized studies, the participants and investigators do not know which group is the experimental one and which is the control: This is the double-blind experiment. When participants do not know but investigators do, this is called the blinded trial. In many surveys, it is often logistically or ethically difficult to "blind" participants, and this may bias the results. One approach is to "blind" the persons administering the survey, as illustrated in Example 2.5.

EXAMPLE 2.5
"Blinding" in Experimental Designs

Two groups of employees have completed 4-week training courses to improve selected business skills. Employees were randomly assigned either to the regular course or to the experimental course. A major objective of the experimental course is the improvement of negotiation skills; this topic is not covered in the regular course. At the end of the 4 weeks, all employees are interviewed by specially trained examiners who rate the employees' skills in setting up contracts for the company. Each employee is rated by two examiners, neither of whom knows whether the employee has participated in the experimental course or the regular course.

To maximize the applicability or generalizability of the results, experiments should probably be conducted in many places with a variety of participants over a number of years.

The technical and financial resources needed for concurrently randomized controlled experiments are high, but the potential for sound conclusions justifies the costs. However, despite their scientific virtues, experimental designs with concurrent controls do not automatically fit all survey situations. The designs are not equipped to provide data for quick decision making. Sometimes, randomization is not ethical if a group is to be denied an experimental intervention that has a reasonable chance of having more benefits than risks. Finally, you cannot assume that randomization alone guarantees that your survey will produce "truth." At the minimum, valid survey findings depend on clearly stated purposes, justified samples, accurate data collection, and appropriate statistical analysis and interpretation.

Guidelines for Experimental Designs Involving Randomly Assigned Concurrent Controls

The following guidelines are recommended when using survey designs with concurrent controls and random assignment:

1. Define the target population.

2. Choose inclusion and exclusion criteria that are theoretically appropriate and practical.

3. If a sample of eligible participants is to be surveyed, use probability sampling (like random sampling) to select it.

4. Use a table of random numbers, computer-generated list, or other means to ensure that the experimental and control groups are randomly constituted.

5. Monitor the effects of potential errors from inadequate implementation of randomization, lack of uniform experimental and control programs, and discovery by participants that they are in the experimental (or control) group.

6. Decide in advance of the survey how you will handle the ethical implications of denying a potentially beneficial intervention to the control group.

7. Be certain that you have the resources to implement and monitor the logistics of a randomized trial or true experiment.

8. Do not rest after you have implemented the design: Check to see that the data collection and analysis methods are equally valid.

CONCURRENT CONTROLS BUT NO RANDOM ASSIGNMENT

Nonrandomized, concurrent controls (quasi-experimental designs) come about when you have at least two already existing groups, one of which is designated experimental (Example 2.6).

EXAMPLE 2.6
Concurrent Controls
but No Random Assignment

1. Studies have shown that children who move many times tend to miss more schooling and are more at risk for significant behavioral problems than are children with stable addresses. Teachers, counselors, and nurses in three schools participated in a program to teach them to survey children who have moved frequently. The purpose of the survey was to guide school and health professionals to anticipate potential problems and, when necessary, to make effective referrals. Two schools were chosen to act as controls. In the control schools, no special intervention was introduced. At the end of 3 years, children whose families met relocation criteria were surveyed in both sets of schools.

2. A nonrandomized trial was used to test a program to reduce the use of antipsychotic drugs in nursing homes. The program was based on behavioral techniques to manage behavior problems and encourage gradual antipsychotic drug withdrawal. Two rural community nursing homes with elevated antipsychotic use were in the experimental group, and two comparable homes were selected as concurrent controls. Residents in both groups of homes had comparable demographic characteristics and functional status, and each group had a baseline rate of 29 days of antipsychotic use per 100 days of nursing home residence.

Concurrent control designs without randomization are easier to implement than experimental designs with randomization. Perhaps their feasibility accounts for the fact that they may be the oldest design, as illustrated in Example 2.7, taken from the Bible (King James version), Daniel 1:11-15.

EXAMPLE 2.7
Concurrent Controls
Without Random Assignment
—The Book of Daniel—

Then Daniel said to Melzar, . . . Prove thy servants, I beseech thee, ten days; and let them give us pulse [seeds from peas and beans] to eat, and water to drink. Then let our countenances be looked upon before thee, and the countenance of the children that eat of the portion of the king's meat: and as thou seest, deal with thy servants.

So he consented to them in this matter, and proved them ten days. And at the end of ten days their countenances appeared fairer and fatter in flesh than all the children which did eat the portion of the king's meat. Thus Melzar took away the portion of their meat, and the wine that they should drink; and gave them pulse.

Random assignment is sometimes infeasible, as it would have been in the case of the "children" who ate the king's meat and those who ate pulse. As another example, suppose you wanted to survey prisoners who participated in a 3-year art therapy program. Each year, 10 prisoners in three facilities will participate in the program; three other facilities have agreed to serve as the control. The primary purpose of the program is to improve prisoners' ability to cope with potentially violent situations by using art as one outlet for emotions like rage and fear. By the end of the third year, 90 prisoners will have participated. In this example, random assignment would probably be logistically complicated and costly, and so you might look for an alternative design.

The use of nonrandomly selected controls, although relatively practical, increases the likelihood that external factors will bias a survey's results. A typical bias associated with nonrandom assignment is selection or membership bias.

Membership bias refers to characteristics that members of groups share simply because they are in the group. The idea is that preexisting groups are usually not assembled haphazardly: they come together precisely because they share similar values, attitudes, behavior, or social and health status. Examples of groups with shared characteristics are people who live in the same neighborhood (they are likely to be similar in their incomes), children who have the same teacher (they may share similar abilities), patients who see a particular physician (they may have a particular medical problem), prisoners at a minimum security facility (they have committed a certain level of crime), and prisoners at a maximum security facility (they also have committed a certain level of crime but it differs from that of prisoners in a minimum security facility). Only random assignment can guarantee that two groups are equivalent from the point of view of all variables that may influence a survey's outcomes.

Membership bias can seriously challenge a survey's accuracy. When you use concurrent controls without random assignment, you should administer a premeasure to determine the equivalence of the groups at the start or at **baseline** on potentially important characteristics. In Example 2.6, the second illustration does this by reporting that residents in each of the two homes had comparable demographic characteristics, functional status, and use of antipsychotics.

The comparability of groups at baseline is often discussed in a table. Example 2.8 shows how this is done. In the example, the characteristics of two concurrent, nonrandomly assigned groups are compared. The groups are participants in a program to teach parenting to young women.

EXAMPLE 2.8
Comparing Baseline
Characteristics in a Table

Characteristics	Experimental ($n = 125$)	Control ($n = 147$)
Infant gender, % male	40.0	42.0
Birthweight, ≤1,500 g, %	24.8	23.8
Maternal age, year, %[a]		
15 - 17	29.6	9.5
18 - 19	32.8	18.4
20 - 24	37.6	72.1
Frequent moving, %	24.8	23.8

a. $p < .001$ for those in the experimental compared with those in the control. (For more about the uses of p in tests of significance, see **How to Analyze Survey Data, Vol. 8 in this series.**)

You can see from the table that the participants in the program differ in their age. If age is an important factor for success in the program, the differences that preexist in the two groups pose a serious problem in this design. A variable that is more likely to be present in one group of subjects than in another or that is related to the outcome of interest and confuses or confounds the results is called a **confounding variable**.

Statistical methods, like analysis of covariance (ANCOVA) or the Mantel-Haenzel chi-square, are available to "control" for the influence of confounding variables when random assignment is not used. As a rule, however, it is better to control for confounders before collecting survey data—that is, as part of design and sampling—than afterward during analysis.

SELF-CONTROLS

A design with self-controls uses a group of participants to serve as its own comparison. Suppose, for example, students were surveyed three times: at the beginning of the year to find out their attitudes toward community service, immediately after their participation in a 1-year course to find out the extent to which their attitudes changed, and at the end of 2 years to ascertain if the change is sustained. This three-measurement strategy describes a design using the students as their own control. In the example, the survey measures the students once before and twice after the intervention (a new course). Designs of this type are also called before-and-after or pretest-posttest designs.

Self-controlled survey designs are prone to several biases. Participants may become excited about taking part in an experiment; they may mature physically, emotionally, and intellectually; or historical events can intervene. For example, suppose a survey reveals that the students in a 2-year test of a school-based intervention acquire important attitudes and behaviors and retain them over time. This desirable result may be due to the new course or to the characteristics of the students who, from the start, may have been motivated to learn and have become even more excited by being in an experimental program. Another possibility is that over the 2-year inter-vention period students may have matured intellectually, and this development, rather than the program, is responsible for the learning. Also, historical or external events may have occurred to cloud the effects of the new course. For example, suppose that during the year an inspired teacher gives several stimulating lectures to the students. The students' outstand-ing performance on subsequent tests may be due as much or more to the lectures as to the program.

The soundness of self-controlled designs is dependent on the appropriateness of the number and timing of measurements. To check retention of learning, should students be tested once? Twice? At what intervals? A program might be considered ineffective just because data were presented too soon for the hoped-for outcomes to occur.

On their own, self-controlled designs are relatively weak. The addition of a control group can strengthen them, as illustrated in Example 2.9.

EXAMPLE 2.9
Combined Self-Control and
Concurrent Control Design to Evaluate
the Impact of Education and Legislation
on Children's Use of Bicycle Helmets

An anonymous questionnaire regarding use of bicycle helmets was sent twice to nearly 3,000 children in three counties. The first mailing took place 3 months before an educational campaign in County 1 and 3 months before the passage of legislation requiring helmets and an education campaign in County 2. The second mailing took place 9 months after completion of the education and combined education-legislation. Two surveys (9 months apart) were also conducted in County 3, the control. County 3 had neither education nor legislation pertaining to the use of bicycle helmets. The table below summarizes the results.

Percentage of Children
Reporting Use "Always" or "Usually"

	Before Intervention	After Intervention
County 1: Education only	8	13*
County 2: Education and legislation	11	37**
County 3: No intervention	7	8

NOTE: The percentages are small and do not add up to 100% because they represent only the proportion of children answering "always" or "usually." Other responses, such as "rarely," constituted the other choices.

*$p < .01$.

$p < .0001$ (for more about p values, see **How to Analyze Survey Data, Vol. 8 in this series).

FINDINGS

The proportion of children who reported that they "always" or "usually" wore a helmet increased significantly ($p < .0001$) from 11% before to 37% in County 2 (education and legislation) and 8% before to 13% ($p < .01$) in County 1 (education only). The increase of 1% in County 3 was not significant.

Education alone and education combined with legislation were relatively effective: either one or both increase the proportion of children reporting helmet use. The education may have taught children to give the socially acceptable responses on the survey, but single education programs alone have not usually encouraged children to give desirable responses to survey questions. The fact that the control group did not improve suggests that Counties 1 and 2's efforts were responsible for the improvements. The addition of the control group adds credibility to the survey results.

HISTORICAL CONTROLS

Surveys that use historical controls rely on data that are available from some other, recorded, source. These data substitute for the data that would come from a concurrent control.

Historical controls include established norms such as scores on standardized tests like the SATs and the MCATs, the results of other surveys conducted with similar groups of people, and vital statistics like birth and death rates. Historical controls are convenient; their main source of bias is the potential lack of comparability between the group on whom the data were originally collected and the group of concern in the survey.

Suppose you were concerned with the proportion of children from birth through age 7 in your county who have a regular source of medical care. You might ask: How do the children in my county, many of whom are poor, compare to other children in the United States with respect to having a regular source of care?

To answer this question, you would follow these four steps:

- Survey the children in your county.

- Find out if comparison data pertaining to U.S. children are available and feasible to obtain.

A good place to find out what is available is to start with city, state, or national health agencies that are responsible for collecting social and health statistics. Another option is to check public and university libraries to find out the type of statistical information they have available to the public and how you get access to it.

■ If information is available and feasible to obtain, use it to create a chart to use as a worksheet to record the information you need for your survey.

Suppose you find useful data from the 1988 U.S. National Health Interview Survey of Child Health. Then you can prepare a chart like the following:

	Under Age 1 (%)	1 - 4 Years (%)	5 - 7 Years (%)
All children			
Family income Under $10,000			
$10,000 - $24,999			
$25,000 - $39,999			
$40,000 or more			

■ Enter your own survey data into the table and apply the appropriate statistical techniques (for recommended statistical methods to use when comparing percentages, see **How to Analyze Survey Data,** Vol. 8 in this series). Consider the following hypothetical example.

Percentage of Children in Hypothetical County (HC) and the United States (US) With a Regular Source of Medical Care

	Under Age 1 (%)		1 - 4 Years (%)		5 - 7 Years (%)	
	HC	US	HC	US	HC	US
All children	89.9	87.2	92.3	84.5	89.5	90.8
Family income under $10,000	83.7	82.4	86.7	88.3	87.6	88.8
$10,000 - $24,999	95.7	92.7	91.3	92.5	88.5	88.3
$25,000 - $39,999	95.3	91.3	96.1	94.6	90.1	89.4
$40,000 or more	95.3	94.4	97.7	96.5	96.7	94.7

SOURCE: Statistics for the U.S. portion obtained from the 1989 U.S. National Interview Survey of Child Health.

WARNING

When interpreting the data in the table, remember that they were collected in 1988, and many changes in health care may have occurred since then.

COMBINATIONS

Experimental designs compare one or more groups. The groups may be surveyed before, during, and after any intervention. Variations on these basic elements are possible. A common design in medical studies is the crossover. In the cross-over, one group is assigned to the experimental group and the other to the control. After a period of time, the experimental and control groups are withdrawn for a washout period. During this time, no treatment is given. The groups are then given the alternative treatment: The first group now becomes the control and the second group the experimental.

The Solomon four-group design is one that combines the randomized control trial with some groups receiving pre- and postmeasures and some receiving only postmeasures. This is illustrated in Example 2.10.

EXAMPLE 2.10
The Solomon Four-Group Design

Group 1	Premeasure	Program	Postmeasure
Group 2	Premeasure		Postmeasure
Group 3		Program	Postmeasure
Group 4			Postmeasure

In this example, Groups 1 and 3 participated in a new program, but Groups 2 and 4 did not. Suppose the new program aimed to improve employees' awareness of health hazards at their place of work. Using the four-group design (and assuming an effective program), the survey should find the following:

1. In Group 1, awareness on the postmeasure should be greater than on the premeasure.

2. More awareness should be observed in Group 1 than in Group 2.

3. Group 3's postmeasure should show more awareness than Group 2's premeasure.

4. Group 3's postmeasure should show more awareness than Group 4's postmeasure.

This design is a randomized controlled trial, and it incorporates self- and concurrent controls. The use of random and nonrandom assignment in the same study is illustrated in Example 2.11.

EXAMPLE 2.11
Random and Nonrandom
Assignment in a Single Study

Four of 14 eligible participating high schools were grouped into two pairs of demographically similar schools. [This is nonrandom assignment.] A 30% sample of 9th-grade classrooms (16 classrooms totaling 430 students) in the first member of the two pairs of schools was selected at random from the total 9th-grade general education enrollment in these two schools to receive a special AIDS-preventive curriculum in the first semester of the academic year. A 20% random sample of 9th-grade classrooms (10 classrooms totaling 251 students) in the second member of the two pairs served as the comparison or control group and received no formal AIDS curriculum at school that semester. Similarly, a 30% sample of 11th-grade classrooms (13 classrooms totaling 309 students) in the second member of the two pairs of schools was selected at random from the total 11th-grade general education enrollment in these two schools to receive the special prevention curriculum in the second semester of the same academic year, and a 20% random sample of 11th-grade classrooms (13 classrooms totaling 326 students) in the first member of the two pairs served as the comparison or control group. A higher proportion of intervention than comparison students was sampled so that more students would be exposed to the special curriculum. The study design also ensured that none of the four participating high schools would be denied implementation of the special curriculum at Grade 9 or 11.

Descriptions (or Observations)

CROSS-SECTIONAL DESIGNS

Cross-sectional designs result in a portrait of one or many groups at one point in time. These designs are used frequently with standard survey-based measurement (that is, mail and self-administered questionnaires and face-to-face and telephone interviews) and are themselves sometimes called survey designs. Example 2.12 gives six illustrative uses of survey-based measurement and cross-sectional designs.

EXAMPLE 2.12
Surveys and Cross-Sectional Designs

1. A face-to-face interview with refugees to find out their immediate fears and aspirations

2. A questionnaire mailed to consumers to find out perceptions of the quality of the goods and services received when ordering by catalogue

3. A telephone interview with patients to find out what has happened since their last surgery

4. A mailed survey with telephone follow-up to find out if residents are prepared properly for emergencies like fire, flood, and earthquake

5. An interview combined with observations to determine how many children use bicycle helmets over a 2-week period

6. Interviews conducted over 1 month to find out teens' views of the quality of their education in 10 schools

Cross-sectional designs provide a portrait of a group during one time period, now or in the past. Sometimes they rely on more than one type of survey measure. In Example 2.12, mail and telephone surveys are used to find out about residents' emergency preparedness, and observations and interviews are combined for data on helmet use among children.

A cross-sectional design that uses random or probability samples is much more likely to have a study population that is **representative** of the target population. For example, suppose you want to conduct a cross-sectional survey about the joys of jogging as perceived by men over 45 years of age. A random sample of 100 men over 45 who jog three or more times each week is more likely to be representative of jogging men over 45 than a selection of the first 100 jogging men who use the Sports Medicine Clinic. Men who come to the clinic may have more injuries, be more "sportsminded," and have more time to visit clinics than a random sample. These characteristics (and others that cannot be anticipated) can affect the applicability of the survey's results to the target: men over 45 years who jog three or more times each week.

Although the result of a cross-sectional design is a group portrait at one point in time, the survey itself may take several weeks or even months to complete. In Example 2.12, to find out about children's use of helmets takes 2 weeks and to uncover teens' views requires 1 month. The longer periods occur with larger samples and when follow-ups are necessary. With very large groups and long periods of data collection, you must define the period to be covered by the survey. For example, consider conducting a year-long survey of the lifestyles of 10,000 people. Over the 12-month period, the very first people surveyed may lose or gain jobs; this factor may influence their lifestyle. Also, during the year, events such as economic recessions and political upheaval may affect people's lifestyles.

To help ensure a uniform set of responses, follow the example of the 1990 U.S. Census and include a time limit, as illustrated in Example 2.13.

EXAMPLE 2.13
Using Time Limits in Surveys

1990 U.S. Census Question

List on the numbered line below the name of each person living here on *Sunday, April 1*, including all persons staying here who have no other home. If EVERYONE at this address is staying here temporarily and usually lives somewhere else, follow the instructions given below.

COHORT DESIGNS

A cohort is a group of people who have something in common and who remain part of the group over an extended period of time. In public health research, cohort studies are used to investigate the risk factors for a disease and the disease's cause, incidence, natural history, and prognosis. They are prospective designs because the direction of inquiry is forward. Cohort designs require two groups: the cohort and the control. They ask "What will happen?" For example, a cohort design may be used in a study to follow the consequences of living with asthma over a 10-year period. To implement the design, people with and without asthma are surveyed and the results compared. (Without a control group, the design is termed a case series.)

Cohort designs sometimes make use of archival data, that is, data from medical, legal, and financial records. For example, in a study of the consequences of living with asthma (and assuming access to complete and accurate records), you might review the medical records of people who developed asthma 10 years ago and follow their recorded progress over time. Notice that, although you are using historical data (the events already happened and are recorded), the direction of inquiry is forward and thus is a prospective design.

Cohorts come in two varieties. Type A focuses on the same population each time survey data are collected, although the samples may be different. Type B, sometimes called a panel study, focuses on the same sample.

- Type A Cohorts: *Different samples from the same population.* With this type of cohort design, you can conduct five surveys of the lifestyles of the class of 1994 over a period of 10 years. Every 2 years, you will draw a sample of 1994 graduates. In this way, some graduates may be asked to complete all five surveys; others will not be chosen to participate at all. Among the most famous cohort studies is the Framingham, Massachusetts, study of cardiovascular disease begun in 1948 to investigate factors associated with heart disease. Over 6,000 people in Framingham agreed to participate in follow-up interviews and physical examinations every 2 years. Some of the children of the original cohort are also being studied.

■ Type B Cohorts: *Same samples.* Type B cohorts or panels are used during elections. Preferences for candidates and views on issues are monitored over time, and the characteristics of supporters and nonsupporters are compared. Type B cohorts are also used to study social, intellectual, and health development in infants and children, as illustrated in Example 2.14.

EXAMPLE 2.14
Cohort Design to Study
Development in Infants and Children

A cohort of infants born in five medical centers was selected for the study if they weighed no more than 2,500 grams (5.5 pounds), were no more than 37 weeks gestational age (the age from conception to birth), and were 40 weeks postconceptual age from January to October. Infants with health or congenital conditions were excluded from the study as were infants whose mothers were under 15 years of age or 25 years or older, could not communicate in English, or were diagnosed with psychiatric illness or alcohol or other drug abuse.

Surveys and assessments were made when each infant was 40 weeks old and 4, 8, 12, 18, 24, 30, and 36 months gestational age. The table below compares the development scores of the infant cohort at 3 years of age.

Characteristic	Intelligence Scores Mean (SD)[a]	Number of Behavior Problems Mean (SD)	Health Rating Index Mean (SD)
Infant gender			
Male	81.0 (17.7)	30.2 (13.5)**	26.7 (5.2)
Female	81.3 (14.6)	25.8 (11.3)	27.7 (4.4)
Birth weight (grams)			
More than 1,500	79.9 (14.9)	29.5 (12.7)	26.4 (5.3)
Less than 1,500	81.6 (16.3)	27.1 (12.3)	27.5 (4.6)
Maternal age (years)			
15 - 17	78.2 (12.0)	29.8 (12.7)	27.0 (4.1)
18 - 19	81.6 (13.3)	29.6 (12.9)	27.4 (5.1)
20 - 24	81.9 (18.0)	26.2 (12.0)	27.3 (4.9)
Family in poverty			
Yes	77.3 (14.2)*	29.5 (13.4)**	27.1 (5.1)
No	87.6 (16.8)	25.0 (10.4)	27.1 (5.1)
Frequent moving			
Yes	80.2 (13.8)	32.0 (13.9)**	27.4 (4.1)
No	81.5 (16.7)	26.3 (11.6)	27.2 (5.0)

a. SD = standard deviation, which is a measure of dispersion or spread around the mean or average.

*$p < .01$—intelligence scores: yes poverty versus no.

**$p < .001$—behavior problems: males versus females; yes poverty versus no; yes moving versus no.

In this cohort of infants, males had significantly more behavior problems than did females. Infants in poverty had significantly lower intelligence scores and more behavior problems. Children who moved frequently had significantly more behavior problems.

Cohort studies sometimes use more than one group. For example, suppose you want to find out if jogging leads to osteoarthritis, a painful condition that affects weight-bearing joints like the knees and lumbar spine. You might take a group of men over 50 years of age, divide them into a "runners" group and a "nonrunners" group, and collect baseline data. After a period of time, say, 5 years, you can measure if any differences exist in the development or progression of the disorder.

Cohort studies can be expensive because they are longitudinal, requiring measurement at several points in time. They are subject to biases from selection. (Those who are chosen and willing to participate may be inherently different from the remainder of the cohort who are not willing.) Type B cohorts— panels—are also prone to loss of data, with incomplete information collected on important variables or no data collected at all after a certain point in time.

CASE-CONTROL DESIGNS

Case-control designs are retrospective. They are used to help explain why a phenomenon currently exists by comparing two groups, one of which is involved in the phenomenon. For example, a case-control design might be used to help understand the social, demographic, and attitudinal variables that distinguish people with frequent headaches from those without.

The cases in case-control designs are individuals who have been chosen on the basis of some characteristic or outcome (such as frequent headaches). The controls are individuals without the characteristic or outcome. The histories of both groups are analyzed and compared in an attempt to uncover one or more characteristics that are present in the cases but not in the controls.

How can you avoid having one group decidedly different from the other, say, older or smarter? **Matching** is often used in case-control designs to guard against confounding variables. For example, in the case-control study of people with frequent headaches, the two groups selected should be similar in age, education, and duration and severity of the headaches. Example 2.15 illustrates the use of case-control designs in surveys.

EXAMPLE 2.15
A Case-Control Design

The National Teacher Corps was created in 1962 to train highly qualified individuals to enter the teaching profession. For the Corps' 30th anniversary, a study was conducted to find out why some people continued to teach and others had changed careers. People who chose teaching as their career (the cases) were matched to the controls on age, gender, educational background, and other social and demographic variables. The controls consisted of people who taught for 2 or fewer years after completion of the Corps' training program.

Eligible participants were mailed a 100-item questionnaire that asked for information on perceptions of current job satisfaction, willingness to take risks, religious preferences, and living arrangements. The academic records of the two groups were also compared before and after participation in the Corps.

Case-control designs are often used by epidemiologists and other health workers to provide insight into the causes and consequences of disease. These designs are generally less time consuming and expensive than cohorts. Matching is intuitively appealing and feasible.

Case-control designs have their problems, however. First, the groups of cases and controls are selected from two separate populations. Because of this, you cannot be certain that the groups are comparable with respect to extraneous factors like motivation, cultural beliefs, and other expectations (some of which you may not know). Also, the data for case-control designs are historical, often coming from inadequate or incomplete records. Data are sometimes obtained by asking people to recall past events and habits. Memory is often unreliable, however, and this introduces mistakes into the survey's data.

Internal and External Validity

A design with external validity produces results that apply to the survey's target population. An externally valid survey of the preferences of airline passengers over 45 years of age means that the findings apply to all airline passengers of that age.

A design is internally valid if it is free from nonrandom error or bias. A study design must be internally valid to be externally valid and to produce accurate findings. To ensure internal validity, you must be aware of and avoid the common risks given in the following checklist.

Internal Invalidity:
Checklist of Risks to Avoid

✓ Maturation.

Maturation refers to changes within individuals that result from natural, biological, or psychological development. For example, in a 5-year study of a preventive health education program for high school students, the students may mature intellectually and emotionally, and this new maturity may be more important than the program in producing changes in health behavior.

✓ Selection.

Selection refers to how people were chosen for the survey and, if they participate in an experiment, how they were assigned to groups. To avoid selection bias, every eligible person or unit should have an equal, nonzero chance of being included.

✓ History.

Historical events may occur that can bias the study's results. For example, suppose a national campaign has been created to encourage people to make use of preventive health care services. If a change in health insurance laws favoring reimbursement for preventive health care occurs at the same time as the campaign, it may be difficult to separate the effects of the campaign from the effects of increased access to care created by more favorable reimbursement for health care providers.

✓ **Instrumentation.**

Unless the measures used to collect data are dependable, you cannot be sure that the findings are accurate. For example, in a before-after design, an easier postmeasure than premeasure will erroneously favor an intervention. Also, untrained but lenient observers or test administrators can rule in favor of an intervention's effectiveness, whereas untrained but harsh observers or test administrators can rule against it.

✓ **Statistical regression.**

Suppose people are chosen for an intervention to foster tolerance. The basis for selection, say, was their extreme views, as measured by a survey. A second administration of the survey (without any intervention) may appear to suggest that the views were somehow softened, but in fact, the results may be a statistical artifact. This is called regression toward the mean and is ubiquitous. Regression effects are the result of factors such as an imperfect test-retest correlation.

✓ **Attrition.**

Attrition is another word for loss of data such as occurs when participants do not complete all or parts of a survey. People may not complete their surveys because they move away, become ill or bored with participation, and so on. Sometimes, participants who continue to provide complete survey data throughout a long study are different from those who do not.

Risks to external validity are most often the consequence of the way in which participants or respondents are selected and assigned. For example, respondents in an experimental situation may answer questions atypically because they know they are in a special experiment; this is called the "Hawthorne" effect. External validity is also a risk just because respondents are tested, surveyed, or observed. They may become alert to the kinds of behaviors that are expected or favored. Sources of external invalidity to avoid are given in the following checklist.

External Invalidity:
Checklist of Risks to Avoid

✓ Reactive effects of testing.

A premeasure can sensitize participants to the aims of an intervention. Suppose two groups of junior high school students are eligible to participate in a program to teach ethics. The first group is surveyed regarding its perspectives on selected ethics issues and then shown a film about young people from different backgrounds faced with ethical dilemmas. The second group of students is just shown the film. It would not be surprising if the first group performed better on a postmeasure if only because the group was sensitized to the purpose of the movie by the questions on the premeasure.

✓ **Interactive effects of selection.**

This occurs when an intervention and the participants are a unique mixture: one that may not be found elsewhere. Suppose a school volunteers to participate in an experimental program to improve the quality of students' leisure time activities. The characteristics of the school (some of which may be related to the fact that it volunteered for the experiment) may interact with the program so that the two together are unique; the particular blend of school and intervention can limit the applicability of the findings.

✓ **Reactive effects of innovation.**

Sometimes, the environment of an experiment is so artificial that all who participate are aware that something special is going on and behave uncharacteristically.

✓ **Multiple program interference.**

It is sometimes difficult to isolate the effects of an experimental intervention because of the possibility that participants are in other complementary activities or programs.

Example 2.16 illustrates how internal and external validity are affected in two different designs.

EXAMPLE 2.16
How the Choice of Design May
Affect Internal and External Validity

Concurrent Controls Without Random Assignment

Description: The Food Allergy Mediation Alliance (FAMA) is a year-long program for people with food allergies. Eligible people can enroll in one of two variations of the program. To find out if participants are satisfied with the quality of the program, both groups complete an in-depth questionnaire at the end of the year, and the results are compared.

Comment: The internal validity is potentially marred by the fact that the participants in the groups may be different from one another at the beginning of the program. More severely allergic persons may choose one program over the other, for example. Also, because of initial differences, the attrition rate may be affected. The failure to create randomly constituted groups will jeopardize the study's external validity by the interactive effects of selection.

Concurrent Controls With Randomization

Description: The Make-A-Wish Trust commissioned an evaluation of three different interventions for visually impaired children. Eligible children were randomly assigned to one of the three interventions, baseline data were collected, and a 3-year investigation was made of effectiveness and efficiency. At the end of the 3 years, the children were examined to determine their functioning on a number of variables including school performance and behavior at home and at school. The children were also interviewed extensively throughout the study. The results of the examinations and interviews were compared with those obtained from a study of visually impaired children who had participated in a similar experiment in another part of the country.

Comment: This design is internally valid. Because children were randomly assigned to each intervention, any sources of change that might compete with the intervention's impact will affect all three groups equally. To improve external validity, the findings from a study of other children will be compared with those from the Make-A-Wish Trust. This additional comparison does not guarantee that the results will hold for a third group of children. Another consideration is that school administrators and staff may not spend as much money as usual because they know the study involves studying efficiency (reactive effects of innovation). Finally, we do not know if and how baseline data collection affected children's performance and interviews (interaction between testing and the intervention).

Eight Commonly Used Study Designs

Design	Benefits	Risks	Potential for Bias or Invalidity
Concurrent controls and random assignment (randomized controlled or control trial; true experiment)	If properly conducted, can establish the extent to which a program caused its outcomes	Proper implementation requires resources and methodologic expertise	*Internal validity:* Excellent *External validity:* If a premeasure is given, possibility of reactive effects of testing; reactive effects of innovation
Concurrent controls without randomization (quasi-experimental)	Easier to implement than a randomized control trial	A wide range of potential biases may occur because, without an equal chance of selection, participants in the program may be systematically different from those in the control group	*Internal validity:* Selection, attrition, cannot be sure about maturation *External validity:* Interactive effects of selection
Self-controls (pretest-posttest)	Relatively easy to implement logistically Provides data on change	Must be certain that measurements are appropriately timed Without a control group, you cannot tell if effects are also present in other groups	*Internal validity:* Maturation, history, instrumentation, and interaction of selection with other factors; regression a possibility *External validity:* Interaction of selection, reactive effects of testing, and possibly reactive effects of innovation

$\rightarrow$

Design	Benefits	Risks	Potential for Bias or Invalidity
Historical controls	Easy to implement; unobtrusive	Must make sure that "normative" comparison data are applicable to participants	*Internal validity:* Selection, attrition, interaction of selection with other factors; cannot be sure about maturation *External validity:* Interactive effects of selection
Solomon four-group	Rigorous design that permits inferences about causes Guards against the effects of the premeasure on subsequent performance	Need to have enough participants to constitute four groups Expensive to implement	*Internal validity:* Excellent *External validity:* Possibility of interaction of selection and reactive effects of innovation
Cross-sectional	Provides baseline information on survey participants and descriptive information about the intervention	Offers a picture of participants and program at one point in time	*Internal validity:* If survey is lengthy, then history and maturation; selection, attrition *External validity:* Only if sample is representative are findings applicable to population

Design	Benefits	Risks	Potential for Bias or Invalidity
Cohort	Provides longitudinal or follow-up information	Can be expensive because they are relatively long-term studies Participants who are available over time may differ in important ways from those who are not	*Internal validity:* Maturation, history, instrumentation, and interaction of selection with other factors; regression a possibility *External validity:* Interaction of selection and the intervention; reactive effects of testing and possibly reaction to innovation
Case-control	Can provide insights into the causes and consequences of disease Generally less time-consuming and expensive than cohorts	The compared groups of cases and controls are selected from two separate populations and you cannot be certain that the groups are comparable with respect to extraneous factors (some of which you may not know) Data often come from records, which may be inadequate or incomplete	*Internal validity:* Selection, attrition, interaction of selection with other factors; cannot be sure about maturation *External validity:* Interactive effects of selection and intervention

Exercises

1. A team of experts spent 5 days interviewing all part-time employees. Which of the following study designs is being used? *Circle one choice.*

Cross-sectional	1
Self-control	2
Concurrent controls without randomization	3
Historical controls	4

2. The goals and aspirations of the 1990 graduates of the three major types of high schools (arts and sciences, vocational, and technical) are followed over 10 years. Each year, the 1990 graduates are interviewed and filmed. Which of the following study designs is being used? *Circle one choice.*

Case-control	1
Cohort	2
Self-control	3
Quasi-experiment	4

3. What are the threats to internal and external validity of these two survey designs?

    a. The ABC Sales Company experimented with a program to help minorities and women get and keep higher-paying jobs. Human resources staff interviewed all employees and examined records to collect data on the program's effectiveness.

    b. An evaluation of three 1-month rehabilitation programs for patients with heart disease was conducted. Patients were free to select the program of their choice. The evaluation team collected information on whether patients' knowledge of their condition and self-confidence had improved. To answer the question, patients in each program were surveyed before and after program participation.

ANSWERS

1. Cross-sectional

2. Cohort

3. a: Internal validity may be affected by historical events, such as new legislation, that may occur at the same time as the program; these events may be more influential than the program. Also, employees may change job ranks naturally over time. Finally, the people who remain employed and in the program may be inherently different (e.g., more skilled) from others who are fired or move away. External validity may be influenced by the reactive effects of innovation.

   b: Selection is a possible risk to internal validity because participants in the two groups may have been different from one another at the beginning of the program. For example, healthier people may choose one program over the other. Also, attrition may be different between the two groups. The external validity is limited by a number of factors including the reactive effects of innovation, interactive effects of selection, and possibly multiple program interference.

Suggested Readings

Brett, A., & Grodin, M. (1991). Ethical aspects of human experimentation in health services research. *Journal of the American Medical Association, 265*, 1854-1857.

This article is an extremely important one because of its implications for experimental designs. The "participants" in experiments and their surveys are human, so the requirements of informed consent apply as do concepts like respect for privacy.

Campbell, D. T., & Stanley, J. C. (1963). *Experimental and quasi-experimental designs for research.* Chicago: Rand McNally.

The classic book on differing research designs. "Threats" to internal and external validity are described in detail. Issues pertaining to generalizability and how to get at "truth" are important reading.

Dawson-Saunders, B., & Trapp, R. G. (1990). *Basic and clinical biostatistics.* East Norwalk, CT: Appleton & Lange.

Chapter 2 discusses study designs in medical research and their advantages and disadvantages. Examples are given of the use of the designs.

71

Fink, A. (1993). *Evaluation fundamentals: Guiding health programs, research, and policy.* Newbury Park, CA: Sage.

Chapter 3 covers the range of designs that are useful in program evaluations. The Evaluation Design Report is discussed as are the roles of independent variables in design and sampling.

Kosecoff, J., & Fink, A. (1982). *Evaluation basics.* Beverly Hills, CA: Sage.

Chapter 4 discusses alternative designs and threats to internal and external validity.

About the Author

ARLENE FINK, PhD, is Professor of Medicine and Public Health at the University of California, Los Angeles. She is on the Policy Advisory Board of UCLA's Robert Wood Johnson Clinical Scholars Program, a health research scientist at the Veterans Administration Medical Center in Sepulveda, California, and president of Arlene Fink Associates. She has conducted evaluations throughout the United States and abroad and has trained thousands of health professionals, social scientists, and educators in program evaluation. Her published works include nearly 100 monographs and articles on evaluation methods and research. She is coauthor of *How to Conduct Surveys* and author of *Evaluation Fundamentals: Guiding Health Programs, Research, and Policy* and *Evaluation for Education and Psychology.*

HOW TO
SAMPLE
IN SURVEYS

THE SURVEY KIT

Purpose. The purposes of this 9-volume Kit are to enable readers to prepare and conduct surveys and become better users of survey results. Surveys are conducted to collect information by asking questions of people on the telephone, face-to-face, and by mail. The questions can be about attitudes, beliefs, and behavior as well as socioeconomic and health status. To do a good survey also means knowing how to ask questions, design the survey (research) project, sample respondents, collect reliable and valid information, and analyze and report the results. You also need to know how to plan and budget for your survey.

Users. The Kit is for students in undergraduate and graduate classes in the social and health sciences and for individuals in the public and private sectors who are responsible for conducting and using surveys. Its primary goal is to enable users to prepare surveys and collect data that are accurate and useful for primarily practical purposes. Sometimes, these practical purposes overlap the objectives of scientific research, and so survey researchers will also find the Kit useful.

Format of the Kit. All books in the series contain instructional objectives, exercises and answers, examples of surveys in use and illustrations of survey questions, guidelines for action, checklists of do's and don'ts, and annotated references.

Volumes in the Survey Kit:

1. **The Survey Handbook**
   Arlene Fink

2. **How to Ask Survey Questions**
   Arlene Fink

3. **How to Conduct Self-Administered and Mail Surveys**
   Linda B. Bourque and *Eve P. Fielder*

4. **How to Conduct Interviews by Telephone and in Person**
   James H. Frey and *Sabine Mertens Oishi*

5. **How to Design Surveys**
   Arlene Fink

6. **How to Sample in Surveys**
   Arlene Fink

7. **How to Measure Survey Reliability and Validity**
   Mark S. Litwin

8. **How to Analyze Survey Data**
   Arlene Fink

9. **How to Report on Surveys**
   Arlene Fink

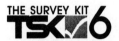

THE SURVEY KIT

TSK✓6

HOW TO SAMPLE IN SURVEYS

ARLENE FINK

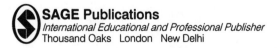

SAGE Publications
International Educational and Professional Publisher
Thousand Oaks London New Delhi

For information address:

SAGE Publications, Inc.
2455 Teller Road
Thousand Oaks, California 91320
E-mail: order@sagepub.com

SAGE Publications Ltd.
6 Bonhill Street
London EC2A 4PU
United Kingdom

SAGE Publications India Pvt. Ltd.
M-32 Market
Greater Kailash I
New Delhi 110 048 India

Printed in the United States of America

Library of Congress Cataloging-in-Publication Data

Main entry under title:

The survey kit.
      p. cm.
    Includes bibliographical references.
    Contents: v. 1. The survey handbook / Arlene Fink — v. 2. How to
ask survey questions / Arlene Fink — v. 3. How to conduct self-
administered and mail surveys / Linda B. Bourque, Eve P. Fielder —
v. 4. How to conduct interviews by telephone and in person / James
H. Frey, Sabine Mertens Oishi — v. 5. How to design surveys /
Arlene Fink — v. 6. How to sample in surveys / Arlene Fink —
v. 7. How to measure survey reliability and validity / Mark S. Litwin —
v. 8. How to analyze survey data / Arlene Fink — v. 9. How to
report on surveys / Arlene Fink.
    ISBN 0-8039-7388-8 (pbk. : The survey kit : alk. paper)
    1. Social surveys. 2. Health surveys. I. Fink, Arlene.
HN29.S724   1995
300′.723—dc20   95-12712

[This book is printed on acid-free paper.

95 96 97 98 99 10 9 8 7 6 5 4 3 2 1

Sage Production Editor: Diane S. Foster
Sage Copy Editor: Joyce Kuhn
Sage Typesetter: Janelle LeMaster

Contents

How to Sample in Surveys:
Learning Objectives

The aim of this book is to guide the reader in selecting and using appropriate sampling methods. The following specific objectives are stated in terms of aspirations for the reader.

■ Distinguish between target populations and samples:

- Identify research questions and survey objectives
- Specify inclusion and exclusion criteria

■ Choose the appropriate probability and nonprobability sampling methods:

- Simple random sampling
- Stratified random sampling
- Systematic sampling
- Cluster sampling
- Convenience sampling
- Snowball sampling
- Quota sampling
- Focus groups

■ Understand the logic in estimating standard errors

■ Understand the logic in sample size determinations

■ Understand the sources of error in sampling

■ Calculate the response rate

1 Target Populations and Samples

A sample is a portion or subset of a larger group called a population. The population is the universe to be sampled. Sample populations might include all Americans, residents of California during the 1994 earthquake, and all people over 85 years of age. Surveys often use samples rather than populations.

A good sample is a miniature version of the population—just like it, only smaller. The best sample is **representative**, or a model, of the population. A sample is representative of the population if important characteristics (e.g., age, gender, health status) are distributed similarly in both groups. Suppose the population of interest consists of 1,000 people, 50% of whom are male, with 45% over 65 years of age. A represen-

1

tative sample will have fewer people, say, 500, but it must also consist of 50% males, with 45% over the age of 65.

Survey samples are not meaningful in themselves. Their importance lies in the accuracy with which they represent or mirror the target population. The target population consists of the institutions, persons, problems, and systems to which or whom the survey's findings are to be applied or **generalized.** Consider the two surveys shown in Example 1.1.

EXAMPLE 1.1
Two Surveys:
Target Populations and Samples

Survey 1

General Purpose: To examine the attitudes of parents regarding the introduction of new dietary and nutritional programs into elementary schools

Target Population: All parents of children in a school district's elementary schools

Sample: 500 of the district's 10,000 parents (100 chosen at random from each of the district's five elementary schools)

Survey 2

General Purpose: To compare the reading habits of different users of the local library

Target Population: All persons who check out books from the library

Sample: Over the course of an allotted 6-month period, first 200 of all who check out books who complete the survey

In the first survey, 500 parents will be sampled, and their responses will be used to represent the views of the target: all parents whose children are in the district's elementary schools. In the second survey, 200 persons will represent the target population of all library users who check out books.

Why should you sample? Why not include all parents and all people who check out books? Sampling is efficient and precise. Samples can be studied more quickly than target populations, and they are also less expensive to assemble. Sampling is efficient in that resources that might go into collecting data on an unnecessarily large number of individuals or groups can be spent on other activities like monitoring the quality of data collection.

Sampling helps focus the survey on precisely the characteristics of interest. For example, if you want to compare older and younger parents of differing ethnicities, sampling strategies are available (in this case, stratified sampling) to give you just what is needed. A sample of the population with precisely defined characteristics is more suitable for many surveys than the entire population.

When selecting a sample, be sure that it is a faithful representation of the target population. No sample is perfect, however, as it usually has some degree of bias or error. The following checklist can be used in helping to ensure a sample whose characteristics and degree of representation can be described accurately.

Checklist for Obtaining a Sample That Represents the Target

✓ Survey objectives are stated precisely.

The objectives are the reasons for doing the survey. Surveys are done to describe, compare, and predict knowledge, attitudes, and behavior. A company may survey its employees to describe and compare educational backgrounds and preferences for work schedules. A school may interview students and use the data to help predict the courses that are likely to have the most influence on future plans.

Survey data are also used to evaluate whether programs and policies have been effective. For example, management may be interested in investigating if employee morale improved 3 years after the firm's reorganization, and a school may want to know how students in a new ethics education program compare with those without such a program in terms of their goals and aspirations. If the employees are given a self-administered questionnaire and the students are interviewed, then the surveys are being used for research purposes. The term "research" is used in a very general way to include systematic inquiries or investigations.

Consider again the surveys of parents' attitudes toward nutrition programs and of the reading habits of library users, as shown in Example 1.2.

EXAMPLE 1.2
General Purposes, Specific Objectives, and Research Questions

Survey 1

General Purpose: To examine the attitudes of parents regarding the introduction of new dietary and nutritional programs into elementary schools

Specific Objective: To describe and compare the attitudes of parents of differing ages, ethnicities, and knowledge of nutrition toward introducing three new dietary and nutrition plans under consideration by the school

Specific Research Questions:

1. What are the attitudes of parents of differing ages toward introducing three new dietary and nutrition plans?
2. What are the attitudes of parents of differing ethnicities toward introducing three new dietary and nutrition plans?
3. Do parents who know more about nutrition differ in their attitudes from other parents?

Survey 2

General Purpose: To compare the reading habits of different users of the local library

Specific Objective: To compare reading habits among local library users of differing ages, gender, and educational attainment

Specific Research Questions:

1. Do differences exist in reading habits among older and younger users?

2. Do differences exist in reading habits among males and females?

3. Do differences exist in reading habits among people of differing educational levels?

The specific research questions are the guide to the specific questions or **items** you will include in the survey. In Survey 1, questions must be included that ask parents their age and ethnicity and test their knowledge of nutrition. In Survey 2, the respondents must be asked their age, gender, education, and reading habits.

EXERCISE

Add at least one possible research question to Surveys 1 and 2 above.

■ POSSIBLE ANSWERS ■

For Survey 1: Do parents of older and younger children differ in their attitudes?

For Survey 2: Which are the most important factors in predicting reading habits: age, gender, and/or educational attainment?

✓ **Eligibility criteria are clear and definite.**

The criteria for inclusion into a survey refer to the characteristics of respondents who are eligible for participation in the survey; the exclusion criteria consist of characteristics that rule out certain people. You apply the inclusion and exclusion criteria to the target population. Once you remove from the target population all those who fail to meet the inclusion criteria and all those who succeed in meeting the exclusion criteria, you are left with a study population consisting of people who are eligible to participate. Consider the illustrations in Example 1.3.

EXAMPLE 1.3
Inclusion and Exclusion Criteria:
Who Is Eligible?

Research Question: How effective is QUITNOW in helping smokers stop smoking?

Target Population: Smokers

Inclusion Criteria:
- Between the ages of 18 and 64 years
- Smoke one or more cigarettes daily
- Have an alveolar breath carbon monoxide determination of more than eight parts per million

Exclusion Criterion: If any of the contraindications for the use of nicotine gum are applicable

Comment: The survey's results will apply only to the respondents who are eligible to participate. If a smoker is under 18 years of age or 65 or over, then the survey's findings may not apply to these people. Although the target population is smokers, the inclusion and exclusion criteria have defined their own world, or study population, as "people who smoke."

Research Question: Are parents satisfied with the new reading curriculum?

Target Population: Parents with children in elementary school

Inclusion Criteria:
- Have a child who has spent at least 6 months in one of the district's elementary schools as of April 15
- English or Spanish speaking

Exclusion Criterion: Inability or unwillingness to participate in a telephone or face-to-face interview in the four weeks beginning May 1

Comment: The target population is parents with children in elementary school. Parents who do not speak English or Spanish or who are unable to participate in an interview are not eligible to be part of the study population.

Both of the above surveys set boundaries for the respondents who are eligible. In so doing, they are limiting the generalizability of the findings. Why deliberately limit applicability?

A major reason for setting eligibility criteria is that to do otherwise is simply not practical. Including everyone under 18 and 65 and over in the survey of smokers requires additional resources for administering, analyzing, and interpreting data from large numbers of people. Also, very young and very old smokers' needs may be different from the majority of adult smokers. For the second survey, including parents who speak languages other than English and Spanish requires translation of the survey, an often difficult and costly task. Setting inclusion and exclusion criteria is an efficient way of focusing the survey on just those people from whom you are equipped to get the most accurate information.

=====

EXERCISE

Directions: Set inclusion and exclusion criteria for the survey of library users described in Example 1.1, Survey 2.

■ POSSIBLE ANSWERS ■

Inclusion Criteria:
- Must use the library within a 6-month period beginning with today's date
- Must check out a book for 24 hours or more
- Must hold a permanent library card

Exclusion Criterion: Not a member of the local community (e.g., relying on interlibrary loans)

=====

✓ Rigorous sampling methods are chosen.

Sampling methods are usually divided into two types. The first is called probability sampling. Probability sampling provides a statistical basis for saying that a sample is representative of the study or target population.

In probability sampling, every member of the target population has a known, nonzero probability of being included in the sample. Probability sampling implies the use of random selection. Random sampling eliminates subjectivity in choosing a sample. It is a "fair" way of getting a sample.

The second type of sampling is nonprobability sampling. Nonprobability samples are chosen based on judgment regarding the characteristics of the target population and the needs of the survey. With nonprobability sampling, some members of the eligible target population have a chance of being chosen, whereas others do not. By chance, the survey's findings may not be applicable to the target group at all.

PROBABILITY SAMPLING

Simple Random Sampling

The first step in sampling is to obtain a **list** of eligible units composing a population from which to sample. If the sample is to be representative of the population from which it is selected, the list or **sampling frame** must include all or nearly all members of the population. In simple random sampling, every subject or unit has an equal chance of being selected from the frame or list. Members of the target population are selected one at a time and independently. Once they have been selected, they are not eligible for a second chance and are not returned to the pool. Because of this equality of opportunity, random samples are considered relatively unbiased. One typical way of selecting a simple random sample is to use a table of random numbers or a computer-generated list of random numbers and apply them to lists of prospective participants.

Suppose a table of random numbers is used to select 10 employees at random from a list containing the names of 20 employees. The 20 names are the target population, and the list of names is the sampling frame. The surveyor assigns each name on the list a number from 01 to 20 (e.g., Adams = 01; Baker = 02; Zinsser = 20). Then, using a table of random numbers (found in practically all statistics books), the surveyor chooses the first 10 digits between 01 and 20. A second way is for the surveyor to use a computer to generate 10 numbers between 01 and 20. Suppose the numbers chosen at random are 01, 03, 05, 06, 12, 14, 15, 17, 19, and 20. Employees' names with the corresponding numbers are included in the sample. For example, Adams and Zinsser with numbers 01 and 20 are included; Baker with number 02 is not.

The advantage of simple random sampling is that you can get an unbiased sample without much technical difficulty. Unfortunately, random sampling may not pick up all the elements in a population that are of interest. Suppose you are conducting a survey of patient satisfaction. Consider also that you have evidence from a previous study that older and younger patients usually differ substantially in their satisfaction. If you choose a simple random sample for your new survey, you might not pick up a large enough proportion of younger patients to detect any differences that matter in your particular survey. To be sure that you get adequate proportions of people with certain characteristics, you need stratified random sampling.

Stratified Random Sampling

A stratified random sample is one in which the population is divided into subgroups or "strata," and a random sample is then selected from each subgroup. For example, suppose you want to find out about the effectiveness of a program to teach men about options for treatment for prostate cancer. You plan to survey a sample of 1,800 of the 3,000 men who have participated in the program. You also intend to divide the men into groups according to their general health status (as indicated by scores on a 32-item test), age, and income (high = +, medium = 0, and low = –). Health status, age, and income are the strata.

The sampling blueprint for the survey of men to find out about their program is given in Example 1.4.

EXAMPLE 1.4
Sampling Blueprint for a
Program to Educate Men in
Options for Prostate Cancer Treatment

Scores and Income	Age (Years)					
	< 55	56 - 65	66 - 70	71 - 75	> 75	Total
25 - 32 points						
High income	30	30	30	30	30	150
Average	30	30	30	30	30	150
Low	30	30	30	30	30	150
17 - 24 points						
High income	30	30	30	30	30	150
Average	30	30	30	30	30	150
Low	30	30	30	30	30	150
9 - 16 points						
High income	30	30	30	30	30	150
Average	30	30	30	30	30	150
Low	30	30	30	30	30	150

Scores and Income	Age (Years)					
	< 55	56 - 65	66 - 70	71 - 75	> 75	Total
1 - 8 points						
High income	30	30	30	30	30	150
Average	30	30	30	30	30	150
Low	30	30	30	30	30	150
Total	360	360	360	360	360	1,800

How do you decide on subgroups? The strata or subgroups are chosen because evidence is available that they are related to the outcome, in this case, the options chosen by men with prostate cancer. That is, proof exists that general health status, age, and income influence a man's choice. The justification for the selection of the strata can come from the literature and expert opinion.

Stratified random sampling is more complicated than simple random sampling. The strata must be identified and justified, and using many subgroups can lead to large, unwieldy, and expensive surveys.

Systematic Sampling

Suppose you have a list of the names of 3,000 customers from which a sample of 500 is to be selected for a marketing survey. Dividing 3,000 by 500 yields 6. That means that 1 of every 6 persons will be in the sample. To systematically sample from the list, a random start is needed. To obtain this, a die can be tossed. Suppose the toss comes up with the number 5. This means that the 5th name on the list is selected first, then the 11th, 17th, 23rd, and so on until 500 names are selected.

Systematic sampling should not be used if repetition is a natural component of the sampling frame. For example, if the frame is a list of names, systematic sampling can result in the loss of names that appear infrequently (e.g., names beginning with X). If the data are arranged by months, and the interval is 12, the same months will be selected for each year. Infrequently appearing names and ordered data (January is always Month 1 and December Month 12) prevents each sampling unit (names or months) from having an equal chance of selection. If systematic sampling is used without the guarantee that all units have an equal chance of selection, the resultant sample will not be a probability sample. When the sampling frame has no inherently recurring order, or you can reorder the list or adjust the sampling intervals, systematic sampling resembles simple random sampling.

Cluster Sampling

A cluster is a naturally occurring unit like a school (which has many classrooms, students, and teachers). Other clusters are universities, hospitals, cities, states, and so on. The clusters are randomly selected, and all members of the selected cluster are included in the sample. For example, suppose that California's counties are trying out a new program to improve emergency care for critically ill and injured children. If you want to use cluster sampling, you can consider each county as a cluster and select and assign counties at random to the new children's emergency care program or to the traditonal one.

The programs in the selected counties would then be the focus of the survey.

Cluster sampling is used in large surveys. It differs from stratified sampling in that you start with a naturally occurring constituency. You then select from among the clusters and either survey all members of the selection or randomly select from among them. With stratified sampling, you create the groups. The difference between the two is illustrated in the two hypothetical cases given in Example 1.5.

EXAMPLE 1.5
Stratified and
Cluster Sampling Contrasted

Case 1: Stratified Sampling

The employees of Microsell were grouped according to their departments, such as sales, marketing, research, and advertising. Ten employees were selected at random from each department.

Case 2: Cluster Sampling

Five of the Foremost Hotel chain's 10 hotels were chosen at random. All employees in the five hotels were surveyed.

Multistage sampling is an extension of cluster sampling in which clusters are selected and a sample drawn from the cluster members by simple random sampling. Clustering and sampling can be done at any stage. Example 1.6 illustrates the use of cluster sampling in a survey of Italian parents' attitudes toward AIDS.

EXAMPLE 1.6
Cluster Sampling and
Attitudes of Italian Parents Toward AIDS

Social scientists from 14 of Italy's 21 regions surveyed parents of 725 students from 30 schools chosen by a cluster sample technique of the 292 classical, scientific, and technical high schools in Rome. The staff visited the schools and selected students by using a list of random numbers based on the school's size. The selected students were given a letter addressed to their parents explaining the goals of the study and stating when they would be contacted.

Cluster sampling and multistage sampling are efficient ways of collecting survey information when it is either impossible or impractical to compile an exhaustive list of the units comprising the target population. For example, it is unlikely that you can readily obtain a list of all patients in city hospitals, members of sporting clubs, and travelers to Europe. You can more easily get lists of hospitals, official sporting clubs, and travel agents.

A general guideline to follow in multistage sampling is to maximize the number of clusters. As you increase the number of clusters, you can decrease the size of the sample within each. For example, suppose you plan to survey patient satisfaction with county hospitals and need a sample of 500 patients. If you include two hospitals, you will need to obtain 250 patients in each, an often logistically difficult task to accomplish when compared to obtaining 50 patients in each of 10 hospitals. In practice, you will have to decide which is more difficult to obtain: cooperation by hospitals or by patients?

NONPROBABILITY SAMPLING

Nonprobability samples are created because the units appear representative or because they can be conveniently assembled. Nonprobability sampling is probably appropriate in at least three situations, as illustrated in Example 1.7.

EXAMPLE 1.7
Three Sample Reasons for
Using Nonprobability Samples

1. *Surveys of Hard-to-Identify Groups.* A survey of the goals and aspirations of members of teenage gangs is conducted. Known gang members are asked to suggest at least three others to be interviewed.

   Comment: Implementing a probability sampling method in this population is not practical because of potential difficulties in obtaining cooperation and completing interviews with all eligible respondents.

2. *Surveys of Specific Groups.* A survey of patients in the state's 10 hospices asks all who are capable and willing to respond about pain and pain management.

   Comment: Because of ethical reasons, the surveyor may be reluctant to approach all eligible patients.

3. *Surveys in Pilot Situations.* A questionnaire is mailed to all 35 nurses who participated in a workshop to learn about the use of a computer in treating nursing home patients with fever. The results of the survey will be used in deciding whether to sponsor a formal trial and evaluation of the workshop with other nurses.

   Comment: The purpose of the survey is to decide whether to formally try out and evaluate the workshop. Because the data are to be used as a planning activity and not to disseminate or advocate the workshop, a nonprobability sampling method is appropriate.

The following are six commonly used nonprobability sampling methods.

Convenience Sampling

A convenience sample consists of a group of individuals that is ready and available, as illustrated in Example 1.8.

EXAMPLE 1.8
A Convenience Sample

Where do low-income people generally obtain mental health services, and how do they pay for them? To answer this question, a survey was conducted over a 2-week period, with interviewers posted in front of five supermarkets and five churches in an urban, low-income neighborhood. During the 2 weeks, 308 people completed the 10-minute survey.

The convenience sample in this survey of use of mental health services consists of all who are willing to be interviewed. People who voluntarily answer the survey's questions may be different in important ways from those who do not, however. For example, they may be more verbal, affecting their interest in and use of mental health services. Because of the potential for bias, the findings from this survey can be applied (and with great caution) only to low-income persons whose age, education, income, and so forth are similar to those in the convenience sample.

Snowball Sampling

This type of sampling relies on previously identified members of a group to identify other members of the population. As newly identified members name others, the sample snowballs. This technique is used when a population listing is unavailable and cannot be compiled. For example, teenaged gang members and illegal aliens might be asked to participate in snowball sampling because no membership list is available. Snowball sampling is not just used with outlaws or unpopular people, as is illustrated in Example 1.9.

EXAMPLE 1.9
Snowball Sampling

A mail survey's aim is to identify the competencies that should be the focus of programs to train generalist physicians for the next 20 years. A list of 50 physicians and medical educators is obtained. Each of the 50 is asked to nominate 5 others who are likely to complete the questionnaire.

Quota Sampling

Quota sampling divides the population being studied into subgroups such as male and female and younger and older. Then, you estimate the proportion of people in each subgroup (e.g., younger and older males and younger and older females). The sample is drawn to reflect each proportion, as illustrated in Example 1.10.

EXAMPLE 1.10
Quota Sampling

An interview was conducted with a sample of boys and girls between the ages of 10 and 15. Based on estimates taken from the school records, the researchers calculated the proportion of children in each subgroup and made this table:

Gender	Age (Years)					
	10	11	12	13	14	15
% Boys	22	16	16	23	10	13
% Girls	12	25	12	24	10	7

Using this table, 22% of the boys and 12% of the girls in the sample should be 10 years old, 16% of the boys and 25% of the girls should be 11 years old, and so on.

For quota sampling to be effective, the proportions must be accurate. Sometimes, this accuracy is elusive. School surveys are sometimes held back by mobile and changing student populations; also, age distributions (such as those in the above table) vary considerably from school to school.

Focus Groups

Focus groups are often used in marketing research to find out what a particular component of the public needs and will consume. They usually consist of 10 to 20 people who are brought together to represent a particular population like teens, potential customers, and members of a particular profession.

Focus groups or variations on them have been used in health and social research when the consumer, client, or patient is the focus of a survey, as illustrated in Example 1.11.

EXAMPLE 1.11
Focus Groups in Surveys

A preliminary version is finally available of a survey of the quality of life of men with prostate cancer. Twelve patients are asked to review the survey questionnaire. The men are asked questions like this: Are all pertinent topics covered? Can you follow the directions easily? How long does the questionnaire take to complete? The results of the focus group's discussion will be used to modify the questionnaire for administration to a large sample of men with prostate cancer.

Focus groups can result in relatively in-depth portraits of the needs and expectations of a specific population. If the group that participates is unique in unanticipated ways (e.g., more educated), its members' responses may not be applicable to the larger population.

A description of commonly used probability and nonprobability sampling methods and their benefits is presented in the following table. Some of the issues that should be resolved when using each method are also discussed.

Commonly Used Probability
and Nonprobability Sampling Methods

Description	Benefits	Issues
Probability Sampling *Simple random sampling* Every unit has an equal chance of selection	Relatively simple to do	Members of a subgroup of interest may not be included in appropriate proportions
Stratified random sampling The study population is grouped according to meaningful characteristics or strata	Can conduct analyses of subgroups (e.g., men and women; older and younger; East and West) Sampling variations are lower than that for random sampling; the sample is more likely to reflect the population	Must calculate sample sizes for each subgroup Can be time consuming and costly to implement if many subgroups are necessary
Systematic sampling Every Xth unit on a list of eligible units is selected. Xth can mean 5th, 6th, 23rd, and so on, determined by dividing the size of the population by the desired sample size	Convenient; use existing list (e.g., of names) as a sampling frame Similar to random sampling if starting point (first name chosen) is randomly divided	Must watch for recurring patterns within the sampling frame (e.g., names beginning with a certain letter; data arranged by month)
Cluster/multistage Natural groups or clusters are sampled, with members of each selected group subsampled afterward	Convenient; use existing units (e.g., schools, hospitals)	

Description	Benefits	Issues
Nonprobability Sampling *Convenience sampling* Use of a group of individuals or units that is readily available	A practical method because you rely on readily available units (e.g., students in a school, patients in a waiting room)	Because sample is opportunistic and voluntary, participants may be unlike most of the constituents in the target population
Snowball sampling Previously identified members identify other members of the population	Useful when a list of names for sampling is difficult or impractical to obtain	Recommendations may produce a biased sample Little or no control over who is named
Quota sampling The population is divided into subgroups (e.g., men and women who are living alone, living with a partner or significant other, not living alone but not living with a partner, etc.) A sample is selected based on the proportions of subgroups needed to represent the proportions in the population	Practical if reliable data exist to describe proportions (e.g., percentage of men over a certain age living alone vs. those living with a partner)	Records must be up-to-date to get accurate proportions
Focus groups Groups of 12 to 20 people serve as representatives of the population	Useful in guiding survey development	Must be certain the relatively small group is a valid reflection of the larger group that will be surveyed

2 Statistics and Samples

Sampling Errors

A good sample is an accurately and efficiently assembled model of the population. No matter how proficient you are, however, sampling bias or error is inevitable.

One major source of error in a sample arises from nonsampling sources. Although this may appear contradictory, the fact is that nonsampling error affects the accuracy of a survey's findings because it mars the sample's representativeness. Nonsampling error occurs because of imprecisions in the definition of the target and study population and errors in survey design and measurement.

Suppose you plan to conduct a survey of the mental health needs of homeless children. One problem you might encounter is that during the time you need for your survey, the needs may change because of historical circumstances. New health policies occurring at the same time as your survey, for example, could produce programs and services that take care of currently homeless children's most pressing needs. One way of avoiding this type of bias, that is, one that comes about because of a change in definition of needs, is to organize the survey so that its duration is not likely to encompass any major historical changes, such as alterations in policies to improve the availability of mental health services. This requires careful timing and an understanding of the political and social context in which all surveys—even small ones—take place.

A second nonsampling problem relates to definitions and inclusion and exclusion criteria. A particular survey's definitions of mental health needs and homeless will necessarily include some children and exclude others. Definitions of key survey concepts should be based on the best available theory and practice; experts may also be asked to comment on them and on the extent to which they are likely to encompass the target population.

Another source of nonsampling bias is nonresponse. Not everyone who is eligible participates; not everyone who participates answers all survey questions. A number of methods can be used to improve the response rate, such as paying respondents for their participation, sending reminder notices that a survey response is due, and protecting respondents with confidentiality and anonymity.

Biases may also be introduced by the measurement or survey process itself. Poorly worded questions and response choices, inadequately trained interviewers, and unreadable survey questionnaires contribute to the possibility of error.

Sampling errors arise from the selection process. A list of names with duplicate entries will favor some people over others, for example. Most typically, selection bias results when nonprobability sampling methods are used and not everyone has a nonzero probability of being chosen. Selection bias is insidious because it can effectively damage the credibility of your survey.

The best way to avoid selection bias is to use probability sampling methods. If you cannot, you must demonstrate that the target and sample do not differ statistically on selected but important variables, such as age, health status, and education. You can get data on these variables from vital statistics (like the census or other federal, state, and local registries) and from published reports. For example, suppose you conduct a survey of low-income women who participate in a statewide project to improve their use of prenatal care services. Without comparison data, you have no way of knowing the extent of bias in your sample, although you can be fairly sure it is there. If use of services increases, you cannot be certain that the program was the cause. The women who participated may have been more motivated to seek care to begin with than were nonparticipants. Useful comparison information may be available in the published literature on prenatal care. With it, you can find out about the patterns of use maintained by women of similar backgrounds.

WARNING

 Be wary of data from other surveys and samples. Although the respondents may be alike in some respects, they may be different in others, which can be the ones that count.

All samples contain errors. Although samples are chosen to exemplify a target population, chance dictates that the two are unlikely to be identical. When you use probability sampling methods, you can calculate how much a sample varies by chance from the population.

If you draw an infinite number of samples from a population, the statistics you produce to describe the sample, like the mean (which is the numerical average), standard deviation, or proportion, will form a normal distribution around the population value. (Additional information about the mean, standard deviation, proportion, and normal distribution can be found in **How to Analyze Survey Data,** Vol. 8 in this series.) For example, suppose that the mean score in a survey of attitudes toward a bond issue is 50. An examination of an infinite number of means taken from an infinite number of samples would find the means clustering around 50. The means that are computed from each sample form a distribution of values. This distribution is called the **sampling distribution.** When the sample size reaches 30 or more participants, the distribution of the sampling means has the shape of the normal distribution. This is true no matter what the shape of the frequency distribution is of the study population, as long as a large number of samples is selected.

The sample means tend to gather closer around the true population mean with larger samples and less variation in what is being measured. The variation of the sample means around the true value is called **sampling error.** The statistic used to describe the sampling error is called the **standard error of the mean.** The difference between the standard deviation and the standard error of the mean is that the standard deviation tells how much variability can be expected among individuals. The standard error of the mean is the standard deviation of the means in a sampling distribution. It tells how much variability can be expected among means in future samples.

When the value of a standard error has been estimated, 68% of the means of samples of a given size and design will fall within the range of 1 standard error of the true population mean; 95% of the samples will fall within 2 standard errors. This is shown in Figure 2.1. When you provide survey results, you report them in terms of how confident you are that the samples fall within the range of 2 standard errors.

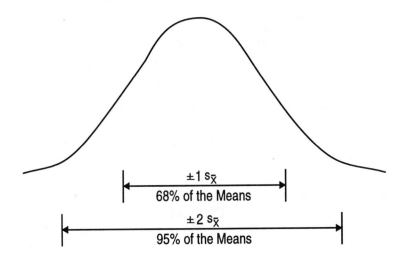

Figure 2-1 Sampling Distribution of the Mean

ESTIMATING THE STANDARD ERROR
FOR SIMPLE RANDOM SAMPLES

Although having a basic understanding of statistical notation is helpful in reading this section, "nontechnically" oriented readers should plow through to the extent possible because of the importance of the logic and principles of sampling that are discussed. Sampling is a complicated activity, and consultation with an expert is advised. However, consultation with the experts is always more satisfying and efficient if the consultee understands the vocabulary and principles.

The formula for estimating the standard error of a mean is calculated from the variance and the size of the sample from which it was estimated:

$$SE = \sqrt{Var/n} \, ,$$

where

$\sqrt{}$	=	square root
SE	=	standard error of the mean
Var	=	variance (sum of the squared deviations from the sample mean over n)
n	=	number of individuals comprising the sample

Surveys typically report proportions or percentages of respondents answering yes or no. For example, 20% of the respondents say "yes" when asked if they understand the difference between the standard deviation and the standard error, and 80% say "no." One way of thinking about the proportion is as the mean of a two-value distribution.

A mean is the average. The formula for calculating the sample mean is

$$\overline{X} = \Sigma X/n,$$

where

$\overline{X}$	=	mean (numerical average)
Σ	=	sum of (Greek letter sigma)
X	=	number of observations (e.g., number of people answering yes)
n	=	sample size (e.g., number of people who answered the question)

Suppose you have two values: 1 = yes and 0 = no. You have 100 people in the sample, and 20 say yes and 80 say no. The mean of the two values—20 and 80—can be calculated this way:

$$\Sigma X = 20 \times 1 + 80 \times 0 = 20;$$
$$\Sigma X/n = 20/100 = .20.$$

A proportion or percentage (e.g., 20% say they do not understand the difference between standard deviations and errors) is a statement about the mean of a 1/0 distribution, and the mean is .20.

The formula for calculating the standard error of a proportion includes the following:

$$p(1 - p),$$

where

$$p \quad = \quad \text{proportion with the characteristic} \\ \text{(e.g., 20% yes)}$$

$$(1 - p) \quad = \quad \text{proportion without the characteristic} \\ \text{(e.g., 80% no)}$$

To calculate the standard error of a proportion, start with the formula for the standard error of the mean ($\sqrt{\text{Var}/n}$). The variation for the proportion is $p(1 - p)$, and so the formula for the standard error of a proportion becomes

$$\sqrt{p(1 - p)/n} \; .$$

With 20% of a 100-person sample understanding the difference between standard deviations and standard errors, the standard error would be

$$\sqrt{p(1 - p)/n} = \sqrt{(.20 \times .80)/100} = \sqrt{.16/100} = .04.$$

If you add .04 to the yes vote and also subtract .04 from it, you have an interval from .24 to .16. You can say that the probability is .68 (1 standard error from the sample mean) that the true population figure is within that interval. If you want to be 95% confident, then you must add 2 standard errors, and the interval now becomes .28 to .12. You can now say that you are 95% confident that the true population mean is between .28 and .12.

The following table gives you the estimated sampling error for a percentage of a sample that has a certain "binomial" characteristic (under 19 years of age or over; male or female) or provides a certain response (yes or no; agree or do not agree). You use the table by finding the connection between the sample size and the approximate percentage for each characteristic or response. The number appearing at the connection is the estimated sampling error at the 95% confidence level.

| Sample Size | Binomial (yes, no; on, off) Percentage Distribution | | | | |
	50/50	60/40	70/30	80/20	90/10
100	10	9.8	9.2	8	6
200	7.1	6.9	6.5	5.7	4.2
300	5.8	5.7	5.3	4.6	3.5
400	5	4.9	4.6	4	3
500	4.5	4.4	4.1	3.6	2.7
600	4.1	4	3.7	3.3	2.4
700	3.8	3.7	3.5	3	2.3
800	3.5	3.5	3.3	2.8	2.1
900	3.3	3.3	3.1	2.7	2
1,000	3.2	3.1	3	2.5	1.9
1,100	3	3	2.8	2.4	1.8
1,200	2.9	2.8	2.6	2.3	1.7
1,300	2.8	2.7	2.5	2.2	1.7
1,400	2.7	2.6	2.4	2.1	1.6
1,500	2.6	2.5	2.4	2.1	1.5
1,600	2.5	2.4	2.3	2	1.5
1,700	2.4	2.4	2.2	1.9	1.4
1,800	2.4	2.3	2.2	1.9	1.4
1,900	2.3	2.2	2.1	1.8	1.3
2,000	2.2	2.2	2	1.8	1.3

Example 2.1 gives an illustration of how to use the tables.

EXAMPLE 2.1
How to Establish Confidence Intervals

In a survey of 100 respondents, 70% answer yes and 30% answer no. According to the preceding table, the sampling error is ±9.2 percentage points. Adding 9.2 and subtracting 9.2 from the 70% who say yes, you get a confidence interval between 79.2% and 60.8%. You can estimate with 95% confidence that the proportion of the sample saying yes is somewhere in the interval.

EXERCISES

1. In a survey of 200 respondents, 60% say yes. What is the confidence interval for a 95% confidence level?
2. In a survey of 150 respondents, 90% say yes. What is the confidence interval for a 95% confidence level?

■ ANSWERS ■

1. 53.1% to 69.8% (interval of 9.8%)
2. About 85% to 95% (interval of about 5%)

Remember that the table only applies to errors due to sampling. Other sources of error, like nonsampling errors or nonresponse, are not reflected in this table. Also, the table only works for simple random samples. For other sampling methods and confidence levels, a more advanced knowledge of statistics is required than is assumed here.

Sample Size: How Much Is Enough?

The size of the sample refers to the numbers of units that need to be surveyed to get precise and reliable findings. The units can be people (e.g., men and women over and under 45 years of age), places (e.g., counties, hospitals, schools), and things (e.g., medical or school records).

The influence of increasing sample size on sampling variation or standard error is shown in Figure 2.2.

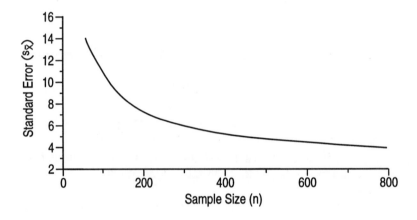

Figure 2-2   Sample Size and Sample Variation

The figure shows that sampling variability decreases as the sample size increases. The gain in precision is greater for each unit increase in the smaller sample size range than in the larger.

When you increase the sample's size, you increase its cost. Larger samples mean increased costs for data collection (especially for interviews), data processing, and analysis. Moreover, increasing the sample size may divert attention from other sampling activities like following up on eligible people who fail to respond. The diversion may actually increase total sampling error. It is very important to remember that many factors affect the amount of error or chance variation in the sample. Besides nonresponse, one of these is the design of a sample. If the sample design deviates from simple random sampling, relies on cluster sampling, or does not use probability sampling, then the total error will invariably decrease the quality of the survey's findings. The size of the sample, although a leading contender in the sampling error arena, is just one of several factors to consider in coming up with a "good" sample.

The most appropriate way to produce the right sample size is to use statistical calculations. These can be relatively complex, depending on the needs of the survey. Some surveys have just one sample, and others have several. Like most survey activities, sample size considerations should be placed within a broad context. The following checklist of factors to account for when considering sample size is useful.

Checklist of Factors to Consider When Calculating Sample Size

✓ **Assemble and clarify all survey objectives, questions, or hypotheses.**

Before you begin to consider the size of the sample, you must decide on the objectives, questions, or hypotheses that the survey is to answer. Consider these:

■ Survey 1: Quality of Life

Objective: To determine if younger and older women differ in their quality of life after surgery for breast cancer

Question: Do younger and older women differ in their quality of life after surgery for breast cancer?

Hypothesis: Younger and older women do not differ in their quality of life after surgery for breast cancer.

■ Survey 2: Fear in School

Objective: To determine if students in urban schools are more fearful of violence or tests

Question: Which do students in urban schools fear more: violence or tests?

Hypothesis: Students in urban schools fear violence more than tests.

■ Survey 3: Use of Mental Health Services

Objective: To determine which of the following reasons account for ethnic/racial differences in the use of mental health services

Question: Which of the following reasons account for ethnic/racial differences in the use of mental health services?

Hypothesis: Lack of knowledge regarding where to go for services predicts underuse of services among African Americans.

■ Survey 4: Attitude Toward Dieting and Exercising

Objective: To determine if a difference exists in attitude toward dieting and exercising and knowledge of health among men and women of differing ages after participation in the company's new and traditional health-promotion/risk-reduction programs

> *Question:* Does a difference exist in attitude toward dieting and exercising and knowledge of health among men and women of differing ages after participation in the company's new and traditional health-promotion/risk-reduction programs?

> *Hypothesis:* After participation in the company's new and traditional health-promotion/risk-reduction programs, differences exist among men and women of differing ages in attitude toward dieting and exercising but not in knowledge of health.

The objectives, questions and hypotheses are illustrations. Little difference exists in how they are stated. Hypotheses, however, require special handling; this is discussed later.

Each objective, question, and hypothesis contains the independent and dependent variables. Independent variables, the "grouping variables," are used to predict or explain the dependent variables. Take the question "Do boys and girls differ in their attitudes toward school?" The grouping or independent variable is gender. The hidden question is whether knowledge of gender predicts attitudes. In statistical terms, the independent variables specify the conditions under which estimates of or inferences about the dependent variable are to be made.

The dependent variables are the attitudes, behaviors, and knowledge the survey is measuring. In statistical terms, they are the variables for which estimates are to be made or inferences drawn. In the question "Do boys and girls differ in their attitudes toward school?" the dependent variable is attitudes toward school.

Independent and dependent variables can be divided into categories or levels. Gender has two categories: male and female. The independent and dependent variables of the four surveys above are described in the following table.

	Independent Variable	**Dependent Variable**
Survey 1	Age of women: older and younger	Quality of life
Survey 2	Students in urban schools	Fear: of violence and tests
Survey 3	Ethnic/racial groups (e.g., African American, Latino, White, Asian Pacific Islander, Chinese, Japanese)	Use of mental health services
Survey 4	Health-promotion programs: new and traditional; gender: male and female; age: from youngest to oldest employee	Attitude toward dieting and exercising; knowledge of the effects of diet and exercise

✓ **Identify subgroups.**

The subgroups refer to the groups in the sample whose survey results must be obtained in sufficient numbers for accurate conclusions. In the four surveys above, the subgroups can be identified by looking at the independent variables. Survey 1's subgroups are older and younger women, Survey 3's are ethnic and racial groups (e.g., African American, Latino), and Survey 4's are new and traditional programs and males and females and youngest to oldest employees. Survey 2 does not specify subgroups.

✓ Identify survey type and data collection needs.

The dependent variables signal the content of the survey. For example, Survey 1's questions will ask respondents about various aspects of their quality of life, Survey 2's will ask about fear in school, Survey 3's about use of mental health services, and Survey 4's about attitudes toward diet and exercise and knowledge of health. For illustrative purposes, assume that Survey 1 is a face-to-face interview, Survey 2 a self-administered questionnaire, Survey 3 a telephone interview, and Survey 4 a face-to-face interview.

Interviews and self-administered questionnaires have specific and general data collection needs. The specific needs will vary according to the survey's situation. For example, the survey about use of mental health services may need to be translated into more than one language, and the survey about fear in school may need to be anonymous. General data collection needs refer to those that are inherent in the survey method itself. For instance, face-to-face interviews require extensive interviewer training and are labor intensive. With mailed questionnaires, although the initial costs of paper and postage may be low, the costs of follow-up and nonresponse may be high.

✓ Check the survey's resources and schedule.

A survey with many subgroups and measures will be more complex and costly than those with few. Consider Example 2.2.

EXAMPLE 2.2
Subgroups, Measures,
Resources, and Schedule

	Subgroups	Type of Survey	Comments
Survey 1: Do younger and older women differ in their quality of life after surgery for breast cancer?	Younger and older women: 2 subgroups	Face-to-face interview	May need time to hire and train different interviewers for younger and older women May have difficulty recruiting sufficient numbers of eligible younger or older women
Survey 2: Are students in urban schools more fearful of violence or tests?	Students in urban schools: 1 group	Self-administered questionnaire	May need time to translate the questionnaire from English into other languages Must decide whether to have confidential or anonymous questionnaires
Survey 3: Which of the following reasons account for ethnic/racial differences in the use of mental health services?	Race/ethnicity: African American, White, Latino, Chinese, Japanese, Southeast Asian, Asian Pacific Islander: 7 subgroups	Telephone interview	May need time to hire and train interviewers who speak many languages

	Subgroups	Type of Survey	Comments
Survey 4: Does a difference in attitude toward dieting and exercising and knowledge of health exist among men and women of differing ages after participation in the company's new and traditional heath-promotion/risk-reduction programs?	Men and women of five differing ages; new and traditional programs: 12 subgroups	Face-to-face interview	Will have to administer one survey with a knowledge and an attitude component or two separate surveys May need time to find or develop the survey

The number of subgroups in Example 2.2 ranges from 1 to 12. Administering a survey to one group is difficult enough; 12 groups increase the difficulty. Relatively more time and other resources are usually needed, especially if you intend to conduct statistical analyses.

To picture the complexity of many survey groups, consider Survey 4 in Example 2.2. This survey has 12 subgroups: new program, traditional program, men of five ages, and women of five ages. This is illustrated in the sampling blueprint given in Example 2.3.

EXAMPLE 2.3
Sampling Blueprint

Years of Age	New Program		Traditional Program	
	Men	Women	Men	Women
20 - 25		*		*
26 - 30				
31 - 40				
41 - 55				
Over 55	*			

NOTE: Asterisks (*) are guides in reading the blueprint. They represent women between 20 and 25 in the new program, women between 20 and 25 in the traditional program, and men over 55 in the new program.

A sampling blueprint provides a pictorial representation of the sampling plan. The blueprint in Example 2.3 is a picture of the groups that are to be surveyed in order to answer the question "Does a difference in attitude toward dieting and exercising and knowledge of health exist among men and women of differing ages (defined in the blueprint as between 20 and 25, 26 and 30, 31 and 40, 41 and 55, and over 55) after participation in the company's new and traditional health-promotion/risk-reduction programs?"

Each of the subgroups is represented by an empty box or **cell**. Three subgroups are marked by an asterisk as examples. To achieve this configuration of subgroups, you can use stratified random sampling. If you were comparing attitudes after participation in the new and traditional program, a statistical rule-of-thumb suggests that you need about 30 people in each group. As soon as you increase the number of cells or subgroups, you also need to increase the sample's size to have at least 30 in each subgroup. This is shown in Example 2.4 in two hypothetical cases. In Case 1, the new and traditional programs are compared, and 60 people are needed. In Case 2, men and women are compared in each program, and 120 people are needed.

EXAMPLE 2.4
More Subgroups and Larger Samples

Case 1

New Program	Traditional Program	Total
Sample = 30	Sample = 30	Sample = 60

Case 2

New Program		Traditional Program		
Men	Women	Men	Women	Total
Sample = 30	Sample = 30	Sample = 30	Sample = 30	Sample = 120

A large number of groups and measures increase the costs of the survey and the time needed to complete it. If the survey's resources and schedule are incompatible with the survey's aspirations, a compromise is necessary.

Calculating Sample Size

The ideal sample is a miniature version of the target population. To achieve this ideal means using techniques to avoid biases due to nonsampling and design errors. Nonsampling errors arise from poor definitions of the target and nonresponse. Design errors occur when sample selection deviates from probability techniques. The ideal sample is also large enough to detect effects or changes. Several different formulas may be used to estimate sample sizes; in fact, a number of books are devoted to the subject.

Suppose a survey is concerned with finding out whether a program is effective in improving the health, education, and quality of life for adolescents. Assume also that one survey objective is to compare the goals and aspirations of adolescents in the program with adolescents who are not in the program. How large should each group of adolescents be? To answer this question, five other questions must be answered.

Checklist of Questions to Ask
When Determining Sample Size

✓ What is the null hypothesis?

The null hypothesis (H_0) is a statement that no difference exists between the average or mean scores of two groups. For example, one null hypothesis for the survey of adolescents is that no difference exists between goals and aspirations (as measured by average survey scores) between adolescents participating in the program and nonparticipants.

✓ **What is the desired level of significance (α level)
related to the null hypothesis involving the mean in
the population (μ₀)?**

NOTE: In hypothesis testing, you use the mean in the
population (μ, or Greek letter mu) rather than the mean in the
sample ($\overline{X}$).

The level of significance, when chosen before the test is
performed, is called the alpha value (denoted by Greek letter
α). The alpha gives the probability of rejecting the null hypothesis when it is actually true. Tradition keeps the alpha
value small—.05, .01, or .001—to avoid rejecting a null hypothesis when it is true (and no difference exists between group
means). The *p* value is the probability that an observed result
(or result of a statistical test) is due to chance (rather than to
participation in a program). It is calculated **AFTER** the statistical test. If the *p* value is less than alpha, then the null is
rejected.

✓ **What chance should there be of detecting an actual
difference? Put another way, what is the power
(1 – β, or Greek letter beta) associated with the
alternative hypothesis involving μ₁?**

When differences are found to exist between two groups,
and, in reality, there are no differences, that is called an alpha,
or Type I, error. When no differences are found between groups,
although in reality there are differences, that is termed a beta,
or Type II, error. These relationships are shown in the following table.

		Truth: Differences Exist	Truth: No Differences Exist
Conclusions From Hypothesis Test	Differences exist (reject null)	Correct	Type I or alpha error
	No differences exist (keep null)	Type II or beta error	Correct

✓ **What differences between the means must be detected to be important? That is, what is a meaningful $\mu_1 - \mu_2$?**

Suppose the survey uses the Goals and Aspirations Scale. This hypothetical scale has 50 points. The first step in the use of this (or another survey searching for differences) is to agree on a difference between means that is important in practical and statistical terms. To decide on importance, you can seek expert guidance and ask a question like "Will a 5-point difference matter? Will 10 points?" (This difference is sometimes referred to as the "effect," and the size of the difference is the "effect size.")

✓ **What is a good estimate of the standard deviation σ in the population?**

The standard deviation (denoted by lowercase Greek letter sigma, or σ) is a common measure of dispersion or spread of data about the mean. Two general rules apply to the standard deviation. First, at least 75% of all values (such as scores) always lie between the mean and 2 standard deviations. If 100 people complete a survey, their mean score is 25, and the standard deviation is 2, then at least 75 respondents will have scores of 25 ± 4. That is, their scores will fall between 21 and 29.

If the distribution of values or observations is a bell-shaped or normal distribution, then 68% of the observations will fall between the mean ±1 standard deviation, 95% of the observations between ±2 standard deviations, and 99% of the observations between ±3 standard deviations.

Estimates of the standard deviation can come from previously done surveys, but before using it, check that the population is similar to your own. If not, the standard deviation is also likely to be different. You can conduct a small pilot test using about 25 people and calculate the standard deviation. Finally, you can have experts give you estimates on the highest and lowest values or scores as the basis for calculating the standard deviation.

The formula for calculating sample size for comparing the means from two independent groups (e.g., adolescents participating in a program to improve their health and education vs. nonparticipants) is given below. This is one of many formulas that might be used in calculating sample size for surveys, as the aim of all formulas is to provide enough survey respondents to produce accurate findings. This formula assumes that the standard deviations in the two populations are equal and the sample sizes are equal in the two groups:

$$\frac{(z_\alpha - z_\beta)\sigma^2}{\mu_1 - \mu_2},$$

where

$\mu_1 - \mu_2$ = magnitude of the difference to be detected between the two groups,

z_α = upper tail in the normal distribution, and

z_β = lower tail in the normal distribution).

These "tails" are defined as

$$z_\alpha = \frac{X - \mu_1}{\sigma/\sqrt{n}} \quad \text{and} \quad z_\beta = \frac{X - \mu_2}{\sigma/\sqrt{n}}.$$

Example 2.5 gives an illustration of the application of the formula.

EXAMPLE 2.5
Calculating Sample Size
in a Survey of Adolescents in
an Experimental and Control Group

Survey Situation

Two groups of adolescents are participating in a program to improve their health, education, and quality of life. At the conclusion of the 3-year program, participants in the experimental and control groups will be surveyed to find out about their goals and aspirations. The highest score on the survey is 100 points. The Type I error or alpha level is set at .05. The probability of detecting a true difference is set at .80. Experts in adolescent behavior say that the difference in scores between the experimental and control groups (the size of the effect) should be 10 points or more. Previous experiments using the survey have revealed a standard deviation of 15 points.

Calculations

For the calculation, let us assume that a standard normal distribution or z distribution is appropriate. The standard normal curve has a mean of 0 and a standard deviation of 1. The two-tailed z value related to $\alpha = .05$ is 1.96 (for more about the standard normal distribution, one- and two-tailed tests, and z values, see **How to Analyze Survey Data**, Vol. 8 in this series; actual z values are obtainable in any elementary statistics book). For $\alpha = .01$, the two-tailed z value is 2.58; for $\alpha = .10$, 1.65; and for $\alpha = .20$, 1.28.

The lower one-tailed z value related to β is $-.84$ (the critical value or z score separating the lower 20% of the z distribution from 80%). Applying the formula

$$(1.96 + 0.84)(15)^2 = 2\left(\frac{42}{10}\right)^2$$

$$2(17.64), \text{ or about } 36.$$

At least 36 adolescents are needed in each group to have an 80% chance of detecting a difference in scores of 10 points.

Sampling Units and the Unit of Analysis

The sampling unit is the individual, group, or other entity that is selected for the survey or assigned to groups. The unit of analysis is the entity whose survey data are examined statistically. Sometimes, sampling and analysis units are the same; at other times, they are not. In simple one-stage sampling, they are the same; in more complex multistage samples, they are not, as illustrated in Example 2.6.

EXAMPLE 2.6
Sampling Units and the Unit of Analysis:
Sometimes the Same and Sometimes Not

Case 1: Sampling Unit and Unit of Analysis Are the Same

Survey Objective: To determine if the program ENHANCE has improved students' attitudes toward school

Sampling Method: Names of 500 eligible students are compiled from school records. From the list, 200 names are randomly selected. Of these, 100 students are randomly assigned to the experimental program and 100 are assigned to the control program.

Survey Instrument: A 10-item self-administered questionnaire. A positive answer to a question means a favorable response.

Statistical Analysis: The number of positive answers on each questionnaire is added to come up with a score. The average score in the experimental and control groups is computed. A comparison is made between each group's average score to test for statistical differences.

Sampling Unit: The student (individual students are selected; individual students are assigned)

Unit of Analysis: The student (each student's questionnaire is scored, and the scores are aggregated and averaged across students)

Case 2: Sampling Unit and Unit of Analysis Are Different

Survey Objective: To determine if the program ENHANCE has improved students' attitudes toward school

Sampling Method: Four elementary schools are selected because they represent the district's 14 schools in terms of enrollment size and family demographies (e.g., socioeconomic indicators). The four schools are grouped into two pairs, AB and CD. A 30% sample of second-grade classrooms (16 classrooms totaling 430 students) in the first members of the two pairs of schools is selected at random from the total second-grade enrollment to receive the experimental program in the first semester. A 20% random sample of second-grade classrooms (10 classrooms totaling 251 students) in the second members of the two pairs serves as the comparison or control group (receiving no formal program). Similarly, a 30% sample of fourth-grade classrooms (13 classrooms totaling 309 students) in the second members of the two pairs of schools is selected at random from the total fourth-grade enrollment to receive the special program curriculum in the first semester, and a 20% random sample of the fourth-grade enrollment (13 classrooms totaling 326 students) in the first members of the two pairs serves as the control. Of the 1,316 students participating, 739 students are assigned to the experimental program and 577 to the control. The sampling strategy provides a greater than 80% power to detect a "small" treatment difference, holding a Type I error at 5%. The sampling strategy can be graphically illustrated as follows:

	Experimental Group		**Control Group**	
Schools	AB	CD	AB	CD
Grade	2	4	4	2
Semester	First	Second	Second	First
% Sample	30	30	20	20
No. Classrooms	16	13	13	10
No. Students	430	309	326	251
Sample size				
Classrooms	29		23	
Students	739		577	

Survey Instrument: A 10-item self-administered questionnaire. A positive answer to a question means a favorable response.

Statistical Analysis: The number of positive answers on each questionnaire is added to come up with a score. The average score in the experimental and control groups is computed. A comparison is made between each group's average score to test for statistical differences.

Sampling Units: The school and the classroom (schools are selected; classrooms are selected and assigned)

Unit of Analysis: The student (each student's questionnaire is scored, and the scores are aggregated across students)

The small number of schools and classrooms in the survey discussed in Case 2 precludes their use as the unit of statistical analysis: Larger samples are needed to detect any existing differences. However, the number of students provides a sample with power greater than 80% to detect a "small" treatment difference, holding a Type I error at 5%.

The sampling method described in Case 2 has several potential biases. First, the small numbers of schools and classrooms may result in initial differences that may strongly influence the outcome of the program. Second, students in each school or classroom may perform as a unit primarily because they have the same teacher or were placed in the classroom because of their similar abilities or interests.

When the unit of analysis is different from the sampling unit, you are often called on to demonstrate statistically or logically that your results are similar to those that would have been obtained had both units been the same. If the analysis finds initial group differences in baseline levels and demographic factors, for example, you may be able to use statistical methods to "adjust" program effects in view of the differences (for more information on statistics, see **How to Analyze Survey Data**, Vol. 8 in this series).

Acceptable Response Rate

All surveys hope for a high response rate. No single rate is considered the standard, however. In some surveys, between 95% and 100% is expected; in others, 70% is adequate. Consider the five cases in Example 2.7.

EXAMPLE 2.7
Five Cases and Five Response Rates

1. The National State Health Interview is completed by a 95% sample of all who are eligible. Health officials conclude that the 5% who do not participate probably differ from participants in their health needs and demographic characteristics. They also decide that the 95% who respond are representative of most of the state's population.

2. According to statistical calculations, the Commission on Refugee Affairs needs a sample of 100 for its mailed survey. Based on the results of previous mailings, a refusal rate of 20% to 25% is anticipated. To allow for this possibility, 125 eligible people are sent a survey.

3. A sample of employees at Uniting Airlines participate in a interview regarding their job satisfaction. A 100% response is achieved.

4. A sample of recent travelers on Uniting Airlines is sent a mailed survey. After the first mailing, a 20% response rate is achieved.

5. Parents are mailed a questionnaire about their knowledge of injury prevention for children. Each parent who sends in a completed questionnaire receives a cash payment within 2 weeks. To receive the payment, parents must complete all 25 questions on the survey. An 85% response rate is obtained.

In the first case described in Example 2.7, 5% of eligible state residents do not complete the interview. These nonrespondents may be very different in their health needs, incomes, and education compared to the 95% who do respond. When nonrespondents and respondents differ on important factors, **nonresponse bias** is introduced. In Case 1, the relatively high response rate of 95% suggests that the respondents are probably similar to most of the state's residents in the distribution of their health problems and demographics. Very high response rates in interviews often are the result of the skills of well-trained interviewers who have the opportunity for feedback and retraining, if needed.

The survey in Case 2 uses past information to estimate the probable response rate. The survey **oversamples** in the hope that the desired number of respondents will participate. Oversampling can add costs to the survey but is often necessary.

Practically all surveys are accompanied by a loss of information because of nonresponse. It is very frustrating and costly to send out a mail survey, for example, only to find that half the addressees have moved. As a guide to how much oversampling is necessary, anticipate the proportion of people who, although otherwise apparently eligible, may not turn up in the sample. For mail surveys, this can happen if the addresses are out-of-date and the mail is undeliverable. With telephone interviews, respondents may not be at home. Sometimes, people cannot be interviewed in person because they suddenly become ill.

In Case 3, a 100% response rate is obtained. Response rates are always highest if the topic is of interest to the respondents or if completion of a survey is considered part of on-the-job or professional obligation to participate in information management.

Unsolicited surveys receive the lowest fraction of responses. A 20% response for a first mailing, as in Case 4, is not uncommon. With effort, response rates can be elevated to 70% or even 80%. These efforts include follow-up mailings and use of graphically sophisticated surveys and monetary and gift incentives like pens, books, radios, music and videotapes, and so on. In some situations, as in Case 4, the adequacy of the response rates can be calculated within a range, say, of 70% to 75%.

In Case 5, parents are paid upon completion of all questions and return of the survey, and a relatively high response rate of 85% is achieved. Incentives of cash or gifts will succeed in a high return rate only if respondents who are contacted are available and able to complete the survey.

Nonresponse to an entire survey introduces error or bias. Another type of nonresponse can also introduce bias: item nonresponse. Item nonresponse occurs when respondents or survey administrators do not complete all items on a survey form. This type of bias comes about when respondents do not know the answers to certain questions or refuse to answer them because they believe them to be sensitive, embarrassing, or irrelevant. Interviewers may skip questions or fail to record an answer. In some cases, answers are made but are later rejected because they appear to make no sense. This can happen if the respondent misreads the question or fails to record all the information called for. For example, respondents may leave out their year of birth and just record the month and date.

Statistical methods may be used to "correct" for nonresponse to the entire survey or just some items. One method involves "weighting." Suppose a survey wants to compare younger (under 25 years of age) and older (26 and older) college students' career goals. A review of school records reveals that younger students constitute 40% of the population, but only 20% return their questionnaires. Using statistical methods, the 20% response rate can be weighted to become the equivalent of 40%. The accuracy of the result depends on the younger respondents being similar in their answers to the nonrespondents and different in their answers from the older students.

Another method of correcting for nonresponse is called "imputation." With imputation, values are assigned for the missing response, using the responses to other items as supplementary information.

The following guidelines can be used to promote responses, minimize response bias, and reduce survey error.

Guidelines for Promoting Responses and Minimizing Response Bias

- Use trained interviewers. Set up a quality assurance system for monitoring quality and retraining.

- Identify a larger number of eligible respondents than you need in case you do not get the sample size you need. Be careful to pay attention to the costs.

- Use surveys only when you are fairly certain that respondents are interested in the topic.

- Keep survey responses confidential or anonymous.

- Send reminders to complete mailed surveys and make repeat phone calls.

- Provide gift or cash incentives.

- Be realistic about the eligibility criteria. Anticipate the proportion of respondents who may not be able to participate because of survey circumstances (e.g., incorrect addresses) or by chance (e.g., they suddenly get ill).

CALCULATING THE RESPONSE RATE

The response rate is the number who respond (numerator) divided by the number of **eligible** respondents (denominator):

Response rate = Respondents/Eligible to respond.

Example 2.8 shows how to calculate the rate.

EXAMPLE 2.8
Calculating the Response Rate

A survey is mailed to 500 women as part of a study to examine the use of screening mammograms in a large health plan. The following eligibility criteria are set:

Inclusion Criteria
- Over 40 years of age

  Current practice restricts routine screening mammograms to women over 40.

- Visited physician in the past year

  If women visited their doctor in the past year, the survey will have access to a relatively recent mailing address.

- Can read and answer all questions by herself

Exclusion Criteria
- Non-English- or non-Spanish-speaking

  Nearly all women in the health plan speak English or Spanish, and the researchers do not have the resources to translate the survey into other languages.

- Diagnosed with dementing illness

  This is a mailed survey. The survey team is unwilling to use a "proxy," that is, someone to answer for the respondent. A proxy may be necessary for many people with dementing illnesses (unless mild). Application of this criterion reduces the complexity of the survey.

- Hospitalized for major physical or mental disorder at the time of the survey

  This criterion is set to avoid undeliverable mail.

The first mailing produces responses from 178 women for a response rate of 35.6% (178/500). After the second mailing, 461 women respond. The survey's response rate is 92.2% (461/500).

Exercises

1. Name the sampling method used in each of these four scenarios.

   a. Two of four software companies are chosen to participate in a new work-at-home program. The five department heads are interviewed in each of the two companies. Six employees are selected at random and complete a self-administered questionnaire by electronic mail.

   b. The rangers at five national parks are each asked to recommend two other rangers.

   c. To be eligible, students must attend a local high school and speak English. Students with poor attendance records will be excluded. All remaining students will be surveyed.

   d. The names of all teens who have been incarcerated within the last 6 months will be written individually on a piece of paper. The names will be placed in a glass jar. A blindfolded referee will selected 10 names to serve on a focus group.

59

2. Draw a sampling blueprint for a survey whose objective is to answer this question:

> How do employees at five companies compare this year and last year in their preferences for work schedules?

3. Review these three sampling plans, and comment on the sources of error or bias.

   a. A self-administered survey to evaluate the quality of medical care is completed by the first 100 patients who seek preventive care. The objective is to find out whether the patients are satisfied with the advice and education given to them. The results are analyzed to identify if any observed differences can be explained by a person's gender, education, or health status.

   b. A questionnaire is mailed to all members of Immunity International. About 60% of the questionnaires are returned. Immunity is pleased with the return rate because most unsolicited mailed surveys rarely receive more than 50% returns on the first try.

   c. Two groups of children are interviewed to find out about their television viewing habits. Both groups have been involved in a program to encourage selective viewing. One program requires more involvement than the other, and it lasts longer also. Is each program equally effective? The plan is to interview at least 100 children in each group for a total of 200 children. These numbers were chosen because a similar program surveyed 200 children and got a very high degree of cooperation.

ANSWERS

EXERCISE 1

1a. Multistage or cluster sampling

1b. Snowball sampling

1c. No sampling. All eligible students will be surveyed. This is the population.

1d. Random sampling

EXERCISE 2

Sampling blueprint:

Companies	This Year	Last Year
1		
2		
3		
4		
5		

EXERCISE 3

3a. This survey of patients' opinions about their medical care uses a convenience sample. Convenience samples sometimes result in groups of people who are markedly different from the target population.

3b. Sampling error is a combination of nonsampling and sampling problems. In this case, the error is a nonsampling error caused by a relatively low return rate (although 60% may be high for unsolicited mailed surveys without follow-ups). Two fifths (40%) of those surveyed did not respond.

3c. A sample of 100 children in each of two groups is decided upon, based on previous sample sizes. To ensure the appropriateness of the sample size for this survey, questions like the following should be answered: How much of a difference between groups is required? What is the desired level of significance related to the null hypothesis? What chance should there be of detecting a true difference (power)? What is the standard deviation in the population? It is possible that the previous survey might serve as a guide to the selection of a sample size for the present survey. Do not automatically assume that the two are identical with respect to their objectives or expectations.

Suggested Readings

Babbie, E. (1990). *Survey research methods*. Belmont, CA: Wadsworth.

A basic survey research primer with example of sampling-in-practice.

Baker, T. L. (1988). *Doing social research*. New York: McGraw-Hill.

A "how to," with examples.

Burnam, M. A., & Koegel, P. (1988). Methodology for obtaining a representative sample of homeless persons: The Los Angeles Skid Row study. *Evaluation Review, 12,* 117-152.

An excellent description of how to obtain a representative sample of an elusive population.

Campbell, D. T., & Stanley, J. C. (1963). *Experimental and quasi-experimental design for research*. Chicago: Rand McNally.

This is a classic book on the designs that are used to structure surveys and the research studies that include them. Because design and sampling interact, this is a valuable sourcebook.

Cook, D. C., & Campbell, D. T. (1979). *Quasi-experimentation: Design and analysis issues for field settings.* Boston: Houghton Mifflin.

This book discusses the issues that arise in fieldwork and quasi-experimentation. It helps bring together issues that link design, sampling, and analysis.

Dillman, D. A. (1978). *Mail and telephone surveys: The total design method.* New York: John Wiley.

The special issues associated with mail and telephone surveys are reviewed in this book.

Frey, J. H. (1989). *Survey research by telephone.* Newbury Park, CA: Sage.

This book contains a good review of the sampling questions that telephone surveys raise.

Henry, G. T. (1990). *Practical sampling.* Newbury Park, CA: Sage.

An excellent source of information about sampling methods and sampling errors. Although statistical knowledge helps, this book is worth reading even if the knowledge is basic.

Kalton, G. (1983). *Introduction to survey sampling.* Beverly Hills, CA: Sage.

This is an excellent discussion of survey sampling. It requires understanding of statistics.

Kish, L. (1965). *Survey sampling.* New York: John Wiley.

This book is a classic and often consulted in resolving issues that arise when implementing sampling designs.

Kraemer, H. C., & Thiemann, S. (1987). *How many subjects? Statistical power analysis in research.* Newbury Park, CA: Sage.

Although this book requires an understanding of statistics, the complexity of statistical power analysis is thoroughly discussed.

Lavrakas, P. (1987). *Telephone surveys.* Newbury Park, CA: Sage.

An important book to read if you are interested in conducting a telephone survey with a sample of people.

Raj, D. (1972). *The design of sample surveys.* New York: McGraw-Hill.

This older book discusses the design and sampling issues associated with large surveys.

Rossi, P. H., Wright, S. D., Fisher, G. A., & Willis, G. (1987). The urban homeless: Estimating composition and size. *Science, 235,* 1336-1341.

A scholarly article on the difficulties of doing research with the urban homeless.

Stuart, A. (1984). *The ideas of sampling.* New York: Oxford University Press.

An interesting addition to a library for the statistically oriented interested in sampling issues.

Sudman, S. (1976). *Applied sampling.* New York: Academic Press.

Discusses issues pertaining to the conduct of large surveys and polls.

Glossary

Alpha The probability of rejecting the null hypothesis when it is actually true. Tradition keeps the alpha value small—.05, .01, or .001 to avoid rejecting a null hypothesis when it is true (and no difference exists between group means).

Cluster A naturally occurring unit like a school (which has many classrooms, students, and teachers). Other clusters include universities, hospitals, cities, states, and so on. The clusters are randomly selected, and all members of the selected cluster are included in the sample.

Convenience sample A group of individuals who are ready and available.

Effect size Differences between the means $(\mu_1 - \mu_2)$

Eligibility criteria Characteristics of the sample (such as age, knowledge, experience) that render an individual appropriate for inclusion into the survey

Exclusion criteria   Characteristics (e.g., too old, live too far away) that rule out certain people from participating in the survey. The survey's findings will not apply to them.

Focus groups   Often used in marketing research to find out what a particular component of the public needs and will consume. They usually consist of 10 to 20 people who are brought together to represent a particular population like teens, potential customers, and members of a particular profession.

Inclusion criteria   Characteristics of respondents who are eligible for participation in the survey

Level of significance   When chosen before the test is performed, is called the alpha value (denoted by the Greek letter α)

Multistage sampling   Extension of cluster sampling in which clusters are selected and then a sample is drawn from the cluster members by simple random sampling

Nonprobability sampling   Some members of the eligible target population have a chance of being chosen for participation in the survey and others do not.

Null hypothesis (H_o)   Statement that no difference exists between the average or mean scores of two groups

p value   Probability that an observed result (or result of a statistical test) is due to chance rather than to participation in a program. It is calculated AFTER the statistical test.

Probability sampling   Every member of the target population has a known, nonzero probability of being included in the sample. Probability sampling implies the use of random selection.

Quota sampling Population being studied is divided into subgroups, such as male and female and younger and older, and then the proportion of people in each subgroup (e.g., younger and older males and younger and older females) is estimated. The sample is drawn to reflect each proportion.

Random sampling Objective means of choosing a sample and is a "fair" way of getting a sample. Members of the target population are selected one at a time and independently. Once they have been selected, they are not eligible for a second chance and are not returned to the pool. Because of this equality of opportunity, random samples are considered relatively unbiased.

Representative sample Model of the population. A sample is representative of the population if important characteristics (e.g., age, gender, health status) are distributed similarly in both groups.

Response rate Number who respond (numerator) divided by the number of eligible respondents (denominator)

Sample Portion or subset of a larger group called a population, which is the universe to be sampled. A good sample is a miniature version of the population.

Sampling distribution Means that are computed from a sample. For example, say the mean score in a survey of attitudes toward a bond issue is 50. An examination of an infinite number of means taken from an infinite number of samples would find the means clustering around 50. The means that are computed from each sample form a distribution of values: the sampling distribution. When the sample size reaches 30 or more, the distribution of the sampling means has the shape of the normal distribution.

Sampling error   Variation of the sample means around the true value. The sample means tend to gather closer around the true population mean with larger sample sizes and less variation in what is being measured.

Sampling frame   List of units that comprise the population from which a sample is to be selected. If the sample is to be representative, then all members of the population must be included on the frame or list.

Sampling unit   Individual, group, or other entity that is selected for the survey or assigned to groups

Snowball sampling   Type of sampling that relies on previously identified members of a group to identify other members of the population. As newly identified members name others, the sample snowballs in size.

Standard deviation   Common measure of dispersion or spread of data about the mean

Standard error of the mean   Statistic used to describe the sampling error. The difference between the standard deviation and the standard error of the mean is that the standard deviation tells how much variability can be expected among individuals. The standard error of the mean is the standard deviation of the means in a sampling distribution. It tells how much variability can be expected among means in future samples.

Stratified random sample   Population is divided into subgroups or "strata," and a random sample is then selected from each subgroup.

Systematic sample   Selecting every nth (5th or 10th or 12th and so on) from a list of eligible survey subjects

Target population   Individuals to whom the survey is to apply. You draw a sample from this group of individuals.

Type I error   Occurs when differences are found to exist between two groups, although in reality there are no differences. Also called an alpha error.

Type II error   Occurs when no differences are found between groups, although in reality there are differences. Also called a beta error.

Unit of analysis   Entity whose survey data are examined statistically

About the Author

ARLENE FINK, PhD, is Professor of Medicine and Public Health at the University of California, Los Angeles. She is on the Policy Advisory Board of UCLA's Robert Wood Johnson Clinical Scholars Program, a health research scientist at the Veterans Administration Medical Center in Sepulveda, California, and president of Arlene Fink Associates. She has conducted evaluations throughout the United States and abroad and has trained thousands of health professionals, social scientists, and educators in program evaluation. Her published works include nearly 100 monographs and articles on evaluation methods and research. She is coauthor of *How to Conduct Surveys* and author of *Evaluation Fundamentals: Guiding Health Programs, Research, and Policy* and *Evaluation for Education and Psychology.*

HOW TO
MEASURE
SURVEY
RELIABILITY
AND VALIDITY

THE SURVEY KIT

Purpose: The purposes of this 9-volume Kit are to enable readers to prepare and conduct surveys and become better users of survey results. Surveys are conducted to collect information by asking questions of people on the telephone, face-to-face, and by mail. The questions can be about attitudes, beliefs, and behavior as well as socioeconomic and health status. To do a good survey also means knowing how to ask questions, design the survey (research) project, sample respondents, collect reliable and valid information, and analyze and report the results. You also need to know how to plan and budget for your survey.

Users: The Kit is for students in undergraduate and graduate classes in the social and health sciences and for individuals in the public and private sectors who are responsible for conducting and using surveys. Its primary goal is to enable users to prepare surveys, and collect data that are accurate and useful for primarily practical purposes. Sometimes, these practical purposes overlap the objectives of scientific research and so survey researchers will also find the Kit useful.

Format of the Kit: All books in the series contain instructional objectives, exercises and answers, examples of surveys in use and illustrations of survey questions, guidelines for action, checklists of do's and don'ts, and annotated references.

Volumes in The Survey Kit:

1. **The Survey Handbook**
   Arlene Fink

2. **How to Ask Survey Questions**
   Arlene Fink

3. **How to Conduct Self-Administered and Mail Surveys**
   Linda B. Bourque and *Eve P. Fielder*

4. **How to Conduct Interviews by Telephone and in Person**
   James H. Frey and *Sabine Mertens Oishi*

5. **How to Design Surveys**
   Arlene Fink

6. **How to Sample in Surveys**
   Arlene Fink

7. **How to Measure Survey Reliability and Validity**
   Mark S. Litwin

8. **How to Analyze Survey Data**
   Arlene Fink

9. **How to Report on Surveys**
   Arlene Fink

THE SURVEY KIT 7
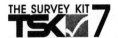

HOW TO MEASURE SURVEY RELIABILITY AND VALIDITY

MARK S. LITWIN

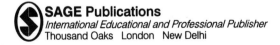

SAGE Publications
International Educational and Professional Publisher
Thousand Oaks   London   New Delhi

For information address:

 SAGE Publications, Inc.
2455 Teller Road
Thousand Oaks, California 91320
E-mail: order@sagepub.com

SAGE Publications Ltd.
6 Bonhill Street
London EC2A 4PU
United Kingdom

SAGE Publications India Pvt. Ltd.
M-32 Market
Greater Kailash I
New Delhi 110 048 India

Printed in the United States of America

Library of Congress Cataloging-in-Publication Data

Main entry under title:

The survey kit.
    p. cm.
    Includes bibliographical references.
    Contents: v. 1. The survey handbook / Arlene Fink — v. 2. How to ask survey questions / Arlene Fink — v. 3. How to conduct self-administered and mail surveys / Linda B. Bourque, Eve P. Fielder — v. 4. How to conduct interviews by telephone and in person / James H. Frey, Sabine Mertens Oishi — v. 5. How to design surveys / Arlene Fink — v. 6. How to sample in surveys / Arlene Fink — v. 7. How to measure survey reliability and validity / Mark S. Litwin — v. 8. How to analyze survey data / Arlene Fink — v. 9. How to report on surveys / Arlene Fink.
    ISBN 0-8039-7388-8 (pbk. : The survey kit : alk. paper)
    1. Social surveys. 2. Health surveys. I. Fink, Arlene.
HN29.S724   1995
300'.723—dc20   95-12712

This book is printed on acid-free paper.

95 96 97 98 99 10 9 8 7 6 5 4 3 2 1

Sage Production Editor: Diane S. Foster
Sage Copy Editor: Joyce Kuhn
Sage Typesetter: Janelle LeMaster

Contents

How to Measure Survey Reliability and Validity: Learning Objectives

The aim of this book is to guide the reader in assessing and interpreting the quality of collected survey data by thoroughly examining the survey instrument used. Also presented are important considerations in coding and pilot-testing surveys. Specific objectives are to:

■ Select and apply reliability criteria, including:

- Test-retest reliability
- Alternate-form reliability
- Internal consistency reliability
- Interobserver reliability
- Intraobserver reliability

■ Select and apply validity criteria, including:

- Content validity
- Criterion validity
- Construct validity

■ Understand the fundamental principles of scaling and scoring

■ Create and use a codebook for survey data

■ Pilot-test new and established surveys

■ Address cross-cultural issues in survey research

1 Overview of Psychometrics

A successful data collection survey is not simply a set of well-designed questions that are written down and administered to a sample population. There are good surveys and bad ones. Bad surveys produce bad data, that is, data that are unreliable, irreproducible, or invalid or that waste resources. Conversely, good surveys yield critical information and provide important windows into the heart of the topic of interest.

Psychometrics is the branch of survey research that enables you to determine how good the survey is. It provides a way to quantify the precision of measurement of qualitative concepts, such as satisfaction. Example 1.1 presents two surveys of hotel guest satisfaction. It is not obvious whether one or the other is better, but they are clearly different. During the course of this book, you will learn how to evaluate their differences.

EXAMPLE 1.1
Two Surveys of Guest Satisfaction

Purpose of the Survey: To assess guest satisfaction at a downtown hotel with a three-item survey at the time of checkout

Survey 1: *Circle one number for each item*

1. Did you enjoy your stay?

   Yes. 1

   No. 2

2. How was the service at the hotel?

   Good. 1

   Bad 2

3. Would you stay here again?

   Yes. 1

   No. 2

Survey 2: *Circle one number for each item*

1. Overall, considering the service, food, and all other aspects of our hotel, how would you describe your stay here?

   Very enjoyable. 1

   Somewhat enjoyable. 2

   Neither enjoyable nor unenjoyable 3

   Somewhat unenjoyable 4

   Very unenjoyable 5

2. How would you describe our service?

More efficient than other hotels I have
stayed in 1
Equally efficient to other hotels I have
stayed in 2
Less efficient than other hotels I have
stayed in 3

3. How likely are you to stay here again?

Highly likely 1
Likely 2
Not sure 3
Unlikely 4
Highly unlikely 5

Which survey is better? Survey 2 appears as though it might produce more useful information because it provides more than just the yes/no type questions used in Survey 1, but you really don't know quantitatively which survey is better. What exactly is meant by *better?* The better survey will more accurately measure guest satisfaction, producing more useful data from which to draw conclusions about the hotel's performance. Strictly speaking, it is difficult to assess the quality of the data you collect. It is easier to assess the accuracy of the survey instrument used to collect that data. This assessment consists primarily of looking at the *reliability* and the *validity* of the survey instrument. Example 1.2 demonstrates that different tools used to measure electrical resistance may produce completely different results. The only way to determine which, if either, is correct is by looking directly at the accuracy of the measurement tools.

EXAMPLE 1.2
Resistance Meters

Two licensed electricians use different resistance meters to measure the ohms in four brand-new circuits during a new product analysis. Pat uses the old meter she has been using for the last 15 years. Jerry uses a new model that he just bought from HomeLine, Inc., a reputable mail order company. After the measurements are taken, Pat's data are 6, 16, 38, and 119 ohms. Jerry's data are 19, 28, 73, and 184 ohms. Because there is no way to determine which, if either, data set is correct, the accuracy of the resistance meters themselves must be assessed. This is done by asking both Pat and Jerry to measure the resistance in a series of quality-control circuits, in which the ohmage is known with certainty in advance. After Pat and Jerry measure the resistance three different times in the quality-control circuits, Pat's meter is found to be more accurate. Therefore, we use her data in the new product analysis of the four new circuits.

The resistance meters in Example 1.2 demonstrate an important concept. Before a survey instrument can be used to collect meaningful data, you must test it to ensure its accuracy. This is true regardless of whether you are dealing with resistance meters, guest satisfaction questionnaires, crime surveys, depression scales, or any other survey instrument. What matters is not how quantitative the data are but how well the survey instrument performs. In the following chapters, this idea is explored in greater detail as the reliability and the validity of survey instruments are discussed.

2 Reliability

In any set of data you collect, there will be some amount of error. Naturally, you want to minimize this error so that the data provide a more accurate reflection of the truth.

In survey research, error comprises two components: random error and measurement error. **Random error** is the unpredictable error that occurs in all research. It may be caused by many different factors but is affected primarily by sampling techniques. To lower the chance of random error, you could select a larger and more representative sample. This increases the cost of the study, so it is often neither practical nor feasible simply to expand the sample. Instead, statistics are used to calculate the probability that a particular result is due to random error. If that probability falls below the limit you set, then you "reject the null hypothesis" and draw inferences about your population. Recall that in statistical analysis a conservative assumption, called the null hypothesis, is made that the two groups of interest do not differ in the particular variable being studied. For instance, in Example 1.1 (Chapter 1), if guest satisfaction between men and women was being compared, the null hypothesis would be that there is no difference. The survey research would be designed to try and reject that null hypothesis, thus allowing inferences to be drawn about differences between male and female hotel guests (for more information on hypothesis testing, see **How to Analyze Survey Data,** Vol. 8 in this series).

Measurement error refers to how well or poorly a particular instrument performs in a given population. No instrument is perfect, so you can expect some error to occur during the measurement process. For example, a stopwatch with a minute hand but no second hand cannot measure a runner's time in a 5-kilometer race to the nearest second. The best it can do is count minutes. Differences in the runner's time of less than 60 seconds will be lost in the measurement error of the stopwatch. The lower the measurement error, the closer the data are to the truth. However, even when random error is thought to be zero, some measurement error will occur. This measurement error reflects the precision (or lack of precision) of the survey instrument itself.

Reliability is a statistical measure of how reproducible the survey instrument's data are. Example 2.1 shows how two different tools used to measure fabric may have very different reliabilities.

EXAMPLE 2.1
Fabric Measurement

Honor Guard Fabric Company sells its fabric by the yard and uses expensive aluminum yardsticks to quantify the amount of each purchase. Dewey Bilkham Fabrics also sells its fabric by the yard but uses tape measures made from inexpensive thin rubber strips to measure its quantities. Fran needs exactly 3 yards of blue cotton fabric to make a slipcover for a favorite living room chair. At Dewey Bilkham, Fran has found over the years that the lengths of measured fabric are inconsistent. Because the rubber tape measures can be stretched to varying degrees depending on the strength of the salesperson, a measured yard may actually be anywhere from 35 inches to 41 inches. At Honor Guard, a measured yard of fabric is always the same length, varying only with the visual acuity of the salesperson. Therefore, Fran goes to Honor Guard to buy fabric, having learned that there a yard is always a yard.

The metal yardsticks are more reliable and have less measurement error than the rubber tape measures. Thus, Honor Guard's results are a more accurate reflection of the truth. Even so, there may still be some degree of measurement error. If the salesperson at Honor Guard doesn't see very well and cannot read the difference between 36 inches and 35 inches, then Fran may still get shorted. Neither the metal yardsticks nor the rubber tape measures are perfectly reliable, so there is always some possibility of measurement error.

No survey instrument or test is perfectly reliable, but some are clearly more reliable than others. When evaluating the value of a data set, begin by looking at the reliability characteristics of the measurement instrument.

Types of Reliability

Reliability is commonly assessed in three forms: test-retest, alternate-form, and internal consistency. Intraobserver and interobserver reliability are also addressed.

TEST-RETEST

Test-retest reliability is the most commonly used indicator of survey instrument reliability. It is measured by having the same set of respondents complete a survey at two different points in time to see how stable the responses are. It is a measure of how reproducible a set of results is. Correlation coefficients, or *r* **values,** are then calculated to compare the two sets of responses (see **How to Analyze Survey Data,** Vol. 8 in this series). These correlation coefficients are collectively referred to as the survey instrument's test-retest reliability. In general, *r* values are considered good if they equal or exceed 0.70. Sometimes, data are not collected from a group of subjects but are recorded by one observer. In this case, test-retest reliability is assessed by having that individual make two separate measurements. These two data sets from the same observer are then compared with each other. The correlation between two data sets from the same individual is commonly known as **intraobserver reliability.** It measures the stability of responses from the same respondent and is a form of test-retest reliability.

In Example 2.2, the measurement of test-retest reliability is demonstrated in a survey item that asks about grand larceny rates in urban centers.

EXAMPLE 2.2
Test-Retest Reliability of a Survey
Instrument Measuring Crime Rates

Ron has designed a new survey instrument to measure grand larceny rates in a group of urban centers at high risk for various types of crime. One of the items on the survey asks the deputy chief of police in each urban center whether grand larceny rates have been mild, moderate, or severe during the past month. To gauge whether respondents' answers to this item are consistent over time, Ron administers the survey instrument once to a sample of 50 deputy police chiefs in different urban centers and records the data. He then administers the identical survey instrument a second time 4 weeks later to the same 50 deputy police chiefs and records those data. Because actual grand larceny rates tend to be stable over short periods of time, Ron expects that any differences in the survey responses will reflect measurement error of the survey instrument and not actual changes in the crime rates. When Ron compares the sets of data from the two different time points, he finds that the correlation coefficient is 0.89. He knows that this item produces responses that are stable over moderate time periods. Therefore, his item has good test-retest reliability because it exceeds 0.70.

Example 2.3 presents a situation where test-retest reliability is low in a survey item that asks about energy levels in the same respondents described in Example 2.2.

EXAMPLE 2.3
Test-Retest Reliability of a
Survey Item Measuring Energy

Ron also wants to assess energy levels in the same deputy police chiefs to find out whether crime rates cause professional burnout among the officers. He designs an item that asks how fresh and energetic they feel today. He administers the same energy question at two time points 4 weeks apart but finds that for this item the correlation coefficient is only 0.32. Ron knows that this item does not produce responses that are stable over time because energy levels are much more likely to change from day to day and from week to week. Various factors may be influencing the changing responses. Perhaps energy levels are not dependent on crime rates in the urban centers. Perhaps energy levels are more related to salary or whether the chief had a chance to eat breakfast. Perhaps there are other factors influencing energy levels in this population. Because Ron does not know what these other factors are, he cannot control for them. Ron is forced to drop this energy item from his survey instrument. Its test-retest reliability is too low.

Test-retest reliability can be calculated not only for single items but also for groups of items. In fact, test-retest reliability is most often reported for entire survey instruments or for scales (more on scales later) within survey instruments. Example 2.4 demonstrates test-retest reliability in a series of written items administered together to measure pain in men undergoing hernia surgery.

EXAMPLE 2.4
Test-Retest Reliability of a Pain Scale

Jackie wants to measure postoperative pain in a group of 12 adult males undergoing hernia surgery. She designs a six-item pain assessment scale, with each item rated from 1 to 10, and then creates a scale score from the sum of the responses to these six items. She administers the survey instrument 2 hours after surgery (Time 1) and again 4 hours after surgery (Time 2), two points when pain levels should be similar. She then compares the two sets of pain scale scores by calculating a correlation coefficient and finds it to be 0.78. She concludes that her pain scale has good test-retest reliability during the immediate postoperative period in this population.

When measuring test-retest reliability, you must be careful not to select items or scales that measure variables likely to change over short periods of time. Variables that are likely to change over a given period of time will produce low test-retest reliability in measurement instruments. This does not indicate that the survey instrument is performing poorly but simply that the attribute itself has changed. Example 2.5 illustrates how to select an appropriate time interval over which to assess test-retest reliability.

EXAMPLE 2.5
Test-Retest Reliability of
Time Intervals in a Survey Instrument
Measuring Anxiety: Two Designs

Design 1

Eric uses a well-known short survey instrument to measure anxiety in a group of college students before and after midterm examinations. He administers the items 4 days prior to the exam (Time 1), 3 days prior to the exam (Time 2), and 2 days after the exam (Time 3). He calculates the correlation coefficient between Times 1 and 2 to be 0.84, the correlation coefficient between Times 1 and 3 to be 0.12, and the correlation coefficient between Times 2 and 3 to be 0.09. The correct test-retest reliability figure to report is 0.84. This reflects the stability of the responses to the survey instrument during a period when Eric would expect the responses to remain fairly stable. Eric deduces that the other two figures represent true changes in anxiety levels and not poor test-retest reliability. Based on his reliable survey instrument, he concludes that anxiety levels go down after exams.

Design 2

Bryan designs his own survey instrument to measure anxiety in the same group of college students at the same time points. His correlation coefficients are 0.34, 0.43, and 0.50, respectively, for Times 1, 2, and 3. Bryan cannot make any sound deductions about anxiety levels because his survey instrument does not have good test-retest reliability.

You can certainly measure characteristics that tend to change over time, but test-retest reliability must be documented over shorter periods to decrease the degree of measurement error attributable to the test itself. When measuring test-retest reliability, you must consider that individuals may become familiar with the items and simply answer based on their memory of what they answered the last time. This is called the **practice effect** and is a challenging problem to address in measures of test-retest reliability over short periods of time. It can falsely inflate test-retest reliability figures.

ALTERNATE-FORM

Alternate-form reliability provides one way to escape the problem of the practice effect. It involves using differently worded items to measure the same attribute. Questions and responses are reworded or their order changed to produce two items that are similar but not identical. You must be careful to create items that address the same exact aspect of behavior with the same vocabulary level and the same level of difficulty. Items must differ *only* in their wording. Items or scales are administered to the same population at different time points, and correlation coefficients are again calculated. If these are high, the survey instrument or item is said to have good alternate-form reliability. One common way to test alternate-form reliability is simply to change the order of the response set. In Example 2.6, two differently ordered response sets are presented for the same item question. Either response set can be used without changing the meaning of the question.

EXAMPLE 2.6
Alternate-Form Reliability
of Response Sets for Depression

The following are equivalent but differently ordered response sets to single items on depression. For each of these three items, the two response sets differ only in their sequence. They are good items for this method of measuring alternate-form reliability.

Item 1: *Circle one number in each response set*

Version A:

How often during the past 4 weeks have you felt sad and blue?

All of the time 1
Most of the time. 2
Some of the time 3
Occasionally 4
Never. 5

Version B:

How often during the past 4 weeks have you felt sad and blue?

Never. 1
Occasionally 2
Some of the time 3
Most of the time. 4
All of the time 5

Item 2: Circle one number in each response set

Version A:

During the past 4 weeks, I have felt downhearted:

        Every day 1
        Some days. 2
        Never 3

Version B:

During the past 4 weeks, I have felt downhearted:

        Never 1
        Some days. 2
        Every day 3

Item 3: Circle one number in each response set

Version A:

During the past 4 weeks, have you felt like hurting yourself?

        Yes. 1
        No. 2

Version B:

During the past 4 weeks, have you felt like hurting yourself?

        No. 1
        Yes. 2

Changing the order of the response set is most effective when the two time points are close together. This approach forces the respondent to read the items and response sets very carefully, thereby decreasing the practice effect. Another way to test alternate-form reliability is to change the wording of the response sets without changing the meaning. In Example 2.7, two items on urinary function are presented, each with two different response sets that collect the same information with different but synonymous wording.

EXAMPLE 2.7
Alternate-Form Reliability of
Response Set Wording on Urinary Function

The following are equivalent but differently worded response sets to two single items on urinary function. The response sets for each item are differently worded but functionally equivalent. This makes them good candidates for use in a test of alternate-form reliability.

Item 1: Circle one number in each response set

Version A:

During the past week, how often did you usually empty your bladder?

1 to 2 times per day	1
3 to 4 times per day	2
5 to 8 times per day	3
12 times per day	4
More than 12 times per day	5

Version B:

During the past week, how often did you usually empty your bladder?

Every 12 to 24 hours 1
Every 6 to 8 hours 2
Every 3 to 5 hours 3
Every 2 hours 4
More than every 2 hours 5

Item 2: Circle one number in each response set

Version A:

During the past 4 weeks, how much did you leak urine?

Never 1
A little bit 2
A moderate amount 3
A lot 4
Constantly 5

Version B:

During the past 4 weeks, how much did you leak urine?

I used no pads in my underwear 1
I used 1 pad per day 2
I used 2 to 3 pads per day 3
I used 4 to 6 pads per day 4
I used 7 or more pads per day 5

Another common method to test alternate-form reliability is to change the actual wording of the items themselves. Again, you must be very careful to design items that are truly equivalent to each other. Items that are worded with different degrees of difficulty do not measure the same attribute. They are more likely to measure the reading comprehension or cognitive function of the respondent. Example 2.8 demonstrates two questions that are *not* equivalent even though they are about the same topic. The items in this example would not provide a good test of alternate-form reliability.

EXAMPLE 2.8
Nonequivalent Item Rewording

The following are differently worded versions of the same item intended to measure assertiveness at work. If you look closely at the wording, you see that they do indeed ask basically the same question. In fact, the response sets are identical. But they are clearly *not* equivalent because their vocabulary levels are profoundly different. They would *not* be good items with which to test alternate-form reliability. The first is a measure of assertiveness, whereas the second is more a measure of reading comprehension.

Item 1: Circle one number

When your boss blames you for something you did not do, how often do you stick up for yourself?

All of the time 1
Some of the time 2
None of the time 3

Item 2: *Circle one number*

When presented with difficult professional situations where a superior censures you for an act for which you are not responsible, how frequently do you respond in an assertive way?

$$\text{All of the time} \dots\dots\dots\dots\dots\dots 1$$
$$\text{Some of the time} \dots\dots\dots\dots\dots 2$$
$$\text{None of the time} \dots\dots\dots\dots\dots 3$$

Despite the same response sets, these two versions are *not* equivalent and therefore *cannot* be used to test alternate-form reliability.

Example 2.9 illustrates two questions that are also differently worded but *are* equivalent and can be used to test alternate-form reliability. Notice that even though the response sets are different, the items are much closer than those shown in Example 2.8.

EXAMPLE 2.9
Equivalent Item Rewording

The following are equivalent but differently worded items that assess loneliness. Notice that although the items are different, they ask about the exact same issue in very similar ways. A high correlation coefficient, or r value, between the responses to these two items would indicate that the item has good alternate-form reliability.

Item 1: *Circle one number*

How often in the past month have you felt all alone in the world?

Every day 1
Some days 2
Occasionally. 3
Never 4

Item 2: *Circle one number*

During the past 4 weeks, how often have you felt a sense of loneliness?

All of the time 1
Sometimes 2
From time to time 3
Never 4

Although the items are worded differently and have different response sets, they effectively measure the same attribute—loneliness.

When testing alternate-form reliability, the different forms may be administered at separate time points to the same population. Alternatively, if the sample is large enough, it can be divided in half and each alternate form administered to half of the group. Results from the two halves are then compared with each other. This technique, called the **split halves method,** is generally accepted as being as good as administering the different forms to the same sample at different time points.

When using the split halves method, you must make sure to select the half-samples randomly. You must also measure the sociodemographic characteristics of both half-samples to make sure there are no group differences that might account for any disparities in the two data sets.

Although all of the preceding examples used two sets of wording or two response sets or two half-samples, there is no rule that limits the number to two. If your sample is large enough, you can use three, four, or more subsamples to test alternate forms of an item. You must check your sample sizes to make sure you have enough statistical power to show a difference in the alternate forms (for an explanation of statistical power, see **How to Analyze Survey Data,** Vol. 8 in this series).

INTERNAL CONSISTENCY

Internal consistency reliability is another commonly used psychometric measure in assessing survey instruments and scales. It is applied not to single items but to groups of items that are thought to measure different aspects of the same concept. Internal consistency is an indicator of how well the different items measure the same issue. This is important because a group of items that purports to measure one variable should indeed be clearly focused on that variable. Although single items may be quicker and less expensive to administer, the data set is richer and more reliable if several different items are used to gain information about a particular behavior or topic. Example 2.10 contains a real scale that is used in medical survey research today. It has been shown to have very high internal consistency reliability.

EXAMPLE 2.10
A Physical Function Scale

In the RAND Medical Outcomes Study (MOS), a large research project conducted in the 1980s, a series of items was developed to measure quality of life in patients with various medical conditions. The most popular survey instrument produced in the MOS is the RAND 36-Item Health Survey, alternatively known as Short Form 36, or SF-36. One of the eight dimensions measured in this survey instrument is physical function. Instead of simply choosing one item to assess physical function, the study's authors determined that it was more useful to ask 10 questions about physical function, as shown below.

Scale for Physical Function

The following questions are about activities you might do during a typical day. Does your health now limit you in these activities? If so, how much?

Circle one number on each line

	Limited a Lot	Limited a Little	Not Limited at All
1. **Vigorous activities,** such as running, lifting heavy objects, participating in strenuous sports	1	2	3
2. **Moderate activities,** such as moving a table, pushing a vacuum cleaner, bowling, or playing golf	1	2	3
3. Lifting or carrying groceries	1	2	3
4. Climbing **several** flights of stairs	1	2	3
5. Climbing **one** flight of stairs	1	2	3
6. Bending, kneeling, or stooping	1	2	3
7. Walking **more than a mile**	1	2	3
8. Walking **several blocks**	1	2	3
9. Walking **one block**	1	2	3
10. Bathing or dressing yourself	1	2	3

It is easy to see how this series of items provides much more information on physical function than a single item, such as the following:

Circle one number for the following item

	Limited a Lot	Limited a Little	Not Limited at All
How limited are you in your day-to-day physical activities?	1	2	3

Internal consistency is measured by calculating a statistic known as Cronbach's coefficient alpha, named for the 20th-century psychometrician who first reported it in 1951. Coefficient alpha measures internal consistency reliability among a group of items combined to form a single scale. It is a statistic that reflects the homogeneity of the scale. That is, it is a reflection of how well the different items complement each other in their measurement of different aspects of the same variable or quality. The formula can be found in any textbook of test theory or psychometric statistics (see also **How to Analyze Survey Data**, Vol. 8 in this series). Example 2.11 provides a demonstration of coefficient alpha calculation. For simplicity, the example contains a scale with three yes/no items, but coefficient alpha can also be calculated for longer scales containing items with more than two responses.

EXAMPLE 2.11
Calculating Internal Consistency

In the RAND 36-Item Health Survey, emotional health is assessed with five items. Suppose we created a smaller mental health scale consisting of the following subset of three items and wanted to test its internal consistency.

Circle one number on each line

During the past month:	Yes	No
Have you been a very nervous person? 1		0
Have you felt downhearted and blue? 1		0
Have you felt so down in the dumps that nothing could cheer you up? 1		0

The response set for each of these items results in a number of points that are summed to form the scale score. A low score reflects poorer emotional health, and a higher score indicates better emotional health. For simplicity, the response sets have been reduced to yes/no answers, with yes = 1 point and no = 0 points.

To calculate coefficient alpha, the scale is administered to a sample of 5 nursing home patients, with the following results obtained:

Patient	Item 1	Item 2	Item 3	Summed Scale Score
1	0	1	1	2
2	1	1	1	3
3	0	0	0	0
4	1	1	1	3
5	1	1	0	2
Percentage positive	3/5 = .6	4/5 = .8	3/5 = .6	

First, you must calculate the sample mean and the sample variance. (These formulas can be found in **How to Analyze Survey Data**, Vol. 8 in this series) Also note the percentage positive responses for each item and that the number of items in the scale is 3.

Calculations

The sample mean score is $(2 + 3 + 0 + 3 + 2)/5 = 2$.

The sample variance is

$$\frac{(2-2)^2 + (3-2)^2 + (0-2)^2 + (3-2)^2 + (2-2)^2}{(5-1)} = \frac{6}{4} = 1.5.$$

Coefficient alpha for a series of dichotomous items is

$$\left[1 - \frac{(\% \text{ positive})_i (\% \text{ negative})_i}{\text{Sample variance}} \right] \left[\frac{k}{k-1} \right],$$

where k = number of items in the scale.

Coefficient alpha is

$$\left[1 - \frac{1 - (.6)(.4) + (.8)(.2) + (.6)(.4)}{1.5} \right] \left[3/3 - 1 \right] = 0.86.$$

The internal consistency coefficient alpha of 0.86 suggests very good reliability in this scale of three dichotomous items.

In Example 2.11, coefficient alpha was calculated for a simple scale of three yes/no items. Most scales contain more than three items, each of which has more than two responses. Coefficient alpha can be calculated for these scales, too, but it is greatly facilitated by a good statistician and a computer.

If a scale's internal consistency reliability is low, it can often be improved by adding more items or by reexamining the existing items for clarity.

Reliability testing of items and scales provides quantitative measurements of how well an instrument performs in a given population. If you develop a new survey instrument, it is imperative to test it for reliability before using it to collect data from which you will draw inferences. One of the major drawbacks of new survey instruments is that they are often nothing more than collections of questions that seem to the surveyors to fit well together. Even when using established survey instruments with long and successful track records, it is important to calculate internal consistency reliability and, if possible, test-retest reliability to document its performance in your population. Established survey instruments typically undergo extensive psychometric evaluation; however, the author's sample population may be quite different from yours. When multicultural issues or language barriers are relevant considerations, it is especially important to conduct reliability testing. If you are collecting data from a group of subjects in whom that survey instrument has not previously been used, you must document the consistency of its psychometric properties, including reliability.

INTEROBSERVER

Interobserver (interrater) **reliability** provides a measure of how well two or more evaluators agree in their assessment of a variable. It is usually reported as a correlation coefficient between different data collectors. When survey instruments are self-administered by the respondent and designed to measure his or her own behaviors or attitudes, interobserver reliability is not used. However, whenever there is a subjective component in the measurement of an external variable, it is important to calculate this statistic. Sometimes, interobserver reliability is used as a psychometric property of a survey instrument; at other times, it is itself the variable of interest. Example 2.12 demonstrates the measurement of interobserver reliability in a survey designed to measure efficiency in the workplace.

EXAMPLE 2.12
Interobserver Reliability of
a Survey Instrument Measuring
the Impact of Job Sharing

Marlene designs a survey instrument to assess the impact of a new job-sharing policy at a newspaper production plant. The policy allows employees with small children to share a 40-hour work-week to allow each worker more time at home. The survey instrument is a questionnaire completed by a "peer judge," who answers a series of 20 questions on the efficiency of the 100-member workforce on each shift. Marlene plans to ask three different workers to act as peer judges and complete the survey instrument by quietly making observations during a regular shift. Marlene will calculate the efficiency score as determined by each peer judge and will then compare the three data sets by calculating correlation coefficients to determine the interobserver reliability of the survey instrument. If the correlations are high, Marlene will know that her survey instrument has high reliability from one observer to another. She may conclude that it can be used by various peer judges to measure the impact of the new policy on efficiency in this workforce. If the correlations are low, Marlene must consider that the survey instrument may be operator dependent, not a good quality for such a survey. She may then conclude that the survey instrument is not stable among different judges. She may decide to assess the new policy's impact by using one judge for all of the work shifts.

In another illustration, Example 2.13 demonstrates that interobserver reliability may be more than a psychometric statistic. It may also be the primary variable of interest.

EXAMPLE 2.13
Interobserver Reliability of a
Research Project on Mammography

Russell is very interested in determining whether mammography is a good test to diagnose early-stage breast cancer. He designs a research project in which he shows the same 10 mammograms to a series of 12 different radiologists. He will ask each radiologist individually to rate each mammogram as suspicious for cancer, indeterminant, or not suspicious for cancer. He will then compare the responses from the 12 radiologists with each other and calculate correlation coefficients. This will provide a measure of interobserver reliability. If the correlations are high, he will conclude that mammography has a high degree of interobserver reliability, but if they are low, he will conclude that the reliability of mammography is suspect. Russell plans to report his findings in the medical literature.

In this example, interobserver reliability is not only a psychometric property of the test but is also an outcome variable of primary interest to the data collector.

Interobserver reliability is often used when the measurement process is less quantitative than the variable being measured. The other forms of reliability previously discussed are more often used when the variable itself is more qualitative. There are, of course, exceptions to this general rule.

Reliability Recap

The following table summarizes the types of reliability and their characteristics along with comments on their use.

Type of Reliability	Characteristics	Comments
Test-retest	Measures the stability of responses over time, typically in the same group of respondents	Requires administration of survey to a sample at two different and appropriate points in time. Time points that are too far apart may produce diminished reliability estimates that reflect actual change over time in the variable of interest.
Intraobserver	Measures the stability of responses over time in the same individual respondent	Requires completion of a survey by an individual at two different and appropriate points in time. Time points that are too far apart may produce diminished reliability estimates that reflect actual change over time in the variable of interest.
Alternate-form	Uses differently worded stems or response sets to obtain the same information about a specific topic	Requires two items in which the wording is different but aimed at the same specific variable and at the same vocabulary level
Internal consistency	Measures how well several items in a scale vary together in a sample	Usually requires a computer to carry out calculations
Interobserver	Measures how well two or more respondents rate the same phenomenon	May be used to demonstrate reliability of a survey or may itself be the variable of interest in a study

Reliability is usually expressed as a correlation coefficient, or r value, between two sets of data. Levels of 0.70 or more are generally accepted as representing good reliability.

3 Validity

Besides determining a survey item's or scale's reliability, you must assess its **validity,** or how well it measures what it sets out to measure. An item that is supposed to measure pain should measure pain and not some related variable (e.g., anxiety). A scale that claims to measure emotional quality of life should not measure depression, a related but different variable. Reliability assessments are necessary, but they are not sufficient when examining the psychometric properties of a survey instrument. Once you document that a scale is reliable over time and in alternate forms, you must then make sure that it is reliably measuring the truth.

Example 3.1 takes another look at the problem of measuring fabric that was explored in Chapter 2's Example 2.1. Before, your concern was with reliability, but now you are concerned with validity.

EXAMPLE 3.1
Fabric Measurement Revisited

Recall from Example 2.1 that Honor Guard Fabric Company uses expensive aluminum yardsticks to measure the length of each piece of fabric it sells. You previously determined that these metal yardsticks are very reliable because they measure out the exact same length of cloth every time. Suppose that during a store audit Honor Guard finds that each of its 1-yard measuring sticks is actually 40 inches long. Every single time the clerk sells a yard of fabric, the measuring sticks reliably count out 40 inches of fabric. Over the years, the company realizes that it has given away thousands of inches of extra fabric because its expensive aluminum measuring sticks are too long. The measurement instruments are reliable but not valid.

Validity must be documented when evaluating new survey instruments or when applying established survey instruments to new populations. It is an important measure of a survey instrument's accuracy.

Types of Validity

Several types of validity are typically measured when assessing the performance of a survey instrument: face, content, criterion, and construct.

FACE

Face validity is based on a cursory review of items by untrained judges, such as your sister, boyfriend, or squash partner. Assessing face validity might involve simply showing your survey to a few untrained individuals to see whether they think the items look OK to them. It is the least scientific measure of all the validity measures and is often confused with content validity. Although the two are similar, face validity is a much more casual assessment of item appropriateness. In fact, many researchers do not consider face validity a measure of validity at all.

CONTENT

Content validity is a subjective measure of how appropriate the items seem to a set of reviewers who have some knowledge of the subject matter. The assessment of content validity typically involves an organized review of the survey's contents to ensure that it includes everything it should and does not include anything it shouldn't. When examining the content validity of medical scales, for example, it is important that actual patients and their families be included in the evaluation process. Clinicians may be unaware of the subtle nuances experienced by patients who live day-to-day with a medical condition. Families also may provide helpful insights into dimensions that might otherwise be overlooked by "experts." This said, it remains important for clinicians to review the items for relevance to and focus on the variables of interest. Content validity is not quantified with statistics. Rather, it is presented as an overall opinion of a group of trained judges. Strictly speaking, it is not a scientific measure of a survey instrument's accuracy. Nevertheless, it provides a good foundation on which to build a methodologically rigorous assessment of a survey instrument's validity.

In Example 3.2, content validity is assessed for a sociological survey on interactions between spouses.

EXAMPLE 3.2
Content Validity of a
Marital Interaction Scale

Josh designs a new scale to collect data on marital interaction as a dimension of health-related quality of life. He develops a series of 16 items about spousal communication, interpersonal confidence, and discussions within the marriage. He plans to use his new scale to assess the impact of social support on a large population of married cancer patients undergoing a difficult and stressful chemotherapy protocol.

Before administering his new scale, Josh asks 15 individuals—3 oncologists, 3 psychologists, 2 social workers, 1 oncology nurse practitioner, 4 cancer patients, and 2 spouses of cancer patients—to review each of the items. He asks these reviewers to rate each item and the scale as a whole for appropriateness and relevance to the issue of marital interaction. He also asks each reviewer to list any areas that are pertinent to marital interaction but not covered in the 16 items. Once all the reviews are complete, Josh studies them to determine whether his new survey instrument has content validity.

If he had wished to assess face validity, Josh might have asked his college roommate or his mother to take a look at the survey and tell him whether the items seemed appropriate. Josh decides to bypass face validity because he has chosen to look more carefully at content validity and knows that face validity is basically worthless.

CRITERION

Criterion validity is a measure of how well one instrument stacks up against another instrument or predictor. It provides much more quantitative evidence on the accuracy of a survey instrument. It may be measured differently, depending on how much published literature is available in the area of study. Criterion validity may be broken down into two components: concurrent and predictive.

Concurrent

Concurrent validity requires that the survey instrument in question be judged against some other method that is acknowledged as a "gold standard" for assessing the same variable. It may be a published psychometric index, a scientific measurement of some factor, or another generally accepted test. The fundamental requirement is that it be regarded as a good way to measure the same concept. The statistic is calculated as a correlation coefficient with that test. A high correlation suggests good concurrent validity. Alternatively, a test may be selected for comparison that is expected to measure an attribute or behavior that is opposite to the dimension of interest. In this case, a low correlation indicates good concurrent validity. The reason why you would not use the established gold standard as your measure of choice is that it may be too cumbersome, expensive, or invasive to apply.

Example 3.3 demonstrates the use of an established scale to assess concurrent validity in a new scale.

EXAMPLE 3.3
Concurrent Validity of
a Pain Tolerance Index

Alisha develops a new four-item index to assess pain tolerance in a group of patients scheduled for surgery. The items draw information from patients' memory of their past experiences with pain. The results from the four items are summed to form a Pain Tolerance Index score. The higher the score, the greater the tolerance for pain. Her index is self-administered and takes about 1 minute for patients to complete. To assess concurrent validity, Alisha administers her four items together with a published pain tolerance survey instrument that has been in use for more than a decade in anesthesiology research. It contains 45 items, requires an interviewer, and takes an average of 1 hour to complete. It is also scored as a sum of item responses. It is generally accepted as the gold standard in the field.

Alisha uses both survey instruments to gather data from a sample of 24 patients. Alisha calculates the correlation coefficient to be 0.92 between the two tests of pain tolerance. She concludes that her index has high concurrent validity with the gold standard. Because hers is much shorter and easier to administer, she convinces the principal investigator in a large national study of postoperative pain to use her more efficient index. Alisha publishes her findings and is awarded a generous academic scholarship as a result of her work.

In Example 3.4, a new survey instrument's validity in measuring water supply is assessed by comparing it with a more standard measure of water supply.

EXAMPLE 3.4
Concurrent Validity of a Water Supply Index

Luis develops an index of overall water supply in desert towns. It is a number calculated from a mathematical formula based on average monthly town rainfall, average monthly depth of the town reservoir, and average monthly water pressure in the kitchen of the local elementary school. The higher the index, the greater the water supply in the town. Luis collects data for 12 consecutive months and uses his formula to calculate a water supply index. During that year, he also records the number of days each month that the Department of Water declares as drought days. At the end of the year, Luis plots his index against the number of drought days for each month. He calculates the correlation coefficient between the two data sets to be −0.81. Because he reasons that these two variables should have an inverse relationship, Luis concludes that his index has good criterion validity.

Although it is important to evaluate concurrent validity, you must make sure to select a gold standard test that is truly a good criterion against which to judge your new survey instrument. It is not helpful to show good correlations with some obscure index just because it happens to be published in a journal or book. Always select gold standards that are relevant, well known, and accepted as being good measures of the variable of interest. When testing concurrent validity, select gold standards that have been demonstrated to have psychometric properties of their own. Otherwise, you will be comparing your new scales to a substandard criterion.

Predictive

Predictive validity is the ability of a survey instrument to forecast future events, behaviors, attitudes, or outcomes. It may be used during the course of a study to predict response to a stimulus, election winners, success of an intervention, time to a clinical endpoint, or other objective criteria. Over a brief interval, predictive validity is similar to concurrent validity in that it involves correlating the results of one test with the results of another administered around the same time. If the time frame is longer and the second test occurs much later, then the assessment is of predictive validity. Like concurrent validity, predictive validity is calculated as a correlation coefficient between the initial test and the secondary outcome.

Example 3.5 demonstrates that the Pain Tolerance Index that was tested for concurrent validity in Example 3.3 may also be tested for predictive validity.

EXAMPLE 3.5
Predictive Validity of
the Pain Tolerance Index

Fourteen years after her initial success, Alisha from Example 3.3 becomes a professor of gynecology at a well-respected research university. She decides to use her Pain Tolerance Index to predict narcotic requirement in patients undergoing a hysterectomy. Having tested her index for reliability and concurrent validity, she now wants to test it for predictive validity. She administers the index to 24 of her preoperative patients and calculates an index score for each individual. Recall that a high score reflects a high tolerance for pain.

Once all the surgeries have been completed, Alisha reviews the medical records. She notes the number of doses of narcotic that were administered for postoperative pain control in each patient. She then calculates a correlation coefficient between the two data elements: index score and number of narcotic doses. When she finds that, the statistic is −0.84. As expected, there is a strong inverse correlation between the Pain Tolerance Index and the amount of narcotic required after surgery. Alisha is pleased to find that her index has high predictive validity in clinical practice. She publishes her results in a national medical journal and is later promoted to the position of chairperson of the gynecology department at the university.

Continuing with this theme, predictive validity can be used in a variety of settings to measure the accuracy of a survey instrument. One of the most well-known survey instruments is the Scholastic Aptitude Test (SAT). In Example 3.6, the SAT is used on a population of college students to predict academic success.

EXAMPLE 3.6
Predictive Validity of SAT Scores

Bob is the dean of students at Brook College, a small liberal arts school in Arizona, and decides to look into whether the SAT scores of entering freshmen predict how well the students will perform during their first semester at Brook. The dean looks back into the registrar's records for the past 5 years and gathers two data elements for each freshman: SAT score and first-semester grade point average. The dean enters the two data sets into his laptop computer and calculates a correlation coefficient between the two. To his surprise, he finds the statistic to be 0.45. The students' SAT scores do not appear to have high predictive validity for early success at Brook College. He immediately writes a memo to the dean of admissions asking that evaluation policies be revised to reflect this important new information.

When Jackie, the dean of admissions at Brook, receives Bob's memo, she decides to do a little investigating of her own. She takes Bob's data and breaks them down year by year. Using the same formula, she calculates correlation coefficients with her own laptop computer and finds that over the past 5 years the predictive validity of SAT scores has been 0.21, 0.36, 0.39, 0.57, and 0.72. Jackie writes a memo back to Bob, suggesting that although SAT scores did not previously have much predictive validity, they have become increasingly more useful in recent years. Jackie proudly sends a copy of her memo to the chancellor for consideration in her upcoming decision on who should be promoted to provost.

Predictive validity is one of the most important ways to measure a test's accuracy in practical applications; however, it is seldom used in longitudinal medical experiments that rely on surveys. Because the time frames are often several years long in such trials, secondary interventions may be implemented during the trial to alter the course of a disease or medical condition. If the final outcomes were compared with a test score from the start of the study, their correlation may be diminished. This would falsely decrease the measured predictive validity of the test and perhaps call into question the statistical qualities of an otherwise valid survey instrument.

Example 3.6 about SAT scores demonstrates that predictive validity (or any other psychometric statistic) may be used in various ways to support different hypotheses. You must be careful with the conclusions you draw from any of these measured psychometric properties. A good exercise is to ask peers in your area who are unfamiliar with your hypothesis to look at a summary of your data and draw conclusions. If enough people draw the same conclusion, you may be somewhat reassured that your inferences are correct. You may also ask peers to take your data and statistics and try to support a point that is opposite to your conclusions. This may open up your mind to different interpretations. It may unhinge your argument, or it may guide your approach to collecting more irrefutable evidence.

CONSTRUCT

Construct validity is the most valuable yet most difficult way of assessing a survey instrument. It is difficult to understand, to measure, and to report. This form of validity is often determined only after years of experience with a survey instrument. It is a measure of how meaningful the scale or survey instrument is when in practical use. Often, it is not calculated as a quantifiable statistic. Rather, it is frequently seen as a gestalt of how well a survey instrument performs in a multitude of settings and populations over a number of years. Construct validity is often thought to comprise two other forms of validity: convergent and divergent.

Convergent

Convergent validity implies that several different methods for obtaining the same information about a given trait or concept produce similar results. Evaluating convergent validity is analogous to measuring alternate-form reliability, except that the former is more theoretical and requires a great deal of work, usually by multiple investigators with different approaches.

Divergent

Divergent (discriminant) validity is another theoretically based way of thinking about the ability of a measure to estimate the underlying truth in a given area. For a survey instrument to have divergent validity, it must be shown not to correlate too closely with similar but distinct concepts or traits. This, too, requires much effort over many years of evaluation.

Validity Recap

Testing a survey instrument for construct validity is more like hypothesis testing than like calculating correlation coefficients. Demonstrating construct validity is much more difficult and usually requires a great deal of effort in many different experiments. Construct validity may be said to result from the continued use of a survey instrument to measure some trait, quality, or "construct." Indeed, over a period of years, the survey instrument itself may define the way we think about the variable. It is difficult to present a specific example of construct validity because its measurement and documentation require such an all-encompassing and multifaceted research strategy.

The following table summarizes the types of validity and their characteristics along with comments on their use.

Type of Validity	Characteristics	Comments
Face	Casual review of how good an item or group of items appear	Assessed by individuals with no formal training in the subject under study
Content	Formal expert review of how good an item or series of items appears	Usually assessed by individuals with expertise in some aspect of the subject under study
Criterion: Concurrent	Measures how well the item or scale correlates with "gold standard" measures of the same variable	Requires the identification of an established, generally accepted gold standard
Criterion: Predictive	Measures how well the item or scale predicts expected future observations	Used to predict outcomes or events of significance that the item or scale might subsequently be used to predict
Construct	Theoretical measure of how meaningful a survey instrument is	Determined usually after years of experience by numerous investigators

Validity is usually expressed as a correlation coefficient, or r value, between two sets of data. Levels of 0.70 or more are generally accepted as representing good validity.

4 Scaling and Scoring

Scales and indexes are not merely collections of reliable and valid items about the same topic. In fact, most established scales represent months or years of work at refining the list of items down to the critical ones that provide a rich view of a single attribute. The most common method used to assess whether different items belong together in a scale is a technique called **factor analysis.** A factor is a hypothesized trait that is thought to be measured with items in a scale. In factor analysis, a computer-executed algorithm is used to test many different possible combinations of items to determine which of them vary together. Factor analysis is used to evaluate and select items from a larger pool for inclusion in a scale or index. The resulting scale is used to produce a score, which in turn is thought to reflect the factor. The factor itself is a theoretical trait or attribute that is only approximated by the scale. Another advanced computer-executed technique called **multitrait scaling analysis** is sometimes used to measure how well a group of items holds together as a scale.

Example 4.1 provides an illustration of how factor analysis might be used to select items for a scale that purports to measure viewer hostility toward sportscasters during Olympic broadcasts.

EXAMPLE 4.1
Factor Analysis of Olympic Sportscasters

Bryant works for United Broadcasting Company (UBC) and wishes to measure television viewer hostility toward the sportscasters at Good Broadcasting System (GBS) during its Winter Olympics coverage. Bryant knows that viewer hostility will be a difficult concept to define, measure, and package into a scale. He begins by administering a reliable 100-item survey to 350 adult viewers on 10 nights of television coverage of the Winter Olympics. The questions cover a wide range of viewer responses, including pleasure, boredom, anger, identification with athletes, patriotism, and exasperation.

After the Games are over, Bryant compiles all his data and enters them into the mainframe computer at UBC. He performs a factor analysis, in which he hypothesizes which items will measure his trait of interest—hostility—and various other traits that the survey might measure. The computer puts out a matrix of statistics, or factor analysis, that examines how well the items hypothesized to measure hostility vary with each other and how well or poorly they vary with the other hypothesized traits. Of the 12 items he has selected, Bryant's factor analysis determines that only 7 of them vary together well enough to form a hostility scale. The other 5 turn out to vary more closely with other hypothesized traits. Bryant presents his hostility scale to the president of UBC, who must decide how to use it against GBS during negotiations for the exclusive rights to cover the upcoming Summer Olympic Games.

One popular way to structure response sets in survey research is called the *Likert scale* method. It involves a series of typically 5 statements that convey various levels of agreement with an item stem. For example, the survey instructions might ask respondents to state how much they agree with the statement "The hotel guest services were satisfactory," using a set of Likert scale responses that reads "strongly agree," "somewhat agree," "neither agree nor disagree," "somewhat disagree," or "strongly disagree." Another item might read "How often do you feel your self-esteem is low?" and uses a Likert scale response set that reads "All of the time," "much of the time," "about half the time," "some of the time," or "none of the time." There are numerous other ways to structure response sets, which are discussed more fully in **How to Ask Survey Questions** (Vol. 2 in this series).

Scoring a survey instrument is usually fairly straightforward and amenable to the creation of computer-driven algorithms. Most established survey instruments have published scoring manuals that instruct the user on how many points to count for each response to each item. It is important to read the scoring rules carefully because many variations exist on how to convert raw scores to standardized scale scores. This allows the researcher to compare different populations from different studies. In some survey instruments, a high score is better; in others, a high score is worse. Some are converted to a standard 0 to 100 range, whereas others may use a range that goes from 0 to 1, 4, 25, and so forth.

When creating a set of scoring rules for your new survey instrument, you must determine whether to use a sum, an average, or some other formula to derive the scale score. Because different items may have different response options, you must decide whether to value each response or each item the same.

Example 4.2 shows how using different scoring techniques can produce very different survey results from the same data.

EXAMPLE 4.2
Scoring of a Beach Quality Index

To select a site for next year's beachfront intramural volleyball tournament, Morgan and Kim design a new two-item index that measures the quality of different beaches. The two items and number of points for each response are as follows:

Circle one number for each item

1. The average summer temperature at this beach is:

$$< 70° \dots\dots\dots\dots\dots\ 0$$
$$70° \text{ to } 80° \dots\dots\dots\dots 1$$
$$> 80° \dots\dots\dots\dots\dots 2$$

2. The average number of clear days per summer month at this beach is:

$$< 7 \dots\dots\dots\dots\dots 0$$
$$7 \text{ to } 13 \dots\dots\dots\dots 1$$
$$14 \text{ to } 20 \dots\dots\dots\dots 2$$
$$21 \text{ to } 25 \dots\dots\dots\dots 3$$
$$> 25 \dots\dots\dots\dots\dots 4$$

After extensive testing of reliability and validity at various sample beaches, they are happy with the survey instrument. However, they disagree on how to carry out the scoring. Morgan wants to score the index by summing the number of points for both items, dividing by 6 (the perfect score for both items), and then reporting the result. Kim wants to score the index by calculating the percentage score for each of the two items and then averaging them together. Kim would divide the number of points in Item 1 by 2 (a perfect score for that item), divide the number of points in Item 2 by 4 (a perfect score for that item), and then calculate a mean score for the two items. Both scores would be reported on a 100-point scale, but they would be calculated differently. To see whether there is a difference in the two methods, they convince the tournament administrator to fly them to Cape Cod, Massachusetts, for a trial.

While on Cape Cod, Morgan and Kim travel to Provincetown and rate the beach at Race Point with scores of 2 and 3, respectively, for the two items. By Morgan's scoring method, Race Point would score $(2 + 3)/6 = 83\%$. By Kim's method, Race Point would score $[(2/2) + (3/4)]/2 = 88\%$.

The reason why Kim's method yields a higher score is that both items are valued equally by scoring them individually and averaging the item results. Race Point has a perfect score on Item 1, so Kim's method values Item 1 more highly. Morgan's method values each item response, not each item, equally. Therefore, the responses in Item 1 are relatively discounted in the total score.

Example 4.2 shows us that seemingly subtle alterations in scoring methods can lead to significant differences in scale scores. Both Morgan's and Kim's methods are correct, but they place different values on the items. When designing a scoring system for a new survey instrument, you must recognize these differences and plan accordingly. Remember, if you score a scale by simply adding up the total number of points from each item, those items with larger response sets will be valued relatively higher than those with smaller response sets. One way of avoiding this problem and valuing all responses equally is to assign increased points to each response in items with smaller response sets. This common technique is demonstrated in Example 4.3.

EXAMPLE 4.3
Beach Quality Revisited

After much discussion, Kim wins the scoring debate with Morgan, and they decide to score their two-item Beach Quality Index in a manner that confers equal weight to each item. The scoring system they produce is this:

	Response	Points Counted
Item 1	0	0
	1	25
	2	50
Item 2	0	0
	1	12.5
	2	25
	3	37.5
	4	50

With this method, scoring is accomplished simply by summing the number of assigned points for each response. Race Point, the beach from Example 4.2, would be scored by adding 50 (Item 1 = 2) and 37.5 (Item 2 = 3) to yield a score of 87.5, which is rounded to 88%—the exact same answer as Kim obtained in Example 4.2.

5 Creating and Using a Codebook

In survey research, coding is the process of going through each respondent's questionnaire and looking for conflicting answers, missing data, handwritten notes, and other variations from the desired "circle one answer" responses. Before recording your survey responses onto a data tape or into a computer file for analysis, you must decide how you are going to categorize the ambiguous answers. No matter how clearly you spell out the instructions to circle only one answer for each item, you will have unclear responses to some items. It may be that the respondent does not correctly follow instructions for your skip patterns or that the respondent circles more than one answer in a response set that is supposed to be mutually exclusive and collectively exhaustive. No matter how thoroughly you think through your items and response sets before testing your survey, there will always be issues that arise during data collection that require you to make subjective decisions or corrections.

Example 5.1 shows one issue that came up during a recent survey of family support systems.

EXAMPLE 5.1
How Many Kids?

In a recent self-administered survey of family support systems in men with emphysema, one seemingly straightforward question caused a moderate amount of confusion in several respondents. The item read:

Circle one number for this item

How many of your children under age 18 live in your home?

> None. 0
> 1 1
> 2 to 4 2
> More than 4 3

Three respondents answered *none* but wrote in the margin that 2 to 4 of their wives' school-aged children from previous marriages lived in the home. During the coding of this survey, the researchers decided to count the wives' young children because stepchildren in the home fulfilled a role similar enough to biological children that there should be no distinction in this study. The research context determined how these children were classified. If the same item had appeared on a survey assessing male fertility, it would not have been appropriate to include the stepchildren. This decision was recorded in the study's codebook for future reference.

The most common data problem is that respondents will skip items either intentionally or by mistake. Usually, you will have to code those items as missing data and decide later how to treat them in the analysis. Occasionally, you can infer the answer to an item from other responses or from other sources, particularly if it is a sociodemographic item, such as age. The best way to handle missing data is to call the respondent and ask for the correct answer to the skipped item. However, this is not always possible. Example 5.2 demonstrates one way to solve the problem of missing data.

EXAMPLE 5.2
Missing Data

In the same survey of family support systems in men with emphysema, the researchers included the following item on family outings:

Circle one number for this item

During the past 4 weeks, how often did you and *all* the other family members who live in your home go out to dinner together?

Not at all.	0
Once or twice	1
Three to five times	2
Six or more times	3

After all the surveys had been returned, they were coded by an undergraduate student research assistant, who found that 15 respondents had failed to answer this item. When he reported this to the study's principal investigator, she asked him to telephone these 15 respondents to try to fill in the missing data. Nine were available and provided answers to this item, but 6 were not reachable despite numerous attempts. The telephone follow-up was also recorded in the study codebook for future reference.

Example 5.2 illustrates that missing data is one of the most problematic areas in survey research. It is critically important to make extensive efforts to minimize the amount of missing data from a survey. Missing data detract from the overall quality of the survey results. They also serve as a quality check on the research methods: The more data that are missing, the poorer the quality of the methodology. Data may be missing for a variety of reasons. Respondents may omit data because they misunderstood skip patterns, failed to grasp the language used, were unable to read the type, tired of a lengthy survey, or for many other reasons. Whatever the explanation, missing data can be devastating to an otherwise well-planned survey project.

In Example 5.3, the value of the codebook is demonstrated when a surveyor makes a decision regarding data after the data had been collected but before they were coded on the survey.

EXAMPLE 5.3
Counting Homicides

Alison, the president of the National Gay and Lesbian Media Coalition (NGLMC), performed a survey to review all articles appearing in daily newspapers in the 50 largest cities in North America during the last 3 years). One of the variables she collected was the number of articles with positive coverage of gay and lesbian issues in each city during each year. She found the article counts to range from none to 455. During the data collection stage of her project, Alison decided to enter the exact number of articles on a blank line next to the question. Later, when she coded the surveys, she decided to collapse the article counts into six groups, which she felt were more meaningful:

Number of Articles	Response Code
0	1
1 to 10	2
11 to 50	3
51 to 174	4
175 to 350	5
> 350	6

Alison made a research decision that she did not need to analyze her data based on the exact number of articles. She recorded the above table in her study codebook for future reference. She knew that if she decided to add more cities to her series several years later, she would not be able to remember where she had drawn the lines between groups. She also knew that her thorough codebook would provide that information.

In some senses, the codebook is a log or documentation of the research decisions that are made during the coding or review of surveys. Despite your best efforts, you will be unable to remember all the small decisions that you make along the way in carrying out the collection, processing, and analysis of survey data. The codebook is a summary of all those decisions. It functions not only as a record but also as a rule book for future analyses with the same or similar data.

The importance of keeping meticulous records cannot be overemphasized. Inevitably in survey research, questions arise about how you collected a data element, where you went for resources, how you documented certain variables, or whether you completed follow-up in a certain way. The only way to guarantee that you can reproduce your methods accurately is to maintain excellent records. This includes your codebook and the way you structured each aspect of your methodology and data analysis.

6 Pilot Testing

Before a new feature film appears in movie theaters, movie studios always show it to sample audiences in various cities to observe their reactions to the characters, plot, ending, and other aspects of the entertainment experience. If some aspect of the film is consistently disliked by these sample audiences, it is usually changed before the movie is released. Similarly, before a new product is introduced into retail stores, manufacturers always test market it to gauge consumer satisfaction. And before buying a new car, you almost always take it for a test drive, even if you are already certain about your choice of models.

Likewise in survey research, one of the most important stages in the development of a new survey instrument involves trying it out on a small sample population. **Pilot testing, or pretesting,** your questionnaire will time and again prove to be worth your energy. Pilot testing almost always identifies errors in a survey's form and presentation. Inevitably, despite extensive thought and planning, errors occur in the final versions of questionnaires. They range from confusing typographical mistakes to overlapping response sets to ambiguous instructions. Usually, the authors are so close to the project that they may overlook even the most obvious of errors. Pilot testing allows the authors a chance to correct these errors before the survey is mass produced or used on a wider scope to gather real data. It allows authors the time and opportunity to redesign problematic parts of the survey before it is actually used. Pilot testing also predicts difficulties that may arise during subsequent data collection that might otherwise have gone unnoticed. At this early stage, most problems are still correctable.

Sometimes, the issues identified during pilot testing are problems of form. For older individuals, many of whom have impaired vision, the type size and font are especially important. Difficulties may also arise with reading comprehension. Many survey respondents are less technically educated than survey researchers. If a survey is written at a level beyond the understanding of its respondents, the resulting data will be spurious or incomplete. Respondents must be able to understand the semantics of the survey items in order to provide honest and thoughtful answers. Likewise, many populations today are not homogeneous in their primary language. Even if a survey is written at a comprehensible level, individuals who are not completely fluent or comfortable with English may answer with data that are not usable.

Language may present significant challenges; however, just because your respondents are not fluent English speakers does not mean you cannot gather data from them. If you are very industrious, you may actually create a foreign-language version of your survey if there is information that you want but is only reliably and validly available in the respondents' native tongue.

In addition, items must be culturally sensitive. Certain areas that are covered in a questionnaire may represent concepts that are unfamiliar to individuals involved in the survey. A more thorough discussion of this potential trap is included in the next chapter. Pilot testing allows many potential impediments to be identified and corrected in advance before too many resources have been expended. You must be careful to avoid these pitfalls when crossing language and cultural barriers in survey research (see Chapter 7 on multicultural issues). Pilot testing will not eliminate any of these problems, but it will identify them so that the researcher can consider the implications and decide prospectively how to handle them.

Example 6.1 demonstrates one of the simple but common problems that is identified when pilot-testing a survey.

EXAMPLE 6.1
Type Size

Ramon was very pleased that his new 10-item questionnaire on attitudes toward aging fits onto one side of a single page. He estimated that it should require about 5 minutes to complete. Before assessing his survey's reliability and validity in a sample of 125 older New Yorkers, Ramon was urged by his professor to conduct a small pilot test with 6 senior citizens. Ramon set up the pilot test by calling the activities office of a local community center and recruiting volunteers.

On the appointed date, the 4 women and 2 men met Ramon at the community center for the short pilot test. To his surprise, Ramon found that the average time they took to complete his survey was 10 minutes. When he queried them as to why, 5 of the 6 stated that they had a great deal of trouble reading the questions, even with their glasses. They had no problems with reading comprehension or with English; they simply could not read the type on the page.

Ramon revised the type size on his survey from 8-point to 12-point type. Instead of fitting onto a single page, the survey now took up two pages. Ramon mailed the new version to his 6 pilot-test respondents and asked for their comments. Each of them replied that it was now much easier to read and complete.

When designing questionnaire layout, authors are often tempted to squeeze as many items as possible onto one or two pages. They think that if a survey looks shorter, it will be easier and quicker to complete. But shortening the length of a questionnaire by making the type size smaller only makes it more difficult to read. If respondents have trouble reading the words on the page, they will not have much energy left to think about the meaning of the questions. Ramon learned in Example 6.1 that sometimes a survey that is a few more pages in length but much easier to read can yield more valuable results than one that fits nicely into a short format. If the type is easier to read, it takes less time to complete two pages than one.

One trick that some researchers have used is creative numbering of the items. Instead of simply numbering questions from 1 to whatever, breaking items into groups or sections may create the illusion that a survey is shorter than it really is. If several items in a survey rely on the same response set, you can turn them into a single item with instructions to circle the column of the correct response. Rather than numbering each item separately, you number the instruction and define the items with letters. This technique is demonstrated in Example 6.2.

EXAMPLE 6.2
Arizona Geological Survey

Eric wishes to collect data on the types of rocks found in the various counties of Arizona. He designs a 40-item questionnaire to be completed by the interior commissioner of each county, but he knows that these individuals are quite busy and may not want to take the time to complete a lengthy survey. After some basic research, Eric discovers that the three most common rock forms in the state are quartz, limestone, and clay. Before sending out his survey, Eric performs a pilot test with two of the commissioners he knows personally. Their main complaint is that 40 items seem like quite a lot. Because Eric does not want to delete any of the items, he revises the numbering system of his survey and mails out his survey.

In his cover letter, Eric introduces his research project and asks for the commissioners' help in complying with a "short 10-item survey." Eric crafts a survey format that relies heavily on grouping similar items together. His first six items are grouped as follows:

Please circle the number corresponding to the most common type of rock at these sites in your county.

	Quartz	Limestone	Clay
Lakes	1	2	3
Hills	1	2	3
Mountains	1	2	3
Suburbs	1	2	3
Forests	1	2	3
Riverbeds	1	2	3

By combining his items together into groups, as shown above, Eric is able to reduce 40 items to 10 items without shortening his survey at all. It simply appears shorter. Eric hopes to find that despite their busy schedules, the county interior commissioners will be cooperative in completing his "short" questionnaire.

Surveys do not have to be filled with page after page of boring and monotonous questions. You can spice up the demeanor of your survey instrument by using some very simple techniques. Varying the response sets into columns for like groups, as in Example 6.2, is one commonly used method. Another is the incorporation of graphics into the response sets. After a series of difficult questions, you can place a few short easy questions to provide a mental break for the respondent.

Another difficulty that presents challenges for survey re-searchers is how to design skip patterns. The instruction "If you answered yes to the previous question, then skip to page 4" may be a wonderful way to use the same questionnaire for different groups, but it may cause you and your respondents untold frustration. Often, pilot testing will identify this type of simple visual problem with your survey's layout and format. At this stage, it can easily be corrected and retested before proceeding to your primary effort at data collection.

Example 6.3 illustrates the problem of the confusing skip pattern, a difficulty that is often identified during pilot testing. At this early stage, it is easily corrected, but if it appeared in the actual survey it could lead to devastating amounts of missing data.

EXAMPLE 6.3
Algebra Attitudes

Kathleen wishes to survey the attitudes of Chicago ninth graders toward different approaches to learning math. She designs a comprehensive questionnaire with several branch points that direct students to different sets of questions. The first item in the questionnaire is as follows:

Circle one letter for Item 1

1. Would you prefer to learn algebra by:

Listening to a teacher present new material
and working problems . . . .   A

Listening to a teacher but working problems
on your own . . . .   B

Reading new material and working problems
all on your own.   C

> *If you answered A, continue with Item 2-11 but skip Items 12-36 and then complete Items 37-50. If you answered B, skip Items 2-11, continue with Items 12-23, skip Items 24-36, and complete Items 37-50. If you answered C, skip Items 2-23 but complete Items 24-50.*

Before taking her survey into the entire school district, Kathleen pilot-tested it in her daughter's ninth-grade class of 30 girls and boys. She found that the students had numerous questions about the skip patterns. Despite their best efforts, the instructions were simply too confusing for them. Kathleen was forced to take her survey back to the drawing board to make it more "user friendly" for these respondents. In her revision, she used graphic images and hand-drawn arrows to direct students through the skip patterns more easily. When she returned to the same class to repeat her pilot test, she found that the students sailed through it without any apparent difficulty.

Pilot testing is not limited to new survey instruments. It is beneficial in even the most well-established survey instruments. Unless you are working with a population that is exactly the same as those in which a survey instrument has been validated, you will probably be introducing some new twist in your particular sample. Pilot testing established survey instruments is extraordinarily helpful in all survey research. You may find for whatever reason that even an established survey instrument does not perform well in your sample. This will afford you the opportunity to select a different survey instrument or even develop your own if you have the time and resources.

Example 6.4 demonstrates another potential problem often identified during pilot testing: the issue of item nonrelevance in your population.

EXAMPLE 6.4
Type A Personalities

The Jenkins Activity Scale is a published and well-established survey instrument that distinguishes individuals with relatively high levels of daily anxiety and compulsion, so-called Type A personalities, from those with lower levels of stress, so-called Type B personalities. It was intended to identify people at risk for heart attacks, strokes, and high blood pressure.

In an effort to find potential clients with certain investment habits, a money management firm decided to mail out this self-administered survey to a national sample of 5,000 members of the American Association of Retired Persons (AARP). The firm has an idea that Type B personalities are more likely to hand over their savings for investments without asking too many questions. After a thorough literature review, the firm's marketing department selected the Jenkins Activity Survey because it was short, easily scored, and well documented to be reliable and valid. The marketing director submitted his proposal to the firm's vice president for growth.

Before committing the firm's resources to this particular survey instrument, the vice president asked her assistant to conduct a small pilot test of the Jenkins Activity Survey with 12 members of the local AARP chapter. Of the 8 surveys that were returned, 7 respondents completed only a small fraction of the items. It turned out that most of the items on the survey referred to respondents' conduct at work, interactions with professional colleagues, and number of vacation days taken from the job. Of the 8 people who replied to the pilot test, only 1 was currently employed. The remainder were retired and could not answer, not surprising given the target audience of retired persons.

The vice president fired the marketing director and hired an expensive outside consulting firm to develop and psychometrically evaluate a new survey instrument that assesses daily anxiety levels in retired persons as a predictor of investment strategies.

Pilot testing is a necessary and important part of survey development. It provides useful information about how your survey instrument actually plays in the field. Although it requires extra time and energy, the pilot test is a critical step in assessing the practical application of your survey instrument.

Checklist for Pilot Testing

✓ Are there any typographical errors?

✓ Are there any misspelled words?

✓ Do the item numbers make sense?

✓ Is the type size big enough to be easily read?

✓ Is the vocabulary appropriate for the respondents?

✓ Is the survey too long?

✓ Is the style of the items too monotonous?

✓ Are there easy questions in with the difficult questions?

✓ Are the skip patterns too difficult?

✓ Does the survey format flow well?

✓ Are the items appropriate for the respondents?

✓ Are the items sensitive to possible cultural barriers?

✓ Is the survey in the best language for the respondents?

7 Multicultural Issues

When designing new survey instruments or applying established ones in populations of different ethnicity, creed, or nationality, you must make sure that your items translate well into both the language and the culture of your target audience. Although you may be able to translate a survey instrument's items into a new language, they may not measure the same dimension in that culture. This is particularly relevant when studying social attitudes and health behaviors. Different cultures have very different concepts of health, well-being, illness, and disease, for example. Therefore, a well-developed concept in one culture may not even exist in another. Even if you start with a well-validated survey instrument in English, various populations within the United States and

69

elsewhere in the world may not approach the concept with the same ideas.

Failing to be attentive to multicultural issues may result in significant bias when collecting data. For example, when classifying ethnicities, survey researchers often categorize all Asians together. For some projects, this may be acceptable; however, many attitudes and behaviors vary tremendously among Chinese, Japanese, Thai, Vietnamese, and other cultures within Asia. By blithely lumping them all into one class, you may overlook differences that are important to your conclusions.

Example 7.1 shows that problems can arise not only from language barriers but also from conceptual differences due to culture.

EXAMPLE 7.1
Elderly Women

Olivia decided to use an established, well-validated, 24-item survey instrument to measure family attitudes in elderly American women of Anglo and Latina descent. To facilitate crossing the potential language barrier, she asked her girlfriend, a native Mexican, to translate the survey into Spanish. After the translation was complete, Olivia administered it to a sample of 300 elderly women, of whom 150 classified themselves as Latina and 150 classified themselves as Anglo-American.

After tabulating her data, Olivia was disappointed to discover that, despite the perfect translation into Spanish, a tremendous amount of data was missing from the Latina respondents' surveys. When she researched the matter more closely, Olivia realized that she had failed to take into account the multicultural issues raised by her project. She found out that the Latina women had a concept of family that was completely different from that of the Anglo-Americans. For example, the Anglos tended to include only parents and children in their concept of family, whereas the Latinas tended to also include grandparents, aunts and uncles, and cousins. The survey instrument had been validated only in Anglo-American populations. Although the words in the survey had been translated quite well into Spanish, the modern philosophy of family in the two groups were so different that most of the Anglo concepts had no real meaning for the Latinas. Therefore, they left many items blank, and Olivia was unable to analyze her data in a useful way.

Exercises

1. Northwest Cable administers a television preference survey to 100 viewers in its southeastern region and presents the following two items at different points in the same survey:

   - How many hours of TV did you watch in the past 7 days?

   - How many programs of what length did you watch during the past 7 days?

   The company is trying to document

   a. Alternate form reliability

   b. Test-retest reliability

   c. Internal consistency reliability

   d. All of the above

2. If Southwest Cable administers a new television preference questionnaire to 50 viewers in its northeastern region on January 15, then repeats the identical survey with the same 50 viewers on February 15, and finds close correlations between the two data sets, its survey instrument can be said to have good

   a. Alternate form reliability

   b. Test-retest reliability

   c. Internal consistency reliability

   d. All of the above

3. When you read that a scale has a coefficient alpha of 0.90, you can be assured that the scale has a high degree of

   a. Alternate form reliability

   b. Test-retest reliability

   c. Internal consistency reliability

   d. All of the above

4. If you were developing a measure of student satisfaction with school lunches in a 750-student elementary school, how might you design an experiment to assess test-retest reliability?

5. Design two different response sets to test alternate-form reliability for the following item from a meteorological survey instrument about regional precipitation:

   *How much rain did your region
   have during the past 4 weeks?*

6. A new survey instrument is published for assessing safety in automobiles. It contains 12 items about a wide range of qualities, such as strength of the seatbelt straps, temperature at which the engine overheats, how well the windshield shatters

during impact, thickness of the steel in the doors, and adequacy of the ventilation system. After the survey instrument is tested in several models, it is determined that the instrument has good test-retest and alternate-form reliability, but its coefficient alpha is only 0.23. What does this mean?

7. The housing office of a large university wants to measure student satisfaction with various aspects of the campus dormitories. After researching the relevant published literature, the housing director cannot find a survey instrument that she thinks is appropriate, so she decides to develop her own. She remembers from her survey research course in college that her index must be reliable and valid. She also remembers that her index must have good content validity. How would you advise her to begin her project?

8. Brian has designed and pilot-tested a new 20-item, self-administered survey instrument that measures religious observance in a group of Midwesterners. How might he go about assessing it for concurrent validity?

9. Obsessions Unlimited is a company that provides personal organization services for individuals who pay a fee in return for individual help in organizing their personal lives. The company is looking for a better way to assess the quality of its applicants for employment as personal organization assistants. The director of personnel wants to devise a screening questionnaire that has excellent predictive validity in selecting assistants who will produce customer satisfaction. He puts together a reliable self-administered index of 20 items, which can be easily completed by applicants for the job. How should he test his index's predictive validity?

Answers

1. Alternate-form reliability

2. Test-retest reliability

3. Internal consistency reliability

4. Because satisfaction with the lunches may be different on any given day, you must administer your survey at separate times on the same afternoon after the lunch in question. For example, you might have students complete a questionnaire right after they return from lunch and again right before school lets out.

5. *Response Set 1:*   In this region, the average total rainfall (to the nearest 10th of an inch) during the past 4 weeks was:

    None

    0.1 to 4 inches

    4.1 to 8 inches

    8.1 to 12 inches

    More than 12 inches

Response Set 2: In this region, the number of days it rained during the past 4 weeks was:

> No days
>
> 1 to 7 days
>
> 8 to 14 days
>
> 15 to 21 days
>
> 22 to 28 days

Response Set 3: In this region, rainfall during the past 4 weeks has been:

> Below average for this time of year
>
> About average for this time of year
>
> Above average for this time of year

6. The survey instrument has low internal consistency reliability. This means that although the items seem to focus on various aspects of the same concept, they may actually be quite different. The author should consider the possibility that the items may not be measuring the same concept.

7. If she wants to ensure content validity, she must tailor her survey instrument to the needs of the students themselves. The best way to start would be to put together a focus group of students presently living in the campus dorms. During this exploratory session, she could get an idea of what issues are important to them. She might then put together a first draft of

her questionnaire and show it to these students for their comments. This would provide initial testing of content validity.

8. To assess concurrent validity, Brian must identify some "gold standard" method of assessing religious observance. He should start by looking in the sociology research literature. Because there may not be such an established measure, he may have to select a measure that appears to be a gold standard. For example, he might use actual attendance at religious services or religious functions during a 4-week period for a randomly selected group of Midwesterners.

9. To test predictive validity of his screening questionnaire, the personnel director must also select an established outcome measure of customer satisfaction. He should administer his questionnaire to all employment applicants over a defined period of time. He should then use the selected outcome measure to document the satisfaction of those customers served by the different employees. By using the results from the screening index to try to predict which employees will have good results on the satisfaction outcomes measure, he can assess the predictive validity of his questionnaire. If those who score well on the screening index also score well on the satisfaction index, then his screening index can be said to have good predictive validity.

Suggested Readings

Fowlern, F. J. (1988). *Survey research methods.* Newbury Park, CA: Sage.

A user-friendly and practical guide to the fundamentals of good survey design.

McDowell, I., & Newell, C. (1987). *Measuring health: A guide to rating scales and questionnaires.* Oxford, UK: Oxford University Press.

A comprehensive guide to the most commonly used health questionnaires, complete with examples of actual items, reliability and validity data, and author addresses for each questionnaire.

Rossi, P. H., Wright, J. D., & Anderson A. B. (1983). *Handbook of survey research.* San Diego, CA: Academic Press, Harcourt Brace Jovanovich.

One of the most complete manuals available on theory, quantitative methods, and practical issues encountered in various aspects of survey research.

79

Tulsky, D. S. (1990). An introduction to test theory. *Oncology, 4,* 43-48.

A thorough, succinct summary of the principles of reliability and validity illustrated with case examples.

Wilkin, D., Hallam, L., & Doggett, M. (1992). *Measures of need and outcome for primary health care.* Oxford, UK: Oxford University Press.

Includes a comprehensive chapter on methods of measurement that covers reliability, validity, scoring, and other practical aspects of survey evaluation.

Glossary

Alternate-form reliability   Measure of survey reproducibility in which a question is worded in two or more different ways and the different versions are compared for consistency in responses.

Codebook   Collection of rules developed when translating survey responses into numerical codes for analysis. For example, a codebook might contain a rule on ethnicity that assigns the number 1 to African Americans, 2 to Anglos, 3 to Asians, 4 to Latinos, and so on. Another rule might assign the number 9 to all items for which data is missing. The codebook is a summary of all such rules to be used as a reference during data analysis.

Concurrent validity   Measure of survey accuracy in which the results of a new survey or scale are compared with the results from a generally accepted "gold standard" test after both tests are administered to the same group of respondents.

Construct validity Theoretical gestalt-type measure of how meaningful a survey instrument is, usually after many years of experience by numerous investigators in many varied settings.

Content validity Measure of survey accuracy that involves formal review by individuals who are experts in the subject matter of a survey.

Convergent validity Measure of survey accuracy that involves using different tools to obtain information about a particular variable and seeing how well they correlate. Evaluating convergent validity is analogous to measuring alternate-form reliability but with different established instruments rather than different wordings of a single item.

Correlation coefficient Statistical measure of how closely two variables or measures are related to each other. Correlation coefficients are usually calculated and reported as r values.

Criterion validity Measure of survey accuracy that involves comparing it to other tests. Criterion validity may be categorized as convergent or divergent.

Divergent validity Measure of survey accuracy that involves using different tools for obtaining information about similar but discrete variables and seeing if they differ.

Face validity Most casual measure of a survey's accuracy, usually assessed informally by nonexperts.

Factor analysis Computer-assisted method used to assess whether different items on a survey belong together in one scale.

Index (see **scale**)

Internal consistency reliability Measure of survey accuracy that reflects how well different items in a scale vary together when applied to a group of respondents.

Interobserver reliability Reproducibility of a set of observations on one variable made by different observers.

Intraobserver reliability Reproducibility of a set of observations on one variable made by the same observer at different times.

Item Question that appears on a survey or in an index.

Measurement error Degree to which instruments yield data that are incorrect due to the measurement process.

Multitrait scaling analysis Advanced computer-assisted method of measuring how well various items go together in a particular scale (similar to **factor analysis**).

Pilot testing During the development phase of a new survey or instrument, the practice of trying out the new survey or index in a small sample one or more times to see how well the survey works, expose errors, and identify areas of difficulty for respondents.

Practice effect Phenomenon in which a respondent becomes familiar with items on a survey or index taken at several time points. Over time, the individual's responses correlate highly with each other simply because that person is remembering previous answers and not because the variable being measured is unchanged.

Predictive validity Measure of survey accuracy in which an item or scale is correlated with future observations of behavior, survey responses, or other events.

Psychometrics   Science of measuring psychological or qualitative phenomena.

r **value**   Statistic that is used to report correlations. (see **correlation coefficient**)

Random error   Degree to which instruments yield data that are incorrect *not* due to the measurement process, but due to uncontrollable fluctuations in responses.

Reliability   Reproducibility or stability of data or observations. When using a survey or index, one wants to achieve high reliability, implying that the data are highly reproducible.

Scale   Series of items that measures a single variable, trait, or domain.

Scaling   Process in which different items are placed together in a single index that pertains to one variable of interest. Factor analysis and multitrait scaling analysis are often used in this process.

Scoring   Conversion of an individual's survey answers into a numerical value for comparison with those of other individuals or of the same individual at different times.

Split halves method   Technique used to assess alternate-form reliability, in which a large sample is equally divided into two smaller samples, each of which is administered a different form of the same question. The responses of the two samples are compared to each other. (see **alternate-form reliability**)

Survey instrument or **Survey**   Series of items that typically contains several scales. A survey may be self-administered or require a trained interviewer. It may be very long or contain a single item. It may be about issues as personal as sexual dysfunction or as impersonal as rainfall.

Test-retest reliability   Measure of the stability of responses over time in the same group of respondents. Many investigators report test-retest reliability by administering the same survey at two different time points (often 4 weeks apart) to the same group of individuals.

Validity   Assessment of how well a survey or index measures what it is intended to measure.

About the Author

MARK S. LITWIN, MD, MPH, is Assistant Professor of Health Services and Surgery/Urology at the UCLA Schools of Public Health and Medicine, where he is involved in teaching, clinical practice, and medical outcomes research. His MD is from Emory University, and his urology training was done at Harvard Medical School's Brigham and Women's Hospital. His MPH is from UCLA, where he received a Robert Wood Johnson Clinical Scholars Fellowship. He has extensive experience in health services research projects, including health-related quality of life, medical resource use, physician payment systems, and other areas of health policy.

THE SURVEY KIT
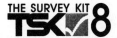
TSK 8

HOW TO
ANALYZE
SURVEY DATA

ARLENE FINK

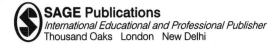
SAGE Publications
International Educational and Professional Publisher
Thousand Oaks   London   New Delhi

For information address:

 SAGE Publications, Inc.
2455 Teller Road
Thousand Oaks, California 91320
E-mail: order@sagepub.com

SAGE Publications Ltd.
6 Bonhill Street
London EC2A 4PU
United Kingdom

SAGE Publications India Pvt. Ltd.
M-32 Market
Greater Kailash I
New Delhi 110 048 India

Printed in the United States of America

Library of Congress Cataloging-in-Publication Data

Main entry under title:

The survey kit.
    p.   cm.
    Includes bibliographical references.
    Contents: v. 1. The survey handbook / Arlene Fink — v. 2. How to
ask survey questions / Arlene Fink — v. 3. How to conduct self-
administered and mail surveys / Linda B. Bourque, Eve P. Fielder —
v. 4. How to conduct interviews by telephone and in person / James
H. Frey, Sabine Mertens Oishi — v. 5. How to design surveys /
Arlene Fink — v. 6. How to sample in surveys / Arlene Fink —
v. 7. How to measure survey reliability and validity / Mark S. Litwin —
v. 8. How to analyze survey data / Arlene Fink — v. 9. How to
report on surveys / Arlene Fink.
    ISBN 0-8039-7388-8 (pbk. : The survey kit : alk. paper)
    1. Social surveys.   2. Health surveys.   I. Fink, Arlene.
HN29.S724   1995
300'.723—dc20   95-12712

This book is printed on acid-free paper.

95 96 97 98 99 10 9 8 7 6 5 4 3 2 1

Sage Production Editor: Diane S. Foster
Sage Copy Editor: Joyce Kuhn
Sage Typesetter: Janelle LeMaster

Contents

How to Analyze Survey Data:
Learning Objectives

Surveys produce observations in the form of narrations or numbers. Narrations are responses stated in the survey participant's own words, which are then counted, compared, and interpreted, often using methods borrowed from communications theory and anthropology.

Numbers, or numerical data, are obtained when, for example, survey respondents may be asked to rate items on ordered, or ranked, scales, say, with 1 representing a very positive feeling and 5 representing a very negative one; in other surveys, participants may be asked to tell their age, height, or number of trips they have taken or books they have read. Survey data that take numerical form are analyzed using statistics, the mathematics of collecting, organizing, and interpreting numerical information.

The aim of this book is to teach you to become better users and consumers of statistics when applied in the analysis of survey data. It hopes to teach the basic vocabulary of statistics and the principles and logic behind the selection and interpretation of commonly used methods to analyze survey data. What the book does *not* do is teach you to be a survey statistician. For that, formal study is recommended, and, when appropriate, statistical consultation. If this book achieves its objectives, you will not only be able to tell the consultant exactly what you need but be able to interpret the data presented to you.

The specific objectives are to enable you to:

■ Learn the use of analytic terms, such as the following:

  – Distribution
  – Critical value
  – Skew
  – Transformation
  – Measures of central tendency
  – Dispersion
  – Variation
  – Statistical significance
  – Practical significance
  – p value
  – Alpha
  – Beta
  – Linear
  – Curvilinear
  – Scatterplot
  – Null hypothesis

■ List the steps to follow in selecting an appropriate analytic method

- Distinguish between nominal, ordinal, and numerical scales and data so as to:

  - Identify independent and dependent variables
  - Distinguish between the appropriate uses of the mean, median, and mode
  - Distinguish between the appropriate uses of the range, standard deviation, percentile rank, and interquartile range
  - Understand the logic in and uses of correlations and regression
  - Learn the steps in conducting and interpreting hypothesis tests
  - Compare and contrast hypothesis testing and the use of confidence intervals
  - Understand the logic in and uses of the chi-square distribution and test
  - Understand the logic in and uses of the t test
  - Understand the logic in and uses of analysis of variance
  - Read and interpret computer output

1 What Statistics Do for Surveys

S tatistics is the mathematics of organizing and interpreting numerical information. The results of statistical analyses are descriptions, relationships, comparisons, and predictions, as expressed in Example 1.1.

AUTHOR'S NOTE: The names of all corporations and survey instruments used in examples throughout this book are fictitious.

EXAMPLE 1.1
Statistical Analysis and Survey Data

A survey is given to 160 people to find out about the number and types of books they read. The survey is analyzed statistically to do the following:

- Describe the backgrounds of the respondents
- Describe the responses to each of the questions
- Determine if a connection exists between the number of books read and travel during the past year
- Compare the number of books read by men with the number read by women
- Find out if gender, education, or income predicts how frequently the respondents read books

Illustrative results are these:

1. *Describe respondents' background.* Of the survey's 160 respondents, 77 (48.1%) were men, with 72 (48%) earning more than $50,000 per year and having at least 2 years of college. Of the 150 respondents answering the question, 32 (21.3%) stated that they always or nearly always read for pleasure.

2. *Describe responses.* Respondents were asked how many books they read in a year and if they preferred fiction or nonfiction. On average, college graduates read 10 or more books, with a range of 2 to 50. The typical college graduate prefers nonfiction to fiction.

3. *Relationship between travel and number of books read.* Respondents were asked how often they traveled in the past year. Frequency of travel was compared to number of books read. Respondents who traveled at least twice in the past year read five or more books.

4. *Comparisons.* The percentage of men and women who read five or more books each year was compared, and no differences were found. On average, women's reading attitude scores were statistically significantly higher and more positive than men's, but older men's scores were significantly higher than older women's.

5. *Predicting frequency.* Education and income were found to be the best predictors of frequency of reading. That is, respondents with the most education and income read the most (one or more books each week).

In the first example, the findings are tallied and reported as percentages. A **tally** or **frequency count** is a computation of how many people fit into a category (men or women, under and over 70 years of age, read five or more books last year or did not). Tallies and frequencies take the form of numbers and percentages.

In the second example, the findings are presented as averages ("on average," "the typical" reader). When you are interested in the center (e.g., the average) of a distribution of findings, you are concerned with **measures of central tendency. Measures of dispersion** or spread, like the range, are often given along with measures of central tendency.

In the third example, the survey reports on the relationships between traveling and number of books read. One way of estimating the relationship between two characteristics is through **correlation.**

In the fourth example, comparisons are made between men and women. The term **statistical significance** is used to show that the differences between them are statistically meaningful and not due to chance.

In the fifth example, survey data are used to "predict" frequent reading. In simpler terms, predicting means answering a question like "Of all the characteristics on which I have survey data (e.g., income, education, type of books read, travel and leisure preferences), which one or ones are linked to frequent reading? For instance, does income make a difference? Education? Income and education?"

What methods should you use to describe, summarize, compare and predict? Before answering that question, you must answer at least four others: Do the survey data come from nominal, ordinal, or numerical scales or measures? How many independent and dependent variables are there? What statistical methods are potentially appropriate? Do the survey data fit the requirements of the methods?

Measurement Scales:
Nominal, Ordinal, and Numerical

A characteristic may be surveyed and measured using nominal, ordinal, and numerical scales. The resulting data are termed nominal, ordinal, or numerical.

NOMINAL SCALES

Nominal scales have no numerical value and produce data that fit into categories such as country of birth or gender. Nominal scales (and the data they yield) are sometimes called categorical scales or categorical data. Two survey questions resulting in nominal or categorical data are presented in Example 1.2.

EXAMPLE 1.2
Survey Questions That Use
Nominal Scales and Produce Nominal Data

1. What is the employee's gender? *Circle one*

Male	1
Female	2

2. Describe the type of lung cancer. *Circle one*

Small cell	1
Large cell	2
Oat cell	3
Squamous cell	4

Both questions categorize the responses. The answer is the "name" of the category into which the data fit. The numbers are arbitrary and have no inherent value. In Question 1, female could be labeled 1 and male 2. The numbers are merely codes.

When nominal data take on one of two values as in the first question (e.g., male or female), they are termed **dichotomous**. Nominal data are also called **categorical**.

ORDINAL SCALES

If an inherent order exists among categories, the data are said to have been obtained from an ordinal scale, as illustrated in Example 1.3.

EXAMPLE 1.3
Survey Questions That Use Ordinal Scales

1. How much education have you completed? *Circle one*

Never finished high school	1
High school graduate but no college	2
Some college	3
College graduate	4

2. Stage of tumor. *Circle one*

Duke's A	1
Duke's B	2
Duke's C	3
Duke's D	4

3. How often during the past month did you find yourself having difficulty trying to calm down? *Circle one*

Always	5
Very often	4
Fairly often	3
Sometimes	2
Almost never	1

Ordinal scales typically are seen in questions that call for ratings of quality (e.g., excellent, very good, good, fair, poor, very poor) and agreement (e.g., strongly agree, agree, disagree, strongly disagree).

NUMERICAL (INTERVAL AND RATIO) SCALES

When differences between numbers have a meaning on a numerical scale, they are called numerical. Age is a numerical variable, and so is weight and length of survival after diagnosis of a serious disease. Numerical data lend themselves to precision, so you can obtain data on age to the nearest second, for example.

You may hear the terms interval and ratio scales. Interval scales have an arbitrary zero point like the Fahrenheit and Celsius temperature scales. The difference, or distance, between 40° and 50° Celsius is the same as the difference between 70° and 80°. But 40° is not twice as hot as 20°, and 0° does not mean no heat at all. Ratio scales, however, have a true zero point, as in the absolute zero value of the Kelvin scale. Practically speaking, ratio scales are extremely rare, and statistically, interval and ratio scales are treated the same; hence the term numerical is a more apt (and neutral) phrase.

Numerical data can be **continuous**—height, weight, age—or discrete—numbers of visits to this clinic, numbers of previous pregnancies. Means and standard deviations are used to summarize the values of numerical measures.

The three measurement scales and their data types are contrasted in the following table.

Measurement Scale and Type of Data	Examples	Comments
Nominal	Type of disease: small-cell, large-cell, oat-cell, and squamous-cell cancer; grade in school: 9th, 10th, 11th, 12th; ethnicity; gender	Observations belong to categories. Observations have no inherent order of importance. Observations sometimes are called categorical.
Ordinal	Ratings of health status (excellent, very good, good, fair, poor) and of agreement (strongly agree, agree, disagree, strongly disagree); rankings (the top 10 movies)	Order exists among the categories—that is, one observation is of greater value than the other or more important.
Numerical	Continuous numerical scales: scores on an achievement test or attitude inventory; age; height; length of survival Discrete numerical scales: number of visits to a physician; number of falls; number of days absent from work or class	Differences between numbers have meaning on a numerical scale (e.g., higher scores mean better achievement than lower scores, and a difference between 12 and 13 has the same meaning as a difference between 99 and 100). Some statisticians distinguish between interval scales (arbitrary 0 point, as in the Fahrenheit scale) and ratio scales (absolute 0, as in the Kelvin scale); these measures are usually treated the same statistically, so they are combined here as numerical.

Independent and Dependent Variables

A **variable** is a characteristic that is measurable. Weight is a variable, and all persons weighing 55 kilograms have the same numerical weight. Satisfaction with a product is also a variable. In this case, however, the numerical scale has to be devised and rules must be created for its interpretation. For example, in Survey A, product satisfaction is measured on a scale from 1 to 100, with 100 representing perfect satisfaction. Survey B, however, measures satisfaction by counting the number of repeat customers. The rule is that at least 15% of all customers must reorder within a year for a demonstration of satisfaction.

Your choice of method for analyzing survey data is always dependent on the type of data available to you (nominal, ordinal, and numerical) and on the number of variables that is involved. Some survey variables are termed **independent,** and some are termed **dependent.**

Independent variables are also called "explanatory" or "predictor" variables because they are used to explain or predict a response, outcome, or result—the dependent variable. The independent and dependent variables can be identified by studying the objectives and target of the survey, as illustrated in Example 1.4.

EXAMPLE 1.4
Targets and Independent Variables

Objective 1: To describe the quality of life of men over 65 years of age with different health characteristics (e.g., whether or not they have hypertension or diabetes) and social backgrounds (e.g., whether they live alone or live with someone; if they are employed or unemployed). The men in the survey had surgery for prostate cancer within the past 2 years.

Target: Men over 65 years of age with differing health characteristics and social backgrounds who have had surgery for prostate cancer within the past 2 years

Independent variables: Age (over 65 years of age), health characteristics (presence or absence of hypertension or diabetes), and social background (living alone or not and employment status)

Dependent variable: Quality of life

Objective 2: To compare elementary school children in different grades in two ways: (a) opinions on the school's new dress code and (b) attitude toward school

Target: Boys and girls in Grades 3 through 6 in five elementary schools

Independent variables: Gender, grade level, and school

Dependent variables: Opinion of new dress code and attitude toward school

Objective 1 has three independent variables and one dependent variable; Objective 2 has three independent and two dependent variables. A next step in the analytic process is to determine whether the survey's data for these variables are nominal, ordinal, or numerical. Look at Example 1.5.

EXAMPLE 1.5
Are Data Nominal, Ordinal, or Numerical?

Survey 1: Men With Prostate Cancer

Independent Variables
- Age (over 65 years of age)
- Health characteristics (presence or absence of hypertension or diabetes)
- Social background (whether living alone or not and employment status)

Characteristics of Survey Questions
- To get age, ask for exact birth date.
- To find out about health characteristics, ask "Do you have any of the following medical conditions? Answer yes or no for each."
- To find out about social background, ask respondents to answer yes or no regarding whether or not they live alone and are presently employed full-time, part-time, or not employed at all.

Type of Data
- Age: Numerical (birth date)
- Health characteristics: Nominal (presence or absence of medical conditions)

- Social background: Nominal (live alone or do not; employed or not)

Dependent Variable
- Quality of life

Characteristics of Survey Questions
- Ask questions that call for ratings of various aspects of quality of life. For example, ask respondents to describe how frequently they feel restless, down in the dumps, rattled, moody, and so on.
- Use categories for the responses, such as all of the time, most of the time, a good bit of the time, some of the time, a little of the time, none of the time.

Type of Data
- Quality of life: Ordinal (May be numerical if statistical evidence exists that higher scores are statistically and practically different from lower scores)

Survey 2: Children, Dress Code, and Attitude Toward School

Independent Variables
- Gender
- Grade level
- Schools

Characteristics of Survey Questions
- To get gender, ask if male or female.
- Ask participants to write in grade level and name of school.

Type of Data
- Gender: Nominal
- Grade level: Nominal
- Name of School: Nominal

Dependent Variables
- Opinion of new dress code
- Attitude toward school

Characteristics of Survey Questions
- To get opinions on new dress code, ask for ratings of like and dislike (e.g., from like a lot to dislike a lot).
- To learn about attitudes, use the Attitude Toward School Rating Scale.

Type of Data
- Opinions of dress code: Ordinal
- Attitudes: Ordinal

When choosing an appropriate analysis method, you begin by deciding on the purpose of the analysis, and then you determine the number of independent and dependent variables and whether you have nominal, ordinal, or numerical data. When these activities are completed, you can choose an analysis method. Example 1.6 shows how this works in two hypothetical cases. (In the example, two statistical methods are mentioned. Their uses are discussed later.)

EXAMPLE 1.6
Choosing an Analysis Method

Survey Objective: To compare scores on the Quality of Life Inventory achieved by men who are employed full-time, part-time, or unemployed and who had surgery for prostate cancer 2 years ago.

Number of Independent Variables: One (employment status)
   Type of data: Nominal (employed full-time, employed part-time, unemployed)

Number of Dependent Variables: One (quality of life)
   Type of data: Numerical (scores)
Name of Possible Method of Analysis: One-way analysis of variance

Survey Objective: To compare boys and girls with differing scores on the Attitude Toward School Questionnaire in terms of whether they do or do not support the school's new dress code

Number of Independent Variables: One (gender)
   Type of data: Nominal (boys, girls)

Number of Dependent Variables: One (support dress code)
   Type of data: Nominal (support or do not support)
Possible Method of Analysis: Logistic regression

In Example 1.6, both choices of analytic method are labeled "possible." The appropriateness of the choice of a statistical method depends upon the extent to which you meet the method's *assumptions* about the characteristics and quality of the data. In the preceding examples, too little information is given to help you decide on whether the assumptions are met.

The aim of the discussion that follows is to guide you in understanding the logic behind the choice of an analytic method. The discussion gives examples of the formulas and use of some of the most commonly accepted statistical procedures and describes their assumptions. The idea is not to turn you into a survey statistician but to guide you in obtaining the information you need to choose the correct analysis. When implementing the analysis, the calculations are only meaningful if they are the ones you need and if the data are available and clean.

The following checklist should be used *before* you choose an analysis method.

Checklist for Choosing a Method to Analyze Survey Data

✓ **Count the number of independent variables.**

✓ **Determine if the data on the independent variables are nominal, ordinal, or numerical.**

✓ **Count the number of dependent variables.**

✓ **Determine if the data on the dependent variables are nominal, ordinal, or numerical.**

✓ **Choose potential data-analytic methods.**

✓ **Screen the survey's objectives (description, relationship, prediction, comparison) against the analysis method's assumptions and outcomes.**

Descriptive Statistics and Measures of Central Tendency: Numerical and Ordinal Data

Descriptive statistics describe data in terms of measures of central tendency. These are measures or statistics that describe the location of the center of a distribution. A **distribution** consists of values (e.g., scores and other numerical values, such as number of years in office, age in years as of today) of a variable or characteristic (e.g., attitudes, knowledge, behavior, health status, and demographics, such as age, income, etc.) and the frequency of their occurrence. For example, in a survey that asks if the respondent is under 25 years of age or 25 years and older, the distribution consists of the ages (with the values: under 25 years and 25 years and older) and the frequency (the number of respondents in each of the two age categories). In a survey that produces scores on a scale from 1 to 10, the distribution of scores consists of the numbers of people who achieve a score of 1, 2, and so on to a score of 10.

Measures of dispersion are descriptive statistics that depict the spread of numerical data. For example, in a survey that produces scores on a scale from 1 to 10, you calculate measures of dispersion to answer questions like "Are most of the scores clustered around a single score, say 5?" and "What is the highest score? The lowest?"

Measures of central tendency are the mean, median, and mode. Measures of dispersion or spread are the range, standard deviation, and percentiles.

MEAN

The **mean** is the arithmetic average of observations. It is symbolized as $\overline{X}$. You calculate the mean by totaling observations (scores or responses) and dividing by the number of observations.

The formula is $\Sigma X/n$. Σ is the Greek letter sigma, and it means to add or sum. X is each individual observation, and n is the total number of observations.

Example 1.7 shows the calculation of the mean.

EXAMPLE 1.7
Calculating the Mean

Students who took the 20-point Attitude Toward Spelling Survey received these 15 scores:

$$-6, -3, -3, 0, 2, 2, 2, 3, 3, 3, 3, 4, 4, 5, 6.$$

The mean $(\Sigma X/n)$ of the scores is

$$(-6) + (-3) + (-3) + (0) + (2) + (2) + (2) + (3) + (3) +$$
$$(3) + (3) + (4) + (4) + (5) + (6) = 25/15 = 1.67.$$

Suppose the 15th student obtained a score of 20 (rather than 6). The mean would be 39/15, or 2.6. The mean is sensitive to extreme values in a set of observations.

You can only use the mean when the numbers you have can be added or when characteristics are measured on a numerical scale like those used to describe height, weight, and scores on a test.

MEDIAN

The median is the middle observation. Half of the observations are smaller and half are larger. No abbreviation or symbol is commonly used for the median. Because it falls in the middle, the median is sometimes considered the "typical" observation.

You determine the median by doing the following:

1. Arrange the observations (scores, responses) from lowest to highest (or vice versa).
2. Count to the middle value. The median is the middle value for an odd number of observations and is the mean of the two middle values for an even number of observations.

Consider this odd number of scores:

$$3, 6, 6, 7, 9, 13, 17.$$

The median is 7 because half of the scores (3, 6, 6) are below 7 and half (9, 13, 17) are above.

Take this even number of scores:

$$-2, 0, 6, 7, 9, 9.$$

The two middle scores are 6 and 7. If you add 6 + 7 and divide by 2, you get the median, 6.5.

EXERCISES

1. Calculate the median for the following:

2, 4, 5, 8, 9, 11.

2. Calculate the median for the following:

3, 9, 7, –2, 6, 7.

■ ANSWERS ■

1. Median is 6.5.
2. Rearrange so that you have 9, 7, 7, 6, 3, –2 for a median of 6.5.

The median is not as sensitive as the mean to extreme values. So, if you have a few "outliers" in the distribution, you will probably want to use the median.

MODE

The mode of a distribution is the value of the observations that occurs most frequently. It is commonly used when you want to show the most "popular" value.

Distribution A		Distribution B	
Score	Frequency	Score	Frequency
34	2	34	0
33	6	33	1
32	8	32	7
31	11	31	21
30	15	30	4
29	18	29	3
28	10	28	7
27	12	27	10
26	8	26	14
25	3	25	23
24	1	24	11
23	0	23	5

Distribution A has a single mode of 29, with 18 responses. This distribution is **unimodal.** Distribution B has two modes, at 25 and 31, so the distribution is **bimodal.**

Distributions: Skewed and Symmetric

When you have a distribution that has a few outlying observations in one direction—a few small values or a few large ones —it is termed **skewed.** A **symmetric** distribution is one in which the distribution has the same shape on both sides of the mean.

Figure 1–1 shows that if the mean and median are equal, the distribution of observations is symmetric (A). If the mean is smaller than the median, the distribution is skewed to the left (B). If the mean is larger than the median, the distribution is skewed to the right (C).

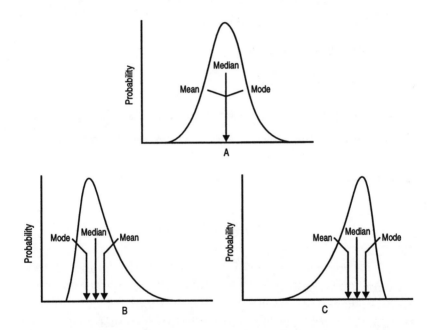

Figure 1–1. Distributions: Skewed and Symmetric
SOURCE: *Statistical First Aid* (p. 32), by R. Hirsch and R. K. Riegelman, 1992, Cambridge, MA: Blackwell Scientific. Copyright 1992 by Blackwell Scientific Publications, Inc. Used with permission.

Checklist for Using the
Mean, Median, and Mode

✓ Use the *mean* when:

- The distribution is approximately symmetric.
- You are interested in numerical values.

✓ Use the *median* when:

- You are concerned with the typical score.
- The distribution is skewed.
- You have ordinal data.

✓ Use the *mode* when:

- The distribution has two or more peaks.
- You want the prevailing view, characteristic, or quality.

Measures of Spread

Suppose you ask a group of people to rate the quality of food at a particular restaurant. You find that the average rating is 3.5 on a scale of 1 (*poor*) to 5 (*excellent*). How close in agreement are the people? Do their ratings cluster around 3 (the middle point), or are the ratings **spread,** with some people assigning ratings of 1 and the remainder 5?

The extent of spread, or the **dispersion** or **variation,** of the observations is described by the range, standard deviation, percentile, and interquartile range.

RANGE

The **range** is the difference between the largest observation and the smallest. Sometimes, the range is expressed by highest and lowest values rather than just the difference between them. Example 1.8 demonstrates how the range is used.

EXAMPLE 1.8
Using the Range

These are the scores achieved by 10 people on the 20-item Survey of Compassionate Behavior:

4, 7, 9, 11, 11, 12, 14, 16, 17, 18.

The range is 14 points. The scores ranged from 4 to 18.

STANDARD DEVIATION

The **standard deviation** is a measure of the spread of data about their mean and an essential part of many statistical tests. Although it is highly unlikely that you will compute a standard deviation by hand, it is useful to see how the standard deviation functions.

The standard deviation (SD) depends on calculating the average distance that the average score is from the mean. The definitional formula is

$$SD = \sqrt{\Sigma \, (X - \overline{X})^2 / (n - 1)}$$

Suppose you had the following 10 scores on the Survey of Compassionate Behavior:

$$7, 10, 8, 5, 4, 8, 4, 9, 7, 8.$$

Here is how to calculate the standard deviation.

- Compute the mean:

1. $\overline{X} = (7 + 10 + 8 + 5 + 4 + 8 + 4 + 9 + 7 + 8)/10 = 7$.
2. Subtract the mean $(\overline{X})$ from each score (X), or $X - \overline{X}$.
3. Square each remainder from Step 2, or $(X - \overline{X})^2$.

Score	Step 2 $(X - \overline{X})$	Step 3 $(X - \overline{X})^2$
7	$(\ 7 - 7) = \ \ 0$	0
10	$(10 - 7) = \ \ 3$	9
8	$(\ 8 - 7) = \ \ 1$	1
5	$(\ 5 - 7) = -2$	4
4	$(\ 4 - 7) = -3$	9
8	$(\ 8 - 7) = \ \ 1$	1
4	$(\ 4 - 7) = -3$	9
9	$(\ 9 - 7) = \ \ 2$	4
7	$(\ 7 - 7) = \ \ 0$	0
8	$(\ 8 - 7) = \ \ 1$	1

4. Sum (Σ) all the squares from Step 3, or $\Sigma(X - \overline{X})^2$:

$$\Sigma(X - \overline{X})^2 = 0 + 9 + 1 + 4 + 9 + 1 + 9 + 4 + 0 + 1 = 38.$$

5. Divide the number in Step 4 by $n - 1$.

$$38/n - 1 = 38/9 = 4.22.$$

A digression: n is the number of scores; n − 1 is used because it produces a more accurate estimate of the true population's standard deviation and has other desirable mathematical properties. The quantity n − 1 is called the **degrees of freedom**, a concept that appears in other statistical formulas and tables. (The term degrees of freedom sounds intuitively meaningful but is in fact a complex statistical concept that is discussed in advanced texts and is well beyond the scope of this book.)

6. Take the square root of the result of Step 5.

$$\sqrt{4.22} = 2.05.$$

The standard deviation squared is called the **variance.** In the above example, the variance is 4.22. This statistic is not used as often as the standard deviation, which has two characteristics that should be kept in mind:

- Regardless of how the survey observations are distributed, at least 75% of them will always fall between the mean plus 2 standard deviations $(\overline{X} + 2SD)$ and the mean minus 2 standard deviations $(\overline{X} - 2SD)$. Suppose the mean of 32 scores is 12 and the standard deviation is 1.2. At least 75% of the 32 scores, or 24 scores, will be between 12 + 2(1.2) and 12 − 2(1.2), or between 14.4 and 9.6.

- Check to see if the distribution of the scores is symmetric (bell-shaped or normal), as shown in Figure 1-2. If so, then the following rules apply:

  About 68% of all observations fall between the mean and 1 standard deviation.

  About 95% of all observations fall between the mean and 2 standard deviations.

  About 99% of all observations fall between the mean and 3 standard deviations.

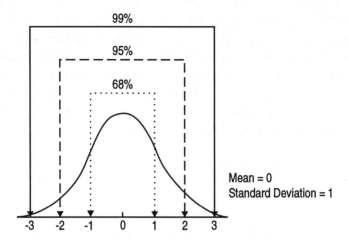

Figure 1–2. Normal Distribution

PERCENTILE

A **percentile** is a number that indicates the percentage of a distribution that is equal to or below that number. To say that a person scored in the 95th percentile means that 95% of others scored the same or below that person. Percentiles are often used to compare an individual value with a set of standards. Obtaining a reading score in the 30th percentile means that, compared to a standard or norm such as statewide scores, 30% have the same or lower scores and 70% have the same or higher scores. The median is the 50th percentile: Half of the distribution is at or above, and half is at or below.

INTERQUARTILE RANGE

A measure of variation that makes use of percentiles is the **interquartile range,** which is the difference between the 25th and the 75th percentile. The interquartile range contains 50%

of the observations. For example, suppose students at the 25th percentile have an average score of 30.2, and those at the 75th have a score of 90.1. The central 50% of the scores, or the interquartile range, is the difference between 90.1 (the 75th percentile) and 30.2 (the 25th). Another way to put it is that 50% of the students achieved scores between 30.2 and 90.1.

Guidelines for Selecting Measures of Dispersion

- *Range.* Numerical (e.g., scores from 1 to 100). The range describes the highest and lowest scores.
- *Standard deviation.* Numerical. Standard deviations describe the spread of means.
- *Percentile.* Ordinal (e.g., ratings on a scale from 1 = *very bad* to 5 = *very good*) or numerical (e.g., scores). The median is the 50th percentile.
- *Interquartile range.* Ordinal or numerical. The interquartile range is the central 50% of a set of observations or the difference between the 75th and the 25th percentile.

Descriptive Statistics and Nominal Data

Survey characteristics that are measured on a nominal scale do not have numerical values, but you can count them and describe how frequently they occur. Typical survey questions producing nominal data are the following:

Did you read these books?

Jane Eyre	Yes	No
Schindler's List	Yes	No

Which best describes your current living status?
   Circle one only.

Living alone	Yes	No
Living with a friend, not related	Yes	No
Living with a relative	Yes	No
Living in a communal arrangement	Yes	No
Other (specify _____)	Yes	No

For each question and its component parts, the choices are yes or no: Yes, I read *Jane Eyre*, or no, I did not; yes, I live alone, or no, I do not; and so on. Nominal survey data are analyzed by using descriptive statistics such as proportion, percentage, ratio, and rate.

PROPORTION AND PERCENTAGE

A **proportion** is the number of observations or responses with a given characteristic divided by the total number of observations. Look at the following table.

Table 1–1
Perceptions of an Experimental and Control Group

Outcome	Experimental Group	Control Group
Felt better	65	73
Felt worse	4	10
Total	69	83

A proportion is a *part* divided by a *whole*. Using the data in Table 1–1, the proportion who felt better in the experimental group is 65 divided by the total number of responses in the experimental group (better and worse), which is 69, or 65/69, or .9420. In the control group, the proportion who felt better is 73/83, or .8795.

A **percentage** is a proportion multiplied by 100%, so the percentage of people who felt better in the experimental group is .9420 × 100%, or 94.2%, while the percentage who felt better in the control is .8795 × 100%, or 87.9% rounded off to 88%.

The proportion is a special case of the mean in which the observations with a given characteristic, say, people who felt better, are assigned the value 1, and the observations without the characteristic, say, people who felt worse, are assigned the value 0. The sum X in the numerator of the formula for the mean is the sum of the 0s and 1s and the denominator is still n (the number of observations). So, the proportion of people (Table 1–1) who felt better is $(65 \times 1) + (4 \times 0)/69$, or .9420.

RATIO AND RATE

A **ratio** is a *part* divided by another *part*. It is the number of observations in a given group with a certain characteristic (e.g., feeling better) divided by the number of observations without the given characteristic (e.g., feeling worse). In Table 1–1, the ratio of feeling better to feeling worse in the experimental group is 65/4, or 16.25. The ratio of feeling better to feeling worse in the control is 73/10, or 7.3.

The **rate** is similar to the proportion except that a multiplier or **base**—1,000, 10,000, 100,000—is used. Rates are always computed over time, say, a year. Using the data in Table 1–1, suppose the experimental group participated in a study for a year, and the base was chosen to be 1,000. The rate of feeling better per 1,000 persons per year is then 65/69 × 1,000, or about 942 persons for each 1,000 per year.

2 Relationships or Correlation

Numerical Data

A relationship is a consistent association between or among variables. Suppose four surveys ask four questions:

1. Are the readers of this magazine also financially well off?
2. Do children who visit the school nurse most often have low self-concepts?
3. Do two observers agree on what they see?
4. Do people who do well in the program read well?

These questions are about relationships. For Question 1, the relationship of interest is between readers and financial well-being; for Question 2, between frequency of visits to the school nurse and self-concept; for Question 3, between what Observers 1 and 2 see; and for Question 4, between success in the program and high reading ability.

When you are concerned with the relationship between two variables, you are ready for correlation analysis. When the two variables are expressed numerically, you use a **correlation coefficient,** sometimes called a Pearson product-moment coefficient (after the statistician who discovered it). The correlation coefficient has a range of +1 to –1.

Consider two variables, X and Y. X is the independent variable, and Y is the dependent variable. A perfect correlation of +1 means that the value of Y increases by the same amount for each unit of increase in the value of X. A correlation of –1 indicates a perfect inverse relationship, in which the value of the dependent variable decreases by the same amount for each unit increase in the value of the independent variable. A correlation coefficient of zero indicates that no relationship exists between the dependent and independent variables. In other words, no consistent (that is, in one direction only) change in the value of the dependent variable occurs for each unit change in the value of the independent variable.

What do correlation coefficients mean? If you examine correlations graphically, you can see that the stronger the correlation (that is, the closer to +1 or to –1), the more it resembles a straight line. This is called a **linear** relationship.

Correlations are described graphically as a **scatterplot** in which the numerical values of the two variables are expressed as points. Figure 2–1a shows a perfect negative correlation (–1) between two variables; Figure 2–1b, a perfect positive correlation (+1); and Figure 2–1c, no correlation at all. As you can see, the correlations of +1 and –1 look like a line. When a correlation is near zero, the shape of the pattern of observations is spread throughout and is somewhat circular. A correlation of .50 tends to be more oval.

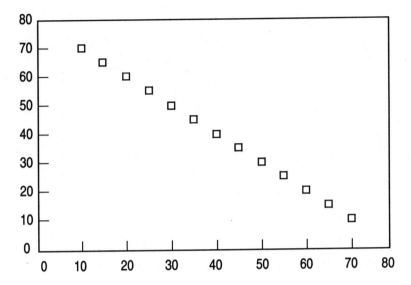

Figure 2–1a. Perfect Negative Correlation

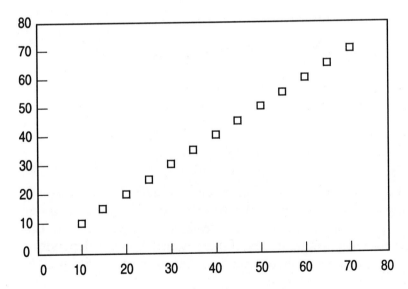

Figure 2–1b. Perfect Positive Correlation

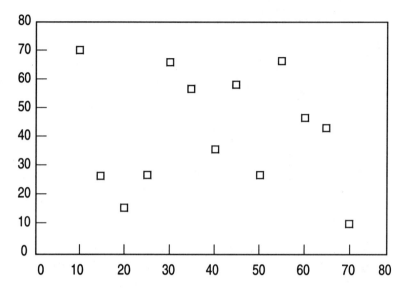

Figure 2–1c. Correlation of Zero

Calculating the Correlation Coefficient

The correlation coefficient is symbolized as r and is usually reported in two decimal places, and the formula for calculating r is

$$r = \frac{\Sigma(X - \overline{X}) (Y - \overline{Y})}{\sqrt{\Sigma(X - \overline{X})^2} \, \sqrt{\Sigma(Y - \overline{Y})^2}}.$$

The data used in the following calculation come from a survey to determine if a relationship exists between years of education and number of books read in the past year. X is the independent variable (years of education). Y is the dependent variable (number of books read in the past year). Ten people participated in the survey.

Respondent	X	Y	$X - \bar{X}$ $(\bar{X} = 9.5)$	$Y - \bar{Y}$ $(\bar{Y} = 11.8)$	$(X-\bar{X})(Y-\bar{Y})$	$(X-\bar{X})^2$	$(Y-\bar{Y})^2$
1	10	12	.5	.2	.1	.2	.04
2	12	14	2.5	2.2	5.5	6.2	4.8
3	5	7	−4.5	−4.8	21.6	20.2	23.0
4	7	9	−2.5	−2.8	7.0	6.2	7.8
5	7	10	−2.5	−1.8	4.5	6.2	3.2
6	12	15	2.5	3.2	8.0	6.2	10.2
7	10	13	.5	1.2	.6	.2	1.4
8	6	8	−3.5	−3.8	13.3	12.2	14.4
9	10	12	.5	.2	.1	.2	.04
10	16	18	6.5	6.2	40.3	42.3	38.4
Sum	95	118			101	100.1	103.3

1. Using the table above to get each Σ in the formula, you see that

$$\Sigma(X - \bar{X})(Y - \bar{Y}) = 101;$$
$$S(X - \bar{X})^2(Y - \bar{Y})^2 = 101.1 \times 103.$$

2. Filling in the formula, you get the following:
   a. $101/\sqrt{100.1}\ \sqrt{103.3}$
      $\sqrt{100.1} = 10.0$ (rounded)
      $\sqrt{100.3} = 10.2$ (rounded)
   b. $101/10 \times 10.2$
      $10 \times 10.2 = 102$
   c. $101/102 = .99$

The correlation coefficient is .99, suggesting a nearly perfect relationship between years of education and number of books read in the past year.

A correlation coefficient measures only a straight-line, or **linear,** relationship. If the distribution of data for either the independent or the dependent variable is skewed or contains outlying values, then you have a **curvilinear** relationship. In this case, a **transformation** of the data is warranted so that you can use conventional statistical methods. (Otherwise, you cannot.) When you transform data, you change the scale of measurement. How do you know if the relationship is curvilinear? You should always plot the relationship. Use the computer to do this unless you have a relatively small sample and the time to plot the relationship by hand on graph paper.

Size of the Correlation

How Large Should a Correlation Be?
A Conservative Rule of Thumb

0 to +.25 (or −.25) = Little or no relationship

+.26 to +.50 (or −.26 to −.50) = Fair degree of relationship

+.51 to +.75 = (or −.51 to −.75) = Moderate to good
relationship

Over +.75 (or −.75) = Very good to excellent relationship

For some social science disciplines, correlations of .26 to .50 are considered quite high, especially if they occur in multiple regression models where one variable is estimated by the use of more than one other variable.

The adequacy of the correlation is largely situational. For example, if the correlation between scores on your new and supposedly efficient attitude inventory and the older, supposedly more cumbersome one is .75, you might feel just fine until you find out that the correlation between someone else's inventory and the older one is .90.

Other than for values of $+1$, 0, and -1, however, correlation coefficients are not easy to interpret. We know, for example, that two variables with a correlation of .50 have a direct but imperfect relationship. Can we say that a correlation of .50 is half that of 1? Actually, to answer this question, you must make use of another statistic: **the coefficient of determination,** or r^2.

The r^2 tells the proportion of variation in the dependent variable that is associated with variation or changes in the independent variable. For a correlation coefficient of .50, the coefficient of determination is $.50^2$, or .25. This means that 25% of the variation in one measure (e.g., number of books read) may be predicted by knowing the value of the other (e.g., years of education)—or the other way around. A correlation of .50 describes an association that is one quarter as strong as a correlation of 1. In the example above (years of education and number of books read) where the correlation coefficient is .99, the coefficient of determination is $.99 \times .99$, or 98%. In this case, 98% of the variation in number of books read can be predicted by knowing years of education—or the other way around.

WARNING

Use correlations to estimate the relationship between two characteristics. Do NOT use them to establish cause and effect, or **causation**. A correlation analysis can show that years of education and numbers of books read are strongly related, but it cannot confirm that people read many books because they have many years of education. For one thing, a preference for reading may be the cause of many years of education, or years of education and number of books may be "caused" by a third factor—for example, a relatively high income.

Ordinal Data and Correlation

The Spearman (the statistician's name) rank correlation, sometimes called Spearman's rho, is often used to describe the relationship between two ordinal or one ordinal and one numerical characteristic, as in Example 2.1.

EXAMPLE 2.1
Using Spearman's Rho

To describe relationships between two ordinal characteristics

Does a relationship exist between ratings of satisfaction and of preferences for leisure time activities?

Does a relationship exist between level of education and ratings of satisfaction?

To describe relationships between one ordinal and one numerical characteristic

Does a relationship exist between level of education and quantity of sports equipment purchased in the past year?

Does a relationship exist between preference ratings and number of trips taken for pleasure?

Spearman's rho is also used with numerical data when the observations are skewed, with respondent outliers. In fact, if the median is the appropriate statistic to measure central tendency, then Spearman's rho is the correct correlation procedure.

The symbol for Spearman's rho is r_s. To calculate r_s, put the data in "rank" order (e.g., from highest to lowest score). Spearman's rho involves tedious computations and should be done by computer.

Spearman's rho ranges from $+1$ to -1, with $+$ and -1 meaning perfect correlation between the ranks rather than the numerical values.

Regression

One of the major differences between correlation and regression is that correlation describes a relationship and regression predicts a value. Regression analysis is concerned with estimating the components of a mathematical model that reflects the relationship between the dependent and independent variables in the population. To make the estimate, you assume that the relationship between variables is linear and that a straight line can be used to summarize the data. Regression is often referred to as linear regression, or simple linear regression. There is, however, nothing simple about regression analysis. Although you should understand its uses and how to interpret the results, you probably need more information than is presented here to actually conduct the analysis or to debate with a statistician the virtues of the alternative regression methods.

A common method for fitting a line to the data or observations is called least squares. Suppose you interview a sample of teenaged mothers to determine the extent to which County A's outreach program was responsible for encouraging them to keep their recommended number of prenatal care appointments. The regression equation would look like this:

Predicted number of visits = a + b (outreach).

This equation can be illustrated graphically, as shown in Figure 2–2.

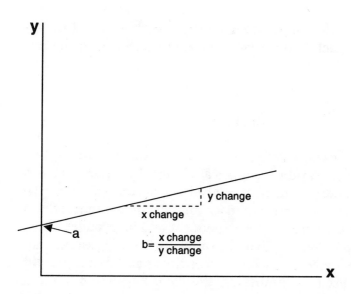

Figure 2–2. Graphic Interpretation of Regression Line

In the figure, you see a Y-axis (vertical) and an X-axis (horizontal). The line intercepts the Y-axis at *a* (called the **intercept**). The slope of the line measures the amount of change in Y for each unit change in X. If the slope is positive, Y increases as X increases; if the slope is negative, Y decreases as X increases. In the example above, in which your interest is the ability to relate prenatal care visits and the county's outreach teen program, *a* is the predicted number of visits without outreach. The slope, *b*, is the change in predicted number of visits for a unit of change in outreach. Stated another way, *b* is the amount of change in number of visits per outreach activity.

In regression, the slope in the population is symbolized by the Greek letter beta, or β_1, called the regression coefficient; β_0 denotes the intercept of the regression line. Also, the values of the Ys provided from the regression equation are predicted rather than actual values. Predicted values are distinguished from actual values by using the symbol $Y_.$. Because not all predictions are perfect, the regression model contains an error term, *e*. This is the amount the actual values of Y depart from the predicted values based on the regression line. The formula for the regression model is

$$Y_. = \beta_0 + \beta_1 X + e.$$

A Note on the Relationship
Between Two Nominal Characteristics

Surveys are usually interested in the significance of the relationship between two nominal variables rather than in just the relationship itself. You are more likely to be concerned with determining if the number of women answering yes to a particular question is statistically different from the number of men answering yes than you are in the extent of agreement between the number of women and men answering yes. Among the techniques for determining the significance of the differences between nominal variables are chi-square and Fisher's exact test. The chi-square distribution is described in Chapter 3. To use it appropriately, the normal distribution and hypothesis testing should be understood first.

The Normal Distribution

The normal distribution is a smooth, bell-shaped curve that is continuous and symmetric around the mean, which is symbolized by μ (Greek letter mu). The standard deviation is symbolized by σ (Greek lowercase letter sigma). The mean ± 1 standard deviation contains approximately 68% of the area under the normal curve; the mean ± 2 standard deviations contains approximately 95% of the area under the normal curve, and the mean ± 3 standard deviations contains approximately 99% of the area under the normal curve.

A normally distributed random variable with a mean and standard deviation can be transformed to a **standard normal,** or **z distribution.** This distribution has a mean of 0 and a standard deviation of 1.

The **z transformation** expresses the deviation from the mean in standard deviation units. Any normal distribution can be transformed to the z distribution by using this formula:

$$z = X - \beta/\sigma.$$

But what is a normal distribution of survey data or observations, and how do you know if you have one? When you study the **population at large,** certain variables like height, weight, blood pressure, and so on are considered normally distributed, that is, with 99% of the observations falling within ± 3 standard deviations of the mean. In actuality, perfectly normal distributions are as rare as perfectly normal people. This is true even for the distribution of height, weight, and blood pressure. Some distributions like these, however, are more normal than others.

Many computer programs will tell you graphically if a distribution is normal. If you prefer, you can plot the data yourself in the form of a histogram or box-and-whisker plot. A histogram uses area to describe the frequency distribution of numerical observations.

If a distribution is normal, then you can use statistical methods that assume normality, such as the *t* test. If not, you must transform the data to make them normal or use statistical methods that are not dependent on normal distributions.

Comparisons: Hypothesis Testing, *p* Values, and Confidence Levels

Surveys often compare two or more groups such as men and women, experimental and control participants, Team A and Team B, and students in the United States and students elsewhere. If differences exist, the magnitude is analyzed for significance. When comparing one nominal independent variable (e.g., experimental and control group) with respect to one numerical dependent variable (e.g., attitudes as measured by a score), a two-sample independent groups *t* test can be used. This statistical test, one of the most common, is illustrated in Example 2.2.

In the example, a survey is conducted after 2 years to find out if an experimental protocol affecting the management practices of a private company has improved the quality and efficiency of the cafeterias in selected schools. A survey is given to participating and nonparticipating schools, and the results are compared. The survey has 100 points; a 15-point difference is needed in favor of the private company for the experiment to be considered a success.

EXAMPLE 2.2
Comparing Two Groups: The *t* Test

Situation

The schools' cafeterias have always been run by employees of the school district. In recent years, the quality and efficiency of the cafeterias have diminished. An outside consulting group is called in to recommend ways to improve the management of the cafeterias. The consultants suggest that a private company, rather than the district, may have the answer. The district agrees. After a bidding process, a contract is awarded to the Great Food Company to manage several school cafeterias. After 2 years, students, teachers, administrators, and other school personnel are surveyed regarding their opinions of the quality of the food and the service and the efficiency of Great Food's operation.

Expectations

A statistically significant difference in opinions will be found favoring Great Food over the district. Opinions will be assessed using the results of a 100-point survey.

Analysis

A *t* test will be applied in comparing the two groups' opinions of quality and efficiency.

In Example 2.2, mention is made of **statistical significance**. This is a very important term. To be significant, differences must be attributable to a planned intervention (e.g., Great

Food's new management efforts) rather than to chance or historical occurrences (e.g., a change in expectations regarding the cafeteria that comes about because most students eat somewhere else).

Statistical significance is often interpreted to mean a result that happens by chance less than once in 20 times, with a p value less than or equal to .05. A p value is the probability of obtaining the results of a statistical test by chance. The null hypothesis states that no difference exists in the means (scores or other numerical values) obtained by two groups. Statistical significance occurs when the null hypothesis is rejected (suggesting that a difference does exist).

The following is a more detailed explanation of these terms and a guide for conducting a hypothesis test and determining statistical significance.

Guide to Hypothesis Testing, Statistical Significance, and p Values

1. *State the null hypothesis.* The null hypothesis (H_o) is a statement that no difference exists between the averages or means of two groups. The following are typical null hypotheses:

- No difference exists between the experimental and the control program's means. For example, no difference exists between privately and publicly managed school cafeterias.

- No difference exists between the sample's (the survey's participants) mean and the population's mean (the population from which the participants were sampled). For example, no difference exists between the sample of teachers chosen to be interviewed and those who were not chosen.

If no difference in means is found, the terminology used is "We failed to reject the null hypothesis." Do not say "We accepted the null hypothesis." Failing to reject the null suggests that a difference probably does NOT exist between the means, say, between the mean opinion scores in School A versus those in School B. If the null is rejected, then a difference exists between the mean opinion scores. Until the data are examined, however, you do not know if School A is favored or if School B is. All you know from the test is that a difference exists in means.

When you have no reason to suspect in advance which of two scores is better, you use a two-tailed hypothesis test. When you have an alternative hypothesis in mind, say, A is better than B, you use a one-tailed test. The tails in hypothesis testing refer to the extreme ends of a statistical distribution. The idea is that if you obtain a statistic that is way out in one or other tail or end of the expected distribution (according to or derived from the null hypothesis distribution), then you reject the null.

2. *State the level of significance for the statistical test (e.g., the t test) being used.* The level of significance, when chosen before the test is performed, is called the alpha value (denoted by the Greek letter α). The alpha gives the probability of rejecting the null hypothesis when it is actually true. Tradition keeps the alpha value small—.05, .01, or .001—because you do not want to reject a null hypothesis when in fact it is true and there is no difference between group means.

The *p* value is the probability that a difference as least as large as the obtained difference would have come about if the means were really equal. The *p* is calculated AFTER the statistical test and is sometimes called the **observed** or **obtained significance level.** If the *p* value, or observed significance, is less than alpha, then the null is rejected.

Current practice requires the specification of exact or obtained p values. That is, if the obtained p is .03, report that number rather than $p < .05$. Reporting the approximate p was common practice when tables in statistics texts were used to find the **critical values** of a distribution. The critical value is the absolute value that a test statistic must exceed for the null hypothesis to be rejected.

Although the computer output for commercially available programs gives exact ps, the practice of giving approximations (.05, .01, .001) has not been eradicated. The merit of using the exact values is that, without them, a finding of $p = .06$ may be viewed as not significant, whereas a finding of $p = .05$ will be.

3. *Determine the critical value the test statistic must attain to be significant.* Each test statistic, such as the mean, t, F, and chi-square, has a distribution. This distribution is called the **sampling distribution.** Its mean is called the **expected value,** and its variability is called the **standard error.**

All test statistic distributions are divided into an area of rejection and an area of acceptance. With a one-tailed test, the rejection area is *either* the upper or the lower tail of the distribution. For a two-tailed test, you have two areas of rejection: one in each tail of the distribution.

Critical values can be found in statistical tables, and these can be found in statistics textbooks. For example, for the z distribution with an alpha of .05 and a two-tailed test, tabular values will show that the area of acceptance for the null hypothesis is the central 95% of the z distribution and that the areas of rejection are the 2.5% of the area in each tail. The value of z that defines these areas is -1.96 for the lower tail and $+1.96$ for the upper tail. If the test statistic is less than -1.96 or greater than $+1.96$, it will be rejected. The areas of acceptance and rejection in a standard normal distribution, using $\alpha = .05$, is illustrated in Figure 2–3.

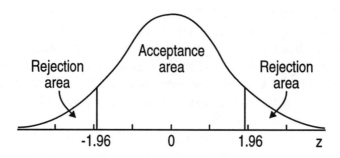

Figure 2–3. Areas of Acceptance and Rejection in a Standard Normal Distribution, Using $\alpha = .05$

4. *Perform the calculation.* Numerous statistical packages are available for making statistical computations. To choose one, read the software reviews in professional journals of education, business, law, statistics, epidemiology, and medicine. Another option is to ask for recommendations. All statistical packages have a manual (and/or tutorial) that teaches how to create data files and give the appropriate commands.

3 Selecting Commonly Used Statistical Methods for Surveys

T his chapter provides a guide to the selection of commonly used data-analytic methods. For simplicity, the guide omits ordinal variables. When independent variables are measured on an ordinal scale, they are often treated as if they were nominal. For example, to predict the outcomes of participation in a program for clients with good, fair, and poor emotional health, rather than treating good, fair, and poor as ordinal variables they can be converted to nominal variables: good (yes or no), fair (yes or no), poor (yes or no).

When dependent variables are measured on an ordinal scale, they are habitually treated as if they were numerical. Suppose the dependent variable in a nutrition program is men's and women's ratings of self-esteem (10 = *very high* and 1 = *very low*). The dependent ordinal variable can, for the sake of the analysis, be regarded as numerical, and mean ratings can be computed.

Before conducting any statistical analysis, check the assumptions in a statistics text or computer manual. If the survey data do not meet the assumptions, look for other statistical methods to use. Even if your data appear to meet the assumptions, check once again after the analysis is performed by studying the computer printout. If you are using correlations or regressions, are the assumptions met concerning linearity? If you are using an independent *t* test, are the variances equal?

Following the guide, the chi-square, *t* test, and analysis of variance (ANOVA) are introduced because of their utility in analyzing survey data. The guide also refers to methods for analyzing data that are not discussed in this book. These methods are complex, but they build upon the principles and assumptions included in this overview. Further information about these methods can be obtained from sources listed in the Suggested Readings section at the end of this book.

General Guide to Data-Analytic Methods in Surveys

Sample Survey Objective	Type of Data		Potential Analytic Method
	Independent Variable	Dependent Variable	
For objectives with one independent and one dependent variable:			
To compare experimental and control counties in children's reported use or failure to use bicycle helmets	Nominal: group (experimental and control)	Nominal: use of helmets (used helmets or did not)	Chi-square; Fisher's Exact Test
To compare experimental and control groups in their attitudes (measured by their scores on the Attitude Survey)	Nominal (dichotomous): group (experimental and control)	Numerical (attitude scores)	One sample *t* test, dependent *t* test, and independent samples *t* test; Wilcoxon Signed-Ranks Test; Wilcoxon Rank-Sum Test (the Mann-Whitney *U*)
To compare teens in the United States, Canada, and England with respect to their attitudes (measured by their scores on the Attitude Survey)	Nominal (more than two values): United States, Canada, and England	Numerical (attitude scores)	One-way analysis of variance (uses the *F* test)
To determine if high scores on the Attitude Survey predict high scores on the Knowledge Test	Numerical (attitude scores)	Numerical (knowledge scores)	Regression (when neither variable is independent or dependent, use correlation)
For objectives with two or more independent variables:			
To compare men and women in the experimental and control programs in terms of whether or not they adhered to a diet	Nominal (gender, group)	Nominal (adhered or did not adhere to a diet)	Log-linear

(continued)

51

General Guide to Data-Analytic Methods in Surveys (continued)

Sample Survey Objective	Type of Data		Potential Analytic Method
	Independent Variable	Dependent Variable	
To compare men and women with differing scores on the Knowledge Test in terms of whether or not they adhered to a diet	Nominal (gender) and numerical (knowledge scores)	Nominal and dichotomous (adhered or did not adhere to a diet)	Logistic regression
To compare men and women in the experimental and control programs with respect to their attitudes (measured by their scores on the Attitude Survey)	Nominal (gender and group)	Numerical (attitude scores)	Analysis of variance (ANOVA)
To determine if age and income and years living in the community related to attitudes (measured by scores on the Attitude Survey)	Numerical (age and income and years living in the community)	Numerical (attitude scores)	Multiple regression
To compare men and women in the experimental and control programs in their attitudes (measured by their scores on the Attitude Survey) when their level of education is controlled	Nominal (gender and group) with confounding factors (such as education)	Numerical (attitude scores)	Analysis of covariance (ANCOVA)
For objectives with two or more independent and dependent variables:			
To compare men and women in the experimental and control programs in their attitude and knowledge scores	Nominal (gender and group)	Numerical (scores on two measures: attitudes and knowledge)	Multivariate analysis of variance (MANOVA)

Reading Computer Output

Suppose an evaluator needs a chi-square analysis. Depending on the statistical program, the output will contain the analysis and additional information. Computer printouts vary in how they present results and in the additional tests and data they provide. Evaluators should become multilingual in output terms so that they can adequately read and talk about a range of statistical programs. Experience helps, and so, in the next few sections, two commonly used statistical techniques are discussed and their corresponding output in one program application are illustrated.

CHI-SQUARE

The **chi-square** (Greek letter chi, χ^2) distribution is the most commonly used method of comparing proportions.

Suppose you survey 208 high school seniors to find out their career preferences. Of this group, 103 have spent a year in a special job training program; the others have not. The survey finds that 40 seniors prefer to go on to college before seeking employment, whereas the remainder prefer to enter the labor force immediately.

The questions you are interested in answering are these:

1. Does a difference exist between program participants and the others in the number or proportion of seniors preferring to continue their education?

2. Does an association (or relationship) exist between being in the program and also preferring to continue in college?

To answer these questions, you could create a table that looks like this:

	Marginal Frequencies		
	Job Program	No Program	Total
Prefer college			40
Do not prefer college			168
Total	103	105	208

The **marginal frequencies** represent the numbers or proportions of seniors in the two survey groups. The **expected frequencies** shown in the table below represent the numbers or proportions of seniors in each **cell,** assuming that no relationship (the null hypothesis) exists between preference and program participation:

	Expected Frequencies		
	Job Program	No Program	Total
Prefer college	20	20	40
Do not prefer college	84	84	168
Total	104	104	208

The expected frequencies refer to the hypothetical distribution if the views of the two groups being compared are alike. So if 40 people prefer college, as the illustrative survey finds, then the expected frequency is 20 in the Job Program group and 20 in the group of nonparticipants.

Chi-square tests enable you to compare the expected frequency in each cell with the frequency that actually occurs (**observed frequencies**). The observed frequencies refer to the survey's data. The differences between observed and expected frequencies are combined to form the chi-square statistic. If a relationship exists between the column and row variables (e.g., whether or not the person is in a program and his or her preference), the two are said to be dependent. In this case, you would decide in favor of differences between the groups.

To assist you in using chi-square tests with two groups (e.g., experimental and control) and a two-pronged **dichotomous** nominal survey outcome (e.g., yes, prefer college or no, do not prefer college), use the following notation:

	Experimental	**Control**	**Total**
Positive	a	b	a + b
Negative	c	d	c + d
Total	a + c	b + d	a + b + c + d = *n*

This is called a 2 × 2 table. The formula for calculating the chi-square for data in a 2 × 2 table is

$$\chi^2(1) = n(ad - bc)^2/(a + c)(b + d)(a + b)(c + d).$$

The (1) refers to the degrees of freedom, a **parameter** that is used also in the *t* distribution. A parameter is the population (as contrasted with a sample) value of a distribution (e.g., the mean of the population is μ, and the standard deviation is σ). The chi-square test is performed as a one-tailed test. If the observed frequencies depart from the expected frequencies by more than the amount that you can expect by chance, you reject the null.

Going back to the example of preference for college when comparing program and nonprogram participants, suppose the 2 × 2 table was filled out to look like this:

	Jobs Program	No Program	Total
Prefer college	80	30	110
Do not prefer college	23	75	98
Total	103	105	208

Using the formula, you would have the following calculations:

$$\chi^2 (1) = n(ad - bc)^2/(a + c)(b + d)(a + b)(c + d).$$

$$\chi^2 = \frac{208[(80)(75) - (30)(23)]^2}{(103)(105)(110)(98)}$$

$$\chi^2 = \frac{208(5310)^2}{116585700}$$

$$\chi^2 = 50.30.$$

The critical value for an α of .01 is 6.635. In other words, 99% of the distribution is below 6.635. (You cannot possibly memorize all critical values; with experience, you will become familiar with many.) Any obtained value above the critical value enables you to reject the null hypothesis that no difference exists between the program and no-program groups. In the example, the obtained statistic is above the critical value, and so the null is rejected. The conclusion is that differences exist between the groups and preference for college is related to program participation.

Chi-square tests can be performed with many numbers of columns and rows. Sometimes, chi-square values are "corrected" with a **continuity correction** or **Yates's correction**.

The correction involves subtracting 0.5 from the absolute value of ad – bc before squaring. Its purpose is to lower the value of the obtained statistic, reducing the risk of a Type I error (rejecting the null when it is true); however, the risk of a Type II error (failing to reject the null when it is false) increases. Finally, when the expected frequencies are small (less than 5), then **Fisher's Exact Test** can be used (for more about this method, consult the appropriate sources in the Suggested Readings section at the end of this book).

Example 3.1 illustrates how to read chi-square output from one sample program (SPSS/PC+). As you can see, besides the significance of the differences, a number of other statistics are also provided. These will vary in importance according to the complexity of the survey and the computer program you use.

EXAMPLE 3.1
Reading Computer Output: Chi-Square

Concern has been raised that unemployed people in Community A do not have adequate access to health care; because of this, they do not get to see physicians when they need to. Does a difference exist in use of services between people who are employed and those who are unemployed? More specifically, does the proportion of people who have a paying job differ from the proportion who do not in terms of whether or not they have seen any doctor (MD) more than once?

Type of Survey: Self-administered questionnaire

Survey Questions:
- In the past year, did you see any MD more than once? (yes or no)
- In the past year, did you have a full- or part-time paying job that lasted 9 months or more? (yes or no)

Independent Variable: Job status (having a full- or part-time paying job or not having one)

Dependent Variable: Use of health services (seeing an MD more than once)

Analysis Method: Chi-square

Computer Output: (sample)

- -

Page 22   SPSS/PC+   6/24/93
a   *b*
Q41C   SEE ANY MD MORE THAN ONCE   by   Q61   PAYING JOB
                          Q61   Page 1 of 1
              Count   °   *c*   *d*
              Row Pct   ° YES   NO
              Col Pct   °   Row
                         °   1.00°   2.00°   Total
Q41C   áááááááááéááááááááééááááááááÇ
e   1.00   °   224 °   631 °   855 *g*
YES   °   26.2 *k* ° 73.8 *k* ° 67.7
                      °   64.6 *l* ° 69.0 *l* °
              úááááááááéáááááááááÇ
f   2.00   °   123 °   284 °   407 *h*
NO   °   30.2 *k* ° 69.8 *k* ° 32.3
                      °   35.4 *l* ° 31.0 *l* °
              ááááááááááéááááááááá₁
              Column   347 *i*   915 *j*   1262 *m*
              Total   27.5   72.5   100.0

- -

Page 23   SPSS/PC+   *p* 6/24/93
   Chi-Square   Value *n*   DF *o*   Significance
- - - - - - - - - -   - - - - - - -   - - - -   - - - - - - - -

q Pearson   2.23778   1   .13467
r Continuity Correction   2.04057   1   .15315
s Likelihood Ratio   2.21574   1   .13661
t Mantel-Haenszel test for   2.23601   1   .13483
     linear association
u Minimum Expected Frequency - 111.909
Number of Missing Observations: 20

- -

Interpretation (refer to corresponding letters marked on computer printout)

a. Q41c refers to the question on the self-administered questionnaire that asks whether the respondent has seen any MD more than once.

b. Q61 refers to the question on the self-administered questionnaire that asks whether the respondent has a paying job.

c. Yes is the column that refers to the positive answer to the question about having a paying job.

d. No is the column that refers to the negative answer to the question about having a paying job.

e. Yes is the row that pertains to the positive answer to the question pertaining to seeing or not seeing any MD.

f. No is the row that pertains to the negative answer to the question pertaining to seeing or not seeing any MD.

g. Total number (855) and percentage (67.7) of people who saw an MD more than once.

h. Total number (407) and percentage (32.3) of people who did not see an MD more than once.

i. Total number (347) and percentage (27.5) of people who have a paying job.

j. Total number (915) and percentage (72.5) of people who do not have a paying job.

k and l. Percentage of people represented in each cell. For example, in the top left-hand cell (Cell a), there are 224 respondents. They represent 26.2% of the 855 who saw any MD more than once and 64.6% of the 347 who also have a paying job.

m. Total number of respondents (1,262).

n. Value refers to the results of the statistical computation.

o. Degrees of freedom.

p. Obtained *p* value. This value is compared to alpha. If it is less, the null is rejected.

q. Pearson is the particular type of chi-square statistic calculated by this particular statistical package.

r. Continuity correction involves subtracting .05 from the difference between observed and expected frequencies before squaring to make the chi-square value smaller.

s. The likelihood ratio is the odds that the results occur in respondents who have seen any MD more than once versus those who have not.

t. Mantel-Haenszel Test for linear association is a log-rank test for comparing two survival distributions. [NOTE: if you do not know what this or any other test means, consult the appropriate sources at the end of this book.]

u. Minimum expected frequency will tell if you have enough observations to proceed with the chi-square test or if you should consider Fisher's exact test.

Conclusion: The obtained significance level is .13467. The null hypothesis (no differences exist between respondents with and without paying jobs in whether or not they saw any MD) is retained.

t TEST

The *t* test's probability distribution is similar to the standard normal distribution, or *z*. It is used to test hypotheses about means and thus requires numerical data. The shape of a *t* distribution approaches the bell shape of a standard normal distribution, which also has a mean of 0 and a standard deviation of 1, as the sample size and degrees of freedom increase. In fact, when the sample has 30 or more respondents, the two curves are very similar, and either distribution can be used to answer statistical questions. Current practice in most fields, however, relies on the *t* distribution even with large samples.

Three situations can arise in which *t* tests are appropriate, as illustrated in Example 3.2.

EXAMPLE 3.2
Three Situations and the *t* Test

Survey 1: Children's Birthday Gifts

Children in McCarthy Elementary School received an average of 4.2 birthday gifts. How does this compare to the results obtained in the national survey of children and birthday gifts?

Type of t: One-sample *t*

Comment: The mean of a group is compared to a **norm,** or standard value (the results of the national survey).

Survey 2: Low-Fat Diet for Men at the Computer Chip Plant

Do average scores on the Feel Good Inventory change for the 50 men after they participate in the Low-Fat Diet Program?

Type of t: Dependent *t*

Comment: The mean of a single group is compared at two times (before and after participation in the Low-Fat Diet Program).

Survey 3: Learning the Ballet

On average, how do men and women compare in their attitudes toward ballet after participation in the ballet exercise program? The highest possible score is 50 points.

Type of t: Independent *t*

Comment: The means of two independent groups are compared.

To apply the *t* test appropriately, the survey data must meet certain assumptions. To use the *t* distribution for one mean (as in Survey 1 above), the assumption is that the observations (e.g., scores) are normally distributed. Some computer programs provide a probability plot that will enable you to certify that the data are consistent with this assumption. Sometimes, you can examine the distribution yourself. If the data are not normally distributed, they can be transformed into a normal distribution. Alternatively, you can decide not to use the *t* and instead use different statistical measures called nonparametric procedures to analyze the data. Nonparametric methods make no assumptions about the distribution of observed values.

A paired design is used to detect the difference between the means obtained by the same group, usually measured twice (as in Survey 2 above). With the paired *t*, the assumption is that the observations are distributed normally. If the survey data violate the assumption, a commonly used nonparametric test for the difference between two paired samples is the **Wilcoxon Signed-Ranks Test.** This method tests the hypothesis that the medians, rather than the means, are equal (consult sources at the end of the book for more information on this test).

The *t* test for independent groups (Survey 3 preceding) assumes that the observations are normally distributed and that the variances of the observations are equal. If the sample sizes are equal, unequal variances will not have a major effect on the significance level of the test. If they are not, a downward adjustment of the degrees of freedom is made (you have fewer), and separate variance estimates are used instead of the combined or "pooled" variance. The statistical test to compare variances is the *F* test; many computer programs perform this test, often in the same program that performs the *t* test. If one of the assumptions of the independent *t* test is violated, an alternative is the nonparametric **Wilcoxon Rank-Sum Test (Mann-Whitney *U*)**. This test assesses the equality of medians rather than means, as does the Wilcoxon Signed-Ranks Test.

Example 3.3 is a sample computer printout for a *t* test from SPSS-PC+.

EXAMPLE 3.3
Reading Computer Output:
Independent Samples *t* Test

County A's health planners are concerned that sicker people may not be using the People's Ambulatory Care (PACE) clinic as often as they should. A survey is conducted to find out if this concern warrants attention.

Type of Survey: Self-administered questionnaire

Survey Questions
- In the past year, did you see any MD more than once? (yes or no)

- The Instrumental Activities of Daily Living (IADL) measure has 20 questions about a person's ability to function and perform various tasks including personal care and home chores. A score of 100 represents maximum functioning.

Independent Variable: Use of health services (seeing an MD more than once at PACE or not)

Dependent Variable: Ability to function (score on the IADL)

Analysis Method: t test

Computer Output: (sample)

- -

Page 97   SPSS/PC+   6/23/93

Independent samples of   Q41D - SEE MD AT PACE CLINIC > 1 TIME
                                  a   *b*
Group 1: Q41 EQ   1.00   Group 2: Q41 EQ   2.00

t-test for: IADL

	c Number of Cases	*d* Mean	*e* Standard Deviation	*f* Standard Error
Group 1	561	75.5246	23.957	1.011
Group 2	311	77.4358	24.112	1.367

i Pooled Variance Estimate   *j* Separate Variance Estimate

g F Value	*h* 2-Tail Prob.	°	t Value	Degrees of Freedom	2-Tail Prob.	°	t Value	Degrees of Freedom	2-Tail Prob.
1.01	.890	°	−1.13	870	.261	°	−1.12	636.61	.262

- -

Interpretation (refer to corresponding letters marked on computer printout)

a. Group 1 answered yes to the question "Did you see an MD at the PACE clinic more than once this year?" The choices were 1 = yes and 2 = no.

b. Group 2 answered no to the question "Did you see an MD at the PACE clinic more than once this year?"

c. Number of cases refers to the number of respondents (sample size) in each group.

d. Mean score obtained on the IADL by each group.

e. Standard deviation of the scores.

f. Standard error of the means.

g. *F* value or statistic obtained in the test to determine the equality of the variances.

h. Probability of obtaining a result like the *F* value if the null is true. If the obtained probability is less than some agreed-on alpha like .05 or .01, the null is rejected. In this case, the probability of .890 is greater than .05, and so the null is retained. The conclusion is that no differences exist in the variances of the two groups.

i. The pooled variance estimate is used when variances are equal. The *p* value is .261, greater than an alpha of .05. The null hypothesis regarding the equality of the group means is retained.

j. The separate variance estimate is used when variances are not equal.

Conclusion: No differences exist in functioning between respondents who saw a doctor at the PACE clinic more than one time and those who did not.

ANALYSIS OF VARIANCE (ANOVA)

Analysis of variance is commonly abbreviated as ANOVA. You use ANOVA to compare the means of three or more groups. For instance, if you want to compare the mean achievement test scores in reading and math of children in Korea, Japan, and Singapore, you use ANOVA.

With ANOVA you ask the question "Does an *overall* difference exist among the groups?" If the results are significant, you can then ask "Which combinations or pairs are responsible for the difference?"

ANOVA guards against multiple Type I errors. A Type I error occurs when you reject the null, when in fact, no difference exists. If you used t tests and an alpha of .05 to compare mean reading scores among children from Singapore, Korea, and Japan, you would need three separate tests: Singapore and Korea, Singapore and Japan, and Japan and Korea.

With three tests, you have a 15% (3% × 5%) chance of incorrectly finding one of the comparisons significant. ANOVA guards against this inflation. It is important to remember, however, that the results of an analysis of variance tell you about the overall or global status of differences among groups. If you find differences, ANOVA does not tell you which groups or pairs of groups are responsible. For that information, you should use post hoc comparisons like Tukey's HSD (honestly significant difference), Scheffé, Neuman-Keuls, or Dunnets procedures. (More information on these techniques can be found in the appropriate sources at the end of the book.)

ANOVA is complex, and whole textbooks have been devoted to it. One-way ANOVAs are used in comparisons involving one factor or independent variable, and two-way ANOVAs are used for two factors. A typical ANOVA table for a one-way analysis of variance is given in Example 3.4.

EXAMPLE 3.4
A Typical ANOVA Table

Source	Degrees of Freedom	Sum of Squares	Mean	F Ratio	p
Between groups					
Within groups					
Total					

ANOVA relies on the F distribution to test the hypothesis that the two variances are equal. The variation is divided into two components: the variation between each subject and the subjects' group mean (e.g., the variation between each participant in the experiment and the experimental group's mean) and the variation between each group mean and the grand mean (the mean of all groups). The sum of squares, mean squares, and degrees of freedom are mathematical terms associated with ANOVA.

Practical Significance:
Using Confidence Intervals

The results of a statistical analysis may be significant but not impressive enough to have practical applications. How can this be? Suppose that after an educational campaign in County A, a 10% increase is reported in the use of bicycle helmets by children. In County B, the control, a 5% increase is reported, and the 5% difference between the two counties is statistically significant. Based on the results, you might be tempted to conclude that the educational campaign is effective. If, however, the expectation was that the campaign was to have reached at least 50% of County A's children, then the 10% achievement level is disappointing. You can conclude that the campaign, although "effective," is too weak to be continued or expanded. With very large samples, even small differences can be significant. When statistical significance alone is inadequate to evaluate survey data, confidence intervals should be used.

Suppose a survey is given to participants of Teach for the World, an international program to encourage the best teachers to participate in the education of children outside their own countries. Because of the complexity of the social and cultural issues involved, eligible teachers are assigned to Program 6, a relatively costly 6-month internship, or to Program 3, which only requires a 3-month internship. Of 800 participants, 480 (60%) respond well to Program 6, and 416 of the 800 (52%) do well in Program 3. Using a chi-square to assess the existence of a real difference between the two treatments, a p value of .001 is obtained. This value is the probability of obtaining by chance the 8-point (60%–52%) difference between teachers in Program 6 and Program 3 or an even larger difference. The point estimate is 8 percentage points, but because of sampling and measurement errors (they always exist), the estimate is probably not identical to the true percentage difference between the two groups of teachers.

A **confidence interval** (CI) provides a plausible range for the true value. A CI is computed from sample data and has a given probability that the unknown true value is located within the interval. Using a standard method, the 95% CI of the 8-percentage-point difference comes out to be between 3% and 13%. A 95% CI means that about 95% of all such intervals would include the unknown true difference and 5% would not. Suppose, however, that given the other costs of Program 6 the smallest practical and thus acceptable difference is 15%, then you can conclude that the 8-point difference between Programs 6 and 3 is not significant from a practical perspective, although it is statistically significant.

The confidence interval and p are related; if the interval contains 0 (no difference), then the p is not significant. However, if much of the interval is above the practical cutoff, then the results can be interpreted as practically inconclusive. For example, if the cutoff were 15% and the CI ranged from -1% to $+25\%$, then much of the interval would fall above the cutoff for practical significance; the survey results would be unclear.

A graphic test for the differences between the means of two independent groups can also be prepared. The 95% CI is calculated and charted. If the means do NOT overlap, differences exist. If the mean of one group is contained in the interval of the second, differences do not exist. If the intervals overlap, but not the means, then you cannot tell if differences exist, and a hypothesis test must be performed. Figure 3–1 shows how charts can reveal differences in independent means.

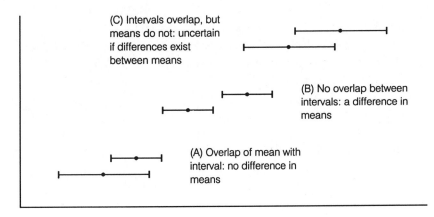

Figure 3-1. Visualizing Differences Between Independent Groups, Using Confidence Intervals

EXERCISE

The following output was obtained from a survey to answer the question, "How do Groups 1, 2, and 3 compare in their attitudes?" A score of 20 was the highest possible; high scores represented the most favorable attitude.

a. What is the null hypothesis?
b. Chart the confidence intervals and tell if the differences among the groups are significant.
c. What is the F probability, and does it agree with the findings you obtained by representing the confidence intervals on a chart?
d. If you find significance, which of the three groups is likely to have contributed most to the finding?

- - - - - - - - - - - O N E W A Y - - - - - - - - - - - -

Variable   DV
by Variable   GROUP

Analysis of Variance

Source	D.F.	Sum of Squares	Mean Squares	F Ratio	F Prob.
Between Groups	2	248.0000	124.0000	8.9793	.0020
Within Groups	18	248.5714	13.8095		
Total	20	496.5714			

- - - - - - - - - - - O N E W A Y - - - - - - - - - - - -

Group	Count	Mean	Standard Deviation	Standard Error	95 Pct Conf Int for Mean	
Grp 1	7	11.0000	3.6056	1.3628	7.6654 To	14.3346
Grp 2	7	8.1429	4.2984	1.6246	4.1675 To	12.1182
Grp 3	7	16.4286	3.1547	1.1924	13.5109 To	19.3462
Total	21	11.8571	4.9828	1.0873	9.5890 To	14.1253

Group	Minimum	Maximum
Grp 1	6.0000	16.0000
Grp 2	4.0000	13.0000
Grp 3	11.0000	19.0000
Total	4.0000	19.0000

---

a. The null hypothesis means that no differences in attitude exist between the mean attitude scores of Groups 1, 2, and 3.

b.

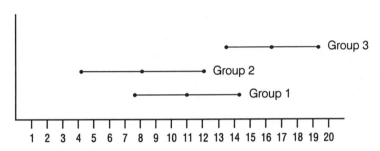

Group 1: Confidence interval 7.67 to 14.33, $\bar{X}$=11.00
Group 2: Confidence interval 4.17 to 12.11, $\bar{X}$=8.14
Group 3: Confidence interval 13.51 to 19.35, $\bar{X}$=16.43

Group 2's mean score is within Group 1's confidence interval. Group 3's interval does not overlap with either group. Statistically significant differences in the means can be seen, and so the null should be rejected.

c. The *F* probability is the observed significance level. It is smaller than the usual alphas (or critical values) of .05 or .01 and is statistically signficant. The graphic and statistical tests agree.

d. ANOVA does not provide information about the group whose mean is responsible for the significant difference. The chart suggests that Group 3 is responsible.

Proceed With Caution:
Screening and Transforming Data

Before analyzing the data, the entire data set should be reviewed. The first step is to screen for outliers and incorrect values. Outliers are observations that are not consistent with the rest of the data set. For example, an outlier might consist of just 1 of 15 teams with uncharacteristically very low job satisfaction scores. Including the team's data might bias the results, but excluding it might also do the same—and the exclusion might be unethical. If you find outliers, you can do the main analysis twice: without and without the outlier. In this way, the effects of the outlier can be determined and the results used in deciding how to handle the outlier.

Screen the data for incorrect values, that is, erroneous statistics. For example, if a survey of satisfaction with a preschool produces data on children who are 10 or 20 years of age, errors in data entry are likely to be present.

Another issue that should be resolved before analysis is what to do about missing values. Missing values refer to data that are not collected from an individual or other sampling unit. Suppose that you survey workers in a nursing home about their satisfaction with their working conditions. Suppose also that of 100 workers only 75 respond to all questions on a self-administered questionnaire. If a complete set of information on all workers is necessary for the analysis, then the sample size must be treated as 75 respondents and not as 100.

Another example of missing values is a failure on the part of all or nearly all people to provide data on a subset of questions pertaining to a particular variable. This can happen, for example, if nearly all workers in the nursing home survey fail to answer one or more questions on the survey of their attitudes. In this situation, you should probably exclude the items from the analysis.

Remember that the appropriate use of certain statistical tests (e.g., one-sample *t*) assumes a normal distribution of data. If data are not normal, they may be transformed or changed from one scale to another. Linear transformations involve a change in the mean and a scaling factor, such as when the *z* transformation is used. With a *z* transformation, the mean of a distribution is expressed as 0, and its standard deviation is 1. Nonlinear transformations result in changing the shape of the distribution so that they become normal. With rank transformations, observations are rank ordered from lowest to highest. The rank transformation is appropriate when observations are skewed.

CODING FOR DATA ANALYSIS

A code has two components: a number for the response (e.g., 1 = yes, and 2 = no, I did not eat any broccoli) and information for the data enterer regarding in which "column" or space to put a respondent's reply. Typical coding strips are shown in Example 3.5.

EXAMPLE 3.5
Typical Coding Strips

A. During the past 7 days, how many times did you eat broccoli?

Circle ONE choice

Once	1	*20*
Two or three times	2	
Four or more	3	
I did not eat any broccoli	4	

B. In the past week, did you eat any of the following?

Circle ONE choice for each food

	Yes (1)	No (2)	
Broccoli	1	2	20
Hamburger	1	2	21
Chicken	1	2	22
Spinach	1	2	23
Potatoes	1	2	24

Or

C. Which of these did you eat in the past week?

Check all that apply

    [ ] Broccoli   20
    [ ] Hamburger   21
    [ ] Chicken   22
    [ ] Spinach   23
    [ ] Potatoes   24
    [ ] I ate none of these. 25

The numbers to the right of the item are the "columns" or places for recording the responses to each item. To the data enterer, it works this way:

Item A: In column 20, place a 1, 2, 3, or 4, depending on the person's response.

Item B: In columns 21, 22, 23, and 24, place a 1 or 2, depending on the person's response.

Item C: In columns 20, 21, 22, 23, and 24, place a 1 if checked or a 2 if not checked.

If an item is left blank, the column must be assigned some number, such as 9 (assuming 8 or fewer choices). If 9 choices or more, can you use another code, say, 99? The answer is yes, but then you must provide for data entry into two columns, and the numbers would be entered as 01, 02 . . . 99. Example 3.6 illustrates coding strips for items with more than 9 choices or a double-digit answer.

EXAMPLE 3.6
More Coding Strips: Items With More Than
9 Choices or With a Double-Digit Answer

D. What was your **total** household **income before taxes** in 1993?

Check ONE only

    [ ] $10,000 or less   *20-21*
    [ ] $10,100 to $12,000
    [ ] $12,100 to $15,000
    [ ] $15,100 to $20,000
    [ ] $21,000 to $30,000
    [ ] $31,000 to $40,000
    [ ] $41,000 to $50,000
    [ ] $51,000 to $70,000
    [ ] $71,000 to $90,000
    [ ] Over $90,000

E. How many people in your household are supported by your total household income? **Write in number of household members**:

___ - ___   *50-51*

DATA ENTRY

Before entering survey data, you must decide on how to file them—in other words, on how to create a data file. For most statistical analyses, you create a rectangular file or a table. In the rectangular file, each horizontal line contains all the data— the data record—for a particular respondent, and each vertical field represents a particular variable (e.g., age). Often, each record in a data file represents individual respondents. Sometimes, however, the record consists of all information for a cluster of individuals or other units (e.g., a classroom or school).

Data can be entered into spreadsheets or forms. Spreadsheets are like rectangular files in which rows represent cases or records and columns represent variables. The form uses the whole computer screen for the case that is being entered and can be structured to look like the original survey instrument. A programmer can help you create tailor-made forms for data entry. Then, you must be sure that data enterers are trained to enter the data quickly and accurately.

THE CODEBOOK

The main purpose of preparing a codebook is to make a data set comprehensible to anyone who would like to use it. The codebook can be begun as soon as the analysis plan is agreed on, but it should be made final after the completion of data screening and cleaning. Usually, the codebook contains a number for each variable, its location (the column in which it can be found), a name for the variable (usually eight or fewer characters in capital letters to accommodate common statistical packages), and a brief description of the meaning of each code. Figure 3–2 is a portion of a codebook for a data set collected from a survey of the postpartum status of women who participated in one of three projects comprising a prenatal care program.

Variable Number	Variable Location (Column)	Variable Name	Description and Comments
1	1-5	PROJID	A five-digit ID project code Use 99999 for missing values
2	6-9	INDIVID	A four-digit ID individual code Use 9999 for missing values
3	10-15	DLIVDATE	Enter month/day/year using 2 digits for each segment. Example: May 20, 1992 = 052092 Use 99 for any missing segment Use 999999 if entire date is missing
4	16-21	FOLLDATE	Use same procedure as for DLIVDATE.
5	22	POSPARVIS	No = 1, Yes = 2, Don't know = 3 Use 9 if missing
6	23-28	VISTDATE	Follow DLIVDATE PROCEDURE If POST-PARTUM VISIT = NO, use 888888; use 999999 if missing
7	36-37	WELVISIT	Use 2 digits: 1 = 01, 2 = 02, etc. Use 00 if none; 99 if missing

Figure 3–2. Portions of a Codebook

Exercises

1. Indicate the type of data likely to be obtained for each of the following:

   a. Ethnicity

   b. Date of birth

   c. Ratings of happiness on a scale from 1 to 5

   d. Preferences

2. Compute the mean, median, and mode for the results of a survey of U.S. eating preferences for Christmas dinner.

First Choice	Number of Respondents
Turkey	10
Prime Rib	9
Ham	6
Lamb	4
Vegetarian	3
Goose	2
Other (e.g., steak)	1

3. A mailed survey with 75 respondents yielded a mean score of 100 and a range of 100 (minimum, 50; maximum, 150). An additional survey with a score of 100 was mailed in after the analysis had been completed. Redo the analysis and report on the mean, range, and sample size.

4. Indicate if each of the following is true or false.

Statement	True?	False?
The sample size has an influence on whether a difference in means is found.		
The obtained p for a t test is the probability that the means of two groups are the same.		
If the obtained p is very large, the means of the two groups are equal. The independent t test is less sensitive to differences than the paired t test.		
The p is calculated before alpha.		
If group sample sizes are equal, unequal variances do *not* cause major problems in the t test.		
If group sample sizes are equal, unequal variances do *not* cause major problems in ANOVA.		

5. For each of the following situations, describe the independent and dependent variables and tell whether they will be described with nominal, ordinal, or numerical data.

Situation	Describe Independent and Dependent Variable	Tell if the Data Are Nominal, Ordinal, or Numerical (interval/ratio)
Patients in the experimental and control groups tell whether pain killers give complete, moderate, or very little relief.		
Participants are divided into four groups: very tall, tall, short, very short. All are surveyed regarding their self-esteem, with a score of 1 meaning very low esteem and 9 meaning very high esteem.		
Residents of the facility are chosen according to whether they have had all recommended vaccinations or not; they are followed for 5 years, and their health status is monitored.		
Men and women with Stage 1, 2, and 3 disease are compared in the quality of life, as measured by scores ranging from 1 to 50.		
Customers of two catalogue companies are surveyed, and their average scores are compared.		

6. Use the following information to select and justify a method of data analysis.

   Question: Does program participation improve participants' ability to be good parents?

   Standard: A statistically significant difference in ability is found in families who have participated in the experimental program as compared to the control program.

   Independent variable: Group membership (experimental vs. control)

   Design: An experimental design with concurrent controls (eligible participants assigned at random to the experimental and control groups)

   Sampling: 100 participants are in each group (a statistically derived sample size).

   Dependent variable: Ability to be a good parent

   Type(s) of data: One important measure is the PARENT, a 50-point survey in which higher scores mean better parents.

   Analytic method: (you fill in)

7. Suppose the survey of the effectiveness of the program to help improve ability to be a parent is concerned with finding out how younger and older persons compare in the experimental and control groups. Assuming the use of the PARENT survey, which produces numerical scores, which statistical method would be appropriate? Explain.

ANSWERS

1. a. Ethnicity: nominal

   b. Date of birth: numerical

   c. Ratings of happiness on a scale from 1 to 5: ordinal

   d. Preferences: cannot tell. If scores, then numerical; ratings, ordinal; yes or no to a list, nominal.

2. Turkey is the mode; data are nominal, so you cannot compute the median or mean.

3. The mean and range stay the same. The sample size increases from 75 to 76.

4.

Statement	True?	False?
The sample size has an influence on whether a difference in means is found.	X	
The obtained p for a t test is the probability that the means of two groups are the same.		X
If the obtained p is very large, the means of the two groups are equal.		X
The independent t test is less sensitive to differences than the paired t test.		X
The p is calculated before alpha.	X	
If group sample sizes are equal, unequal variances do *not* cause major problems in the t test.	X	
If group sample sizes are equal, unequal variances do *not* cause major problems in ANOVA.		X

5.

Situation	Describe Independent and Dependent Variable	Tell if the Data Are Nominal, Ordinal, or Numerical (interval/ratio)
Patients in the experimental and control groups tell whether pain killers give complete, moderate, or very little relief.	Independent variable: group; dependent variable: pain relief	Independent variable is nominal; dependent variable is ordinal.
Participants are divided into four groups: very tall, tall, short, very short. All are surveyed regarding their self-esteem, with a score of 1 meaning very low esteem and 9 meaning very high esteem.	Independent variable: height; dependent variable: self-esteem	Independent variable is ordinal; dependent variable is numerical.
Residents of the facility are chosen according to whether they have had all recommended vaccinations or not; they are followed for 5 years, and their health status is monitored.	Independent variable: having or not having recommended vaccinations; dependent variable: health status	Independent variable is nominal; there is not enough information to determine the dependent variable.
Men and women with Stage 1, 2, and 3 disease are compared in the quality of life, as measured by scores ranging from 1 to 50.	Independent variable: gender and stage of disease; dependent variable: quality of life	Independent variables are nominal and ordinal; dependent variable is numerical.
Customers of two catalogue companies are surveyed, and their average scores are compared.	Independent variable: catalogue company; dependent variable: satisfaction	Independent variable is nominal; dependent variable is numerical.

6. *Analysis:* A two-sample independent groups *t* test

   Justification for the analysis: This *t* test is appropriate when the independent variable is measured on a categorical scale and the dependent variable is measured on a numerical scale. In this case, the assumptions of a *t* test are met. These assumptions are that each group is normally distributed (or has a sample size of at least 30) and that group variances are equal.

7. If the survey's aim is to find out how younger and older persons in the experimental and control groups compare in ability to be good parents, and assuming that the statistical assumptions are met, then an analysis of variance is an appropriate technique.

Suggested Readings

Afifi, A. A., & Clark, V. (1990). *Computer-aided multivariate analysis.* New York: Van Nostrand Reinhold.

A textbook on multivariate analysis with a practical approach. Discusses data entry, data screening, data reduction, and data analysis. Also explains the options available in different statistical packages.

Braitman, L. (1991). Confidence intervals assess both clinical and statistical significance. *Annals of Internal Medicine, 114,* 515-517.

This brief article contains one of the clearest explanations anywhere of the use of confidence intervals and is highly recommended.

Dawson-Saunders, B., & Trapp, R. G. (1990). *Basic and clinical biostatistics.* Englewood Cliffs, NJ: Prentice Hall.

A basic and essential primer on the use of statistics in medicine and medical care settings. Explains study designs, how to summarize and present data, and discusses sampling and the main statistical methods used in analyzing data.

Fink, A. (1993). *Evaluation fundamentals: Guiding health programs, research, and policy.* Newbury Park, CA: Sage.

Chapter 7 discusses basic statistical methods. Although the examples and exercises have been tailored to program evaluation, many are applicable to surveys because survey data are often used in evaluation studies.

Norusis, M. J. (1983). *SPSS introductory statistics guide.* Chicago: SPSS, Inc.

This manual accompanies a statistical package for the social sciences. It contains an overview and explanation of the logic behind most of the statistical methods commonly used in the social sciences. The manual also presents and explains statistical output.

Siegel, S. (1956). *Nonparametric statistics for the behavioral sciences.* New York: McGraw-Hill.

A classic textbook on nonparametric statistics.

Glossary

Analysis of covariance (ANCOVA)   Special type of analysis of variance or regression used to control for the effect of a possible confounding variable.

Analysis of variance (ANOVA)   Statistical technique to determine if there are differences between two or among three or more groups on one or more variables. The F test is used in ANOVA.

Area of acceptance and **area of rejection**   Components of a test statistic (e.g., the t). With a one-tailed hypothesis test, the rejection area is *either* the upper or the lower tail of the distribution. For a two-tailed test, you have two areas of rejection: one in each tail of the distribution.

Categorical scales   Like nominal scales in that there is no numerical value. Categorical scales yield data that classify people, for example, as under and over 25 years of age and readers (or not readers) of Spanish-language newspapers.

Cell   Counts or values in a table.

Censored observation   One whose value is unknown usually because the participant has not been in the survey long enough for the outcome of interest to occur.

Chi-square   Used to test the null hypothesis that nominal characteristics are not associated. The chi-square tests the null hypothesis that proportions are equal.

Code   Term used to describe computer-ready data. A code has two components: a number for the response (e.g., 1 = yes and 2 = no to the statement "I did not eat any broccoli") and information for the data enterer regarding which "column" or space to put a respondent's reply.

Codebook   Record of the terms used to instruct the computer in data entry and data analysis. Usually, the codebook contains a number for each variable, its location (the column in which it can be found), a name for the variable (usually eight or fewer characters in capital letters to accommodate common statistical packages), and a brief description of the meaning of each code.

Coefficient of determination (r^2)   Square of the correlation coefficient. It tells the proportion of variation in the dependent variable that is associated with variation or changes in the independent variable. For a correlation coefficient of .50, the coefficient of determination is $.50^2$, or .25. That means that 25% of variation in one measure may be predicted by knowing the value of the other.

Confidence interval   Plausible range for the true value, computed from sample data, and has a given probability that the unknown true value is located within the interval.

Contingency table Used to display counts or frequencies for two or more nominal variables.

Continuity correction (see **Yates's correction**)

Correlation Extent of association between and among variables.

Correlation coefficient (*r*) Measure of the linear relationship between two numerical measurements made on the same set of persons, places, or things. It ranges from −1 to +1, with 0 meaning no relationship.

Critical value (of a distribution) Absolute value that a test statistic must exceed for the null hypothesis to be rejected. These values are compiled into statistical tables.

Curvilinear relationship Distribution of data for either the independent or dependent variable is skewed or contains outlying values.

Degrees of freedom, or *n* − 1 Concept that appears in many statistical formulas and tables. The term sounds intuitively meaningful, but in fact, it is a complex statistical concept beyond the scope of this book.

Dependent *t* test (also called a paired *t* test or a one-sample *t* test) Statistical method for comparing the difference or change in a numerical variable that is observed for two paired or matched groups. It is also used with before-and-after measures on the same group.

Dependent variables Those whose values are responses, outcomes, or results. They are predicted by the independent variables. They are also called response variables.

Descriptive statistics   Describe data in terms of measures of central tendency.

Dichotomous variables   Nominal variables that have two outcomes only, such as male and female and dead and alive.

Distribution   Values (e.g., scores and other numerical values like number of years in office, age in years as of today) of a variable or characteristic (e.g., attitudes, knowledge, behavior, health status, demographics like age, income, etc.) and the frequency of their occurrence.

Expected frequencies   Those that are observed in a contingency table if the null hypothesis is true.

Expected value   Mean of a sampling distribution of a test statistic (e.g., the t).

Fisher's Exact Test   Used to test the null hypothesis that nominal characteristics are not associated. It is used when the sample size is too small for a chi-square test.

Frequencies   Like tallies in that they take the form of numbers and percentages.

Frequency count   Computation of how many people fit into a category (men or women, under and over 70 years of age, read five or more books last year or did not).

Independent samples t (sometimes called two-sample t)   Used to test the null hypothesis.

Independent variables   Also called "explanatory" or "predictor" variables because they are used to explain or predict a response, outcome, or result—the dependent variable.

Intercept Where the regression line intercepts the Y-axis at *a* on a graphic description of the mathematical model.

Interval scale Type of numerical scale that has an arbitrary zero point like the Fahrenheit and Celsius temperature scales. The difference, or distance, between 40° and 50° Celsius is the same as the difference between 70° and 80°. But 40° is not twice as hot as 20°, and 0° does not mean no heat at all. The statistical methods used in most surveys are the same for interval and ratio scales.

Level of significance When chosen before the test is performed, it is called the alpha value (denoted by the Greek letter α). The alpha gives the probability of rejecting the null hypothesis when it is actually true. Tradition keeps the alpha value small—.05, .01, or .001—because you do not want to reject a null hypothesis when, in fact, it is true and there is no difference between group means.

Likelihood ratio Odds that a given level of test result (e.g., a score of 90 on the Heart Test) would be expected from someone (e.g., a patient) with and without a problem (e.g., heart disease).

Linear Straight line.

Linear regression (of *Y* on *X*) Process of determining a regression or prediction equation to predict *Y* from *X*.

Logistic regression Technique used when the dependent variable is dichotomous.

Log-rank test Statistical method for comparing two survival curves when there are censored observations.

Mann-Whitney U (See **Wilcoxon Rank-Sum Test**)

Mantel-Haenszel Chi-Square Test Used to test two or more 2×2 tables.

Marginal frequencies (probabilities) Row and column frequencies in a contingency table. They are the frequencies listed on the margins of the table.

Mean Arithmetic average of observations. It is symbolized as $\overline{X}$.

Measures of central tendency Used when you are interested in the center (e.g., the average) of a distribution of findings. These measures are the mean, median, and mode.

Measures of dispersion Descriptive statistics that depict the spread of numerical data. Common measures of dispersion are range, standard deviation, and percentiles.

Median Middle observation. Half the observations are smaller and half are larger. No abbreviation or symbol is used for the median.

Mode of a distribution Value of the observations that occurs most frequently. It is commonly used when you want to show the most "popular" value.

Multiple regression Method for determining a prediction equation to predict Y from a set of variables, $X_1, X_2 \ldots X_n$.

Multivariate analysis of variance (MANOVA) Statistical method that provides a holistic test when there are multiple dependent variables and the independent variables are nominal.

Nominal scale Used to describe characteristics that have no numerical values (e.g., gender, ethnicity).

Normal distribution   Smooth, bell-shaped curve that is continuous and symmetric around the mean, symbolized by the Greek letter μ, or mu.

Null hypothesis (H_o) No difference exists in the means (scores or other numerical values) obtained by two groups. Statistical significance occurs when the null hypothesis is rejected (suggesting that a difference does exist).

Numerical scales   Used for characteristics that can be assigned numerical values. Age, height, and scores on a test are numerical data. Interval and ratio scales are two types of numerical scales.

Observed frequencies   Counts actually obtained in a study.

One-sample t test   Also known as a paired t test or a dependent t test.

One-tailed test   One in which the alternative hypothesis specifies a deviation from the null in one direction. The critical region is located in both tails of the distribution of the test statistic.

One-way ANOVA   Used to test for differences when you have one dependent variable with numerical data. ANOVA uses the F statistic.

Ordinal scales   Used for characteristics that have an underlying order among them, although the order may be arbitrary. Examples of ordinal scales are these: frequently, often, sometimes, rarely, never; strongly agree, agree, disagree, and strongly disagree.

Paired t test   Also called a dependent t test or a one-sample t test.

Parameter is the population value of a distribution such as the mean mu, μ.

Percentile   Number that indicates the percentage of a distribution that is equal to or below that number. To say that a person scored in the 95th percentile means that 95% of others scored the same or below that person. Percentiles are often used to compare an individual value with a set of standards.

Proportion   Number of observations or responses with a given characteristic divided by the total number of observations. A proportion is a *part* divided by a *whole.*

p **value**   Probability of obtaining the results of a statistical test by chance. The *p* value is the probability that a difference at least as large as the obtained difference would have come about if the means were really equal. The *p* is calculated *AFTER* the statistical test and is sometimes called the observed or obtained significance level. If the *p* value or observed significance is less than alpha, then the null is rejected.

Range   Difference between the largest observation and the smallest. Sometimes, the range is expressed by highest and lowest values rather than just the difference between them.

Ratio   A *part* divided by another *part.* It is the number of observations in a given group with a certain characteristic (e.g., feeling better) divided by the number of observations without the given characteristic (e.g., feeling worse).

Ratio scales   Those with a true zero point (as in the absolute zero value of the Kelvin scale). The statistical methods used in most surveys are the same for interval and ratio scales.

Regression   Predicts a value. Regression analysis is concerned with estimating the components of a mathematical model that reflects the relationship between the dependent and independent variables in the population. To make the estimate, you assume that the relationship between variables is linear and that a straight line can be used to summarize the data. Regression is often referred to as linear regression or simple linear regression. Regression differs from correlation in that correlations are used to describe relationships rather than predict values.

Sampling distribution Distribution of a test statistic (e.g., the mean, t, F, and chi-square). Its mean is called the *expected value*, and its variability is called the *standard error*.

Scatterplots Graphical depictions of the relationship (correlation) between variables. In a scatterplot, the numerical values of the two variables are expressed as points.

Skewed distribution A few outlying observations in one direction —a few small values or a few large ones.

Spearman rank correlation (sometimes called **Spearman's rho**) Often used to describe the relationship between two ordinal or one ordinal and one numerical characteristic. The symbol for Spearman's rho is r_s.

Standard deviation Measure of the spread of data about their mean and an essential part of many statistical tests. The standard deviation (SD) depends on calculating the average distance that the average score is from the mean. The standard deviation is symbolized with the Greek letter sigma, or σ.

Standard error Variability of a sampling distribution (e.g., the t).

Standard normal distribution (or **z distribution**) Mean of 0 and a standard deviation of 1.

Statistical significance Result that occurs by chance within specified limits, say, 1 time in 20, with a p value less than or equal to .05. Statistical significance occurs when you reject the null hypothesis.

Statistics Mathematics of organizing and interpreting numerical information. The results of statistical analyses are descriptions, relationships, comparisons, and predictions.

Symmetric distribution One in which the distribution has the same shape on both sides of the mean.

Tally Computation of how many people fit into a category (men or women, under and over 70 years of age, read five or more books last year or did not). Tallies (like frequencies) take the form of numbers and percentages.

Transformation of data Changing the scale of measurement.

Two-tailed test One in which the alternative hypothesis specifies a deviation from the null in either direction. The critical region is located in both tails of the distribution of the test statistic.

Variable Characteristic that is measurable, such as weight and satisfaction with health care.

Variance Standard deviation squared.

Wilcoxon Rank-Sum Test (the **Mann-Whitney U**) Nonparametric test for comparing two dependent samples with ordinal data or with numerical observations that are not normally distributed. This test assesses the equality of medians rather than means (as does the Wilcoxon Signed-Ranks Test).

Wilcoxon Signed-Ranks Test   Nonparametric test for comparing two independent samples with ordinal data or with numerical observations that are not normally distributed.

Yates's correction (also called a **continuity correction**)   Refers to the process of subtracting 0.05 from the absolute value of ad-bc before squaring. Its purpose is to lower the value of the obtained statistic, reducing the risk of a Type I error (rejecting the null when it is true); however, the risk of a Type II error (failing to reject the null when it is false) increases.

z distribution (or **standard normal distribution**)   Mean of 0 and a standard deviation of 1.

z transformation   Expresses the deviation from the mean in standard deviation units. Any normal distribution can be transformed to the z distribution.

About the Author

ARLENE FINK, PhD, is Professor of Medicine and Public Health at the University of California, Los Angeles. She is on the Research Advisory Board of UCLA's Robert Wood Johnson Clinical Scholars Program, a health research scientist at the Veterans Administration Medical Center in Sepulveda, California, and president of Arlene Fink Associates. She has conducted evaluations throughout the United States and abroad and has trained thousands of health professionals, social scientists, and educators in program evaluation. Her published works include nearly 100 monographs and articles on evaluation methods and research. She is coauthor of *How to Conduct Surveys* and author of *Evaluation Fundamentals: Guiding Health Programs, Research, and Policy* and *Evaluation for Education and Psychology*.

HOW TO
REPORT
ON SURVEYS

THE SURVEY KIT

Purpose: The purposes of this 9-volume Kit are to enable readers to prepare and conduct surveys and become better users of survey results. Surveys are conducted to collect information by asking questions of people on the telephone, face-to-face, and by mail. The questions can be about attitudes, beliefs, and behavior as well as socioeconomic and health status. To do a good survey also means knowing how to ask questions, design the survey (research) project, sample respondents, collect reliable and valid information, and analyze and report the results. You also need to know how to plan and budget for your survey.

Users: The Kit is for students in undergraduate and graduate classes in the social and health sciences and for individuals in the public and private sectors who are responsible for conducting and using surveys. Its primary goal is to enable users to prepare surveys and collect data that are accurate and useful for primarily practical purposes. Sometimes, these practical purposes overlap the objectives of scientific research, and so survey researchers will also find the Kit useful.

Format of the Kit: All books in the series contain instructional objectives, exercises and answers, examples of surveys in use and illustrations of survey questions, guidelines for action, checklists of do's and don'ts, and annotated references.

Volumes in The Survey Kit:

1. **The Survey Handbook**
   Arlene Fink

2. **How to Ask Survey Questions**
   Arlene Fink

3. **How to Conduct Self-Administered and Mail Surveys**
   Linda B. Bourque and *Eve P. Fielder*

4. **How to Conduct Interviews by Telephone and in Person**
   James H. Frey and *Sabine Mertens Oishi*

5. **How to Design Surveys**
   Arlene Fink

6. **How to Sample in Surveys**
   Arlene Fink

7. **How to Measure Survey Reliability and Validity**
   Mark S. Litwin

8. **How to Analyze Survey Data**
   Arlene Fink

9. **How to Report on Surveys**
   Arlene Fink

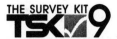

THE SURVEY KIT

TSK 9

HOW TO
REPORT
ON SURVEYS

ARLENE FINK

SAGE Publications
International Educational and Professional Publisher
Thousand Oaks London New Delhi

For information address:

 SAGE Publications, Inc.
2455 Teller Road
Thousand Oaks, California 91320
E-mail: order@sagepub.com

SAGE Publications Ltd.
6 Bonhill Street
London EC2A 4PU
United Kingdom

SAGE Publications India Pvt. Ltd.
M-32 Market
Greater Kailash I
New Delhi 110 048 India

Printed in the United States of America

Library of Congress Cataloging-in-Publication Data

Main entry under title:

The survey kit.
    p.   cm.
    Includes bibliographical references.
    Contents: v. 1. The survey handbook / Arlene Fink — v. 2. How to ask survey questions / Arlene Fink — v. 3. How to conduct self-administered and mail surveys / Linda B. Bourque, Eve P. Fielder — v. 4. How to conduct interviews by telephone and in person / James H. Frey, Sabine Mertens Oishi — v. 5. How to design surveys / Arlene Fink — v. 6. How to sample in surveys / Arlene Fink — v. 7. How to measure survey reliability and validity / Mark S. Litwin — v. 8. How to analyze survey data / Arlene Fink — v. 9. How to report on surveys / Arlene Fink.
    ISBN 0-8039-7388-8 (pbk. : The survey kit : alk. paper)
    1. Social surveys. 2. Health surveys. I. Fink, Arlene.
HN29.S724   1995
300'.723—dc20   95-12712

This book is printed on acid-free paper.

95 96 97 98 99 10 9 8 7 6 5 4 3 2 1

Sage Production Editor: Diane S. Foster
Sage Copy Editor: Joyce Kuhn
Sage Typesetter: Janelle LeMaster

Contents

How to Report on Surveys:
Learning Objectives

A survey's report consists of a summary and explanation of its findings, methods, and significance. Reports are of interest to the public, students in education and the social and health sciences, scientists and policymakers, and individuals in business and government and in the public and private sectors.

Surveys have a long history starting with the ancient Hebrews and Romans who used polls—one kind of survey—to collect census information for taxation purposes. In recent times, surveys have become one of the most popular methods of collecting data on nearly all of society's woes and wishes. Proper reporting of the results of these surveys is a skill that is almost comparable to composing a readable business letter or conveying information by telephone or electronic mail.

The aim of this book is to teach you the basic skills needed to prepare and interpret accurate and useful survey reports. Its specific objectives are to:

■ Prepare, interpret, and explain lists, pie charts, and bar and line charts

■ Prepare, interpret, and explain tables

■ Identify survey report contents for:

    – Oral presentations

    – Written presentations

    – Technical and academic audiences

    – General audiences

- Prepare slides

- Prepare transparencies

- Explain orally the contents and meaning of a slide or transparency

- Explain in writing the contents and meaning of a table or figure

- Explain orally and in writing the survey's objectives, design, sample, psychometric properties, results, and conclusions

- Review reports for readability

- Review reports for comprehensiveness and accuracy

1 Lists, Charts, and Tables: Presenting the Survey's Results

A survey's report can be written and/or oral and presented to large and small groups. The report's effectiveness and usefulness depend to a large extent on the clarity of its presentation. Lists, charts, and tables are used to maximize clarity.

AUTHOR'S NOTE: The names of all corporations and survey instruments used in examples throughout this chapter are fictitious.

Lists

Lists are used to state survey objectives, methods, and findings. The following examples of these uses of lists come from a formal talk about a survey of the use of mental health services in a large American city.

==

1. To State Survey Objectives

   Mental Health Services Questionnaire: Purposes

   TO FIND OUT ABOUT:

   ■ Accessibility

   ■ Satisfaction

   ■ Barriers to use

2. To Describe Survey Methods

   Seven Tasks

   ■ Perform literature review

   ■ Pose study questions

   ■ Set inclusion and exclusion criteria

   ■ Adapt the Prevention in Psychological (PIP)
     Function Survey

   ■ Pilot test and revise the PIP

   ■ Train interviewers

   ■ Administer the PIP

3. To Report Survey Results or Findings

PIP's Results

✓ **62% state that services are almost always inaccessible.**

- No difference between men and women
- No difference between younger and older respondents

✓ **32% of users are almost always satisfied.**

- Men more satisfied
- No difference between younger and older respondents

✓ **25% of potential users named at least one barrier to use.**

- Limited access to transportation most frequently cited barrier

---

Lists are simple to follow and so are very useful in survey reports. However, they typically need explanation in oral reports. One of the results illustrated in the example above is that no difference in satisfaction was found between younger and older respondents. The speaker must explain "younger" and "older" to the audience as these terms can vary from person to person.

Other terms, like inclusion and exclusion criteria (also in List 2), may need explanation. In written reports, lists can be used as a "table." For example, a report might use the second list above and precede it with a statement like "Table X lists the seven tasks that were needed to complete this survey of mental health use in an urban American city."

The following guidelines are helpful if you use lists in a survey report.

Guidelines for Using Lists
in Survey Reports

1. *Use only a few words to express each idea.* Use short words, phrases, or sentences.

   Poor

   ### The Literature Review

   We conducted a review of the literature to find out about the barriers to use of mental health services by low-income residents of U.S. inner cities.

   Better

   ### The Literature Review

   Purpose: Identify barriers to use of mental health services

   Focus: Low-income residents of U.S. inner cities

2. *Be consistent.* Each part of the list should be just words, just phrases, or just sentences. Use the same part of speech to start. Use the same capitalization and punctuation in all lists.

Poor

One year's experience
Interviewers must be willing to drive within inner cities to
    conduct interviews in respondents' places of residence.

Better

- One year's experience
- Willing to drive within inner cities
- Willing to conduct interviews in respondents' residences

3. *Leave blank spaces between the elements of the list to make it easier to read.*

4. *Use marks (bullets, checks) to set apart elements of the list.* For example, bullets are used in the "better" example for Item 2.

5. *In a single presentation, keep the symbols consistent.* For example, use checks for main headings and bullets for secondary headings.

6. *Have no more than four items on the list in a slide and no more than eight in a handout.*

7. *Use colors and drawings sparingly and keep them consistent.* If you use blue for bullets and red for checks at the beginning of the report, stay with that color scheme until the end.

Pie Charts

A figure is a method of presenting data as a diagram or chart. Pie charts are one type of figure. They are used to show survey data as proportions, that is, percentages or numbers that are part of a whole. For example, you can use a pie chart to describe a survey's responses in percentages, as illustrated in Figure 1–1.

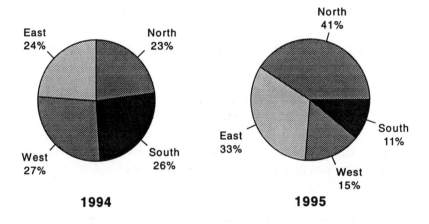

Figure 1–1. City Responses: A Survey of Mental Health Service Use
SOURCE: Telephone interviews.

The pie chart is given a title and an explanation of the source of data—telephone interviews. As you can see from the pies, the response rates in all parts of the city were fairly equal proportionately in 1994 (ranging from 23% to 27%). In 1995, the northern part of the city substantially increased its responses, and the proportions throughout the city were no longer similar.

If you want to emphasize one "slice" of the pie, make it the darkest or lightest pattern or separate it from the rest. In Figure 1–2, the northern part of the city's increased response rate is emphasized by separation.

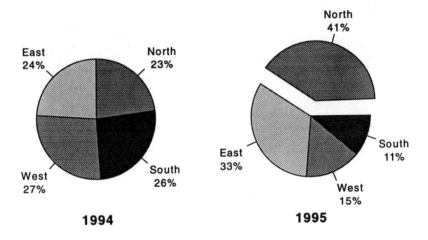

Figure 1–2.   City Responses: A Survey of Mental Health Service Use
SOURCE: Telephone interviews.

To emphasize change in proportions, use two pies. If you want to show growth, make the second pie larger than the first. If you want to show decline, make the second pie smaller. In Figure 1–3, pies are used to show the impact after one year of a maternal and infant health program on costs of care for hourly workers at Smith and Zollowitz, Inc.

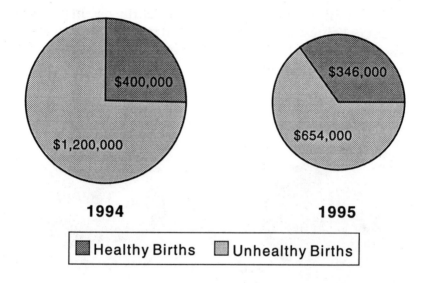

Figure 1–3.   Efficient Baby Care
SOURCE: Smith and Zollowitz, Inc. Reprinted with permission.

Looking at the two pies, you can conclude that the maternal and infant health program reduced the costs of caring for healthy and unhealthy births. The information in these pies comes from Smith and Zollowitz, Inc., and this is specified along with the statement that the pies are reprinted with permission. If data come from a source other than your own survey, you must put the origin directly on the figure. You have an ethical (and sometimes legal) obligation to name your source. Sometimes, you may have to request written permission to use copyrighted or proprietary information. The authors of the pie (or any other graphic illustration) will tell you exactly how they want to be acknowledged. Most U.S. federal government publications allow you to reprint data without receiving explicit permission to reprint. Of course, you are obligated to name the source of information. If in doubt, call the government agency directly.

The following guidelines are useful for the construction and use of pie charts.

Guidelines for Preparing Pie Charts

- Use pies to express proportions or percentages.
- Give the pie a relatively short title. Sometimes, a subtitle helps.
- Give the source of the data (e.g., telephone interviews or the ABC Company).
- Use no more than eight slices.
- If necessary, group the smallest slices together and label them "other."
- To emphasize a slice, separate it from the remainder of the pie or make it the darkest (or brightest) color or pattern.
- To emphasize changes over time, use larger pies to show growth and smaller ones to show shrinkage.
- Name the source of information for the pie. If the entire pie is reprinted from some other source, acknowledge it the way the authors want you to. Sometimes, you will have to get formal permission in writing to reprint the pie in your report.

WARNING

Do NOT use patterns on adjacent slices that create optical illusions.

Do NOT put red and green slices next to each other because about 5% of the population cannot distinguish red from green.

Bar and Line Charts

Bar charts (or graphs) depend on an *X*-axis and a *Y*-axis. The vertical axis is the *Y* and represents the unit of measurement or dependent variable, such as dollars, scores, or number of people responding. On the *X*-axis, you can put nearly all types of data, including names, years, time of day, and age. The *X*-axis usually has data on the independent variable.

Bar charts are often used in survey reports because they are relatively easy to read and interpret. Figure 1–4 shows the results of a 5-year study of curriculum preferences in five schools. Notice that the chart has a title, both the *X*-axis and the *Y*-axis are labeled, and the source of data is given.

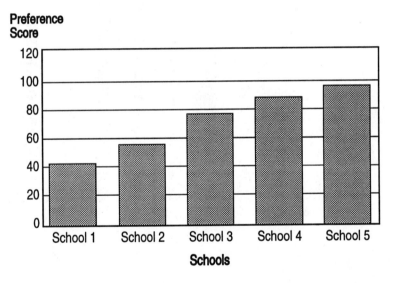

Figure 1–4. Curriculum Preferences in Five Schools
SOURCE: 1995 Curriculum Survey for Teachers.

The chart shows that Schools 1 and 5 appear different in their preference scores, with School 1 at just above 40 and School 5 at just under 100.

Bar charts can be used for many survey purposes, including comparing groups and studying changes over time. Figure 1–5 compares job satisfaction for clerical and technical workers over a 10-year period. Because two groups (clerical workers and technical workers) are involved, a key (or legend) to the meaning of the bars is given. Also, the company that sponsored the survey is named.

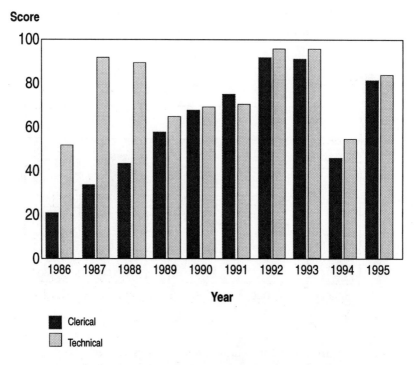

Figure 1–5. Job Satisfaction: A 10-Year Study
SOURCE: Satisfaction Inventory (higher scores are more positive).
NOTE: Study sponsored by the L. L. Green Company.

The chart shows that clerical workers' satisfaction has been lower than technical workers' for 9 of the 10 years. Only in 1991 were the positions reversed and clerical workers seemed more satisfied than technical workers.

You might complain that the use of 10 sets of bars clutters the chart. For more than six or seven bars, you can show the chart horizontally, as in Figure 1–6.

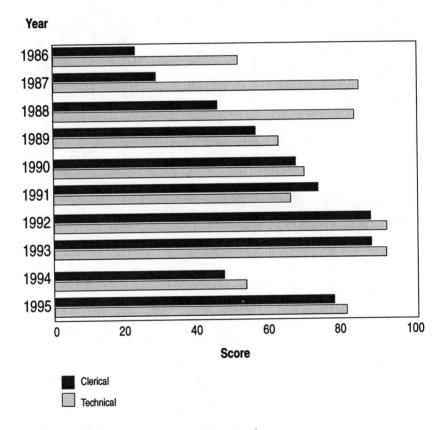

Figure 1–6. Job Satisfaction: A 10-Year Study
SOURCE: Satisfaction Inventory (higher scores are more positive).
NOTE: Study sponsored by the L. L. Green Company.

The same information can be presented in a line (Figure 1–7).
Note also that to reduce the clutter, the years are grouped in
units of two.

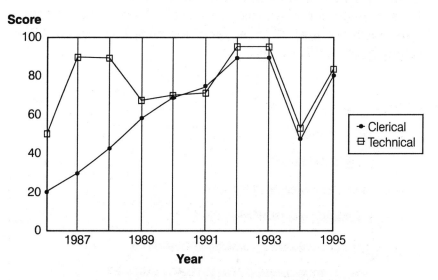

Figure 1–7. Job Satisfaction: A 10-Year Study
SOURCE: Satisfaction Inventory (higher scores are more positive).
NOTE: Study sponsored by the L. L. Green Company.

Keep bar and line charts simple. Use no more than four or
five lines in any single chart.

Bar and line charts can be misleading, so be careful not to compromise your results. For example, 1,000 people were asked their opinions regarding use of national parks. The opinions were compiled into scores. Compare the report of opinions in June, July, and August on the next two bar charts (Figures 1–8 and 1-9).

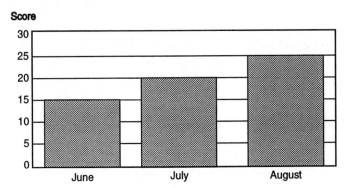

Figure 1–8. Opinion of National Park Reserves: A Survey of 1,000 Park Users SOURCE: Parks Department Annual Summer Questionnaire (high scores are most positive), U.S. Department of the Interior, Division of Parks and Land Management.

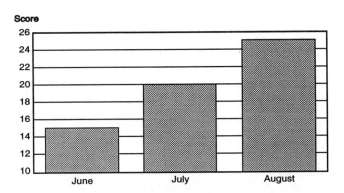

Figure 1–9. Opinion of National Park Reserves: A Survey of 1,000 Park Users SOURCE: Parks Department Annual Summer Questionnaire (high scores are most positive), U.S. Department of the Interior, Division of Parks and Land Management.

In Figure 1-8, the opinions do not *appear* to be as different from one another as they do in Figure 1-9, even though a close reading of the data show that the two contain identical scores. Two features of the charts change the purely visual interpretation. First, Figure 1-8 has a "zero" starting point; Figure 1-9 does not. Omitting the zero makes the change look greater than it is. If your chart does not start with zero, this should be indicated.

The second reason why the charts look different is that the values chosen for the Y-axis greatly affect the graphic presentation of data. Look at Figures 1-10 and 1-11.

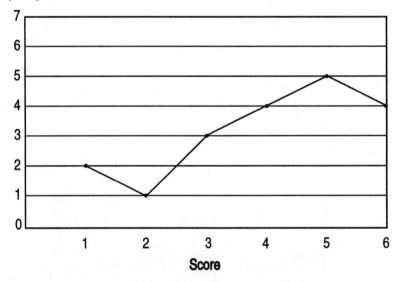

Figure 1-10.   Children and the Dress Code
SOURCE: Dress Up and Dress for Education (DUDE) Survey.
NOTE: Children were asked their opinion of a new dress code. The chart shows the number or frequency of children, with scores ranging from 1 to 6. Higher scores are more positive.

Frequency

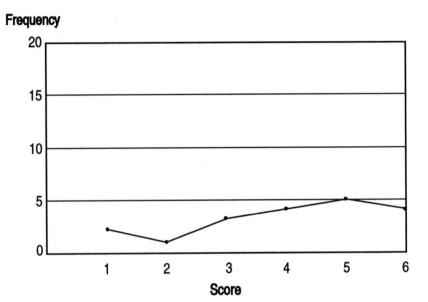

Figure 1–11. Children and the Dress Code
SOURCE: Dress Up and Dress for Education (DUDE) Survey.
NOTE: Children were asked their opinion of a new dress code. The chart shows the number or frequency of children, with scores ranging from 1 to 6. Higher scores are more positive.

Change appears less dramatic when the Y-axis has many points separating each value (in Figure 1–11, five points separate each frequency value) than it does when the Y-axis has few points (in Figure 1–10, one point separates each frequency value).

The magnitude of change can also be maximized or minimized by the choice of starting time. Look at Figures 1–12 and 1–13.

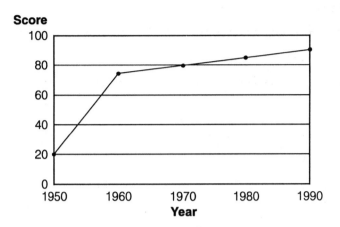

Figure 1–12. Changes in Beliefs
SOURCE: Belief Inventory.

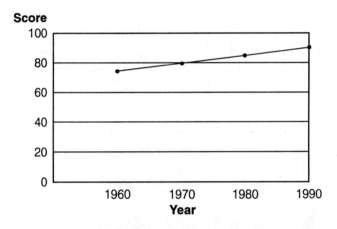

Figure 1–13. Changes in Beliefs
SOURCE: Belief Inventory.

Figure 1–12 shows that the biggest change in beliefs scores occurred in 1950. Figure 1–13 does not show this; the scores look fairly consistent over time.

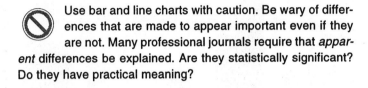

WARNING

Use bar and line charts with caution. Be wary of differences that are made to appear important even if they are not. Many professional journals require that *apparent* differences be explained. Are they statistically significant? Do they have practical meaning?

Look at the next two illustrations. They represent the results of a survey comparing changes in eating, smoking, and dietary habits among students. Some of the students were in the Health Assessment and Prevention Program for Youth (HAPPY), and some were in a control health program. Figure 1–14 suggests that changes (for better and worse) took place for all behaviors, including whether or not students ate fast food and stopped smoking. Figure 1–15 explains the differences. Using statistical tests, the changes in smoking and exercise are not statistically significant (with $p < .05$ as the level of significance). Notice also that figures, when used in scholarly publications, place their associated explanations underneath.

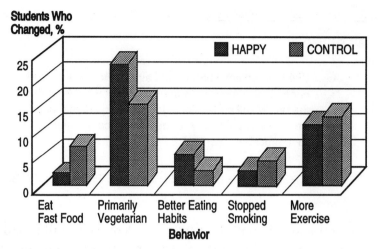

Figure 1–14. HAPPY Versus Control
SOURCE: Health Assessment and Prevention Program for Youth.

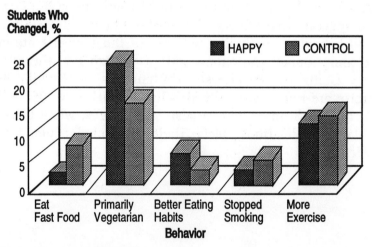

Figure 1–15. HAPPY Versus Control
SOURCE: Health Assessment and Prevention Program for Youth.
NOTE: Health-promotion-related behavior changed from baseline to follow-up. Results of chi-square tests for each behavior were $p < .05$ for eating fast foods, for primarily vegetarian, and for better eating habits; $p < .10$ for stopped smoking; and $p < .60$ for more exercise.

A list of guidelines for constructing and using bar and line charts follows.

Guidelines for Preparing Bar and Line Charts

- Give each chart a title.
- Explain the meaning of the values on the X-axis and Y-axis.
- Clarify the context of the survey. (For example, it was conducted at the XYZ Company.)
- Give the source of information.
- Use bar charts to compare groups or show changes over time. The bars should be vertical. If using more than six bars, consider a horizontal chart or use lines.
- Provide a key, or legend, to special shadings or types of lines, if more than one group or time period is depicted in a chart. For example, the key for the results of a survey of two groups might indicate that the results for Group 1 are represented by a dotted line and those for Group 2 by squares.
- Keep charts as uncluttered as possible. For example, instead of printing all years in a 10-year study, group them by twos. Use no more than four or five lines in a chart.
- Use line charts to compare survey results over many points in time.
- Choose the values for the Y-axis so that the results are accurate reflections of the survey's findings. If you do not start at zero, indicate this directly on the chart.
- Choose accurate starting times when illustrating change.
- Explain the meaning of the differences that appear on the chart. Are they statistically significant?
- Place explanations of the figure underneath it.

Tables

Tables are used to summarize data about respondents and their responses and to compare survey results over time. Suppose you are responsible for surveying students in an experiment to find out if their health habits can be improved through a teen-based program called the Health Assessment and Prevention Program for Youth (HAPPY). Students in three high schools are randomly assigned to HAPPY or a control health program. The survey's main objectives are to describe and compare the students in each program and to compare their health habits (e.g., willingness to exercise regularly) before entering the program, immediately after, and 2 years later. If you achieve the survey's objectives, you will produce tables that look like these "shells."

1. *Description of Students in HAPPY and the Control Program*

The table will contain the number (*n*) and percentage of the sample (%) in HAPPY and in the control program that are different ages (years), go to different high schools, are male or female, and speak primarily English, Russian, Spanish, or some other language at home.

Characteristics	HAPPY		Control	
	n	%	*n*	%
Age (years)				
Under 13				
13 - 15				
16 - 17				
Over 17				
High school				
Grant				
Lincoln				
Clinton				
Gender				
Female				
Male				
Primary language spoken at home				
English				
Russian				
Spanish				
Other (specify)				

$\rightarrow$

2. *Changes Over Time in HAPPY and the Control Program:*
Willingness to Exercise Regularly

The shell table below is set up to compare scores on a
25-question Exercise Inventory.

Timing	HAPPY Scores	Control Scores
Before HAPPY		
Immediately after		
Two years after		

When should tables be used? Tables are especially useful in
written reports because the reader can spend time with them.
Technically oriented people also like them in oral presentations. Actually, little information is available to conclusively
guide you in the choice of charts versus tables. If you need to
make a visual impact, then charts are appropriate. If you want
to illustrate your points with numbers, then tables are appropriate. Often, survey reporters offer a variety of tables and
charts in a single report.

The following guidelines are useful when preparing tables
for survey reports.

Guidelines for Preparing Tables

- *Column headings are determined by the most important comparison.* For example, if you are comparing boys and girls to find out if age and city make a difference in their responses to a survey, you will have two main column headings: boys and girls.

If you are describing the characteristics (e.g., age or educational level) of users and nonusers of seat belts, the values (e.g., numbers and percentages of persons with the differing characteristics) go in the columns.

Characteristics	Users		Nonusers	
	n	%	*n*	%
Age (years) Under 18				
18 - 25				
26 - 35				
36 - 45				
46 and over				
Gender Male				
Female				

	Users		Nonusers	
Characteristics	n	%	n	%
Years using				
Less than 1				
1 - 3				
4 - 6				
Over 6				

- *If appropriate and possible, put statistical values in ascending (largest values) to descending order.* The table below describes the results of a nationwide survey of 734 people who were asked whether they preferred basketball or baseball.

Statistical Values in Order:
The National Sports Preferences Survey[a]

	Number of People Choosing		
Region	Baseball	Basketball	Total
Northeast	140	124	264
South	100	52*	152
West	89	138**	227
North Central	45	46	91
Total	374	360	734

a. Survey administered by the Center for Sports and Health, Washington, D.C.
*$p = .003$; **$p = .002$.

Note that in this table the preferences for baseball are in descending order. The choice of which values to place first depends on the points being emphasized. If the survey's focus was on preferences for basketball, then the first cell of the table under "Region" would have been West.

- *Use a standardized set of symbols to call the reader's attention to key aspects of the table, such as statistical significance.* For example, in the previous table, the superscript "a" comes first and tells you the source of data. The next two symbols (asterisks) tell you the *p* values, a statistic that helps you decide if the results you found in the survey are the consequence of a program or of chance. To find sets of symbols, check out the tables in journals that are appropriate to your field of study or interest.

2 Talking About the Survey

Learn About the Listeners

A typical concern of anyone who has to report on a survey is how simple or technical to be. The first task is to estimate the needs of the audience. In general, one of three scenarios is likely:

> *Scenario 1:* The audience consists of nontechnical people. They want to know what the survey found, if the findings are important, and how to use them. They are not interested in the methodological details and in statistics and tables.

Scenario 2: The audience consists of technical people. They want details on the survey's methods. What was the response rate? How was the sample chosen? Were differences found in the demographic characteristics of respondents and nonrespondents?

Scenario 3: The audience is mixed. Some are interested in statistics and tables, and others are not.

How can the needs of all of the groups be met? The good news is that certain reporting principles apply to all audiences. These include the general topics that should be included in the talk and the need for simplicity and variation. The amount of time spent on various aspects of the talk and the depth of coverage varies. If you are unsure of the composition of the audience or you are fairly certain it is mixed, then prepare a relatively nontechnical talk and be prepared to augment it for the more technical types with a discussion period or with written handouts.

All talks are enhanced with visual aids. The most common are overhead transparencies and slides.

Overhead Transparencies and Slides

Overhead transparencies are acetate sheets onto which letters or figures have been transferred. They can be prepared by using water-soluble or permanent-ink felt-tip pens, photocopying typed or computer-generated materials, or generating direct copies from a laser printer. You need a special projector to use overheads. Slides are usually 35 mm (2-inch × 2-inch) and also need a special projector.

Both overheads and slides have advantages and disadvantages, as shown in the following table.

	Overheads	Slides
Advantages	Can be prepared quickly and economically	Compact: easily carried and stored
	Speaker faces audience, facilitating discussion	Suitable for any size audience
	Easy to carry and store	Projectors are readily available
	Uses ordinary room lighting	Tend to be considered "professional"
	Can make additions or deletions during the talk	
	Can change the order during the talk	
Disadvantages	Projectors are large and heavy	Relatively expensive
	Projectors may block the listeners' view of the screen	Need extra time for designing
	Can be messy if frequent erasures are made	Need extra time to process
	Mechanics of keeping overheads in focus may distract listeners	Need a really darkened room: inhibits discussion and note taking
		No changes of any sort possible during the talk

The following guidelines can assist when preparing overheads. Illustrations of transparencies in use are given in the next section, Talking About Surveys.

Guidelines for Preparing
Overhead Transparencies

■ Each transparency should contain only one main idea, table, or figure. Complex transparencies force the listeners to focus on the overhead and not the talk or to give up on the overhead and listen to the talk.

■ Use the 6 × 6 rule: 6 words per line and 6 lines per transparency.

■ Limit yourself to about 7.5 × 9.5 inches on an 8.5-x-11-inch overhead.

■ Use simple letter styles and fonts like Helvetica, Roman, and Courier. Letters should be about 3/8 inches high or 18-point type.

■ Use upper- and lowercase letters.

■ Colors are useful to emphasize a point, illustrate similarities and differences between points, and show the actual color of an object. Color can be added by using colored sheets (overlays) or felt-tip marking pens.

■ Make sure that the projector does not block the listeners' view of the screen.

■ Before you discuss a transparency, check the screen to make sure that the machine is focused and that the overhead is straight.

Use the following guidelines to prepare slides. Illustrations of slides in use are given in the next section, Talking About Surveys.

Guidelines for Preparing Slides

- Limit each slide to one main concept.
- Allow the listener 1 to 2 minutes per slide. The exception to this is when you have similar slides in a sequence, such as lists, pies, or graphs, or with the same format.
- If you adapt information from a textbook or other survey, check to see if it needs to be simplified.
- Prepare slides using the features of word processing or graphic programs. Special slide-preparation software can also be used.
- Use no more than 7 to 9 lines of text per slide and no more than 6 or 7 words per line.
- To emphasize points, underline titles, use bullets or check marks, number each point, or use contrasting colors to separate points.
- Use phrases, not complete sentences.
- Highlight key words by underlining, using different type size, alternative spacing, or different colors, or putting them in a circle or box.
- If you have "down time" with no appropriate slides, use a filler. These often consist of an opaque, blank slide or the title of the presentation. Do not use cartoons as the filler because they are distracting in the middle of a talk. (If you use cartoons to lighten the presentation, make sure the audience can see the caption.)

- Use handouts to summarize information and provide technical details and references. Make sure that your name, the name of the presentation, and the date are on each page of the handout. Do not distribute handouts until you are finished speaking *unless* you refer to them during your talk.

- In general, upper- and lowercase letters are easier to read than all uppercase.

- Round numbers to the nearest whole number. Try to avoid decimals, but if you must, round to the nearest tenth (32.6%, *not* 32.62%).

- Limit tables to 5 rows and 6 columns.

- If graphs are used, make sure that both the X- and the Y-axes are clearly labeled.

- Make sure that *all* information on the slide is discussed in the talk.

- The minimum height of the letters should be .5 mm. Use the largest letters possible to fill the area available.

- Use bold type.

- Use slides that have a blue or black background with white lettering.

- Use no more than four colors per slide.

- Avoid these color combinations: green, blue, and gray; black, blue, and brown; and white and yellow.

- Review the slides before you talk. Nothing is more embarrassing than misspelled words and upside-down slides. Place a mark or spot in the lower left corner of each slide mounting. When slides are in the projector, rotate each slide so that the mark is on the outer right edge facing you. You should load the slide tray yourself to make sure you have all the slides you need in the order you want them.

Talking About Surveys: Step by Step

When talking about a survey, remember the preacher's proverb:

> First, you tell 'em what you're gonna tell 'em, then you tell 'em, then you tell 'em what you told 'em, and then you tell 'em what to do with it.

What *you're gonna tell* is the introduction, *telling* is the methods and results, *what you told* is the conclusion, and *what to do* are the implications, recommendations, or next steps.

TALKS AND TITLES

The title should be brief and understandable to listeners and clearly limit the topic. Phrases like "a report of," "an analysis of," or "the use of" should be avoided because they add words but do not clarify much.

Poor

   An Analysis of a Survey of Boys' and Girls' Attitudes to the New Dress Code

   A Report of a Survey of Boys' and Girls' Attitudes to the New Dress Code

Better

   Boys' and Girls' Attitudes to the New Dress Code

Poor

> The Use of a Survey in Comparing Boys' and Girls' Attitudes toward the New Dress Code

Better

> Comparing Boys' and Girls' Attitudes toward the New Dress Code

Alternative

> Attitudes toward the New Dress Code: Comparing Boys and Girls

The talk should include the names of persons who made sufficiently large contributions to the survey's purposes, methods, and write-up so that if called upon, they too could report on it (even if they would need some assistance to do so). In some cases, you are ethically (and legally) bound to mention who sponsored (paid for) the survey. You may also want to include the geographic location of the report and the date. The following are sample slides showing authors and acknowledgments.

Authors (slide)

**ARE WE SATISFIED
WITH OUR WORK?**

**A COMPARISON OF FULL-TIME
AND PART-TIME EMPLOYEES**

Prepared by the Work Study Team

Presented by Martin Federman

Los Angeles, California

Acknowledgments (slide)

```
ACKNOWLEDGMENTS

Technical Foundation
Work and Leisure Corporation
```

HOW TO INTRODUCE THE TALK

The introduction should point out the purposes of the talk and address the topics that will be covered or the questions that will be answered. It helps also to tell the listener the order that your talk will follow. The following are two slides showing a presentation's purposes and questions and an overhead with the talk's order.

Purposes of the Talk (slide)

```
Objectives

◆ Present Survey Results
◆ Offer Recommendations
◆ Discuss Next Steps
```

Questions Answered by the Talk (slide)

Questions

◆ **Differences in satisfaction between**
  - **Full-time and part-time**
  - **Men and women?**
  - **Managers and engineers?**

Questions

◆ **Characteristics of**
  - **Most Satisfied?**
  - **Least Satisfied?**

Order of the Talk (transparency)

What to Expect

◆ **Background: Why Survey Satisfaction**
◆ **Who Participated**
◆ **How Chosen**
◆ **The Survey: Contents and Statistical Properties**
◆ **Findings**
◆ **Conclusions and Recommendations**

The introduction to an oral presentation also consists of the information you think listeners should have to put the survey in its proper context. The background can include some or all of the following:

1. *Why the survey was done.* What is the problem or issue that the survey's data are supposed to help resolve?

2. *The setting in which it takes place.* The setting includes the political, social, and educational environment. Survey information can be used to help describe current status, monitor changes, and recommend future programs and policies. For example, if a survey has been conducted to help management decide how to reorganize a department, your presentation will discuss the current organization and review the issues pertaining to reorganization that the survey is specifically designed to help resolve.

3. *Unique features.* A survey can be unique in many ways. It may be the first of its kind in the organization, the first to involve the participation of certain members of an organization, or the first to reach a special group of respondents. Also, the findings may be unusual: either going against the conventional wisdom ("We all thought we would find that . . . ") or going against the findings of other surveys and studies ("A survey of children's feelings about strict dress codes directly contradicts our results. . . ").

The introduction to a talk is especially challenging because you can lose or win the audience during it. To encourage listening, several techniques are advocated:

Ask a question that will be answered during the presentation. For example, for a talk on work satisfaction, you might ask the audience "Do you think younger and older employees differ in their satisfaction?" "What about the bosses? How satisfied are they, do you think?"

Make a controversial statement that will be supported by the survey's findings. For example, you might say, "A number of studies have shown that more generous maternity leave policies are associated with greater work satisfaction, but we did not find this to be true."

Relate the survey's topic or findings to a current event.

Tell a relevant personal experience.

Tell a humorous anecdote related to the topic of the survey.

Refer to a previous talk or to its topic.

OVERVIEW OF THE SURVEY

Provide a brief overview of the survey to focus the listeners and help them get a feeling for its size and scope. Concentrate on the following:

- *Type of survey* (telephone or face-to-face interviews, mailed or self-administered questionnaires, reviews of records, observations, or other)

- *Number of participants and response rate* (Example: "More than 100 people participated, giving us about 86% of all who were eligible.")

- *How long the survey took* (Example: "We conducted 15-minute interviews over a 6-month period.")

- *Survey's general contents* (Example: "Of the 50 questions, nearly all asked about satisfaction with work, although about 10 focused on demographic questions like age and income.")

Think of the overview as part of the introduction. That is, you are providing the context for the survey. Later on in your talk, you will go into greater detail about the contents and responses.

Next, tell the audience the specific characteristics and contents of the survey. You will probably want to illustrate one or more questions.

Characteristics (slide)

```
┌─────────────────────────────────────────┐
│ ┌───────────────────────────────────────┐ │
│ │                                       │ │
│ │         Survey Characteristics        │ │
│ │                                       │ │
│ │   ◆ 25 Questions                      │ │
│ │                                       │ │
│ │   ◆ Mailed Questionnaire              │ │
│ │                                       │ │
│ │   ◆ One Follow-up Mailing             │ │
│ │                                       │ │
│ │   ◆ $10 per Each Completed Survey     │ │
│ │                                       │ │
│ └───────────────────────────────────────┘ │
└─────────────────────────────────────────┘
```

Content (slide)

```
┌─────────────────────────────────────────┐
│ ┌───────────────────────────────────────┐ │
│ │                                       │ │
│ │            Survey Content             │ │
│ │                                       │ │
│ │   ◆  5 Questions:  Mental Health      │ │
│ │                                       │ │
│ │   ◆  5 Questions:  Physical Health    │ │
│ │                                       │ │
│ │   ◆ 10 Questions:  Social Functioning │ │
│ │                                       │ │
│ │   ◆  5 Questions:  Demographic        │ │
│ │                                       │ │
│ └───────────────────────────────────────┘ │
└─────────────────────────────────────────┘
```

Sample Question (transparency)

```
┌─────────────────────────────────────────────┐
│                                             │
│            Sample Question:                 │
│           Social Functioning                │
│                                             │
│  During the past month, how often did you   │
│  feel isolated from others?                 │
│                                             │
│                          (Circle One)       │
│       Always                  1             │
│       Very often              2             │
│       Fairly often            3             │
│       Sometimes               4             │
│       Almost never            5             │
│       Never                   6             │
│                                             │
└─────────────────────────────────────────────┘
```

TALKING ABOUT PSYCHOMETRICS

Psychometrics is a branch of measure development that deals with the design, administration, and interpretation of quantitative assessments. Some surveys are designed to quantitatively assess constructs. In measurement language, a construct is a relatively abstract variable as contrasted with a variable that is operationalized in terms of measurable or quantifiable indicators. Depression is an example of a mental health construct. You can operationalize it by asking a series of questions linked to depression and including inability to sleep, mood, frequency of crying, feelings of isolation, and so on. The questions asked in the survey define or operationalize the construct. But does the survey consistently distinguish among people who are depressed and those who are not? If it does, it is valid (and reliable). When a survey claims to measure depression, or any other construct for that matter, its reliability and validity must be quantitatively demonstrated.

Reliability refers to the consistency of a score and the extent to which a measure is free from random error. Validity means the extent to which a measure measures what it is supposed to and does not measure what it is not supposed to. A scale is an aggregation of one or more questions ("items") that cluster together and can be scored as one measure. Sometimes, a survey has several scales. For example, a survey of health might use scales for physical health and for emotional health. A score on one scale is independent of a score on the other (for a more complete discussion on surveys and psychometrics, see **How to Measure Survey Reliability and Validity,** Vol. 7 in this series).

To describe the key psychometric properties of a survey—reliability, for example—a transparency might be appropriate.

> *Scenario:* Facing Each Act With Resolve (FEAR) is a self-administered questionnaire to measure ability to cope with natural disasters like floods, fires, and earthquakes. FEAR has three scales: Concern, Coping, and Satisfaction With Coping. Internal consistency reliability is calculated. This is a method for estimating score reliability from the correlations among the items in the scale. Coefficient alpha is an internal consistency reliability coefficient.

The following transparency is prepared.

Internal Consistency Reliability Coefficient (*N* = 300)			
Scale	**No. Items**	**Mean**	**Reliability Coefficient**
Concern	10	73	.92
Coping	2	93	.71
Satisfaction With			
Coping	1	61	.63

**HIGH SCORES MEAN MORE CONCERN
AND BETTER COPING AND SATISFACTION**

Highest Score = 100 Points

When you have a transparency or slide that contains a table, **you must explain the title, the headings, and any other contextual or organizing information** before you describe the data in the table and, when appropriate, offer interpretations. You must not assume that the audience can routinely read tables, much less read yours.

Listen in on the following report.

EXPLAINING A TABLE

Explain the title. "The next slide gives the internal consistency reliability coefficients for the FEAR questionnaire. The coefficients were computed based on the scores of 300 respondents."

Explain the headings. "The first column contains the three FEAR scales [points to the appropriate place on the screen]:

Concern, Coping, and Satisfaction With Coping. The next column contains the mean score [points to the appropriate place on the screen]. The third column contains the reliability coefficient for each scale [points to the appropriate place on the screen]."

Explain any other information necessary for the listener to follow the talk. "High scores are the most positive, with the highest possible score on all scales being 100 points."

Explain the contents of the table. "As you can see, the Concern Scale has 10 items, with a mean score of 73. Reliability is .92. Coping has 2 items, with a mean score of 93 and a reliability coefficient of .71. Satisfaction With Coping has 1 item, a mean of 61, and a reliability of .63."

Interpretation. "We concluded that the internal consistency reliability coefficients were sufficiently high for our purposes."

TALKING ABOUT DESIGN

A design is a way of arranging the environment in which a survey takes place. The environment consists of the individuals or groups of people, places, activities, or objects that are to be surveyed.

Some designs are relatively simple. A fairly uncomplicated survey might consist of a 10-minute interview on Wednesday with 50 parents to find out if they support the school bond issue, and if so, why. This survey provides a cross-sectional portrait of one group's opinions at a particular time, and its design is called cross-sectional.

More complicated survey designs use environmental arrangements that are experiments, relying on two or more groups of participants or observations. When the views of randomly constituted groups of 50 parents each are compared, the survey design is experimental.

Experimental designs are characterized by arranging to compare two or more groups, at least one of which is experimental. The other is a control (or comparison) group. An experimental group is given a new or untested, innovative program, intervention, or treatment. The control is given an alternative. A group is any collective unit. Sometimes, the unit is made up of individuals (e.g., men who have had surgery, children who are in a reading program, or victims of violence). At other times, the unit is self-contained (e.g., a classroom, company, or hospital).

Two types of experimental designs are commonly used. The first is called a concurrent control design in which participants are randomly assigned to groups. Concurrent means that each group is assembled at the same time. For example, when 10 of 20 schools are randomly assigned to an experimental group while at the same time 10 are assigned to a control, you have a randomized controlled trial, or true experiment.

A second type of experimental design uses concurrent controls, but the participants are *not* randomly assigned. These designs are called nonrandomized controlled trials, quasi-experiments, or nonequivalent controls.

Other experimental designs include the use of self-controls, historical controls, and combinations. Self-control survey designs require premeasures and postmeasures and are called longitudinal or before-after designs. Historical controls make use of data collected from participants in other surveys. Combinations can consist of concurrent controls with or without pre- and postmeasures.

A second category of survey design is descriptive (sometimes called observational). These designs produce information on groups and phenomena that already exist. No new groups are created. A very common descriptive design is the cross-section.

Cross-sections provide descriptive data at one fixed point in time. A survey of American voters' current choices is a cross-sectional survey. Cohorts are forward-looking designs that provide data about changes in a specific population. Suppose a survey of the aspirations of athletes participating in the 1996 Olympics is done in 1996, 2000, and 2004. This is a cohort design, and the cohort is 1996 Olympians. Case controls are retrospective studies that go back in time to help explain a current phenomenon. At least two groups are needed. Suppose you survey the medical records of a group of smokers and of a group of nonsmokers of the same age, health, and socioeconomic status and then compare the results. This is a case-control design. A design is internally valid if it is free from nonrandom error or bias. A study design must be internally valid to be externally valid and to produce accurate findings (for more about survey design, see **How to Design Surveys,** Vol. 5 in this series).

When making oral presentations, you may want to visually explain the design. One relatively simple way to do this is to use the "organization chart" function of a computer graphics program.

Consider the following example of the hypothetical use of a survey entitled FEAR, which measures ability to cope with natural disasters like fires, floods, and earthquakes. People are eligible to join a program to combat their fears (Program Combat) or a control group if they are over 18 years of age, are willing to attend all 10 group sessions, and can converse comfortably in English. The control consists of a 1-hour film. The design is an experimental one using concurrent controls without randomization because participants choose which of the two (the program or the control) is more convenient and likely to be more effective for them.

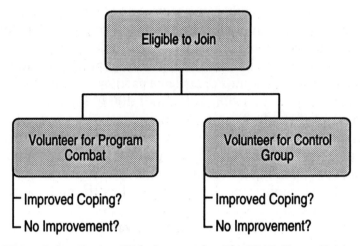

Figure 2–1. Coping With Catastrophe: The FEAR Survey Design

When you present the audience with a figure (including pie, bar, and line graphs), you must explain it. You cannot assume that the audience will automatically comprehend it. Listen to this explanation:

> The FEAR survey design is an experimental design. Specifically, it uses concurrent controls without randomizing participants. The very top box [point, if appropriate] represents all participants who were eligible for the experimental or control groups. You probably recall that to be eligible, people had to be over 18, willing to attend 10 sessions, and comfortable speaking English. Participants could choose which of the two aspects of the experiment they preferred. This is shown in the diagram [point, if appropriate]. At the conclusion of the experiment, we surveyed everyone in both groups and compared whether they perceived that their abilities to cope had improved or not. This is shown on the third level of the diagram [point, if appropriate]. As you can see, neither group improves.

TALKING ABOUT SAMPLING

A sample is a portion or subset of a larger group called a population. Surveys often use samples rather than populations. A good sample is a miniature version of the population— just like it, only smaller. The best sample is representative or a model of the population. A sample is representative of the population if important characteristics (e.g., age, gender, health status) are distributed similarly in both groups. Suppose the population of interest consists of 150 people, 50% of whom are male, with 45% over 65 years of age. A representative sample will have fewer people, say, 75, but it must also consist of 50% males, with 45% over 65.

Survey samples are not meaningful in themselves. Their importance lies in the accuracy with which they represent or mirror the target population. The target population consists of the institutions, persons, problems, and systems to which or whom the survey's findings are to be applied or generalized.

The criteria for inclusion into a survey consist of the characteristics of individuals that make them eligible for participation; the exclusion criteria consist of characteristics that rule out certain people. You apply the inclusion and exclusion criteria to the target population. Once you remove from the target population all those who fail to meet the inclusion criteria and all those who succeed in meeting the exclusion criteria, you are left with a study population consisting of people who are eligible to participate.

How large should a sample be? The size of the sample refers to the number of units that needs to be surveyed to get precise and reliable findings. The units can be people (e.g., men and women over and under 45 years of age), places (e.g., counties, hospitals, schools), and things (e.g., medical or school records).

The most sensible way to produce the right sample size is to use statistical calculations. These can be relatively complex, depending on the needs of the survey. Some surveys have just one sample, and others have several (for a more complete discussion, see **How to Sample in Surveys,** Vol. 6 in this series).

In an oral talk, you should consider providing a description of the inclusion and exclusion or eligibility criteria, the sampling method or design, and the sample size, as illustrated in the following two survey scenarios.

> *Scenario 1:* This is a handout for a report of the inclusion and exclusion criteria used in a survey to find out which is most effective in getting adults to stop smoking: nicotine gum alone, nicotine gum and a support group, or a support group alone.

ELIGIBILITY

Target Population: **Patients who smoke**

Inclusion Criteria:

- **Between the ages of 18 and 64 years**
- **Smoke one or more cigarettes daily**
- **Alveolar breath CO determination of more than eight parts per million**

Exclusion Criterion:

- **Any contraindications for nicotine gum**

Scenario 2: These are two transparencies to report on sample selection and size in a survey of high school students who participated in a project to favorably modify their acquired immunodeficiency syndrome (AIDS)-related knowledge and beliefs. For the survey, schools were paired so that one urban and one suburban high school were joined. High schools A and C are urban; B and D are suburban.

HOW SAMPLE WAS CHOSEN

	Experimental		Control	
Schools	AB	CD	AB	CD
Grade	9	11	11	9
% Sample	30%	30%	20%	20%
# Classrooms	16	13	13	10
# Students	430	309	326	251

SAMPLE SIZE

	Experimental	Control
Classrooms	29	23
Students	739	577

EXERCISE

Suppose you are asked to describe the contents of the preceding two transparencies ("How Sample Was Chosen" and "Sample Size"). Write out the talk you will give.

■ SUGGESTED ANSWER ■

The first transparency shows how the sample was chosen from four schools. The four were divided into two pairs: Schools A and B were one pair, and C and D were the second. Both pairs participated in the experimental and control groups, but as you will see, if the 9th grade was in the experimental group, the 11th grade in that pair was in the control. (Point to the screen.)

The table shows you the schools, the grade in each school, the percentage sample of that grade, the number of classrooms, and the number of students.

Ninth- and 11th-grade students participated. If 9th-grade students were in the experimental group in Schools AB, then 11th-grade students were in the control in CD. A 30% sample was taken of all experimental grades as was a 20% sample of the control. (Point to the screen.)

The next slide shows the total sample size of classrooms and students. As you can see, 29 classrooms were involved in the experimental group and 23 in the control group. This means 739 students were involved in the experimental group and 577 in the control group.

TALKING ABOUT DATA ANALYSIS

Surveys produce observations in the form of narrations or numbers. The narrations consist of responses stated in the survey participant's own words. Narrations are counted, compared, and interpreted, often using methods borrowed from communications theory and anthropology.

Survey data also take numerical form. For example, in some surveys, respondents may be asked to rate items on ordered or ranked scales, say, with 1 representing a very positive feeling and 5 representing a very negative one. In other surveys, they may be asked to tell their age, height, or number of trips they have taken or books they have read. The analysis of numbers or observations that take numerical form is done using "statistics." The results of statistical analyses are descriptions, relationships, comparisons, and predictions, and these are the most common types of analyses done for surveys.

Reporting the analysis methods and the results of the analysis often provide the greatest challenge in an oral report. Differences exist in the amount of detail that you can present in a written report and in a visual aid. In a written report, you are often expected to provide detailed tables and figures. In an oral report, the detail cannot be on the visual aid. You must verbalize it with or without the help of a handout.

The following tables are examples of the same data, dangers in the home, presented in two ways: as an in-text table for a written report and as a handout or slide for an oral report.

For a Written Report

	% Experimental Homes[a]	% Control Homes[a]	p[b]	Adjusted Odds Ratio	95% CI[c]
Living room					
Rugs (tripping danger)	22.5	35.2			
Peeling paint	10.6	14.5			
Floor in need of repair	4.9	3.7			
Any problems	28.5	40.2	< .001	0.55	0.45, 0.68

→

	% Experimental Homes[a]	% Control Homes[a]	p[b]	Adjusted Odds Ratio	95% CI[c]
Hall					
Rugs (tripping danger)	9.3	15.8			
Peeling paint	4.3	10.2			
Floor in need of repair	2.4	2.0			
Any problems	13.0	20.1	< .001	0.54	0.41, 0.71
Bedroom					
Rugs (tripping danger)	12.2	14.7			
Peeling paint	6.8	9.2			
Floor in need of repair	3.1	2.1			
Any problems	16.9	17.8	.02	0.73	0.55, 0.95
Kitchen					
Rugs (tripping danger)	16.2	16.0			
Peeling paint	10.6	11.3			
Floor in need of repair	7.8	3.5			
Any problems	25.5	21.3	.24	1.15	0.91, 1.45

a. Percentages are based on the evaluation of 902 homes in the experiment and 1,060 in the control.
b. Logistic regression adjusted for the presence of children 5 years of age and younger and adults over 70 years of age.
c. CI = confidence interval.

For an Oral Report (either handout or slide)

DANGER IN THE HOME: 902 Experimental and 1,060 Controls		
	E, %	**C, %**
Living Room	28.5	40.2*
Hall	13.0	20.1*
Bedroom	16.0	17.8
Kitchen	26.5	21.3
*p < .001		

The table for the written report contains three more columns than does the one for the oral report. Also, the table in the written report contains more detailed information comparing specific dangers (rugs, peeling paint, floor in need of repair) in each room. The essential information is in both tables: the comparison groups (experimental and control), the size of each group, and whether or not the differences between groups are statistically significant. A statistically significant difference between groups suggests that differences are likely to be the result of participation in the experiment rather than a chance finding. You can also use the table for the written report as a handout. (More information on how to do and interpret statistical analyses for surveys is found in **How to Analyze Survey Data,** Vol. 8 in this series.)

3 The Written Report

A useful written report provides enough clearly explained information so that at least two interested individuals can agree on the survey's objectives, methods, and conclusion. If the report is being submitted to a funding agency, such as the government or a foundation, the composition and format may be set for you. In most situations, you are on your own in deciding what to include and how long the report should be. The following is a checklist of the contents to consider in preparing the report.

Checklist of Contents for a Survey Report

✓ **List the title, authors, sponsors, location of report, and date.**

Make sure the report has a brief, clear title. Tell who prepared the report. If appropriate, distinguish between preparation of the report and conduct of the survey. Specify the sponsor of the survey: Who asked for it? Who paid for it? In what town, city, state, or province was the report written? What is the date of the report?

✓ **In the introduction, state the need or problem to be solved and the research questions to be answered or hypotheses to be tested.**

✓ **List the survey's characteristics.**

- *Type of survey instrument(s)* (e.g., mailed self-administered questionnaire, face-to-face-interview, observation, record review, telephone interview). Tell why the particular type was chosen. For example, was the survey available and previously validated? Were interviews more appropriate than self-administered questionnaires? Why?

- *Contents*

  Number of questions

  Description of content of questions

  Descriptions of response types (e.g., ratings from 1 to 5, with 1 = *most positive* and 5 = *most negative*)

  Description of scales (e.g., Attitude Toward Academics is a 20-question survey with two different scales of 10 questions each; one scale surveys attitudes toward school and the other measures attitudes toward reading)

■ *Psychometric characteristics*

Scales

— Content

— How questions are scored

— How questions are combined into scales

Reliability

— How established (stability, equivalence, homogeneity, and inter- and intrarater)

— Adequacy of reliability for survey's uses

— Adequacy of description and methods for establishing reliability

Validity

— How established (content, face, criterion, construct, convergent)

— Adequacy of validity for survey's uses

— Adequacy of description and methods for establishing validity

■ *Administration and other logistics*

Characteristics of survey administrators (e.g., education, experience)

Description of training activities for interviewers and other data collectors

Characteristics of quality assurance methods to ensure that survey is administered and interpreted in a uniform way by everyone who administers it

Length of time to complete each survey

Length of time for entire survey to be completed

- *Relevant literature and other surveys on the same topics*

✓ **Explain the survey methods.**

- *Design*

  Experimental or descriptive

  Limits on internal and external validity

- *Sample*

  If a population, explain

  If a sample, how selected (probability sample or convenience sample)

  If more than one group, how assigned

  How sample size was chosen

  Potential biases (e.g., because of how sample was chosen or assigned, sample size, and missing data from some or all respondents on some or all survey questions)

- *Analysis*

✓ **Relate results to the survey's objectives, research, or study question.**

✓ **State conclusions.**

- Summary of important points

- How findings compare to other surveys (yours and surveys done elsewhere)

✓ **State implications (meaning) and recommendations (next steps).**

Academic and Technical Survey Reports

Basically, two types of survey reports are the most common. The first consists of the academic survey report. This is a report prepared for specific rather than general audiences. The audiences can be in universities, business, and government, and the expectation is that a great deal of technical detail will accompany the results and recommendations. Below are two illustrations of what, for the sake of convenience, are called academic or technical survey reports.

Illustration 1: The Competencies of Generalist Physicians
A national survey is conducted of a representative sample of program directors and faculty in academic medicine who are pediatricians, general internists, and geriatricians. The survey is designed to find out the most important competencies for generalist physicians to acquire and sustain in medical school, as residents, and 7 years into their practice. The results will be used in guiding curriculum development policy.

Illustration 2: Drug-Exposed Babies
The state commissioned a survey of 56 county welfare service agencies to learn about the caseload and nature and quality of services given to drug-exposed babies. The report was prepared by the Statistics Branch of the Welfare Agency and will be used to devise a minimal data set and also as a basis for making decisions regarding welfare services in the state.

Survey Reports for General Audiences

The second type of survey report is designed to reach a general audience. Do not mistake "general" for "not too bright."

General audiences may consist of the public in general, but they may also contain people who can run businesses, schools, and government. You should assume that a general audience is very smart but not an expert in the specific topic covered by the survey. Examples of reports for general audiences are given below.

Illustration 1: Drug-Exposed Babies

A report of a survey of the state's welfare services for newborns exposed to drugs is given to both branches of the legislature and to the press.

Illustration 2: Satisfied Employees

A report of a survey of employee satisfaction is given to the company's Board of Directors and to all employees.

Illustration 3: Quality of Life of College Seniors at Technical University (TU)

A report of a survey given to all college seniors is written for the Office of Student Affairs at TU. It is available to all students and members of the faculty.

Contents of Reports

Technical reports or components of them often serve as the basis of reports for more general audiences. Because of this, they tend to be longer and more comprehensive. Also, their organization is usually different. In technical reports, the conclusions and recommendations are placed after the methods. In general survey reports, the main findings are almost always placed up front. Examples of tables of contents and lengths of each chapter are given in the following outline.

Table of Contents for a Technical Report

Executive Summary
Title page: Authors, geographic location of survey report, date

Acknowledgments: Sponsors of the survey; data collectors; participants; research, field, and technical assistance

Text of summary

The Report
Title page: Authors, geographic location of survey report, date

Acknowledgments: Sponsors of the survey; data collectors; participants; research, field, and technical assistance

Table of contents

List of tables

List of figures

1. *Introduction*—5 to 10 pages

   Need or problem to be solved

   How survey fits into the context of others previously done

   Survey objectives

   Research questions/hypotheses: Description of main outcomes and independent variables

   Limitations imposed by scope and focus of survey

   ■ Comment: Tell about the particular need or problem the survey's data will help resolve. Survey data are used to describe the current status and inform program development and policymaking. For example, a company might sponsor a survey of employees' satisfaction to find out how things stand now or to determine if new programs (such as work-at-home programs) or policies (such as a change in supervisory practices) are needed. If the survey is part of a research study, state the hypothesis or research questions. For which independent and dependent variables will the survey's data be used? What are the survey's specific purposes?

Keep the introduction relatively brief. Most readers want to quickly get into the body of the text. Save comments and background literature to help support your conclusions and recommendations. Tell the reader what the survey covers and excludes either here or later in the conclusions. For example, if the survey is about parents' attitudes, you might say something like this: "We interviewed parents in English and Spanish. We restricted the questions to attitudes toward the dress code and new library and counseling programs."

2. *The Survey*—20 pages

Type (e.g., interviews, mailed questionnaire)

Number of questions for entire survey and all subscales

Description of content

Administration: Time to administer, time to complete, duration of data collection

Relevant literature and other surveys

- Comment: The reader should have a clear idea of the characteristics of the survey: its type, length, contents, and time to complete. Give example questions. Make the entire survey form available to readers by listing in a table the questions and response formats, placing the survey in an appendix, or telling how it can be obtained. If appropriate, give the theoretical framework for the survey. Suppose the survey is about consumer preferences. Do the questions come from a psychological theory regarding how people make choices and take risks? Are some or all of the questions based on the work of others or other surveys? If so, describe and cite those sources.

3. *Design*—3 to 5 pages

   Description

   Justification

   Limitations and threats to internal and external validity

   ■ Comment: Describe the design (experimental? descriptive?) Why was the design selected? Also, tell the design's impact on external and internal validity. (Limitations can be described here or later in the conclusions.)

4. *Sampling*—2.5 pages

   Inclusion and exclusion criteria

   Sampling methods: Description, explanation, and justification

   Sample size: Explanation and justification

   Potential biases resulting from sampling methods

   ■ Comment: Describe who was eligible to participate and how they were selected (at random? by volunteering?). Justify the choice of method. How was the sample size arrived at? Did all who were eligible agree to participate? Did all who agreed also complete all survey questions? What biases are introduced into the survey's responses because of the nature of the sampling methods and sample? (You may prefer to answer this in the conclusions.) A bias is a systematic error that affects the accuracy and applicability of the survey's findings. For example, people who do not complete the entire survey may be different in important ways from those who do. They may be more verbal (perhaps more educated) or more motivated and interested in the survey topic.

5. *Psychometrics:* Reliability and Validity—1 paragraph to
   20 pages

   Reliability: How ensured (including pretesting, training,
       and quality assurance activities) and how calculated

   Validity: How ensured and established

   ■ Comment: Many surveys are fairly simple and do not have
   sophisticated psychometric properties. For example, a 10-
   item questionnaire to find out customer preferences probably does not warrant the extensive psychometric validation
   that a survey of health status does. However, even short,
   relatively simple surveys should be administered in a standardized way with assurances that the respondents understand the questions and can provide reliable information. A
   one-paragraph description of reliability and validity can
   suffice for relatively simple surveys.
       Many surveys consist of many scales, all purporting to
   measure attitudes, values, and opinions. The data from
   these surveys are used to make important decisions that
   affect large numbers of people. For more complex surveys, it
   is very im- portant that information about reliability be
   provided. Not only do you want to prove that the data are
   reliable and valid, you must also demonstrate that you have
   used a high-quality method and described it adequately.

6. *Results*—15 pages

   Response rate

   Description of respondents

   Outcomes for each survey objective, research question, or
       hypothesis

   ■ Comment: The results or findings tell what the survey data
   suggest or show. For example, if you are comparing men and
   women at three points in time regarding their beliefs, as measured by the BELIEF Questionnaire, you will answer these
   questions:

1. What do men believe at Time 1? Time 2? Time 3?
2. Do men change significantly in their beliefs over time?
3. What do women believe at Time 1? Time 2? Time 3?
4. Do women change significantly in their beliefs over time?
5. How do the changes observed in men and women compare?

Do not interpret the results for the reader in this section. Just report the data that were obtained from the survey. Interpretation comes next—in the conclusions.

The following is an example of how to write up the results of survey data that have been analyzed statistically:

Table A contains data from a study of Program CAREER whose purpose is to prepare college students for entry into the job market. For the study, Program CAREER students are compared to other students who do not participate in a special program. Both groups, totaling 500 participants and nonparticipants, are surveyed before and after Program CAREER begins. To make the comparisons, scores are averaged for surveys of knowledge, beliefs, self-reliance, and risk-taking behaviors. The averages are tested for differences using a statistical method called a t test. In this case, the test is used to examine differences in the observed change score (after the program minus before) for each measure.

Table A
Before-and-After Mean Scores (standard deviations) and
Net Change Scores, by Program Group (N = 500 students)

Survey Measures	Program CAREER Students		No-Program Students				
	Before Program CAREER	After Program CAREER	Before Program CAREER	After Program CAREER	Net Difference	t	p
Knowledge	75.6 (11.8)	85.5 (8.8)	78.8 (10.9)	81.2 (9.6)	7.50	8.9	.0001*
Beliefs							
Goals	2.5 (1.1)	2.1 (1.0)	2.5 (1.1)	2.3 (1.1)	−0.15	1.5	.14
Benefits	3.5 (0.7)	3.8 (0.7)	3.7 (10.7)	3.8 (0.7)	0.19	4.7	.0001*
Barriers	4.4 (0.6)	4.5 (0.6)	4.4 (0.6)	4.4 (0.6)	0.09	1.2	.22
Values	5.4 (0.9)	5.5 (0.8)	5.5 (0.9)	5.5 (0.9)	0.09	0.7	.50
Standards	2.8 (0.6)	2.9 (0.6)	2.8 (0.6)	2.8 (0.6)	0.12	3.0	.003*
Self-reliance	3.7 (0.7)	3.9 (0.7)	3.7 (0.7)	3.8 (0.7)	0.10	2.2	.03*
Risk-taking behavior	1.5 (2.5)	1.3 (2.3)	1.0 (2.0)	1.3 (2.4)	−0.48	2.8	.006*

*Statistically significant.

More information on how to do and interpret statistical tests like the *t* test is found in **How to Analyze Survey Data, Vol. 8 in this series.**)

Before you write the results, answer these questions for yourself:

1. *What do the columns represent?* In this example, the columns give data on the mean scores and standard deviations (in parentheses) for CAREER and No-Program students before and after the program. The net difference in scores and the *t* statistic and *p* value are also shown. (**How to Analyze Survey Data** provides more information on the standard deviation, *t* statistic, and *p* values.)

2. *What do the rows represent?* In this case, the rows show the specific variables that are measured—for example, knowledge and goals.

3. *Are any data statistically or otherwise significant?* In this case, knowledge, benefits, self-reliance, and risk-taking behavior are statistically significant, as indicated by an asterisk. (To be significant, differences must be attributable to a planned intervention, such as Program CAREER, rather than to chance or historical occurrences, such as changes in vocational education that are unrelated to Program CAREER.) Statistical significance is often interpreted to mean a result that happens by chance less than once in 20 times, with a *p* value less than or equal to .05. A *p* value is the probability of obtaining the results of a statistical test by chance. (**How to Analyze Survey Data** provides more information on the meaning and uses of statistical significance.)

4. *Can these data stand alone?* In this example, you cannot tell because no other information is given. Sometimes, one table is compared to another or some of the data in one table are compared to another.

Here's how to write up the results.

> Table A presents the before-and-after means and the observed net change scores for each of the eight survey measures for the 500 Program CAREER and comparison students. Significant effects favoring Program CAREER were observed for five of the eight measures: knowledge, beliefs about benefits and standards, self-reliance, and risk-taking behaviors.

7. Conclusions—10 pages

What the results mean

Applicability of the results to other people and settings

- Comment: This is the place to summarize and interpret the results. Are they good? Bad? How do they fit into the context of other surveys? Do they support or contradict other people's findings? You can also discuss some or all of the limitations of the survey's design, sampling, scope, and focus. Remind the reader that your findings hold for the group that was surveyed but may or may not be applicable to other settings (e.g., offices, schools, towns).

8. Recommendations—10 pages

- Comment: Some surveys are conducted to provide data to decision makers or makers of policy who then determine what to do with the findings. In this situation, recommendations are not called for. When recommendations are required, be careful not to go beyond your survey or the findings. That is, be sure that if you recommend an activity you have evidence that it will work. Did the survey ask about the activity? Can you cite a reference that suggests that the activity is likely to be effective?

References

Appendixes
The survey itself; additional technical information, including methods for selecting samples, determining sample size; complex or detailed statistics

Body of report: Maximum 115 pages

Table of Contents for a General Report

Executive Summary
Title page: Authors, geographic location of survey report, date
Acknowledgments: Sponsors of the survey; data collectors; participants; research, field, and technical assistance
Text of summary

The Report
Title page: Authors, sponsors, geographic location, date
Acknowledgments: Sponsors of the survey; data collectors; participants; research, field, and technical assistance
Table of contents
List of tables
List of figures

1. *Introduction*—2 pages
Need or problem to be solved
How survey fits into the context of others previously done
Survey objectives
Limitations imposed by scope and focus of survey

2. *Summary of Major Findings or Results*—10 pages

3. *Survey Content*—1 page

4. *Participation Rates*—1 page

5. *Other Methods: Administration, Reliability, and Validity*—
   1 page

6. *Conclusions and Recommendations*—10 pages

References

Appendix (Same as for the technical report; can make this a separate volume)

Body of report: 25 pages

A NOTE ON REPORT LENGTH

A report that is 300 pages long is unlikely to be read in its entirety. Sometimes, very long reports are prepared as documentation of the development and validation of important surveys, especially those that are used in research. Generally, though, reports need not be longer than 100 to 125 pages, and most can be 25 to 50.

THE EXECUTIVE SUMMARY

An executive summary provides all potential users with an easy-to-read report of the survey's major objectives, characteristics, findings, and recommendations. The summary usually varies in length from 3 to 15 pages. Executive summaries are often required and always advisable.

Three rules govern the preparation of the summary:

- Include only the most important objectives, characteristics, findings, and recommendations.
- Avoid jargon.

  Poor: We used a ***cluster sampling strategy*** in which schools were assigned at random . . .

  Better: We assigned schools at random . . .

  Poor: We established ***concurrent validity by correlating scores*** on Survey A with those on Survey B.

  Better: We examined the relationship between scores on Surveys A and B.

- Use active verbs.

  Poor: The use of health care services ***was found*** to be more frequent in people under 45 years of age.

  Better: The survey found more frequent use of services by people under 45 years of age.

  Poor: ***It is recommended*** that the FLEX Hours Work Program be implemented within the next 3 months.

  Better: We recommend the implementation of the FLEX Hours Work Program within 3 months.

Reviewing the Report for Readability

After writing a survey report, review it for readability. The conventional wisdom believes that most people are comfortable reading below their actual level. For general audiences, ease of reading is especially important. Here is one formula:

1. Take a 100-word sample of the survey report.
2. Compute the average number of words in each sentence. If the final sentence in your sample runs beyond 100 words, use the total number of words at the end of that sentence to compute the average.
3. Count the number of words in the 100-word sample with more than two syllables. Do not count proper nouns or three-syllable word forms ending in -ed or -es.
4. Add the average number of words per sentence to the number of words containing more than two syllables and multiply the sum by 0.4.

- Example: Suppose a 100-word passage contains an average of 20 words per sentence and 10 words of more than two syllables. The sum of these is 30. Multiplying 30 by 0.4 gives you a score of 12. This means that the passage requires a 12th-grade reading level.

Reviewing the Report for Comprehensiveness and Accuracy

The following tabular "scoring" sheets are provided as a guide to the preparation and review of written and oral survey reports. All tables use the same scale:

4 = Definitely yes
3 = Probably yes
2 = Probably no
1 = Definitely no
0 = No data; uncertain
NA = Not applicable

INTRODUCTION AND BACKGROUND	4	3	2	1	0	NA
Are the survey's main objectives or guiding questions stated measurably?						
If the survey is part of a research study, are the research questions or hypotheses stated precisely?						
Is a description given of how the survey fits into the context of previous surveys done locally?						
Is a description given of how the survey fits into the context of previous surveys done elsewhere?						
Are the people or agencies that commissioned the survey acknowledged?						
Are the actual writers of the report acknowledged?						
Are the people or agencies responsible for conducting the survey acknowledged?						
Is an explanation provided of the problem or need the survey's data are to resolve?						
Other?						

SURVEY CONTENT	4	3	2	1	0	NA
Is the total number of questions given?						
Is the content of the survey adequately described?						
Is the number of questions given for each scale or subscale?						
Is the content described adequately for each scale?						
Are the response choices adequately described?						
Is the time for administration specified?						
Is the time needed for individuals to complete the survey given?						
Is the relevant literature included?						
Other?						

DESIGN AND SAMPLING	4	3	2	1	0	NA
Is the design described adequately?						
Is the design justified?						
If a sample, are sampling methods adequately described?						
If a sample, are the survey's participants randomly selected?						
If more than one group, are the survey's participants randomly assigned?						
If the unit that is sampled (e.g., students or employees) is not the population of main concern (e.g., teachers or managers), is this addressed in the report (e.g., in the analysis or discussion)?						
If a sample, and a nonrandom sampling method is used, is evidence given regarding the similarity of the groups at baseline?						
If groups are not equivalent at baseline, is this problem adequately addressed in the analysis or the interpretation?						
Are criteria given for including all sampling units (e.g., students, teachers) and whoever else is studied?						
Are criteria given for excluding units?						
Is the sample size justified, say, with a power calculation?						
Is information given on the number of participants in the source population?						

DESIGN AND SAMPLING	4	3	2	1	0	NA
Is information given on the number of participants eligible to participate?						
Is information given on the number who agreed to participate?						
Is information given on the number who refused to participate?						
Is information given on the number who dropped out or were lost to follow-up before completing the survey?						
Is information given on the number of respondents who completed all questions?						
Is information given on the number on whom some data are missing?						
If observations or measures are made over time, is the time period justified?						
Are reasons given for individuals or groups who dropped out?						
Are reasons given for missing data?						
Are the effects on generalizability of choice, equivalence, and participation of the resultant sample explained?						
Are the effects on internal validity of choice, equivalence, and participation of the resultant sample explained?						
Other?						

RELIABILITY AND VALIDITY	4	3	2	1	0	NA
Are the independent variables defined?						
Are the dependent variables defined?						
Are data provided on the survey's reliability for each variable?						
Are data provided on the survey's validity for each variable?						
Are the methods for ensuring reliability (e.g., quality assurance and training) described?						
Are the methods for ensuring reliability adequate?						
Are the methods for ensuring validity described?						
Are the methods for ensuring validity adequate?						
Are the scoring methods adequately described?						
Are the scaling methods described?						
Are the scaling methods adequate?						
Is the survey's administration adequately described?						
Is information provided on methods for ensuring the quality of data collection?						
Is the duration of the survey justified?						

$\rightarrow$

RELIABILITY AND VALIDITY	4	3	2	1	0	NA
Is the duration sufficient for the survey's objectives?						
Are the effects on the survey's generalizability and practicality of the selection, reliability, validity of data sources, and the length of data collection explained?						
Other?						

DATA ANALYSIS	4	3	2	1	0	NA
Are statistical methods adequately described?						
Are statistical methods justified?						
Is the purpose of the analysis clear?						
Are scoring systems described?						
Are potential confounders adequately controlled for in the analysis?						
Are analytic specifications of the independent and dependent variables consistent with the survey's research questions or hypotheses?						
Is the unit of analysis specified clearly?						
Other?						

REPORTING	4	3	2	1	0	NA
Are references given for complex statistical methods?						
Are complex statistical methods described in an appendix?						
Are exact p values given?						
Are confidence intervals given?						
Are the results of the analysis clearly described?						
Are the survey's findings clearly described?						
Do the conclusions follow from the survey's results?						
Are the survey's limitations discussed adequately?						
Does the validity of the findings outweigh the limitations?						
Other?						

Exercises

1. Create a pie chart from the following information.

Thirty-four counties were surveyed about the actions they take after a mother tests positive for drugs and the child is referred to Child Protective Services. The findings are that 5% of the children received no services, 20% remained at home with informal supervision, dependency petitions were filed for 64%, and other actions taken for 11%.

2. Present the following information in a slide format. In so doing, include the percentage as well as the number of counties.

Drug testing for women and infants was done under four conditions: mandatorily without mother's consent, tested with consent, anonymous testing, and other protocols. Of 28 counties that responded to the survey, 15 used mandatory testing, 10 only tested if mothers consented, 9 used other protocols, and 2 used anonymous testing. Some counties conducted tests under more than one condition.

3. Draw a bar chart, using the data in Table X below.

Table X
Major Causes of Adolescent Mortality, 1985
(10-19 years old)

Cause	% Mortality
Motor vehicle accidents	38
Natural causes	27
Suicide	10
Other vehicle/injury	10
Homicide	9
Drowning	4
Fires	2

SOURCE: "Trends and Current Status in Childhood Mortality: United States, 1900-1985," by L. Fingerhut and J. Kleinman, *Vital and Health Statistics*, Series 3, No. 26 (DHHS Publication No. 89-1410). Hyattsville, MD: National Center for Health Statistics, 1989.

4. Write the text for the table on page 54 in Chapter 2.

5. Write the text for Table Y, which shows the results of a survey of high school students' knowledge and beliefs especially as they pertain to welfare reform. A statistically significant result is $p < .05$.

Table Y
Baseline and Follow-up Mean, (*SD*),
and Net Change Scores for Outcomes,
by Treatment Group (*N* = 860 students)

Outcome	Experimental Group		Control Group		Net Difference	*t*	*p*
	Pre	Post	Pre	Post			
Knowledge	75.6 (11.6)	85.5 (8.8)	78.8 (10.9)	81.2 (9.6)	7.50	8.9	.0001
Attitude toward reform	2.5 (1.1)	2.1 (1.0)	2.5 (1.1)	2.3 (1.1)	−0.15	1.5	.14
Beliefs	3.5 (0.7)	3.8 (0.7)	3.7 (0.7)	3.8 (0.7)	0.19	4.7	.0001
Risk-taking behavior	4.4 (0.6)	4.5 (0.6)	4.4 (0.6)	4.4 (0.6)	0.09	1.2	.22
Values	5.4 (0.9)	5.5 (0.8)	5.5 (0.9)	5.5 (0.9)	0.09	0.7	.50
Self-efficacy	2.8 (0.6)	2.9 (0.6)	2.8 (0.6)	2.8 (0.6)	0.12	3.0	.003
Political preferences	3.7 (0.7)	3.9 (0.7)	3.8 (0.7)	3.8 (0.7)	0.10	2.2	.03
Religiosity	1.5 (0.5)	1.3 (2.3)	1.3 (2.4)	1.3 (2.4)	−0.48	2.8	.006

ANSWERS

1.   Actions After Referral to Child Protective Services
             (*N* = 34 Counties)

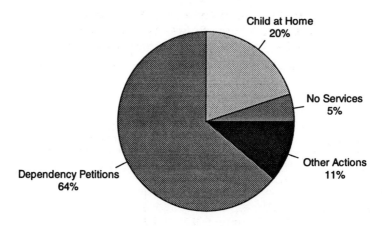

Child at Home
20%

No Services
5%

Other Actions
11%

Dependency Petitions
64%

2.

CONDITIONS OF DRUG TESTING
FOR WOMEN AND INFANTS
(28 COUNTIES)

Conditions	Number	%
Mandatory	15	54
Mother's Consent	10	36
Other Protocols	9	32
Anonymous	2	7

SOME COUNTIES REPORTED
MORE THAN ONE CONDITION

3. ### Major Causes of Adolescent Mortality—1985
(10-19 Years Old)

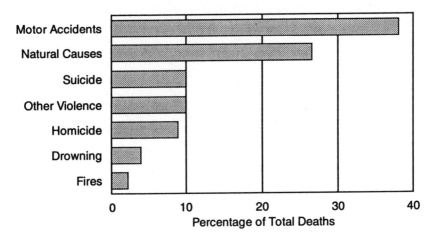

Percentage of Total Deaths

4. Table X compares dangers in the living room, hall, bedroom, and kitchen. The survey found that the living room and hallway areas of the experimental homes were signficantly less likely to have tripping dangers from loose floor coverings and peeling paint than were the same areas in control homes. The differences were smaller in the experimental and control homes for the bedrooms, and no statistically meaningful differences were obtained between both groups for the kitchen.

5. Table Y presents the pre- and postsurvey means and observed net change scores for each of eight outcomes for 860 students. Significant effects favoring the experiment were observed for five (knowledge, beliefs, self-efficacy, political preferences, and religiosity) of the eight outcomes.

Suggested Readings

Bailar, J. C., & Mosteller, F. (1988). Guidelines for statistical reporting in articles for medical journals. *Annals of Internal Medicine, 108,* 266-273.

The title of this article suggests that it is primarily appropriate for articles in medical journals. However, others can benefit from the discussion on figures and tables and the merits of confidence intervals and exact p values.

Bates, E. S., & Abemayor, E. (1991). Slide presentation graphics using a personal computer. *Archives of Otolaryngology and Head and Neck Surgery, 117,* 1026-1030.

An evaluation of four graphics programs for making slides. Although out of date in terms of technology and cost, the criteria used by the authors are still relevant.

Fink, A. (1993). *Evaluation fundamentals: Guiding health programs, research, and policy.* Newbury Park, CA: Sage.

This book devotes a chapter to written and oral reports. Examples are given of complete reports, executive summaries, and abstracts.

Lin, Y.-C. (1989). Practical approaches to scientific presentation. *Chinese Journal of Physiology, 32,* 71-78.

Describes the purposes, language, and style of oral presentation, with particular emphasis on using slides in scientific presentations.

Pfeiffer, W. S. (1991). *Technical writing.* New York: Macmillan.

Provides useful tips on the details of putting together formal reports. Discusses the cover and title page, table of contents, and executive summary. It also contains rules for preparing charts and giving oral presentations. Its orientation is for business, but many of the lessons can be adapted to health evaluation.

Spinler, S. (1991). How to prepare and deliver pharmacy presentations. *American Journal of Hospital Pharmacy, 48,* 1730-1738.

Provides extremely useful tips on the preparation and use of slides. Also discusses how to rehearse and then deliver an oral presentation.

About the Author

ARLENE FINK, PhD, is Professor of Medicine and Public Health at the University of California, Los Angeles. She is on the Policy Advisory Board of UCLA's Robert Wood Johnson Clinical Scholars Program, a health research scientist at the Veterans Administration Medical Center in Sepulveda, California, and president of Arlene Fink Associates. She has conducted evaluations throughout the United States and abroad and has trained thousands of health professionals, social scientists, and educators in program evaluation. Her published works include nearly 100 monographs and articles on evaluation methods and research. She is coauthor of *How to Conduct Surveys* and author of *Evaluation Fundamentals: Guiding Health Programs, Research, and Policy* and *Evaluation for Education and Psychology*.